PSYCHOPHARMACOLOGY, SEXUAL DISORDERS AND DRUG ABUSE

PSYCHOPHARMACOLOGY, SEXUAL DISORDERS AND DRUG ABUSE

Proceedings of the Symposia held at the VIII Congress of the Collegium Internationale Neuro-Psychopharmacologicum Copenhagen, August 14–17, 1972

Editors:

T. A. BAN, J. R. BOISSIER, G. J. GESSA, H. HEIMANN, L. HOLLISTER,
H. E. LEHMANN, I. MUNKVAD, HANNAH STEINBERG, F. SULSER,
A. SUNDWALL and O. VINAŘ

1973

NORTH-HOLLAND PUBLISHING COMPANY,
AMSTERDAM — LONDON
AVICENUM, CZECHOSLOVAK MEDICAL PRESS, PRAGUE

65593

© NORTH-HOLLAND PUBLISHING COMPANY — 1973

All Rights Reserved. No part of this publication may be reproduced, stored in a retrieval system, or transmitted in any form or by any means, electronic, mechanical, photocopying, recording or otherwise, without the prior permission of the Copyright owner.

Library of Congress Catalog Card Number: 73-86075
ISBN North-Holland: 0 7204 41390
ISBN American Elsevier: 0 444 105603

Publishers:

NORTH-HOLLAND PUBLISHING COMPANY,
AMSTERDAM
NORTH-HOLLAND PUBLISHING COMPANY, LTD.,
LONDON
AVICENUM, CZECHOSLOVAK MEDICAL PRESS,
PRAGUE

Sole distributors for the U.S.A. and Canada:

AMERICAN ELSEVIER PUBLISHING COMPANY, INC.
52 VANDERBILT AVENUE, NEW YORK, N.Y. 10017

Printed in Czechoslovakia by Polygrafia, Prague

PREFACE

In June 1971 a programme committee consisting of experts in all aspects of psychopharmacology met in Copenhagen in order to prepare the programme for the eighth congress of the Collegium Internationale Neuro-Psychopharmacologicum (C.I.N.P.). For two days the state of psychopharmacology was surveyed and themes considered of current interest were chosen. It was decided that the meeting would include subjects of general interest to all psychopharmacologists in plenary sessions, while those of more special interest should be dealt with in symposia, several of which should be given simultaneously. The time allotted and the accommodation available limited the number of plenary sessions and symposia, and it was thought desirable to reserve some time for free communications. Judging from the free communications given, the choice of subjects proved appropriate; only one additional subject, namely the testing of drugs, was the topic for an appreciable number of free communications.

After the preparatory meeting the members of the programme committee approached a series of outstanding specialists, and asked each of them to be responsible for a plenary session or a symposium, by arranging the programme, choosing and inviting the appropriate speakers and acting as chairman during the session.

The congress was held at the Royal Danish School of Pharmacy, Copenhagen, from Monday, 14th to Thursday, 17th August, 1972. The planned programme consisting of 4 plenary sessions, 13 symposia and 167 free communications of which 90 were presented in a scientific exhibition, was adhered to.

The abstracts of the meeting were published as a supplement to *Psychopharmacologia*, vol. 26, 1972. The free communications have been published in full in various journals on psychology, psychopharmacology, pharmacology, and psychiatry according to the choice of the authors. This book contains most of the papers given in the plenary sessions and the symposia. They comprise an excellent review of the most intensively studied aspects of psychopharmacology at the beginning of the nineteen-seventies.

In my capacity of president for C.I.N.P. from 1970 to 1972 as well as chairman of the organizing committee of the 8th congress I have the honour on behalf of all participants to convey my most cordial thanks to all who have helped, the programme committee, the chairmen who have arranged and edited the sessions, Professor Votava who carried out the general editorial work, and last but not least to the authors of the articles for their excellent contributions.

Copenhagen, 1973

Erik Jacobsen

CONTENTS

PREFACE V
(E. JACOBSEN)

NEW APPROACHES TO THE DISCOVERY OF PSYCHOACTIVE DRUGS
(Editor: HANNAH STEINBERG)

A. PLETSCHER: New biochemical approaches to the discovery of psychoactive drugs 3

T. M. ITIL: Quantitative pharmaco-EEG — a new approach to the discovery of a psychotropic drug 13

JOYCE J. KAUFMAN: Quantum chemical and theoretical techniques for the understanding of action of psychoactive drugs 31

P. DENIKER et J. R. BOISSIER: Les échanges du pharmacologue et du psychiatre 43

P. ETEVENON and J. R. BOISSIER: Quantitative and computer EEG analysis in animal neuropharmacology 49

H. RENNERT und G.-E. KÜHNE: Beiträge der Pharmakopsychiatrie zur Entwicklung nosologischer Modelle 55

SOCIAL IMPLICATIONS OF PSYCHOPHARMACOLOGY
(Editor: H. E. LEHMANN)

R. JUNGK: Zukünftige Gesichtspunkte über die mögliche soziale Verwendbarkeit der Psychopharmakologie 59

M. SCHOU and P. C. BAASTRUP: Personal and social implications of lithium maintenance treatment 65

O. H. ARNOLD: Veränderungen des depressiven Erlebens unter Lithium-Dauertherapie . . 69

N. BOHAČEK: Social aspects of psychopharmacology 75

A. HORDERN: Tranquillity denied 81

Z. BÖSZÖRMÉNYI: Ego-strength changes during pharmacotherapy 85

R. ROPERT: Certains aspects sociaux de l'emploi des neuroleptiques à action prolongée: à propos d'une enquête auprès des psychiatres français sur l'introduction de ces médicaments 91

TRAINING MODELS IN PSYCHOPHARMACOLOGY
(Editor: T. A. BAN)

T. A. BAN: Psychopharmacology in the teaching of psychiatry 99

B. MÜLLER-OERLINGHAUSEN and H. HELMCHEN: Postgraduate training in psychopharmacology 105

P. KIELHOLZ: Training models in psychopharmacology 109

O. J. Rafaelsen: WHO training course in psychopharmacology for teachers in medical schools 113
J. J. Lopez Ibor and J. J. Lopez–Ibor Aliño: Training models in psychopharmacology . . 115
D. J. Smeltzer, W. Knopp, D. L. Hunter, R. Mako and F. M. Smeltzer: A computer program to assist independent study of the clinical use of psychotropic drugs 119

DRUG EFFECTS IN NORMALS: CORRELATIONS WITH PHARMACOLOGICAL AND CLINICAL EFFECTS
(Editor: H. Heimann)

H. Heimann: Methodological principles for psychobiological comparison of the effects of psychotropic drugs 127
W. P. Koella: Neurophysiological foundation of behaviour 135
G. Stille und K. Dixon: Korrelation pharmakodynamischer Effekte in verschiedenen Höhen biologischer Organisation 143
D. Bente: Differentielle und generelle Wirkungen psychotroper Pharmaka auf das menschliche EEG 149
W. Janke: Methodologische Aspekte zur Relevanz von Psychopharmaka-Untersuchungen an Gesunden für die Pharmakotherapie 157
H. P. Huber: Zur persönlichkeitsspezifischen Wirkung psychotroper Substanzen auf der Neurotizismusdimension 165
P. Dietsch, F. Albrecht und H. J. Mönikes: Versuch zur Darstellung einer neuroleptischen Behandlung mit EMD 16139 an gesunden Versuchspersonen 171
Z. Böszörményi und Gy. Solti: Eine neue Methode zur Auswertung der Psychotropenwirkung bei normalen Versuchspersonen 177

BIOCHEMICAL FINDINGS IN MENTAL ILLNESS. SCHIZOPHRENIC DISORDERS
(Editor: I. Munkvad)

D. Richter: The nature of the schizophrenic psychoses 185
E. H. Ellinwood, Jr. and A. Sudilovsky: The relationship of the amphetamine model psychosis to schizophrenia 189
Elisabeth Bock and O. J. Rafaelsen: Proteins in blood and cerebrospinal fluid in schizophrenic patients. A preliminary report 205
H. H. Berlet: Tryptophan metabolism and schizophrenia 209
K. Inanaga and M. Tanaka: Effects of L-DOPA on schizophrenia 229
P. Laduron: N-methylation of biogenic amines in the brain with 5-methyltetrahydrofolic acid as the methyl donor: a possible implication in schizophrenia 235

STRATEGY OF TREATMENT OF CHRONIC PATIENTS (PHARMACOLOGICALLY)
(Editor: O. Vinař)

O. Vinař: Whom do neuroleptic drugs help? 247

F. Eckmann: Langjährige Behandlung mit Neuroleptika bei chronisch schizophren kranken Männern 257

R. P. De Buck: Relative safety and efficacy of high and low dose administration of fluphenazine-HCl to psychotic patients 265

K. J. Linden, M. Knaack und W. Edel: Die Kombination von Rating Scales und Handschrifttest zur Objektivierung und Quantifizierung neuroleptischer Effekte. Eine Doppelblindstudie mit Fluspirilene und Penfluridol 273

J. Simeon, B. Saletu, G. Viamontes, M. Saletu and T. Itil: Clinical and neurophysiological investigations of combined thioridazine—d-amphetamine maintenance therapy and withdrawal in childhood behavior disorders 279

T. A. Ban and H. E. Lehmann: Niacin in the treatment of schizophrenias: alone and in combination 293

R. R. Fieve, J. Mendlewicz and J. L. Fleiss: Dominant X-linked transmission in manic-depressive illness: linkage studies with the XGa blood group 301

J. Mendlewicz, R. R. Fieve and F. Stallone: Genetic aspects of lithium prophylaxis in bipolar manic-depressive illness 309

E. T. Mellerup, P. Plenge and O. J. Rafaelsen: Lithium effects on carbohydrate and electrolyte metabolism 319

P. Grof, E. Loughrey, B. Saxena, L. Daigle and J. Quesnell: Lithium stabilization and weight gain 323

W. Werner: "Technical failures" in lithium prophylaxis 329

S. Kanowski and B. Mueller-Oerlinghausen: Need for additional medication in outpatients during three years of prophylactic lithium treatment 335

LONG-TERM EFFECTS OF PSYCHOTROPIC DRUGS
(Editor: Hannah Steinberg)

Hannah Steinberg and M. Tomkiewicz: Long term after-effects of psychoactive drugs on animal behaviour 343

J. P. von Wartburg, M. M. Ris and T. G. White: A possible role of biogenic aldehydes in long-term effects of drugs 355

O. Tesařová: The role of personality factors in the development of depressive conditions in the course of psychopharmacotherapy 363

J. Cochin: Tolerance to the narcotic analgesics. A long-term phenomenon 369

Z. Votava: Tolerance and withdrawal effects after one week administration of perphenazine in rabbits 377

I. Møller-Nielsen, B. Fjalland, V. Pedersen and M. Nymark: Development of tolerance in animals by repeated administration of neuroleptics 383

J. Metyšová: Changes in central effects of several neuroleptics after their repeated administration 387

V. Hansen, J. Ravn and C. Rud: Long-term treatment of psychiatric patients with clopenthixol. Analysis of laboratory investigations 391

STRIATUM AND NEUROLEPTICS
(Editor: J. R. Boissier)

J. R. Boissier et E. Baum: Anatomie et physiologie comparées du système extra-pyramidal. Aspect cholinergique 395

N.-E. Andén, H. Corrodi, K. Fuxe and U. Ungerstedt: Action of neuroleptics on the nigro-neostriatal dopaminergic pathway 407

R. Papeschi and I. Munkvad: Relation of the effect of neuroleptics in animals to pharmacological parkinsonism and antipsychotic action in man 415

A. Villeneuve, K. Jus, A. Jus and J. Gautier: Neuroleptics and dyskinesias 431

P. Deniker et D. Ginestet: Effets thérapeutiques et effets extra-pyramidaux des neuroleptiques chez l'homme 441

DRUGS FOR TREATMENT OF SEXUAL DISORDERS
(Editor: G. L. Gessa)

G. L. Gessa and A. Tagliamonte: Role of brain monoamines in controlling sexual behaviour in male animals 451

B. J. Meyerson, M. Eliasson, L. Lindström, A. Michanek and A. Ch. Söderlund: Monoamines and female sexual behaviour 463

W. Lichtensteiger: Interactions between tubero-infundibular dopamine neurons and the pituitary-gonadal axis 473

C. Kordon: Effect of drugs interfering with central neurotransmitters on pituitary gonadotropic regulation 481

O. Benkert: Pharmacological experiments to stimulate human sexual behaviour 489

Ursula Laschet and L. Laschet: Antiandrogens in sexual disorders: influence of cyproterone acetate on the human neuro-endocrine system 497

H. Steinbeck and F. Neumann: Regulation of sexual behavior 503

M. Da Prada, M. Carruba, A. Saner, R. A. O'Brien and A. Pletscher: The action of 5,6-dihydroxytryptamine and L-DOPA on sexual behaviour of male rats 517

CHOLINERIC MECHANISMS IN THE CENTRAL NERVOUS SYSTEM
(Editor: A. Sundwall)

B. Karlén, G. Lundgren, I. Nordgren and B. Holmstedt: Ion pair extraction in combination with gas phase analysis of acetylcholine 525

J. Schuberth and A. Sundwall: Biosynthesis and compartmentation of acetylcholine in the brain 533

M. Israel: Synthesis and release of acetylcholine in nerve electroplaque junctions from *Torpedo marmorata* 547

E. Heilbronn: Release of low molecular substances from cholinergic vesicles as a consequence of phospholipase A_2 attack 551

P. C. Emson and F. Fonnum: Application of microchemical analysis to the characterization of neurons from the brain of *Helix aspersa* 555

G. Pepeu and A. Nistri: Effects of drugs on the regional distribution and release of acetylcholine: functional significance of cholinergic neurons 563

METABOLISM OF CNS STIMULATING DRUGS
(Editor: F. Sulser)

L. G. Dring and J. Caldwell: The metabolism of the amphetamines in man and laboratory animals 577

F. Cattabeni, G. Racagni and E. Costa: Methamphetamine, fenfluramine and their metabolites: identification and subcellular localization in rat brain homogenates 585

T. B. Vree, J. Th. M. van der Logt, P. Th. Henderson and J. M. van Rossum: Metabolism of cyclohexylisopropylamines in man in comparison with amphetamines 595

Elaine Sanders-Bush and F. Sulser: p-Chloramphetamine: studies on the biochemical mechanism of its action on cerebral serotonin 607

R. W. Fuller, B. B. Molloy and C. Parli: The effect of β,β-difluoro substitution on the metabolism and pharmacology of amphetamines 615

T. Lewander and J. Jonsson: Drugs and certain conditions interfering with the metabolism and excretion of amphetamine in the rat 625

E. Costa: Pharmacological implications of the changes of brain monoamine turnover rates elicited by (+) amphetamine and some chemically related compounds 637

A. Randrup, I. Munkvad and J. Scheel-Krüger: Mechanisms by which amphetamines produce stereotypy, aggression and other behavioural effects 659

J. M. Davis, D. S. Janowsky, M. Khaled El-Yousef and H. J. Sekerke: The psychopharmacology of methylphenidate in man 675

PSYCHOPHARMACOLOGY OF CANNABIS
(Editor: L. Hollister)

R. D. Miller, R. W. Hansteen, H. E. Lehmann, L. Reid, L. Lonero, C. Adamec, L. Theodore and B. Jones: The commision's experimental studies of acute effects of marijuana, Δ^9-THC and alcohol in humans 685

O. J. Rafaelsen, P. Bech, J. Christiansen and L. Rafaelsen: Cannabis and alcohol: effects on simulated car driving and psychological tests. Correlation with urine metabolites 689

D. Ladewig and V. Hobi: The effects of Δ^9-THC on simulated driving performance 693

S. Fisher, R. C. Pillard and R. W. Botto: Hypnotic susceptibility during cannabis intoxication 699

A. Dittrich and B. Woggon: Experimental studies with Δ^9-tetrahydrocannabinol in volunteers — subjective syndromes, physiological changes and after-effects 701

M. Fink, J. Volavka, R. Dornbush and P. Crown: Effects of cannabis on human EEG and heart rate — evidence of tolerance development on chronic use 703

L. E. Hollister: Human pharmacology of marihuana: what next? 705

S. Szara: Δ^9-Tetrahydrocannabinol — potential precursor of "False Hormones"? 707

AUTHOR INDEX 711

SUBJECT INDEX 713

NEW APPROACHES
TO THE DISCOVERY OF PSYCHOACTIVE DRUGS

Chairmen: Hannah STEINBERG and L. JULOU

Associate chairman: T. HALLAS-MØLLER

ACKNOWLEDGEMENTS

Help from the following is gratefully acknowledged: the Foundations' Fund for Research in Psychiatry, F. Hoffmann–La Roche & Co. and Mrs. E. Lawrence.

NEW BIOCHEMICAL APPROACHES TO THE DISCOVERY OF PSYCHOACTIVE DRUGS

A. PLETSCHER

Research Department, F. Hoffmann-La Roche & Co. Ltd., Basel

In recent years, evidence has accumulated that various neurohumoral transmitters, for example noradrenaline (NA), dopamine (DA), 5-hydroxytryptamine (5-HT), acetylcholine, glycine, γ-aminobutyric acid (GABA), are essential for the function of the central nervous system (CNS). Interference with neurohumoral transmitters in the brain has also been shown to be at least partly responsible for the action of many modern psychotropic drugs. This paper deals with the pharmacological changes of the neurohumoral transmitters belonging to the class of aromatic monoamines (catecholamines and 5-HT). How various kinds of psychotropic drugs used in therapy interfere with these transmitters in the CNS is first briefly reviewed. Some new approaches which might lead to the development of future psychotropic agents will then be discussed.

Today's psycho-neurotropic drugs

Many modern psychotropic drugs used in human therapy can be classified according to the mechanism by which they interfere with neurohumoral transmitters. These drugs change the metabolism of cerebral monoamines in the following ways (Fig. 1).

1. *Reserpine-like* drugs cause a depletion of cerebral monoamines, probably by impairing their presynaptic storage at the level of the storage organelles. The drugs act on 5-HT, NA as well as on DA, causing the concentration of the monoamines in the synaptic cleft to decrease.

2. *Amantadine* is thought to liberate DA from intraneuronal, but extragranular stores. Therefore, the DA concentration in the synaptic cleft would increase. The drug also seems to release NA from extragranular sites of noradrenergic nerve endings (26).

3. *Amphetamine and related drugs* also liberate catecholamines from sites located outside the storage organelles (extragranular store) of the nerve endings. These drugs furthermore seem to inhibit the re-uptake of monoamines at the level of the presynaptic membrane and to interfere with the oxidative deamination of the monoamines. The cerebral content of the catecholamines in the synaptic cleft might therefore increase, at least in some areas of the CNS.

4. *Tricyclic antidepressants* (imipramine-type) inhibit the re-uptake of liberated monoamines at the level of the presynaptic membrane, probably increasing the content of

monoamines located in the synaptic cleft. The tricyclic antidepressants interfere with the uptake of catecholamines as well as of 5-HT. The antidepressants with a tertiary amine group seem to preferentially affect the 5-hydroxytryptaminergic neurons, whereas the secondary amines are likely to act more markedly on noradrenergic neurons (10, 11).

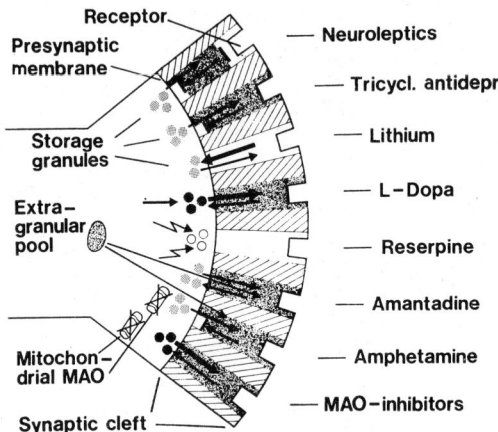

Fig. 1. Mode of action of psycho-neurotropic drugs at the monoaminergic nerve ending: schematic representation of current views.

5. *Neuroleptics* (chlorpromazine- and haloperidol-type) enhance the turnover of catecholamines, especially of DA. Evidence suggests that this effect is the consequence of a primary blockade of catecholaminergic receptors which leads to a positive feedback on catecholamine synthesis (tyrosine or phenylalanine hydroxylase) (4). The turnover of 5-HT does not seem to be markedly enhanced by the classical neuroleptics.

6. *Lithium* has been claimed to enhance the re-uptake of NA into the adrenergic nerve endings of the CNS (12), which causes a decrease in NA located within the synaptic cleft (20).

7. *Monoamine oxidase (MAO) inhibitors* increase the cerebral content of monoamines. Their action bears on 5-HT as well as on catecholamines and is probably due largely to the inhibition of the oxidative deamination, a major metabolic pathway of aromatic monoamines. Hence, the total content of cerebral monoamines (presynaptically and in the synaptic cleft) increases.

8. *L-DOPA*, the precursor of DA, causes an increases of this amine in the brain, mainly in the extrapyramidal centers. In cases of DA deficiency (e.g. in Parkinson's syndrome), L-DOPA may at least partly replete the missing DA in the basal ganglia.

This classification of psychotropic drugs is not absolute as one type of drug may influence the monoamine metabolism in several ways. Neuroleptics, for instance, block catecholaminergic receptors and also inhibit the re-uptake of catecholamines at the presynaptic membrane. L-DOPA, besides increasing the cerebral content of DA, diminishes that of 5-HT and S-adenosylmethionine, and drugs like MAO inhibitors and reserpine not only influence the monoamine content but also interfere with the monoamine turnover. It is likely that some of the therapeutic effects of the psychotropic drugs are directly or indirectly connected with their influence on biogenic monoamines. Other mechanisms seem also to be involved, e.g. a direct influence on receptor sites, interferences with other neurohumoral transmitters such as GABA and acetylcholine, and changes of the electrolyte balance (e.g. by lithium (13)).

New approaches

1. Enhanced catecholamine turnover without catalepsy

In animals the action of neuroleptic drugs on cerebral DA turnover is in general associated with a cataleptic effect which may have a similar origin as the extrapyramidal motor disturbances seen in man. The cataleptic effect is thought to be due to a blockade of dopaminergic receptors in the extrapyramidal brain centers which leads to an increased DA turnover. It has not yet been proved whether the interference with the extrapyramidal brain centers is responsible for the antipsychotic action of neuroleptics in schizophrenia. Nevertheless, the search for new neuroleptic drugs has been based mainly on their cataleptogenic action in animals.

A chemical congener of chlorpromazine, clozapine,*) has been developed recently

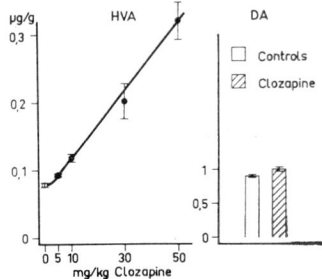

Fig. 2. Content of homovanillic acid (HVA) and dopamine (DA) in rat brain (without cerebellum, pons and medulla oblongata) 2 hours after i.p. administration of various doses of clozapine. In the DA experiments the dose of clozapine was 50 mg/kg. The animals were kept normothermic by elevating the environmental temperature to 32°C. HVA and DA were estimated by spectrophotofluorimetric procedures. The values are expressed in µg/g wet tissue and represent averages with SEM of 3—10 and 3 experiments for HVA and DA, respectively. The point 0 on the abscissa indicates the concentration of HVA in control rats (6).

which seems to have antipsychotic action in schizophrenia, apparently without producing major disturbances of the extrapyramidal functions. In animals, clozapine is practically devoid of a cataleptogenic action (2, 3, 6, 24, 25), but it markedly enhances the DA turnover. In the rat, for instance, the drug increases the cerebral content of homovanillic acid (HVA), the main metabolite of DA (Fig. 2), but causes no change in the cerebral DA concentration and does not interfere with the outflow of HVA from the brain. The drug also enhances the disappearance of striatal DA caused by α-methyltyrosine, an inhibitor of the DA synthesis (Table 1) (6).

The reason for the dissociation of the increased DA turnover from the cataleptogenic action remains to be further investigated. Based on the above and other findings, a tentative hypothesis has been put forward. Clozapine may induce a blockade of DA receptors which might be of the surmountable type, whereas the blockade caused by the classical neuroleptics seems to be insurmountable. On this assumption, the clozapine-induced receptor blockade may be overcome by the increased liberation of DA from

---

*) 8-chloro-11-(4-methyl-1-piperazinyl)-5H-dibenzo-(b, e) (1, 4) diazepine.

Table 1

Effect of clozapine on the disappearance of cerebral dopamine induced by α-methyl-p-tyrosine (αMT; inhibitor of tyrosine hydroxylase)

Treatment	DA content (%)
Clozapine	100 ± 2
α-MT	50 ± 1
Clozapine + α-MT	38 ± 1

Normothermic rats. Clozapine (50 mg/kg) and αMT (300 mg/kg) were injected i.p. 3 h and 2 h respectively before sacrifice. The figures are averages with S.E. of 3 experiments and represent percentages of normal controls (= 100). Absolute dopamine values of controls: 0.903 ± 0.012 (4 experiments). For details of experimental procedure see Fig. 2 (6).

dopaminergic nerve terminals resulting from the feedback activation of DA neurons. The reversal of the receptor blockade by DA possibly prevents catalepsy.

The significance of the increased DA turnover for the antipsychotic action of neuroleptic drugs in schizophrenia remains to be further investigated. Provided that the clinical results of clozapine are confirmed, the antipsychotic action of neuroleptics may have no causal connection with the extrapyramidal disorders. It cannot, however, be excluded that the antipsychotic effect is correlated with an increase of the DA turnover in the basal ganglia.

2. Cortical spreading depression

Unilateral application of 25% KCl to the dura of the rat cerebral cortex induces a depolarization wave which spreads to the whole ipsilateral, but not to the contralateral cortex (Fig. 3). During this depolarization, called spreading depression (SD), the electrical

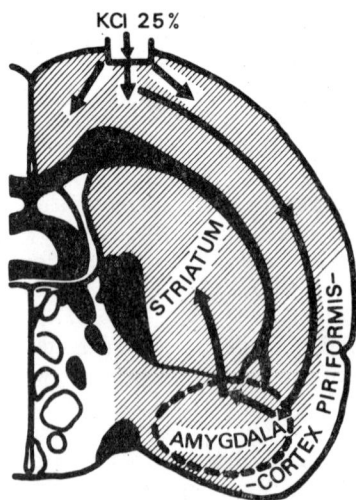

Fig. 3. Spreading depression: depolarization wave induced by epidural application of 25 % KCl in the right cerebral cortex.

activity of the cortex and the striatum is markedly diminished. The cerebral turnover of DA and NA (21) also shows an increase on the side homolaterally to the KCl application. For instance, after unilateral application of 25 % KCl the endogenous HVA markedly rises and the α-methyltyrosine-induced decrease of DA is enhanced in the homolateral striatum compared to the contralateral striatum and to untreated controls (19) (Table 2). Epidural application of 20 % NaCl neither causes SD nor enhances the striatal DA turnover. The 5-hydroxyindoleacetic acid of the striatum homolaterally to the KCl application does not show a significant increase indicating that the rise of HVA is not due to a nonspecific inhibition of the outflow of phenolcarboxylic acids from the brain.

The possible reasons for the increased DA turnover in SD have been discussed elsewhere (19). Suppression of an inhibitory pathway from the striatum to the substantia nigra may be of importance for activating the DA neurons in the latter structure.

Recent experiments indicate that the changes induced by SD can be influenced by drugs. During SD diazepam further enhances the HVA rise in the homolateral but not in the contralateral striatum (7). Hexobarbital is without this effect (Table 2). Diazepam does not change the DA content indicating that the effect on HVA in the homolateral

TABLE 2

Cerebral homovanillic acid (HVA) in spreading depression and effect of diazepam and phenobarbital.

I.p. injection of	HVA content of hemisphere	
	Left	Right
Saline	0.095 ± 0.004[a]	0.149 ± 0.006[b]
Diazepam	0.099 ± 0.005[c]	0.180 ± 0.007[d]
Phenobarbital	0.093 ± 0.003[e]	0.125 ± 0.006[f]

Diazepam (10 mg/kg), phenobarbital (50 mg/kg) or saline was injected i.p. 30 min before the epidural application of 25 % KCl on the right cerebral cortex. One hour after KCl, the rats were sacrificed, and two pooled left (L) or right (R) cerebral hemispheres (without cerebellum, pons and medulla oblongata) were analyzed for HVA by a spectrophotofluorimetric method. Hypothermia of diazepam- and phenobarbital-treated rats was prevented by keeping the animals at an environmental temperature of 32°C. The concentration of HVA is expressed in µg/g wet weight. The values represent means with SEM obtained from 5—8 experiments (7, 19).

P values: a : b, c : d, e : f, d : b < 0.01
f : b $< 0.05; > 0.01$

striatum is due to an additional enhancement of the DA turnover. In normal animals kept strictly normothermic, diazepam affects the content neither of DA nor HVA in the brain. Whether the effect of diazepam in normothermic animals during SD is due to additional suppression of the inhibitory striato-nigral pathway (see above) or whether the drug stimulates an activating striato-nigral projection remains to be investigated. Present experiments indicate that the cerebral monoamine turnover may be more sensitive to the action of drugs during SD than under normal conditions. Therefore, SD might be a convenient method for investigating certain types of drug such as minor tranquilizers.

During SD certain drugs also induce typical behavioural changes. Apomorphine

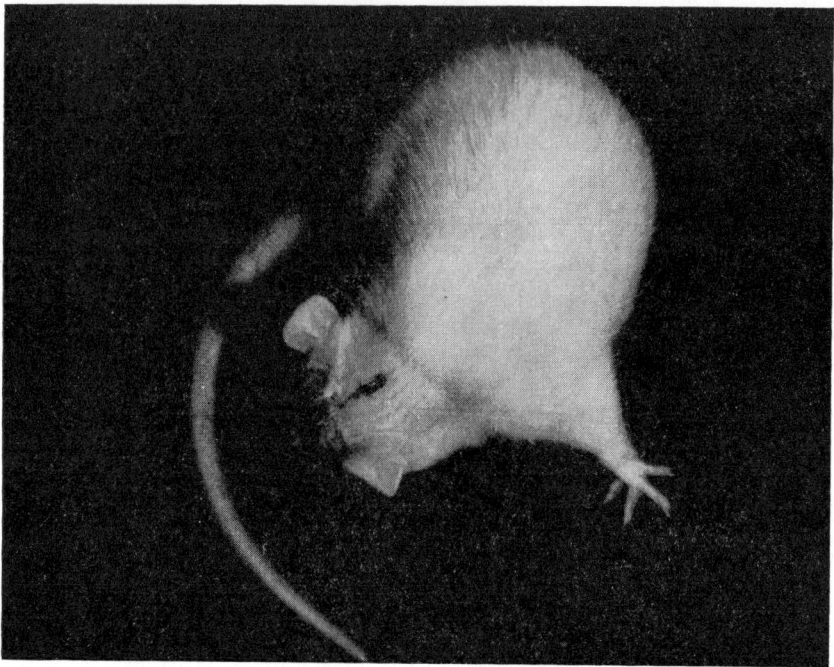

Fig. 4. Rat with epidural application of 25 % KCl on the right cerebral cortex. Dextrorotation due to i.p. injection of 5 mg/kg apomorphine.

injection into animals with unilateral SD causes the animals to rotate towards the side of the KCl application (Fig. 4). A similar form of behaviour is seen in rats given apomorphine after unilateral coagulation of the striatum (1). The rotatory behaviour in both conditions is probably the consequence of the unilateral inactivation or destruction, respectively, of striatal neurons and may result from the predominant stimulation by apomorphine of the dopaminergic receptors of the intact striatum. Reversible inactivation of striatal neurons by unilateral SD may therefore be a relatively simple method for the screening of central dopaminergic drugs.

3. 5-HT and sexual behaviour

The physiological role of 5-HT in the CNS is not fully understood. Good evidence exists that the amine has a function in sleep control. Furthermore, it may be involved in the regulation of pain and mood. Another function of cerebral 5-HT has recently been proposed, control of sexual behaviour. This claim is based on experiments with *p*-chlorophenylalanine, an inhibitor of 5-HT synthesis which rather selectively lowers the 5-TH content of the brain (18, 22, 23, 27). Thus, animals kept in isolation for some days and then injected with *p*-chlorophenylalanine show marked sexual stimulation concomitantly with the decrease of cerebral 5-HT. For instance, the mounting frequency of these animals is markedly increased. The mounts are characterized by the typical coital position followed by pelvic thrusts. In addition, other signs of sexual stimulation are observed, such as penile erection, grooming, scratching and licking the genitals.

Recently, another experimental tool has become available, 5,6-dihydroxytryptamine (5,6-DHT). This compound, when administered into the cerebral ventricles of rats, seems to preferentially destroy 5-hydroxytryptaminergic nerve terminals in the CNS, lowering the cerebral 5-HT content in a relatively selective way, especially in the spinal cord (8, 9). Concomitantly with the 5-HT decrease, the animals show marked sexual stimulation after being kept in isolation prior to the 5,6-DHT administration. Their sexual behaviour resembles that seen after *p*-chlorophenylalanine (14). Injection of the 5-HT precursor 5-hydroxytryptophan to animals pretreated with 5,6-DHT or *p*-chlorophenylalanine reestablishes normal cerebral 5-HT levels and also normalizes sexual behaviour (Table 3).

TABLE 3

Effect of 5,6-dihydroxytryptamine (5,6-DHT) alone and in combination with 5-hydroxytryptophan (5-HTP) on brain amines and sexual behaviour of male rats

Experiment	Cerebral amines (%)			Mounting animals (number in %)	
	5-HT	DA	NE	$\geq 1 \times$	$> 10 \times$
Controls	100 ± 2	100 ± 2	100 ± 4	0	0
5,6-DHT	49 ± 4	93 ± 1	92 ± 3	63	36
5,6-DHT + 5-HTP	104 ± 9	106 ± 3	83 ± 3	0	0

5,6-DHT (50 µg) was injected into the cerebral ventricles. 5-HTP (100 mg/kg) was administered i.p. 9 h after 5,6-DHT. Nine hours after the administration of 5,6-DHT the behaviour of the rats was watched for 3 h and immediately afterwards the animals were sacrificed to measure the brain amines by spectrophotofluorimetric methods. The experiments with 5,6-DHT were carried out on 70 animals, those with 5,6-DHT + 5-HTP and controls on 30 animals each. The brain amines are indicated in percent of controls (= 100) and represent averages with SEM(14).

The experiments with 5,6-DHT which decreases the cerebral 5-HT by a different mechanism of action than *p*-chlorophenylalanine thus confirm that a selective diminution of 5-HT in the CNS leads to sexual stimulation in animals.

In patients with Parkinson's syndrome, chronic administration of L-DOPA has been reported to cause hypersexuality in some instances. In animals, L-DOPA, especially in combination with an inhibitor of extracerebral decarboxylase, is known to selectively decrease the cerebral content of 5-HT (5, 17). Such animals show marked sexual stimulation. In fact, in rats pretreated with the decarboxylase inhibitor Ro 4-4602[*]) and then given two doses of L-DOPA, the mounting frequency is considerably increased, and the other behavioural effects typical of sexual stimulation (pelvic thrusts, penile erection, grooming, licking, scratching) are observed. At the same time, the cerebral 5-HT is decreased (Table 4). Repeated administration of L-DOPA alone (e.g. 8 i.p. doses of 100 mg/kg each with a time interval of 4 h) also induces sexual stimulation and some decrease of cerebral 5-HT. The latter is, however, less marked than that seen with the combination of Ro 4-4602 + L-DOPA (15).

---

[*]) [N-(DL-seryl)-N^1-(2, 3, 4-trihydroxybenzyl)hydrazine] . HCl

TABLE 4

Effect of L-DOPA combined with Ro 4-4602 (inhibitor of extracerebral decarboxylase) on the cerebral 5-hydroxytryptamine (5-HT) content and the sexual behaviour of male rats

		Sexual behaviour	
Drugs	Brain 5-HT	Average mounts per animal	% of animals mounting > 10 ×
Ro 4-4602	99 ± 1	0.9	0
Ro 4-4602 + L–DOPA	43 ± 3	16	38

In the experiments regarding sexual behaviour, Ro 4-4602 (50 mg/kg) was administered i.p. 75 min before the start of the observation period. Two doses of L-DOPA-methylester (each corresponding to 50 mg/kg of the free amino acid) were injected i.p. 45 min and immediately before the observation period. During the observation period, which lasted 3 h, the number of typical mounts was counted. The experiments with Ro 4-4602 alone were performed on 70 animals, those with the combination L-DOPA + Ro 4-4602 on 90 animals. The 5-HT was measured in the brain (without cerebellum) by a spectrophotofluorimetric method 30 min after Ro 4-4602 and 60 min after the last dose of L-DOPA. The 5-HT values represent averages with SEM of 8 experiments each carried out with a pool of two brains. The values are indicated as a percentage of untreated controls (= 100) (15).

These and other findings [e.g. with MAO inhibitors (16)] indicate that 5-HT is involved in the regulation of sexual behaviour in animals and possibly also in man. The mechanism of action of 5-HT is not yet known. Furthermore, the role of other brain amines, e.g. catecholamines, remains to be elucidated. According to available data, it appears that sexual behaviour can be altered by preferential changes of the 5-HT content of the CNS. Therefore, a selective interference with the 5-HT content or with the 5-HT receptors in certain areas of the CNS might present a new approach for designing drugs which regulate sexual behaviour.

SUMMARY

The first part deals with some current concepts regarding the changes of the monoamine metabolism in the central nervous system induced by various clinically used psycho-neurotropic drugs, i.e. reserpine and similar drugs, amantadine, amphetamine-like compounds, tricyclic antidepressants, neuroleptics, lithium, monoamine oxidase inhibitors, and L-DOPA. In a second part, some possible new experimental approaches characterized by changes of the monoamine metabolism in the central nervous system are outlined which might help in the design of psychoneurotropic drugs. The following effects seem to be of interest: (1) increase of cerebral catecholamine turnover without cataleptic action (new type of neuroleptics), (2) enhancement of the catecholamine turnover and induction of rotatory behaviour during spreading depression (minor tranquillizers and dopamine receptor stimulants, respectively), and (3) selective alterations of the 5-HT content and of 5-hydroxytryptaminergic receptors (control of sexual behaviour).

ACKNOWLEDGEMENTS

This work is the result of collaboration with Drs. G. Bartholini, M. Carruba, M. Da Prada, W. Haefely, M. Jalfre, H. H. Keller, R. A. O'Brien, L. Pieri and A. Saner.

REFERENCES

1. ANDÉN, N.-E. (1971) Monoamines and synaptic transmission. In: Symposium Bel-Air IV, Monoamines, Noyaux Gris Centraux et Syndrome de Parkinson, p. 61 (Georg & Masson) Genève/Paris.
2. ANGST, J., BENTE, D., BERNER, P., HEIMANN, H., HELMCHEN, H. and HIPPIUS, H. (1971) Das klinische Wirkungsbild von Clozapin (Untersuchung mit dem AMP-System). Pharmakopsychiat. **4**, 201.
3. ANGST, J., JAENICKE, U., PADRUTT, A. and SCHARFETTER, Ch. (1971) Ergebnisse eines Doppelblindversuches von HF 1854 (8-Chlor-11-(4-methyl-1-piperazinyl)-5HT-dibenzo (b, e) (1,4)diazepin) im Vergleich zu Levomepromazin. Pharmakopsychiat. **4**, 192.
4. BAGHI, S. P. and ZARYCKI, E. P. (1972) Chlorpromazine stimulation of catecholamine formation from phenylalanine in brain. Fed. Proc. **31**, 579.
5. BARTHOLINI, G., DA PRADA, M. and PLETSCHER, A. (1968) Decrease of cerebral 5-hydroxytryptamine by 3,4-dihydroxyphenylalanine after inhibition of extracerebral decarboxylase. J. Pharm. Pharmacol. **20**, 228.
6. BARTHOLINI, G., HAEFELY, W., JALFRE, M., KELLER, H. H. and PLETSCHER, A. (1972) Effects of clozapine on cerebral catecholaminergic systems. Brit. J. Pharmacol. **46**, 736.
7. BARTHOLINI, G., KELLER, H., PIERI, L. and PLETSCHER, A. (1972) The effect of diazepam on the turnover of cerebral dopamine. In: Studies of Neurotransmitters at the Synaptic Level. Adv. Biochem. Psychopharmac., Vol. 6 (Raven Press) New York.
8. BAUMGARTEN, H. G., BJÖRKLUND, A., LACHENMAYER, L., NOBIN, A. and STENEVI, U. (1971) Long-lasting selective depletion of brain serotonin by 5,6-dihydroxytryptamine. Acta Physiol. Scand., Suppl. **373**, 1.
9. BAUMGARTEN, H. G., LACHENMAYER, L. and SCHLOSSBERGER, H. G. (1972) Evidence for a degeneration of indoleamine containing nerve terminals in rat brain induced by 5,6-dihydroxytryptamine. Z. Zellforsch. **125**, 553.
10. CARLSSON, A. (1970) Structural specificity for inhibition of (^{14}C)-5-hydroxytryptamine uptake by cerebral slices. J. Pharm. Pharmacol. **22**, 729.
11. CARLSSON, A., CORRODI, H., FUXE, K. and HÖKFELT, T. (1969) Effect of antidepressant drugs on the depletion of intraneuronal brain 5-hydroxytryptamine stores caused by 4-methyl-α-ethyl-meta-tyramine. Europ. J. Pharmacol. **5**, 357.
12. COLBURN, R. W., GOODWIN, F. K., BUNNEY, W. E. and DAVIS, J. M. (1967) Effect of lithium on the uptake of noradrenaline by synaptosomes. Nature, **215**, 1395.
13. COPPEN, A. (1967) The biochemistry of affective disorders. Brit. J. Psychiat. **113**, 1237.
14. DA PRADA, M., CARRUBA, M., O'BRIEN, R. A., SANER, A. and PLETSCHER, A. (1972) The effect of 5,6-dihydroxytryptamine on sexual behaviour of male rats. Europ. J. Pharmacol. **19**, 288.
15. DA PRADA, M., CARRUBA, M., SANER, A., O'BRIEN, R. A. and PLETSCHER, A. (1972) The action of 5,6-dihydroxytryptamine and L-Dopa on sexual behaviour of male rats. C.I.N.P. Congress, Copenhagen, 1972. Avicenum, Czechoslovak Medical Press, Praha.
16. DEWSBURY, D. A., DAVIS, H. N. jr. and JANSSEN, P. E. (1972) Effects of monoamine oxidase inhibitors on the copulatory behavior of male rats. Psychopharmacologia, **24**, 209.
17. EVERETT, G. M. and BORCHERDING, J. W. (1970) L-Dopa: effect on concentrations of dopamine, norepinephrine, and serotonin in brains of mice. Science, **168**, 849.
18. GESSA, G. L. (1970) Brain serotonin and sexual behavior in male animals. Ann. intern. Med. **73**, 622.
19. KELLER, H. H., BARTHOLINI, G., PIERI, L., and PLETSCHER, A. (1972) Effect of spreading depression on the turnover of cerebral dopamine. Europ. J. Pharmacol. **20**, 287
20. SCHANBERG, S. M., SCHILDKRAUT, J. J. and KOPIN, I. J. (1967) The effects of psychoactive drugs on norepinephrine-^{3}H metabolism in brain. Biochem. Pharmacol. **16**, 393.
21. SCHANBERG, S. M., SCHILDKRAUT, J. J., KRIVANEK, J. and KOPIN, I. J. (1968) Effect of cortical spreading depression on norepinephrine-^{3}H metabolism in brain stem. Experientia, **24**, 909.
22. SHEARD, M. H. (1969) The effect of p-chlorophenylalanine on behavior in rats: relation to brain serotonin and 5-hydroxyindoleacetic acid. Brain Res. **15**, 524.

23. SHILLITO, E. E. (1969) The effect of p-chlorophenylalanine on social interactions of male rats. Brit. J. Pharmacol. **36**, 193.
24. STILLE, G. and HIPPIUS, A. (1971) Kritische Stellungnahme zum Begriff der Neuroleptika (anhand von pharmakologischen und klinischen Befunden mit Clozapin). Pharmakopsychiat. **4**, 182.
25. STILLE, G., LAUENER, H. and EICHENBERGER, E. (1971) The pharmacology of 8-chloro-11-(4-methyl-1-piperazinyl)-5H-dibenzo[b,e][1,4]diazepine (clozapine). Farmaco, Ed. prat. **26**, 603.
26. STRÖMBERG, U. and SVENSSON, T. H. (1971) Further studies on the mode of action of amantadine. Acta pharmac. toxicol. **30**, 161.
27. TAGLIAMONTE, A., TAGLIAMONTE, P., GESSA, G. L. and BRODIE, B. B. (1969) Compulsive sexual activity induced by p-chlorophenylalanine in normal and pinealectomized male rats. Science, **166**, 1433.

A. P., Research Department, F. Hoffmann-La Roche & Co. Ltd., Basel, Switzerland

QUANTITATIVE PHARMACO-EEG — A NEW APPROACH TO THE DISCOVERY OF A PSYCHOTROPIC DRUG*)

T. M. ITIL

Missouri Institute of Psychiatry, University of Missouri School of Medicine, St. Louis

Although BERGER, the discoverer of electroencephalography, demonstrated 40 years ago that a series of CNS effective drugs, administered orally or parenterally, produce characteristic changes in the scalp-recorded electroencephalogram (EEG), this method seldom has been used systematically in the development of psychotropic drugs. With a few exceptions such as FINK, BORENSTEIN, GOLDSTEIN, and PFEIFFER, most investigators apply the EEG in psychopharmacology to determine drug-induced CNS "side effects". Based on the experience that all psychopathologically effective drugs produce systematic changes in the EEG and on the hypothesis that there are close correlations between EEG and behavior alterations, we have systematically applied this method in the diagnosis and prognosis of psychiatric syndromes, in objective evaluation of patients' behavior, and in the development of new psychotropic drugs. In this report we discuss the application of scalp recorded computerized electroencephalogram (CEEG) in the development of new psychotropic drugs.

During the first ten years of our research we collected a large amount of data on the EEG effects of drugs using the visual evaluation technique. In the subsequent five years we replicated our findings using quantitative techniques, and in the last three years we have been applying quantitative EEG as a predictive method in new drug evaluations.

CLASSIFICATION OF PSYCHOTROPIC DRUGS BASED ON "VISUAL" EVALUATION

The EEG classifications of psychotropic drugs based on the visual evaluation of records done by FINK (5), FINK et al. (8), BORENSTEIN et al. (2, 3), and ITIL (12, 16) not only are similar to each other but, more important, are in agreement with the classification based on the clinical use of these compounds. By administering in the same subjects up to 25 different psychotropic drugs on an acute, intravenous basis and taking into consideration the dosage, rate and route of administration, and "individual reactivity" of the subjects, we have established that every drug which is proven to be effective in human behavior also produces significant EEG alterations. Among the tested phenothiazine derivatives, we initially were able to establish four electroencephalographical reaction

---

*) Supported, in part, by the Psychiatric Research Foundation of Missouri.

types (12): (1) phenothiazines which produce low voltage fast EEGs with some slow waves (promethazine reaction type), (2) phenothiazines which induce high voltage rhythmical slow waves and decrease of fast activity (chlorpromazine reaction type), (3) phenothiazines which produce high voltage rhythmical alpha activity and some slow waves (piperazine reaction type), and (4) phenothiazines which produce relatively high voltage slow waves with superimposed fast beta activity (levomepromazine reaction type). Our clinical and EEG investigations have demonstrated that "promethazine EEG reaction type" drugs have a marked sedative effect but no substantial antipsychotic properties, while the "piperazine reaction type" drugs are sedative to a lesser degree but are very effective in schizophrenia. Furthermore, we observed that phenothiazines which produce "chlorpromazine reaction type" EEG alterations (the majority of aliphatic phenothiazines) have sedative properties, produce extrapyramidal side effects, and are predominantly effective in psychomotor agitation of different etiology. Drugs which produce "levomepromazine reaction type" EEG alterations, such as levomepromazine and some of the piperidyl phenothiazines (e.g., thioridazine) have mood elevating effects in addition to sedative properties and, therefore, are also beneficial in the treatment of depressive syndromes (13). We reported that imipramine, a then relatively unknown non-phenothiazine compound, induced EEG alterations similar to that of the "levomepromazine reaction type" (12).

We applied this EEG classification for the first time in testing a series of phenothiazines. In this study we predicted that butaperazine, a piperazine phenothiazine, would be more effective than the other four tested piperazines in the treatment of schizophrenic patients, since it produced the most marked alpha activity in the EEG (1). The subsequent clinical investigations confirmed our prediction. Today, butaperazine is one of the most commonly used neuroleptics in Germany.

In a later classification of psychotropic drugs, we included some new compounds (13). We observed that lorusil, padisal, and some morpholino phenothiazine derivatives, as well as some bi- and tricyclic derivatives such as benadryl and benactyzine, also show a "promethazine-type EEG reaction". The newly tested piperazine derivatives such as trifluoperazine, thioproperazine and fluphenazine showed "piperazine-type EEG reactions," and were also effective in schizophrenia. Amitriptyline, which showed the "levomepromazine EEG reaction type," was found to be effective in depression.

Although by using thiopental activation we were further able to demonstrate that drugs effective in schizophrenia produce EEG alterations different from those effective in depressive syndromes, neither our findings nor the similar findings of FINK and BORENSTEIN could stimulate sufficient interest to promote EEG as a significant method in developing new drugs. The major criticisms of EEG drug research have been the lack of knowledge of the origin of brain waves, unknown factors regarding the metabolism of drugs, limitation of scalp recording techniques, physiological fluctuations of EEG frequency and amplitude distributions, and, last but not least, relatively "unscientific" evaluations of EEG records without quantification. Disregarding the critics, we systematically collected further EEG and drug data and replicated our studies using the quantitative method of evaluation.

CLASSIFICATION OF PSYCHOTROPIC DRUGS BASED ON QUANTITATIVE EEG

One of the first and most important findings in quantitative EEG research was the discrimination of chlorpromazine, a neuroleptic, from imipramine, a thymoleptic, by FINK (4) using analog frequency analyzer. Although the two drugs seemed similar, the differences in clinical effectiveness were confirmed by the differences in alterations of brain function. Later, GOLDSTEIN and BECK (11), using the amplitude integration technique (DROHOCKI), and ULETT et al. (26), using analog frequency analyzer, demonstrated differences in EEG alterations after some minor and major tranquilizers. Using

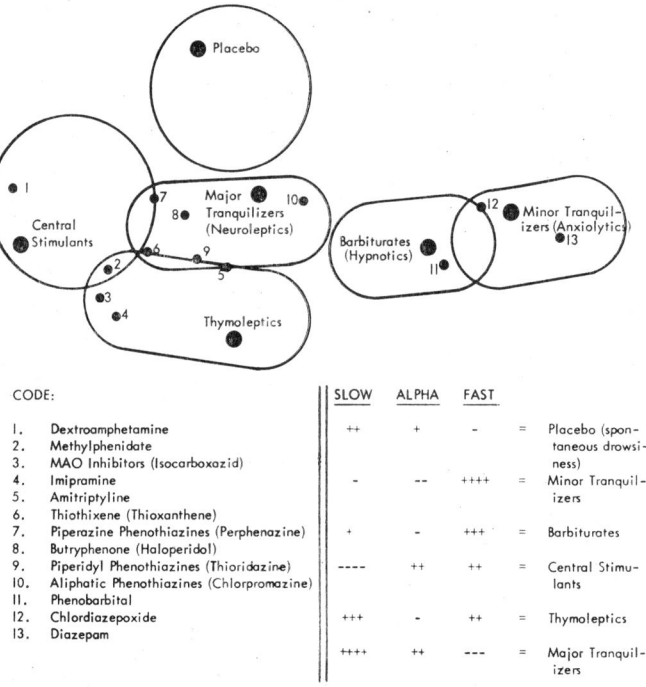

Fig. 1. Classification of psychotropic drugs based on visual evaluation. Minor tranquilizers produce most fast activity while major tranquilizers produce the most slow waves. Central stimulants markedly decrease slow waves and major tranquilizers markedly decrease fast activity. Thymoleptics produce slow and fast waves. After placebo, due to relaxed setting, patients are getting drowsy with the result of increase of slow waves in the EEG.

digital computer period analysis and analog frequency analyzers with FINK and SHAPIRO, we advocated the significance of quantitative EEG in psychopharmacology (6, 7). We demonstrated that the most important representatives of minor and major tranquilizers and antidepressants (chlordiazepoxide, chlorpromazine, and imipramine, respectively) indeed produce statistically significant different EEG alterations in normal volunteers and in psychiatric patients (16, 17).

In a study just completed, we investigated 13 psychotropic drugs with known clinical effectiveness and placebo in three matched groups of normal male volunteers. Based on our visual evaluation of psychotropic drugs, we predicted five different EEG reaction types which include minor tranquilizers, barbiturates, central stimulants, thymoleptics, and major tranquilizers (Fig. 1). The evaluation of digital computer analyzed EEG data demonstrated that minor tranquilizers (diazepam and chlordiazepoxide) decreased slow waves and increased fast activities, particularly in the frequency range of 20—40 cps

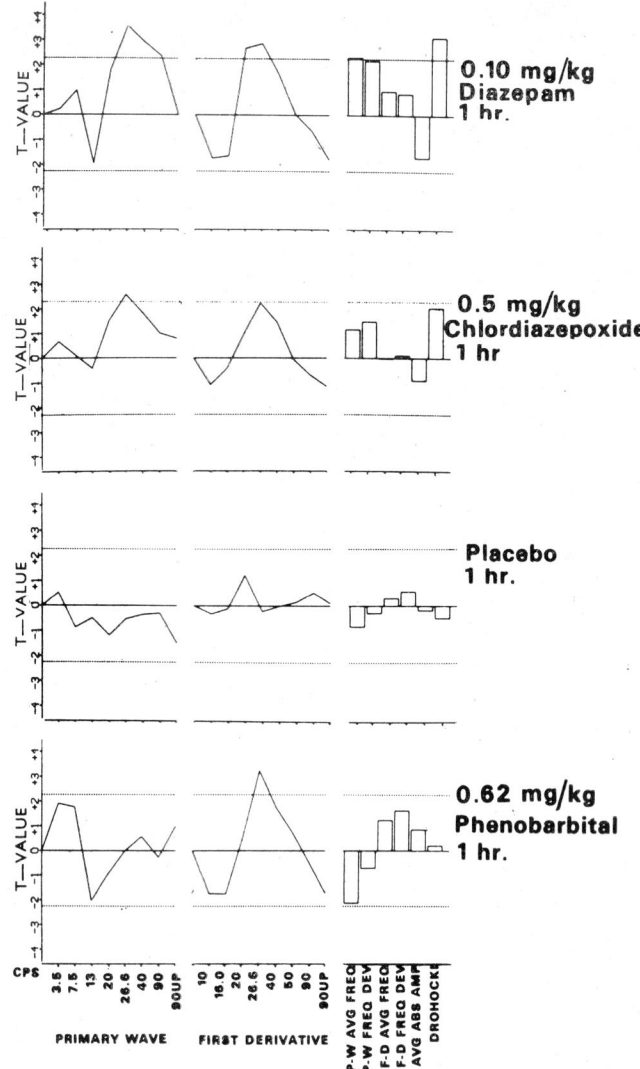

Fig. 2. EEG profiles of minor tranquilizers based on digital computer period analysis. Twenty-two computer analyzed EEG variables are shown on the abscissa; t-values of the changes of these variables from the predrug state to 1 hour after administration are shown on the ordinate. The dotted line implies statistical significance at the level of $P < 0.05$. Sample size = 10. EEG recording combination: right occipital to right ear (recording was done during reaction time measurements). As can be seen, chlordiazepoxide, but particularly diazepam, increased fast activity both in primary wave and first derivative measurements. Changes occurred in the average frequency, frequency deviation, amplitude and amplitude variability (DROHOCKI) in the same direction with both minor tranquilizers. Placebo did not produce any significant changes. Phenobarbital also increased fast activity in the first derivative measurement. In the primary wave measurement a marked increase of slow waves is seen.

(minor tranquilizer EEG profile) (Fig. 2). Thioridazine, perphenazine, and chlorpromazine increased slow waves and decreased fast activity (major tranquilizer CEEG profile) (Fig. 3). Interestingly, up to the third hour after administration, thioridazine, which is generally accepted as a neuroleptic, produced CEEG alterations similar to those of other neuroleptic drugs while later the CEEG changes showed a similarity to those induced by amitriptyline. Both tricyclic antidepressants (imipramine and amitriptyline)

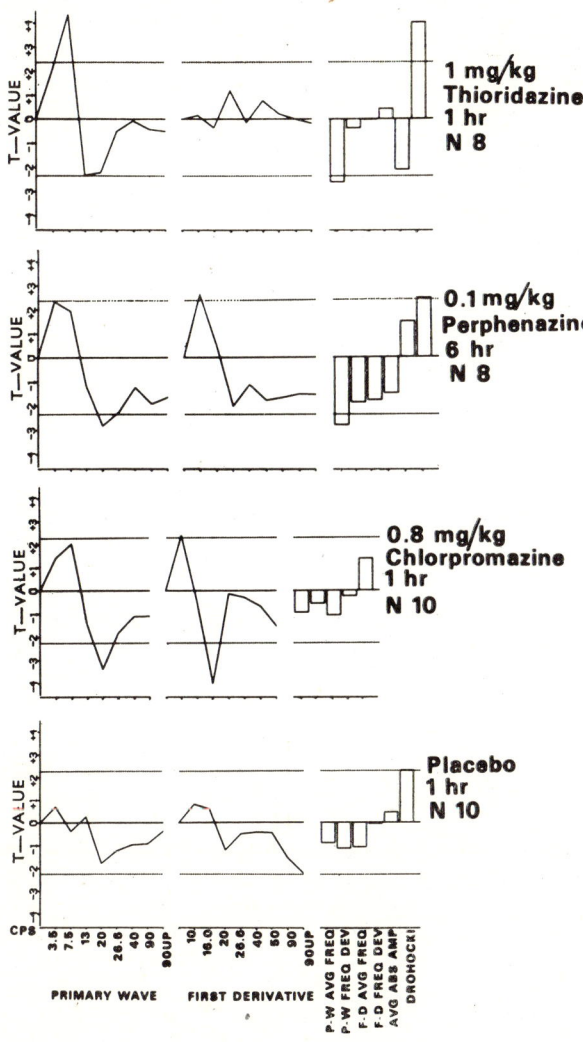

Fig. 3. EEG profiles of major tranquilizers based on digital computer period analysis. Thioridazine, perphenazine, and chlorpromazine increased slow waves and decreased fast activity in primary wave measurements. Similar profiles in the first derivative measurements were seen after perphenazine and chlorpromazine. The significant changes occurred 1 hour after thioridazine and chlorpromazine and 6 hours after oral administration of perphenazine. EEG recording combination: right occipital to right ear (N = 10) (abscissa and ordinate are the same as in Fig. 2).

increased both slow and fast activity in the EEG (thymoleptic CEEG profile) (Fig. 4). Isocarboxazid, a thymoleptic-effective MAO inhibitor, decreased slow waves and fast activity, and increased alpha waves in the primary wave measurements, but also increased slow waves in the first derivative measurements. Therefore, from the EEG point of

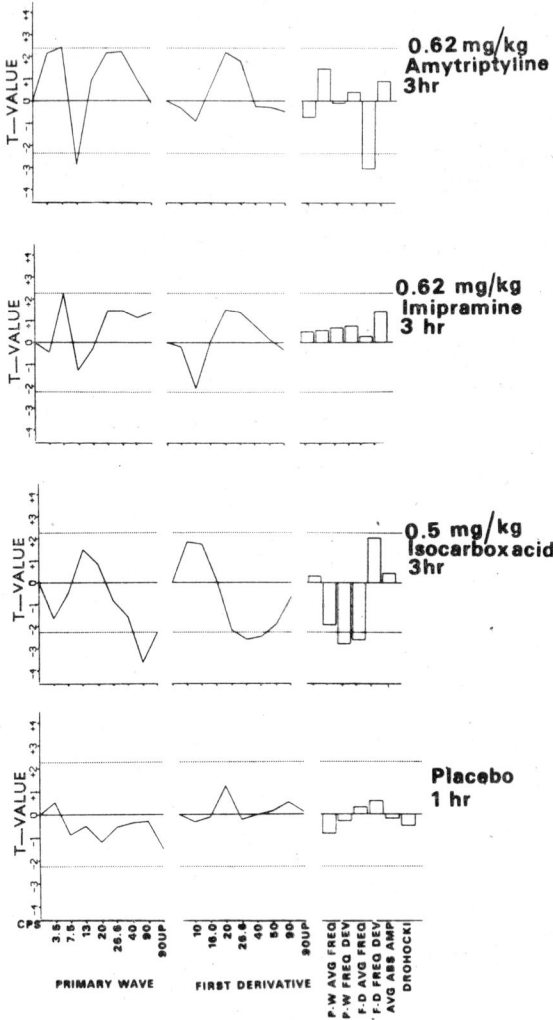

Fig. 4. EEG profiles of thymoleptics based on digital computer period analysis. Amitriptyline and imipramine increased slow waves as well as fast activity, decreased alpha waves in the primary wave measurements, decreased slow and increased fast activity in the first derivative measurements. Amitriptyline produced more slow waves than imipramine, suggesting more sedative properties in equimolar dosages. Isocarboxacid decreased slow and increased fast activity in the primary wave measurements which suggests central stimulatory properties. An increase of slow waves in the first derivative measurements also suggests, however, some central inhibitory properties. This discriminates this component from CNS stimulants (see Fig. 5). Recording was done from right occipital to right ear ($N = 10$).

view this compound can be classified between tricyclic antidepressants and central stimulants. Dextroamphetamine and methylphenidate decreased slow waves and increased fast activity in the EEG (CNS stimulants CEEG profile) (Fig. 5).

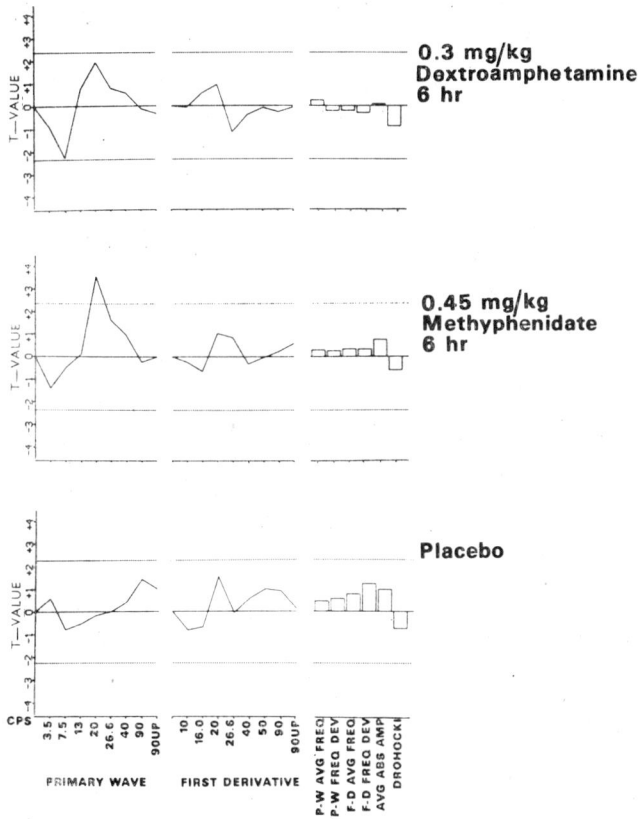

Fig. 5. EEG profiles of CNS stimulants based on digital computer period analysis. Both dextroamphetamine and methylphenidate markedly decreased slow waves and increased fast activity 6 hours after oral administration. In contrast to minor tranquilizers no marked changes occurred in first derivative measurements (superimposed activity). Recording was done from right occipital to right ear (N = 9).

QUANTITATIVE PHARMACO-ELECTROENCEPHALOGRAPHY

The process involving the use of digital computer analyzed EEG and statistical procedures for the establishment of the central effectiveness of a new compound in humans, the prediction of its clinical usefulness and an estimation of the effective dosage range after single oral administration has been called "quatitative pharmaco-electroencephalography" (18—21). While in previous studies we had applied EEG as a retrospective approach in the classification of psychotropic drugs with known clinical effectiveness, quantitative pharmaco-electroencephalography has been used in Phase 1 and pre-Phase 1 trials in the development of new psychotropic drugs. Using quantitative pharmaco-electroencephalography, in the last three years we have predicted the clinical effectiveness of a series of compounds.

I. *Quantitative pharmaco-electroencephalography studies with compounds predicted by pharmacology as "psychotropic"*

The type of clinical effectiveness of a series of compounds which already had been predicted based on animal models could be confirmed with the use of quantitative pharmaco-electroencephalography in humans.

A. *CEEG prediction of a major tranquilizer*

1. *SQ-11,290*

SQ-11,290, a derivative of dihydrodibenzoxazepine heterocycle (4-[3-(7-chloro-5,11-dihydrodibenz[b, e] [1,4]-oxazepin-5-yl) propyl]-1-piperazine ethanol dihydrochloride), was predicted, using animal pharmacology, to be effective in anxiety syndromes, schizophrenic pathology, manic disorders, and agitated states. The single effective oral dosage range was estimated to be 5.0—1,000 mg. Quantitative pharmaco-electroencephalography demonstrated that this compound indeed has obvious effects on human brain function (19). The EEG profile of SQ-11,290 was similar to that of the "chlorpromazine reaction type" with an increase of slow waves and decrease of fast activity and, therefore, it was predicted that SQ-11,290 would be an effective major tranquilizer. The single effective dosage was predicted to be 25—50 mg. Subsequent clinical investigations have confirmed that SQ-11,290 is indeed a neuroleptic with effective daily dosages of 100 mg (4 × 25 mg) (19).

B. *CEEG prediction of minor tranquilizers*

1. *Chlorazepam*

Chlorazepam is actually not a new compound but rather a chemical entity resulting from the combination of diazepam and chloralhydrate in equimolar proportions. The chloralhydrate element represents 36.8% of the molecular weight of this compound. Qualitatively, chlorazepam behaves much like its diazepam moiety. On a milligram-to-milligram basis in animal studies, chlorazepam was found to be more potent than diazepam. By quantitative pharmaco-electroencephalography, it was demonstrated that chlorazepam indeed has a significant central effect in man (19). The types of changes induced by chlorazepam are almost identical to those produced by diazepam (Fig. 6). Chlorazepam differed from diazepam only during the first hour recording, when chlorazepam produced more EEG changes. Later, diazepam induced more EEG alterations than chlorazepam. The subsequent clinical study confirmed this prediction based on quantitative pharmaco-electroencephalography. In a double-blind study a group of anxiety subjects treated with chlorazepam showed improvement similar to a group given diazepam; however, the chlorazepam group received 45% less diazepam. This indicated that a minimum amount of chloralhydrate does indeed potentiate diazepam effects on the EEG as well as on anxiety syndromes (19).

2. SCH-12,041

SCH-12,041 is a synthetic compound with a chemical structure related to those of chlordiazepoxide, diazepam, and oxazepam (7-chloro-1,3-dihydro-5-phenyl-1-[2,2,2-trifluoroethyl]-2H-1,4-benzodiazepin-2-one) and is different from diazepam only in the trifluoroethyl substituent at position 1. Based on animal studies, it was predicted that SCH-12,041 may be a useful psychopharmacological agent in man, possibly as an anticonvulsant, minor tranquilizer, and/or muscle relaxant.

Single dose trials using quantitative pharmaco-electroencephalography have shown that in single oral dosages of 20—240 mg SCH-12,041 produces significant EEG changes

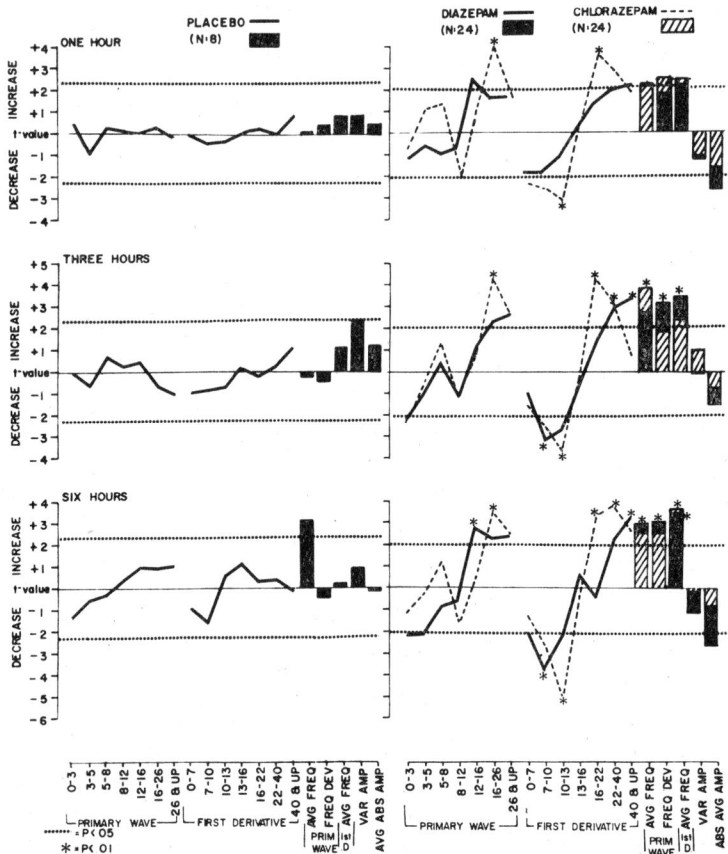

Fig. 6. Changes in EEG period analysis measurements 1, 3 and 6 hours after oral administration of placebo, diazepam and chlorazepam. Nineteen computer EEG measurements are shown on the abscissa and t-values of these measurements from pre- to postdrug (or placebo) period on the ordinate; EEG leads were placed from right occipital to right ear. Diazepam dosage range: 1—20 mg (mean 6.4 mg), chlorazepam dosage range: 1—20 mg (mean 6.4 mg). During recordings 1, 3 and 6 hours after administration, in comparison to predrug levels, both diazepam and chlorazepam produced significantly more fast waves in the primary wave as well as first derivative measurements. A significant increase of average frequencies and frequency deviation also occurred. The only major difference between the two drugs is the increase of slow waves with chlorazepam and a decrease after diazepam, particularly during the first hour after administration.

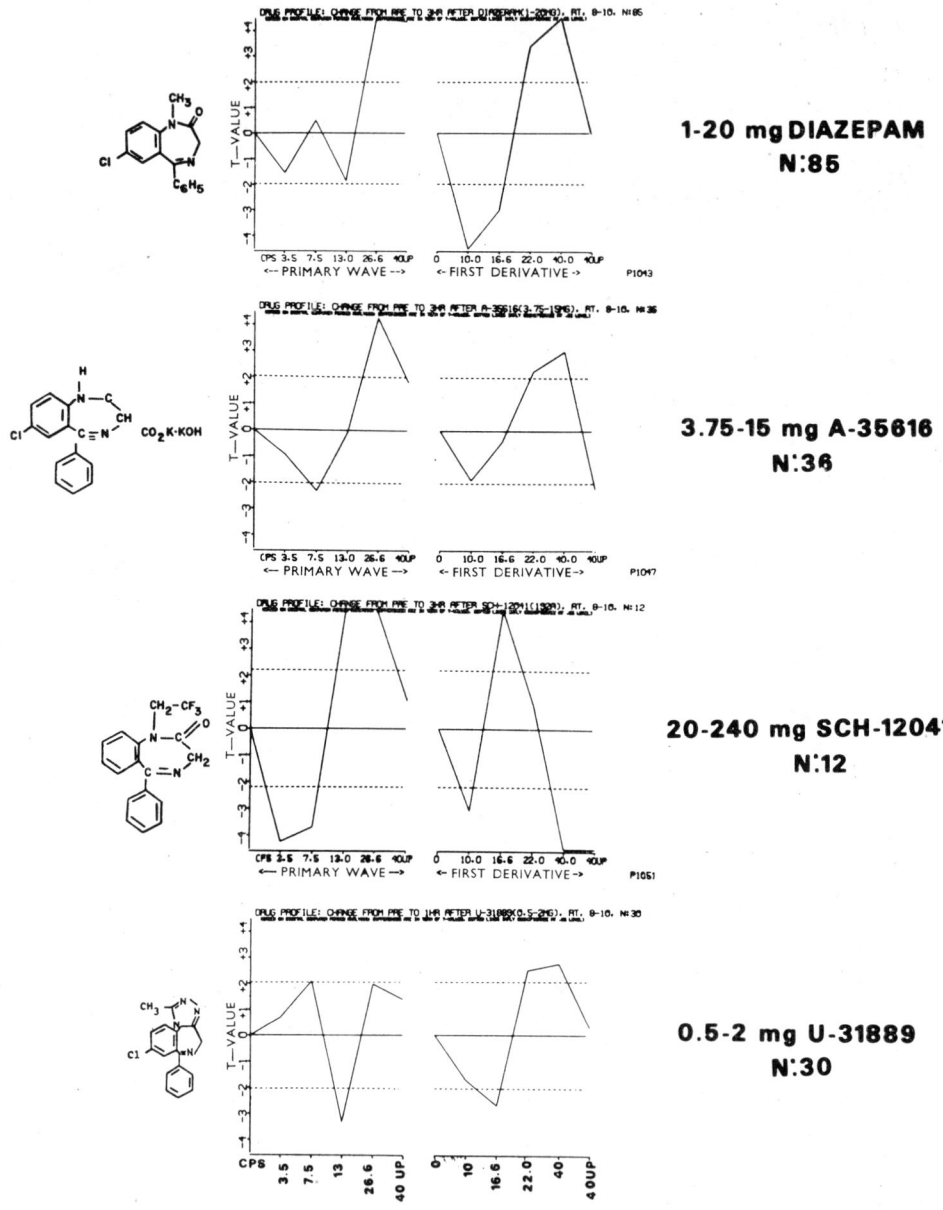

Fig. 7. Prediction of anxiolytic drugs based on digital computer EEG profiles. Ten EEG measurements are shown on the abscissa and t-values of the EEG measurements from pre- to postdrug period on the ordinate. EEG leads were placed from right occipital to right ear. Dosages of 1.0—20 mg diazepam produced a significant increase of fast activity and decrease of slow waves in both primary wave and first derivative measurements (sample size = 85). A-35,616 (clorazepate dipotassium) and SCH-12,041 (halazepam) in oral dosages of 3.75—15 mg and 20—240 mg, respectively, produced changes almost identical in quality to those of diazepam. Accordingly, both compounds have been predicted as "anxiolytic" (minor tranquilizer).

characteristic for minor tranquilizers (Fig. 7). In dosages of 1.0—20 mg, however, the EEG changes did not reach the level of the statistical significance as was the case after placebo, indicating that this dosage range does not induce significant changes in brain function. The single clinically effective dosage of SCH-12,041 was predicted to be 30—40 mg based on EEG dose response studies. The clinical trials confirmed the anxiolytic effects of SCH-12,041 (18).

3. *A-35,616*

Abbott-35,616 is a new diazepam analog, dipotassium clorazepate (7-chloro-2,2-dihydroxy-5-phenyl-3-carboxy-2,3-dihydro-1H-1,4-benzo[f] diazepin, dipotassium). Quantitative pharmaco-electroencephalography demonstrated that single oral dosages of this compound produce EEG changes (increase of fast activity and decrease of slow waves) which are characteristic of all presently known minor tranquilizers (Fig. 7). EEG changes after A-35,616 occurred earlier than diazepam but lasted a shorter time. The minimum single clinically effective dosage was estimated as 7.5 mg. Clinical studies with this compound have demonstrated that A-35,616 is indeed an anxiolytic drug similar to diazepam.

4. *U-31,889*

U-31,889 is a new triazolobenzodiazepine derivative (phenyl-4H-triazolo[4,3-a] [1,4]benzodiazepine). Although it has been predicted by animal pharmacology to be an anxiolytic drug, the compound was given to us in order to investigate its hypnotic properties. Our study, using digital computer period analysis of the all-night sleep, clearly demonstrated that U-31,889 has a profile similar to that of an anxiolytic drug, with increasing 20—40 cps fast activities. Interestingly, particularly in high dosages (1 and 2 mg), U-31,889 also increases slow waves, an effect similar to amitriptyline. The effective single dosage of U-31,889 was estimated to be 0.5 mg. The subsequent clinical trial demonstrated that in daily dosages of 2 mg (4 × 0,5 mg) U-31,889 is an effective anxiolytic (23).

C. *CEEG prediction of antidepressants*

1. *SCH-12,650*

SCH-12,650 is a 2-[p-chlorophenyl-2-(pyridyl)-hydroxymethyl] imidazoline maleate. The single dose trials using quantitative pharmaco-electroencephalography demonstrated that this compound has an EEG profile similar to that of imipramine (Fig. 8). SCH-12,650

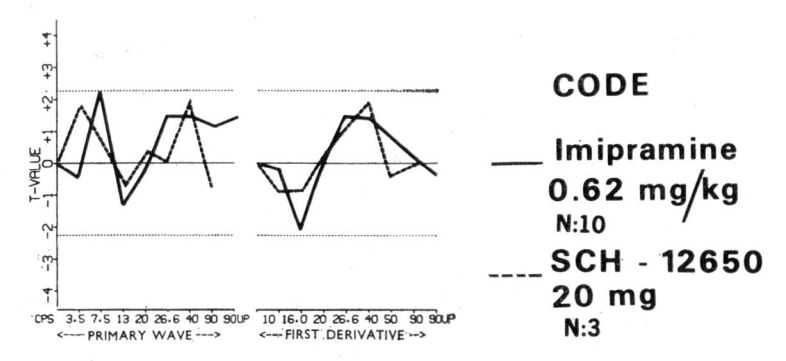

Fig. 8. EEG profiles of imipramine and SCH-12,650 based on digital computer period analysis. Three hours after 20 mg oral administration, SCH-12,650 produces changes very similar to imipramine (0.62 mg/kg) with an increase of slow and fast activity in the first derivative measurements.

was predicted to be a thymoleptic with a single effective dosage of 20 mg. An open clinical trial in depressive subjects confirmed our prediction: SCH-12,650 was found to have antidepressant effects with obvious centrally stimulatory properties.

2. *OI-77*

OI-77, a new tricyclic (5-methylaminoacetyl-6-methyl-5,6-dihydrophenanthridine hydrochloride) showed a profile similar to imipramine in pharmaco-electroencephalographical trials. An open clinical trial in depressive patients showed that OI-77 is an antidepressive drug with clinical efficacy and side effects similar to imipramine (24).

D. *CEEG prediction of an "antiaggressive" drug*

1. *SCH-12,679*

SCH-12,679 (d-7,8-dimethoxy-3-methyl-phenyl-2,3,4,5,-tetrahydro-1H-3-benzazepine acid maleate) is a new compound with no close chemical similarity to any other drug in

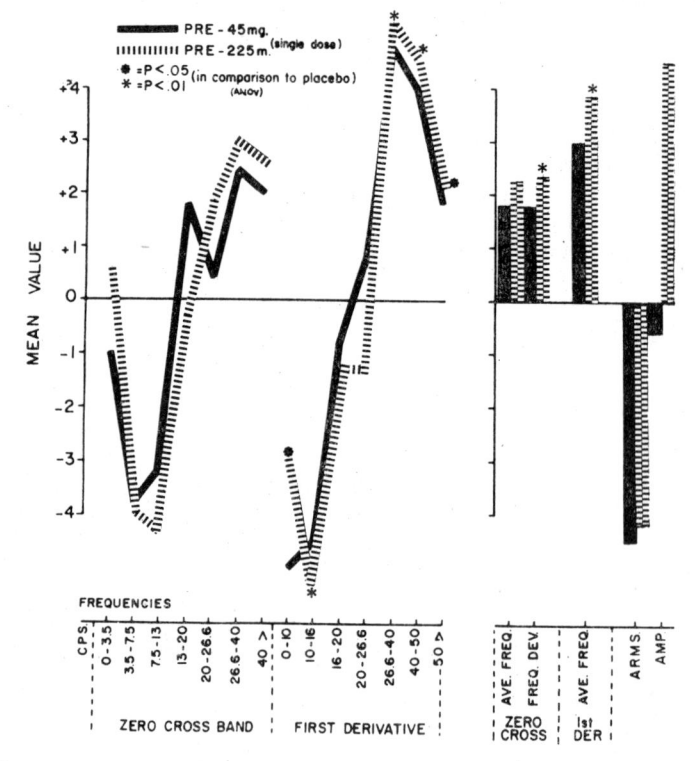

Fig. 9. EEG profile of SCH-12,679 based on digital computer period analysis. EEG measurements are shown on the abscissa and mean values of the EEG measurements from predrug to 3 hours after oral drug administration on the ordinate. EEG leads: right occipital to right ear, 10-minute resting recordings pre- and postdrug period. Both 45 mg and 225 mg of SCH-12,679 produced a decrease of slow waves and an increase of fast activity. Particularly in the first derivative measurements, both the decrease of slow waves and increase of fast activity reached the level of statistical significance with 225 mg. With decrease of slow waves and increase of fast activity the SCH-12,679 profile is similar to those of minor tranquilizers and CNS stimulants. However, in contrast to minor tranquilizers, it induces less fast activity in the primary wave measurements, and in contrast to CNS stimulants it induces more fast activity in the first derivative measurements. Accordingly, SCH-12,679 presents a new type of EEG profile (N=10).

therapeutic use. The most striking feature of its pharmacological profile lies in the specificity of its tranquilizing activity. No other major tranquilizer or known antianxiety drug approached the wide separation observed with SCH-12,679 between potential pharmacological and side effect doses. In mice and monkeys, SCH-12,679 reduces aggressive behavior over wide dose ranges and with no signs of neurological (extrapyramidal) symptoms or sedation. Quantitative pharmaco-electroencephalography demonstrated that after single oral dosages SCH-12,679 has a central effect in man, and the types of EEG changes suggest that the drug has no similarity to the EEG profiles of presently available minor or major tranquilizers. Single doses of 45 mg and up produce fast activity and decrease slow waves (Fig. 9). In contrast to the typical minor tranquilizer profile, SCH-12,679 also increased very fast beta activity of over 50 cps. Clinical investigations have shown that SCH-12,679 had no minor or major tranquilizer effects (25) but exhibited a "new" clinical profile. SCH-12,679 was found, however, to be effective in aggressive outbursts of behaviorally disturbed, mentally retarded adolescents without producing sedation (23).

II. *Quantitative pharmaco-EEG studies with compounds not predicted by animal pharmacology as "psychotropic"*

In fact animal pharmacology had already predicted the psychotropic properties and clinical activity of the above-mentioned compounds. However, we were able recently to test the predictive value of our method on a series of compounds which had not been predicted by animal pharmacology to have any psychotropic properties.

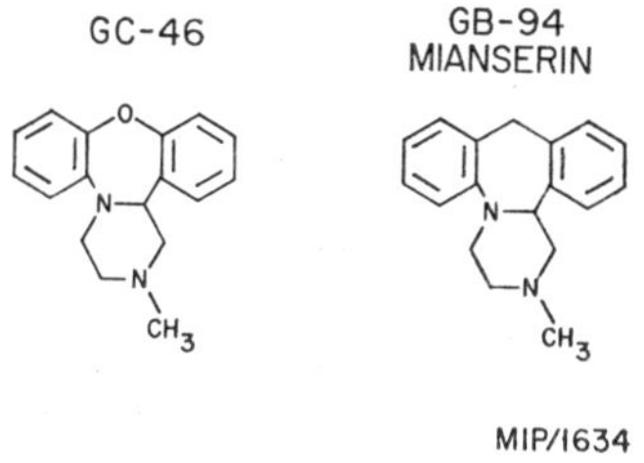

Fig. 10.

In recent investigations, we were able to confirm the reports of some investigators regarding the serotonin hypothesis in mania and the therapeutic effects of antiserotonin compounds in manic patients (20). In the search for potent antiserotonin compounds with less toxic effects to investigate in manic patients, we received two compounds which belong to a known group of "tetracyclic" compounds: GB-94 (mianserin hydrochloride) (1,2,3,4,10,14b-hexahydro-2-methyl-dibenzo [c,f] pyrazino-[1,2-a] azepine monohydrochloride) and GC-46 (2[N]-methyl-1,3,4,14b-tetrahydro-2H-pyrazino[1,2-d] dibenzo [b,f][1,4] oxazepine) (Fig. 10). These "tetracyclics" were developed by structural modification of the phenbenzamine molecule in order to enhance its antiserotonin activity (27). Based on animal pharmacology, both compounds indeed have potent peripheral antiserotonin properties but less CNS effects (sedative properties) than the control compound (cyproheptadine). Both drugs were predicted to be effective in the treatment of allergic conditions, hay fever, asthma and migraine. Since, however, the clinical testing did not show any superiority to existing antiallergic drugs, clinical trials with these compounds were discontinued many years ago.

As usual, before the clinical trials in manic patients, we studied the effects of these drugs in normal volunteers after oral administration of different doses (Phase 1 trials) using quantitative pharmaco-electroencephalography. In the pilot EEG trials we were able to determine that both compounds produce significant changes in the EEG. The types of EEG alterations were similar to those induced by existing tricyclic antidepressant compounds (increased slow waves and increase of superimposed fast beta activity) which we called the "thymoleptic EEG reaction type" (13, 14) (Fig. 11). We observed that equimolar doses of GB-94 produced more EEG changes than GC-46 and predicted that GB-94 would have clinical effects similar to those of amitriptyline, and GC-46 to those

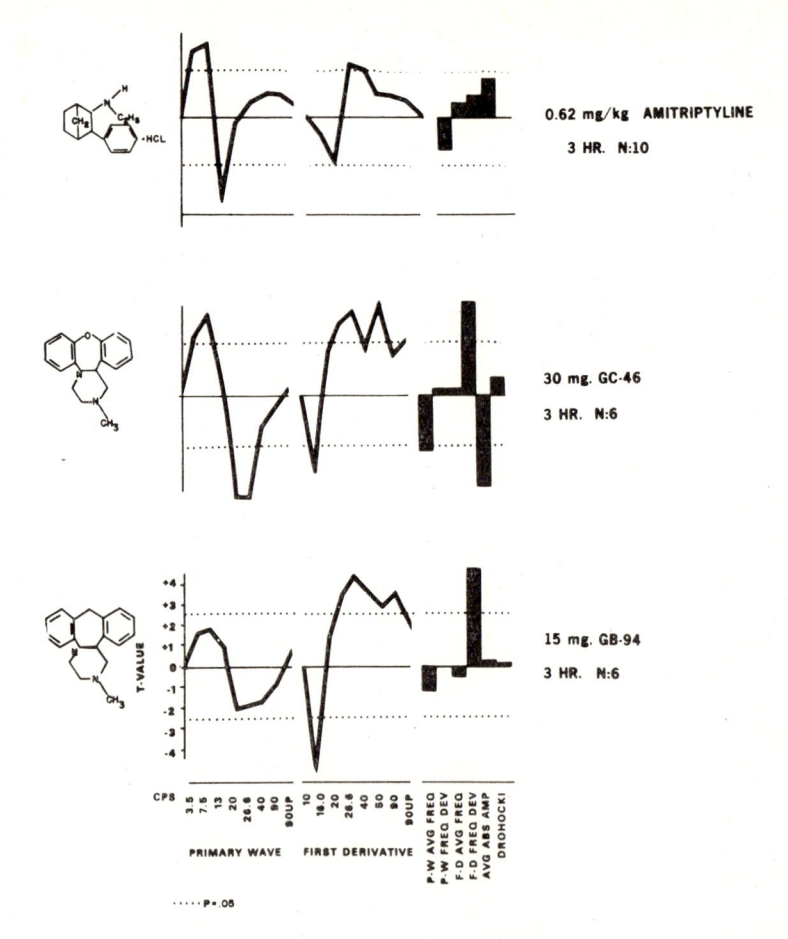

Fig. 11. EEG profiles of thymoleptic drugs (based on digital computer analysis). Three hours after 0.62 mg/kg amitriptyline an increase of slow and an increase of fast activity is seen, which is the typical thymoleptic CEEG profile. 30 mg GC-46 and 15 mg GB-94 both showed an increase of slow waves and decrease of fast activity (only up to 40 cps) in the primary wave measurements (some similarity to major tranquilizers), but a marked decrease of slow and a significant increase of fast activity in first derivative measurements, very similar to tricyclic thymoleptics. Both compounds, but particularly GB-94, resemble amitriptyline more than imipramine.

of imipramine (22). We established the effective dose of GB-94 as 10—20 mg single dose (Fig. 12). The subsequent double-blind controlled trial with amitriptyline demonstrated that in daily dosages of 30—55 mg, GB-94 is indeed an antidepressive compound with a psychopathological effect similar to amitriptyline (22). Based on three different rating scales, it was established that GB-94 had a significant effect on several symptoms of depressive patients. Depressive mood, sadness, feeling of inadequacy, deprivation, hopelessness, low self-esteem, insomnia and irritability showed statistically significant

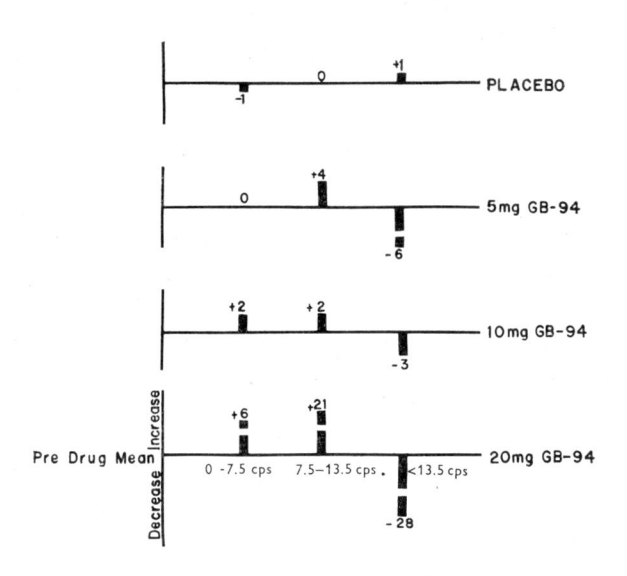

Fig. 12. EEG dose response curves of GB-94 based on digital computer period analysis. Three EEG measurements are shown on the abscissa and changes from predrug to 1 hour after drug administration are shown on the ordinate. While placebo did not produce marked changes, after GB-94, particularly in the 0—7.5 cps frequency band, a dose-related increase is seen.

improvement. None of the 51 symptoms on the Side Effects Rating Scale showed a significant worsening during GB-94 treatment. In contrast, some symptoms such as restlessness, insomnia, sadness and irritation did show significant improvement. The effect of chronic administration of GB-94 on the EEG was similar to that seen in single dose trials with an increase of slow waves and slow beta activity (only in first derivative) (Fig. 13). As expected, the control compound, amitriptyline, produced similar clinical and EEG alterations. During the first week of evaluation GB-94 was effective on more symptoms (rapid onset of antidepressive effects), while during the third week amitriptyline was more effective. However, the differences between the two compounds were not at the level of statistical significance (discriminant analysis) in any of the clinical or EEG data or in any of the evaluation periods. In further trials in schizophrenic patients GB-94 was found to be effective only in paranoid schizophrenics while the other schizophrenics showed significant deterioration with a worsening of total psychopathology. Accordingly, GB-94 could not be classified as a major tranquilizer (neuroleptic). The pilot trial in anxiety subjects showed that GB-94 is effective predominantly in depressive symptomatology. Improvement of some anxiety symptoms has been considered a secondary effect and, therefore, GB-94 also could not be classified as a typical anxiolytic.

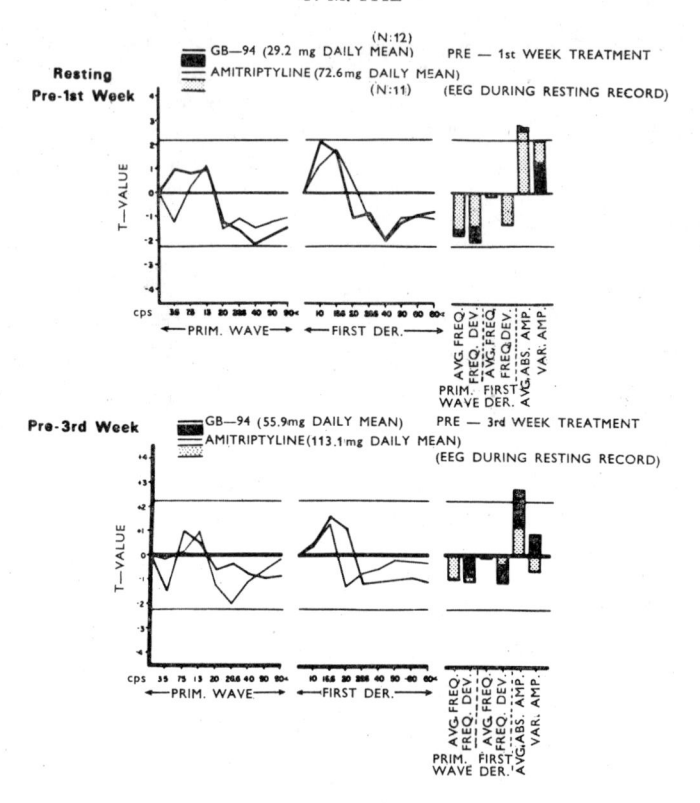

Fig. 13. EEG profiles of GB-94 and amitriptyline based on digital computer period analysis. Twenty-two CEEG measurements are shown on the abscissa and t-values from predrug to the first and third weeks of the treatment on the ordinate. In each time period (predrug, first and third weeks) the t-test changes of the CEEG measurements in a 20-minute resting record (right occipital to right ear lead) were computed in comparison to the predrug period. As can be seen, both amitriptyline and GB-94 produce very similar changes with an increase of slow waves and decrease of fast activity in the primary wave and first derivative measurements. During the first week amitriptyline did not increase very slow waves in the primary wave measurements. During the third week of treatment the CEEG changes were qualitatively similar (particularly in the first derivative measurements); however, the degree of the changes compared to the first week was less. The changes reached levels of statistical significance (dotted line implies 0.05 level) in more CEEG measurements during the first week than during the third week of the treatment period (due to filtering of the activities above 40 cps the typical pattern of the increase of fast activity with thymoleptics was not seen in these profiles).

Conclusion

Because of the lack of knowledge about the mode of action of psychotropic drugs and the failure to find a biochemical explanation of their clinical effectiveness, the development of new psychotropic drugs based on animal model is arbitrary and limited. The basic approach is a retrospective one. The primary effort in animal pharmacology is on investigating compounds similar to widely used drugs with well-known clinical applications. As a result, clinical investigators receive dozens of so-called "new drugs" which are, in fact, merely better or worse copies of successfully marketed compounds. Therefore, it is understandable that most new psychotropic drugs were discovered by chance in clinical practice. In spite of the lack of basic knowledge regarding the origin of the bioelectrical activity of the brain, electrophysiological methods such as electroencephalogram and evoked potential techniques with the application of computer analysis seem to be promising approaches in early evaluation of new drugs (Phases 1 and 2). The prediction of the antidepressive properties of cyclazocine, a narcotic antagonist (8, 9), and the discovery of GB-94 are examples which suggest that the application of "human CEEG model" in drug trials may add new dimensions to the "animal pharmacology model" in exploring the psychotropic effects of drugs. In recent years we not only have demonstrated that compounds with similar clinical effectiveness have similar CEEG profiles, but also have established significant correlations between certain psychopathological syndromes and quantitative EEG patterns. Although our approach is also retrospective, it is not limited to the known CEEG profiles. New CEEG profiles of fenfluramine (10) and SCH-12,679 (21) are indicative of new clinical applications. Max Fink's and our studies clearly demonstrate that the computerized EEG is an extremely useful method of predicting the CNS effects of new compounds, determining clinically effective dose ranges and establishing the "bioavailability" of psychotropic drugs.

Summary

Using quantitative pharmaco-electroencephalography, with the aid of computer analysis of the EEG and statistical processing of the data, the previous classification of psychotropic drugs by the "visual" evaluation technique was confirmed. Subsequently, the clinical uses of one major tranquilizer, four anxiolytics, two thymoleptics and one "antiaggression" drug were predicted. Although the CEEG predictions of clinically effective dosage ranges were more accurate than those of animal pharmacology, the psychotropic properties of all these compounds already had been predicted by "animal model." However, recently we discovered the psychotropic properties of a new compound (GB-94) using the EEG model alone. In fact, even after we had established the clinical usefulness of this compound, the animal model failed to show any pharmacological or neurochemical properties of the existing psychotropic drugs. This clearly demonstrates a fact already known: retrospective animal pharmacology has a limited usefulness in the development of new drugs. Quantitative electroencephalography seems to be very promising not only in predicting the psychotropic properties of a compound but, equally important, in determining effective dosage ranges and establishing "bioavailability" of psychoactive drugs, and therefore it is a very useful method in early testing of new compounds.

REFERENCES

1. Bente, D. and Itil, T. M. (1960) EEG-Veränderungen unter chronischer Medikation von Piperazinyl-Phenothiazine-Derivaten. Med. Exp. (Basel) **2**, 132.
2. Borenstein, P., Dujo, Ph. and Chiva, M. (1965) A propos de la classification des substances psychotropes selon leurs effets sur l'electroencephalogramme. Ann. medicopsychol. (Paris) **123**, 429.
3. Borenstein, P., Cujo, Ph., Kramarz, P. and Champion, C. (1969) A propos de certains aspects electroencephalographiques de l'action des psychotropes. Sem. Hop. Paris **19**, 1332.
4. Fink, M. (1961) Quantitative electroencephalography and human psychopharmacology: I: Frequency spectra and drug action. Med. exp. (Basel) **5**, 364.
5. Fink, M. (1963). Quantitative electroencephalography in human psychopharmacology. II: Drug patterns. In: Glaser, G. (Ed.), EEG and Behavior, p. 177. New York: Basic Books.

6. FINK, M., SHAPIRO, D. M., HICKMAN, C. and ITIL, T. M. (1966): Quantitative analysis of the electroencephalogram by digital computer methods. III: Applications to psychopharmacology. Publication No. 3. St. Louis: Psychiatric Research Foundation of Missouri.
7. FINK, M., SHAPIRO, D., HICKMAN, C. and ITIL, T. (1968): Digital computer analyses in psychopharmacology. In: KLINE, N. and LASKA, E. (Eds.), Computers and Electronic Devices in Psychiatry, p. 109. New York: Grune and Stratton.
8. FINK, M., ITIL, T., ZAKES, A. and FREEDMAN, A. (1969) EEG patterns of cyclazocine, a narcotic antagonist. In: KARCZMAR, A. and KOELLA, W. (Eds.), Neurophysiological and Behavioral Aspects of Psychologic Drugs, p. 62. Springfield, Ill.: Charles C. Thomas.
9. FINK, M., SIMEON, J., ITIL, T. M., and FREEDMAN, A. M. (1970) Clinical antidepressant activity of cyclazocine — a narcotic antagonist. Clin. Pharmacol. Ther. **11**, 41.
10. FINK, M., SHAPIRO, D. M. and ITIL, T. M.(1971) EEG profiles of fenfluramine, amobarbital and dextroamphetamine in normal volunteers. Psychopharmacologia (Berlin) **22**, 369
11. GOLDSTEIN, L. and BECK, R. (1965) Amplitude analysis of the electroencephalogram. Int. Rev. Neurobiol. **8**, 265.
12. ITIL, T. M. (1961) Elektroencephalographische Befunde zur Klassifikation neuro- und thymoleptischer Medikamente. Med. exp. (Basel) **5**, 347.
13. ITIL, T. M. (1964) Elektroencephalographische Studien bei Psychosen und Psychotropen Medikamenten. Istanbul: Ahmet Sait Matbaasi.
14. ITIL, T. M. (1968) Electroencephalography and pharmacopsychiatry. In: FREYHAN, F. A., PETRILOWITSCH, N. and PICHOT, P. (Eds.), Clinical Psychopharmacology, Modern Problems of Pharmacopsychiatry, Vol. I, p. 163. Basel/New York: Karger.
15. ITIL, T. M. (1971) Quantitative pharmaco-electroencephalography in assessing new antianxiety agents. In: VINAR, O., VOTAVA, Z. and BRADLEY, P. B. (Eds.), Advances in Neuro-Psychopharmacology, p. 199. Amsterdam: North-Holland Publishing Co.
16. ITIL, T., SHAPIRO, D. and FINK, M. (1968) Differentiation of psychotropic drugs by quantitative EEG analysis. Agressologie, **9**, 267.
17. ITIL, T., SHAPIRO, D. M., FINK, M., KIREMITCI, N. and HICKMAN, C. (1969) Quantitative EEG studies of chlordiazepoxide, chlorpromazine and imipramine in volunteer and schizophrenic subjects. In: EVANS, W. O. and KLINE, N. S. (Eds.), The Psychopharmacology of the Normal Human, p. 219. Springfield, Ill.: Charles C. Thomas.
18. ITIL, T., GANNON, P., CORA, R., POLVAN, N., AKPINAR, S., ELVERIS F. and ESKAZAN, E. (1971) SCH-12,041, a new antianxiety agent (quantitative pharmaco-electroencephalography and clinical trials). Physicians' Drug Manual (PDM) **3**, 26.
19. ITIL, T. M., GÜVEN, F., CORA, R., HSU, W., POLVAN, N., UCOK, A., SANSEIGNE, A. and ULETT, G. A. (1971) Quantitative pharmacoelectroencephalography using frequency analyzer and digital computer methods in early drug evaluations. In: SMITH, W. L. (Ed.), Drugs, Development and Brain Functions, p. 145. Springfield, Ill.: Charles C Thomas.
20. ITIL, T. M., POLVAN, N. and HOLDEN, J. M. C. (1971) Clinical and electroencephalographic effects of cinanserin in schizophrenic and manic patients. Dis. nerv. Syst. **32**, 193.
21. ITIL, T. M., STOCK, M. J., DUFFY, A. D., ESQUENAZI, A., SALETU, B. and HAN, T. H. (1972) Therapeutic trials and EEG investigations with SCH-12,679 in behaviorally disturbed adolescents. Curr. ther. Res. **14**, 136.
22. ITIL, T. M., POLVAN, N. and HSU, W. (1972) Clinical and EEG effects of GB-94, a "tetracyclic" antidepressant (EEG model in discovery of a new psychotropic drug). Curr. ther. Res. **14**, 395.
23. ITIL, T. M., SALETU, B., MARASA, J. and MUCCIARDI, A. N. (1972) Digital computer analyzed awake and sleep EEG (sleep prints) in predicting the effects of a new triazolobenzodiazepine (U-31, 889). Pharmacopsychiat. **5**, 225.
24. ITIL, T. M., CORA, R., HSU, W., CIG, E. and SALETU, B. (1972) Clinical, toxicological and electroencephalographical effects of a new tricyclic antidepressant, OI-77 (in press).
25. KESKINER, A., ITIL, T. M., HAN, T. H., SALETU, B. and HSU, W. (1971), Clinical, toxicological and electroencephalographic study with SCH-12,679 in chronic schizophrenics. Curr. ther. Res. **13**, 714.
26. ULETT, G. A., BOWERS, C. A., HEUSLER, A. F., QUICK, R., WORD, T. and WORD, A. (1964) A study of the behavior and EEG patterns of patients receiving tranquilizers with and without the addition of chlordiazepoxide. J. Neuropsychiat. **5**, 558.
27. VAN DER BURG, W. J., BONTA, I. L., DELOBELLE, J., RAMON, C. and VERGAFTIG, B. (1970) A novel type of substituted piperazine with high antiserotonin potency. J. med. Chem. **13**, 35.

T. M. I., Missouri Institute of Psychiatry, University of Missouri School of Medicine, 5400 Arsenal St., St. Louis, Mo. 63139, U.S.A.

QUANTUM CHEMICAL AND THEORETICAL TECHNIQUES FOR THE UNDERSTANDING OF ACTION OF PSYCHOACTIVE DRUGS*)

Joyce J. KAUFMAN

Division of Anesthesiology, Department of Surgery, and Department of Chemistry, The Johns Hopkins University School of Medicine, Baltimore, Maryland

Introduction

There are two potentially fruitful areas in which theoretical chemists can contribute to the field of "molecular medicine". The first, is to perform quantum chemical calculations of the molecular electronic wave functions of the endogenous biochemical or exogenous drug molecules in order to characterize the molecular conformations, reactivities and interactions of these molecules as completely as possible. Our group is deeply involved in this and some results on the antipsychotic drugs will be discussed later.

The second area, a novel one, yet intimately connected to the first, is bringing to bear on molecular medical problems concepts of topological and topographical analyses and systems analysis. Developing such analyses led us to a fundamental understanding of the mechanism of anti-psychotic drugs including their bizarre side effects. Similar analysis has also indicated a possible mechanism by which narcotics, such as morphine or heroin, cause physical addiction and how this addiction might be reversed without ever employing maintenance on narcotics or narcotic antagonists.

What is a molecular quantum chemical calculation? Basically, it is solving for the motion of the electrons in the field of the nuclei which comprise the molecule. In principle, all one needs to know about a molecule to perform such a calculation is of what atoms is the molecule composed and its molecular geometry. Even if one does not know exactly where the atoms are located, because quantum chemistry is based on the variational principle, the geometrical conformation with the lowest total molecular energy is the most preferred conformation of the molecule. Thus, quantum chemistry can give the conformation of a molecule even if its crystal structure has not been determined. Also, quantum chemistry can tell us which other low energy conformations are practically possible, as some of these may prove important in solution.

Quantum chemical calculations can also give the electronic charge distribution at each atom and between the atoms. This charge distribution is intimately related to how a molecule behaves and what type of reactions and interactions it can undergo. The more similar the charge distributions of two related molecules, the more probable it is that these molecules will interact in the same way.

---

*) This research was supported in part by NIMH under Grant No. ROI MH18967-02.

There seem to be two main criteria governing whether or not a drug will be effective for a specific purpose. The first is the conformation of the drug, or at least of the vital part of it which is intimately connected to receptor site interaction. If the atoms are not in the correct spatial orientation, they will not fit into the receptor site and, thus, will be ineffective.

The second important factor is the electronic distribution on the atoms of a drug. To interact with a receptor site, the drug must have a charge distribution compatible with requirements for interacting with the receptor site. Where an effective drug has been found, a related drug with a similar charge distribution in the part of the molecule vital for pharmacological action, will have a reasonable probability of acting in the same way. Where a drug is thought to act by blocking the receptor site of an endogenous molecule, then the more closely the conformation and the electronic distribution of the vital part of the drug resemble those of the endogeneous molecule, the more probable it is that the drug will block the receptor site.

Other factors which influence drug effectivity, such as transport and metabolism, are secondary to the molecular conformation and electronic charge distribution for understanding the mechanism of drug action.

Topological analysis deals with connections between atoms. Often a common topological pattern of atoms is buried within a series of much larger molecules. Topographical analysis deals with patterns of atoms which are in the same spatial positions relative to one another (although not necessarily topologically related). Our use of systems analysis in this pharmacological context most closely resembles war game analysis. One is told all the observed facts about an opponent and from these a deterministic model is constructed. An initial move is made and the final outcome is deduced from following the appropriate pathways in the deterministic model.

ANTIPSYCHOTIC DRUGS

The late DR. DANIEL EFRON, Chief of the Pharmacology Division of the National Institutes of Mental Health persuaded and inspired me to perform theoretical investigations on neuroleptic drugs, particularly chlorpromazine. The fundamental question to be asked was how such drugs might act? This seemed a logical start to trying to sort out the myriad of observed structure-activity relationships of widely varied families of antipsychotic drugs and their congeners.

The neuroleptic drugs cover a wide and apparently diverse class of compounds, most of which have a similar mode of action. These molecules are quite large from the quantum chemical point of view and one would like to focus on the conformational and electronic properties of the portions of the molecules vital for pharmacological action rather than have to analyse results for the entire molecule.

One research effort concentrated on quantum chemical computations of a series of neuroleptics (promazines, perazines and piperidopromazines) to investigate their conformations and electronic distributions. By characterizing the electronic structure of these molecules, certain similar indices could point to structures in common.

A second path of research investigated how the concepts of topological and topographical analyses and systems analysis could be applied to unravelling the mechanism of action of such drugs.

Two papers were instrumental in leading us to formulate an overall picture of the action of neuroleptic drugs, including their bizarre side effects. One was by SNYDER (6) postulating that chlorpromazine blocks the dopamine receptor and the other was the fine work of SEDVALL and NYBÄCK (23) on the ^{14}C-tyrosine experiments in the presence of neuroleptics.

A. *Topological and topographical conformational similarities among neuroleptic drugs and biogenic amines*

The antipsychotic phenothiazines and butyrophenones were postulated by SNYDER (6) to alter dopamine metabolism in the brain in such a way to suggest that these drugs may act by blocking dopamine receptors. It was suggested that dopamine may be superimposable upon a portion (the *a* ring bearing the Cl substituent) of the known X-ray structure of chlorpromazine.

It also seems to us that while there could be involvement of the *a* ring as supposed by SNYDER, it is equally probable that the opposite *c* ring is also involved at some point interfering in the dopamine pathway. Many phenothiazines with very bulky substituents in the 2-position are effective tranquilizers (28) yet the *a* ring bearing these substituents could scarcely fit into any receptor sites that would be conformationally appropriate for dopamine. (It is quite possibly the involvement of the *c* ring of chlorpromazine which causes a number of the well defined side effects.)

In order to see most clearly the conformational similarities, space filling CPK molecular models were constructed for chlorpromazine, perazine and the biogenic amines. Using a technique, developed previously by another member of our group (31), the models were mounted in a frame and photographed from all six sides relative to a fixed point.

JANSSEN had originally proposed in 1964 (8) that the fundamental structure necessary for neuroleptic action was

This proposal was criticized by JOULOU in 1965 (11) on the grounds that it did not include such classes as tetrabenazine, the piperazinic derivatives of indole (which, however, are more closely related structurally to reserpine)

and dibenzothiazepines

JANSSEN later reexamined these classes and other effective neuroleptics and in 1969 (9) postulated that all that seems necessary is the fundamental structure

This structure alone can correlate the antipsychotic activity of the three major classes of neuroleptics: 4-phenylbutylamines (such as the butyrophenones), 3-anilinopropylamines (such as the phenothiazines) and 3-phenoxypropylamines (such as spiramide). Neuroleptics of these three classes seem to be able to adopt only one S-shaped common conformation and JANSSEN expected, therefore, that it is in this conformational state that they interact with receptor molecules (10).

Our topological examination indicated that the dibenzothiazepines do fit into the customary classification

JANSSEN indicated there were exceptions such as the ethylaminoindoles, which could have a three carbon chain or benzoquinolizines which could have a two carbon chain. However, our careful examination of the stereotopology of the ethylaminoindoles (which are topologically related to Rauwolfia alkaloids) indicates that the three carbon chain is probably not effective of itself but rather because the three carbon atoms and the attached nitrogen are sitting where they would have been had there been an extra carbon between them and the first aromatic ring

The tetrabenzazines do not fit the general pattern. In this particular case because of the rigidity of the structure the N must be in an orientation relative to the ring closely resembling that of the biogenic amines which have only a two carbon chain.

Interestingly enough, just the pattern recognition of this type allowed us to detect a misprint in Compound 55, piperidochlorpromazine in USDIN and EFRON (28) which as drawn showed a pattern

$$\text{Ph-N(CH}_3\text{)-(CH}_2)_2-C\underset{C-N}{\overset{C-C}{\langle\ \rangle}}C\ |\ CH_3$$

(with 4 carbons attached to the ring N atom)

The structure should really be

$$\text{Ph-N(CH}_3\text{)-(CH}_2)_2-C\underset{N-C}{\overset{C-C}{\langle\ \rangle}}C\ |\ CH_3$$

which does meet the necessary topological requisites. (This misprint has been corrected in the second edition — 29).

What significance has the nitrogen which is part of the phenothiazine ring? Is it an essential part of the antipsychotic drug structure? We believe that chemically it is not vital but as it is conformationally rigid, holds the

$$-C-C-C-N\langle\begin{smallmatrix}R\\R\end{smallmatrix}$$

side chain in a specific position relative to the ring at least at the position of attachment. This hypothesis explains the effectiveness of the thioxanthene class of antipsychotic drugs.

The C—C linkage is conformationally rigid and serves the same purpose as the $\overset{\vee}{\underset{|}{N}}$ in attaching the side chain in a certain conformational position relative to the ring.

B. *Theoretical results*

We have performed quantum chemical calculations with varying degrees of rigor for neuroleptic drugs. We are finishing an *ab initio* LCAO-MO-SCF calculation for promazine and chlorpromazine (12, 25) to use as a standard against which to compare the results of less rigorous computations. Semi-rigorous computational techniques derived by us earlier (13) are being tested for the large drug molecules (26). We extended the derivation of the INDO method to included orbitals and parameters for second-row elements (14). A number of molecular orbital calculations have been carried out by more conventional techniques to establish the conformational preferences of the side chains of promazine and its Cl and CF_3 derivatives, perazine and its Cl and CF_3 derivatives and piperidopromazine and its Cl and CF_3 derivatives (12). [The reference conformations were the crystallographically determined ones for chlorpromazine (19) and thiethylperazine (20)]. In each case for the vital rotation around the N_1-C_{13} bond (the one connecting the alkyl side chain to the phenothiazine ring) the lowest calculated total energy was at the crystallographic conformation.

As may be observed in the prototype, Fig. 1 (E_{total} vs N_1-C_{13} rotation angle for chlor-

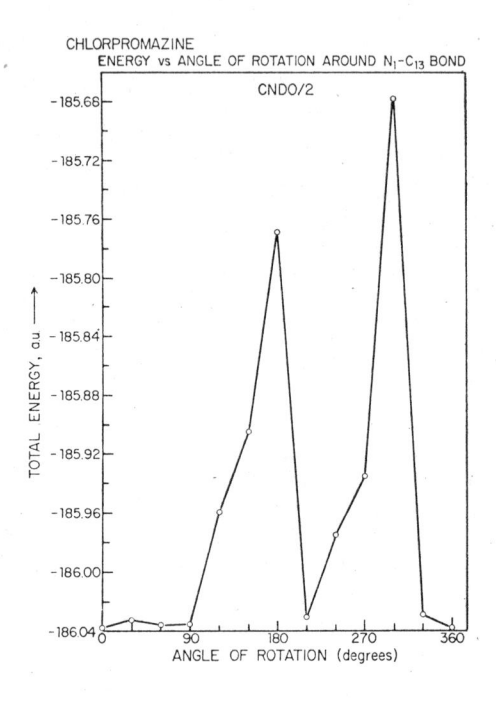

Fig. 1. Conformation for the angle of rotation (abscissa) and total energy (ordinate) for chlorpromazine.

promazine), there are other low lying possible conformations as well as some which are so high in energy as to be inaccessible. (Conformational possibilities for the rotations in the side chain itself indicate low lying energy conformations in addition to the crystallographic one.)

The individual molecular orbital energy levels and the electron density distributions were calculated for each conformation of each molecule.

C. *Systems analysis*

The idea that the neuroleptic drugs are involved in the dopamine pathway has been convincingly demonstrated by the experimental observation that in the presence of neuroleptic drugs, there is an increased synthesis and turnover in brain ^{14}C-dopamine and ^{14}C-norepinephrine upon injection of ^{14}C-tyrosine (23). The dopamine is thought to be involved in the antipsychotic effect and the norepinephrine in the sedative effect. An independent similar study with ^{14}C-tyrosine in the presence of morphine showing increased turnover in the ^{14}C-norepinephrine but less certainly in the dopamine (18) confirms the role of norepinephrine in narcotic action and probably also in the sedative effect.

There are at least four major side effects of the phenothiazine tranquilizers which vary in a regular manner with the ionization potentials of the phenothiazines. The hypothermic and the anti-histamine effects vary directly and the anti-emetic and anti-adrenaline effects vary inversely with the ionization potentials. With the experimentally demonstrated involvement of phenothiazines in the dopamine and norepinephrine pathways, it now becomes clear that the basis of these side effects is that the phenothiazines or their metabolites are also mimicking and becoming involved, to a greater or lesser extent, in those and in several other biogenic amine pathways. (Space limitations do not permit the details to be presented here. A more complete manuscript is available from the author on request.)

The involvement of phenothiazine with adrenergic mechanisms indicates one possible source of the hyperpigmentation and retinal pigmentation sometimes observed as undesirable side effects on protracted chlorpromazine treatment.

Melanin may be formed during the oxidation of tyrosine or tryptophan; the usual mechanism is the enzymatic oxidation of tyrosine to 3,4-dihydroxphenylalanine (DOPA) and the further oxidation of this intermediate to melanin, a dihydroxy indoxylic acid occurring in polymerized form (27). Since it has been observed that there is an increased synthesis and turnover of ^{14}C-dopamine and ^{14}C-norepinephrine in the presence of neuroleptic drugs, it is logical to presume that there is some involvement of DOPA in this pathway, possibly an increased synthesis of DOPA. If some of this DOPA is preferentially oxidized to melanin, rather than decarboxylated to dopamine, this would explain the increased pigmentation. One reason for preferential oxidation of the DOPA rather than decarboxylation could be a deficiency in the individual of the enzyme L-aromatic amino acid decarboxylase (which decarboxylates DOPA to dopamine). It is known that inactivation of the enzyme tyrosinase (which catalyses the production of melanin from tyrosine and *in vitro* is concerned with the production of epinephrine from tyrosine) by a copper chelating agent is effective in blocking such melanin production (5).

This phenomenon has interesting implications in possible understanding and therapy of the disease retinitis pigmentosa. We conjecture that this disease is endogenously caused by the same mechanism that causes retinal pigmentation exogenously induced by certain neuroleptics, and thus may be amenable to the same treatment.

The source of the anti-histamine effect of phenothiazine is quite clearly involvement in the histamine system by blocking histamine receptors. The antipsychotic phenothiazines were developed from the antihistamines. The sedative property of antihistamines now becomes clear in our framework. The antihistamines must also affect the rate of synthesis and turnover of norepinephrine which causes the sedative effect. A simple ^{14}C-tyrosine experiment could easily prove or disprove this theory.

The origin of the hypothermic effect of the phenothiazines is less obvious because the basic cause of hypothermia itself is still the subject of speculation. However, it has been proposed that tryptaminergic mechanisms in the hypothalamus are involved in thermoregulation (3). The effects on body temperature of 5-hydroxytryptamine (5-HT) or procedures influencing hypothalmic 5-HT have strengthened this idea (4). Thus, in our framework, a possible cause of hypothermia is involvement of phenothiazine or a metabolite in the 5-HT pathway. Phenothiazines interfere with heat loss as well as heat conservation, suggesting a central hypothalamic action (1).

Other possibilities for species active in the side effects as well as in the antipsychotic effects occur to us based on the recent observation of the presence of the major metabolite 7-hydroxychlorpromazine and the metabolite 8-hydroxychlorpromazine in the brain (22).

Earlier work has shown that the introduction of hydroxy or methoxy group(s) to the chlorpromazine molecule reduces pharmacological activity. Of the compounds tested, 7-hydroxy-chlorpromazine and 3-hydroxychlorpromazine showed pharmacological activity most similar to chlorpromazine (21). Recent experiments have shown that the 7-hydroxylated and desmethylated derivatives are about as effective as the parent compound in accelerating both accumulation and disappearance of ^{14}CoA from ^{14}C tyrosine in mouse brain (24).

We hypothesize that as the hydroxy or methoxy groups are added to the molecule in the c ring, the c ring is then mainly involved in the biogenic amine pathways. It begins to resemble a catechol nucleus and thus attaches to a receptor site appropriate for this structure.

From the many different physiological effects caused by each individual biogenic amine, it is reasonable to assume that more than one type of receptor site occurs for each of them. How the molecule must be oriented to fit into this site must determine the subsequent physiological effect or reuptake. The same holds true for the phenothiazines or other neuroleptics. With which specific receptor site a part of the drug molecule interacts, governs when the neuroleptic will exhibit an antipsychotic effect or one of the other side effects. As the molecule becomes metabolized its pattern of interaction will change as portions of the molecule may become available for different receptor interactions.

Now that the antipsychotic efficiency of a large number of neuroleptic drugs is well established, it seems obvious that the choice of drug will be governed mainly by the absence of undesirable side effects and its duration of action.

JANSSEN (9) has introduced a new class of antipsychotically active compounds, long-acting neuroleptic drugs derived from N-[4:4-(bis-4'-fluorophenyl)-butyl] piperidine. They are reported to be more effective, more predictable, less likely to induce unwanted effects, and much easier to prescribe, administer and take because of their long and regular duration of action. The extremely long duration of action of these compounds is due to the fact that they metabolize very slowly; brain concentrations being more easily maintained than with the older neuroleptics. In our framework, this is very easy to understand. The F atoms are in the positions which would be 3- or 7- in chlorpromazine if one considers the C atom attached to the two phenyl rings in place of the ring N of chlorpromazine. Chemically it is known that an F atom attached to an aromatic ring is quite inert and, so has little tendency to be metabolized. Thus, the OH-derivative will not form readily. Forming an OH-derivative has been shown to make a drug less effective as an antipsychotic possibly because it induces the drug to become involved in biogenic pathways other than the dopamine pathway.

In conclusion, from this topological study the antipsychotic effectivity of a wide variety of neuroleptics becomes very clear. This study also indicates the basis for the observed side effects of these drugs and the probable influence of metabolism of these drugs. This framework should help make more systematic the choice of new drugs to be synthesized or screened.

NARCOTICS

A very similar situation prevails with the narcotics. For several years we have been collaborating with the Maryland Centre for Psychiatric Research in an effort to understand on a molecular basis narcotic addition and how to control it. A special interest of that group has been in the area of narcotic antagonists.

As experts in the field admitted not yet understanding how narcotics work, we had to read the available pharmacological evidence and many theories and to construct, bit by bit, an operational theory for the mechanism of action. It was helpful to have been working on the antipsychotic drug mechanism at the same time. There were a few scattered observations that reserpine blocked the action of morphine and chlorpromazine could potentiate morphine action. Thus it was obvious that there were some common pathways being affected by both narcotics and anti-psychotics.

The recent ^{14}C-tyrosine experiments (18), gave indisputable evidence that the norepinephrine pathway was being affected by narcotics as well as being involved in side effects of anti-psychotic action. The acetylcholine pathway has also been shown to be involved in narcotic action but in a different way (2).

WAY (17, 30) has demonstrated that an increase in brain 5-HT accompanies the development of tolerance and physical dependence, strongly suggesting that their development is closely involved with the biosynthesis of 5-HT.

A. *Topological analysis*

There are five main classes of clinically useful analgesics for man (7). These are, in order of their historical rise: (1) the opium alkaloids and their derivatives; (2) pethidine and its congeners, originated by EISLEB and SCHAUMANN; (3) methadone and its cognates, due to BOCKMUHL and EHRHARDS; (4) the morphinans and relatives, discovered by GREWE; and the last and very important class, (5) the 6,7-benzomorphans, originated by EVERETT L. MAY.

Almost all of the strong narcotic analgesics in these five classes of drugs have three or four structurally similar characteristics. They have: (1) a quaternary carbon atom; (2) an aromatic nucleus linked to this carbon; (3) a tertiary amino group with two saturated carbon atoms away from the quaternary carbon atom; and, (4) a phenolic hydroxyl group situated *meta* to the quaternary carbon — if the tertiary nitrogen is a part of a fused piperidine ring system.

Although the phenolic group is not an essential feature in the rigid compounds like morphine, morphinans and benzomorphans, it always gives more active compounds when present.

These structure-activity correlations, although interesting as an *ex post facto* analysis, are, according to pharmacologists, lacking in any predictive capacity. They indicate, however, the important functional portions of the molecule for derivation of useful quantum chemical indices.

The similarities and differences to the anti-psychotics should be noted. For narcotics the aromatic ring should be connected to a quaternary carbon which is then connected to an alkyl substituted nitrogen by a two atom chain. There must also be a phenolic OH-group. This should immediately indicate a similarity to the catechol portion of the biogenic amines. We have calculated wave functions for such narcotics as morphine which has 110 valence electrons.

B. *Systems analysis*

The most vital problem we could investigate was not minute examination of the structure activity between close narcotic congeners, but rather, how does a narcotic cause addiction. And, were there any new concepts which could be used to cure physical addiction?

After intensive systems analysis, the following hypothetical cause emerges for narcotic addiction. We postulate that a narcotic blocks the receptor site of a biogenic amine for one or more of the other normal neurotransmitters; the ^{14}C experiments indicate that the norepinephrine receptor is certainly one of the major ones involved. There is a known physiological phenomenon called negative feedback. If a receptor site is blocked, there is, somehow, a transmission of this information to the presynapse. Essentially, this information reports that no signal is being received at the postsynapse. This, in turn, causes an increased synthesis and release of the neurotransmitter whose receptor site is blocked.

When an addict is under the influence of a narcotic, certain receptor sites are blocked. This causes an increase in the rate of synthesis and release of that neurotransmitter. However, the receptor sites remain blocked by the narcotic for a time, and the increased synthesis and release of the neurotransmitter has little effect during that period. Once the narcotic begins to wear off, the law of mass action serves to unblock the receptor site. Unfortunately, the presynapse must still be synthesizing and releasing a large excess of the neurotransmitter, which must cause many of the severe withdrawal symptoms. Earlier, in the section on antipsychotics we mentioned that a drug resembling a biogenic amine must be able to mimic many other biogenic amines and get involved in many pathways, so certainly a loose biogenic amine can do the same. Indeed, tracing back from the observed withdrawal symptoms to the probable causal biogenic amine effect would lead one to the same conclusion. There would be a reversible alteration in the body's natural rate of synthesis and release of neurotransmitter because as the receptors became unblocked, the negative feedback would cease. Gradually the presynapses would return to a normal rate of synthesis and release of neurotransmitter. This is, indeed, observed. By keeping an addict off narcotics for a short time he can be broken of any physical dependence and the withdrawal symptoms disappear. This has little to do with his psychological dependence. Psychiatrists involved in treating hard-core narcotic abusers say that the vast majority of these individuals have a long underlying history of psychosis which precedes their addiction.

However, this postulated mechanism of addiction by negative feedback induced increased synthesis and release of normal neurotransmitter does lend some hope for developing a new method of treatment which might be especially valuable for the young addict, perhaps accidentally hooked, who wishes to be cured. Getting rid, somehow, of the excess neurotransmitter still being synthesized and released upon narcotic withdrawal, should ameliorate most of the severe withdrawal symptoms. This might be done either by stimulating the rate of production of the metabolizing enzyme, or by adjusting the enzyme balance further up the biogenic amine pathway to lessen the rate of enzymatic synthesis of the offending neurotransmitter.

ACKNOWLEDGEMENTS

This research was supported in part by NIMH under Grant No. R01 MH18967-02 and performed in collaboration with them. We especially acknowledge the inspiration of the late Dr. Daniel H. Efron and the stimulating conversations with Drs. Jerome Levine, Albert A. Manian and Earl Usdin.

The narcotics research was performed in collaboration with Drs. John. C. Krantz and Albert A. Kurland of the Maryland Center for Psychiatric Research.

References

1. DOMINO, E. F., HUDSON, R. D. and ZOGRAFI (1968) Substituted Phenothiazine: Pharmacology and Chemical Structure. In: Drugs Affecting the Central Nervous System. Editor, BURGER, A., Marcel Dekker, Inc., New York.
2. DOMINO, E. F. (July 1972) Private communication.
3. FELDBERG, W. and MYERS, R. D. (1963) A New Concept of Temperature Regulation by Amines in the Hypothalamus. Nature, 200, 1325.
4. FELDBERG, W. (1968) Recent Advances in Pharmacology, 4th Edition. Editors, ROBSON, J. M., STACEY, R. S. J. and A. Churchill, Ltd., London; (1968) Symposium or 5-Hydroxytryptamine, Editors, PAASMEN, M. K. and KLINGE, E. Ann. Med. exp. Biol. Fenn. 46, 361.
5. GREINER, A. C. and NICHOLSON, G. A. (1965) Schizophrenia — Melanosis, Cause or Side-Effect with? Lancet 2, 1165.
6. HORN, A. and SNYDER, S. (1971) Chlorpromazine and Dopamine: Conformational Similarities that Correlate with the Antischizophrenic Activity of Phenothiazine Drugs. Proc. nat. Acad. Sci. 68, 2325.
7. JACOBSON, A. E., MAY, E. L. and SARGENT, L. J. (1970) Analgetics in Medicinal Chemistry, Part II, 3rd Edition. Editor, BURGER, A., Wiley-Interscience. New York.
8. JANSSEN, P. A. J., IVe Reunion du Collège International de Neuro-Psychopharmacology, Birmingham, 31/8—3/9/64.
9. JANSSEN, P. A. J. (September 1969) Recent Developments in the Field of Neuroleptic Drugs. Paper presented before the Division of Medicinal Chemistry, 158th National Meeting of the American Chemical Society. New York.
10. JANSSEN, P. A. J. (1970) The Neuroleptics. Editors BOBON, D. P., JANSSEN, P. A. J. and OBON, J. B. Karger, S., Basel, München, Paris, New York.
11. JULOU, L., DUCROT, R. and FOUCHE, J. (1965) Atti Convegni Farmitalia, Etude de quelques relations entre la structure chimique et l'activité neuroleptique. Agiornamento in psiconeurofarmacologia, p. 20. Milano.
12. KAUFMAN, JOYCE, J. and KERMAN, E. (1972) Quantum Chemical Calculations on Antipsychotic Drugs and Narcotic Agents. Int. J. quant. Chem. 6S, 319.
13. KAUFMAN, JOYCE, J. (1965) Semi-rigorous LCAO-MO-SCF Methods for Three-Dimensional Molecular Calculations. J. chem. Phys. 43, S152.
14. KAUFMAN, JOYCE, J. and PREDNEY, R. (1972) Extension of INDO Formalism to d Orbitals and Parameters for Second Row Atoms. Int. J. quant. Chem. 6S, 231.
15. KAUFMAN, JOYCE, J. and MANIAN, A. A. (1972) Topological Conformational Similarities among Antipsychotic Drugs, Narcotics and Biogenic Amines: A Summary. Int. J. quant. Chem. 6S, 375.
16. LEVINE, I., EFRON, D. H. and KAUFMAN, JOYCE, J. (September 1971) Private communication.
17. LOH, H. H., SHEN, F. and WAY, E. L. (1969) Inhibition of Morphine Tolerance and Physical Dependence Development and Brain Serotonin Synthesis by Cycloheximide. Biochem. Pharmacol. 18, 2711.
18. LOH, H. H., HITZEMAN, R. J., CRAVES, F. B. and WAY, E. L. (1971) Reported to the Committee on the Problems of Drug Dependence. Toronto.
19. McDOWELL, J. J. H. (1969) The Crystal and Molecular Structures of Chlorpromazine. Acta Cryst. B25, 2175.
20. McDOWELL, J. J. H. (1970) The Crystal and Molecular Structure of Thiethylperazine, a Derivative of Phenothiazine. Acta Cryst. B26, 954.
21. MANIAN, A. A., EFRON, D. H. and GOLDBERG, M. E. (1965) A Comparative Pharmacological Study of a Series of Monohydroxylated and Methoxylated Chlorpromazine Derivatives. Life Sci. 4, 2425.
22. MANIAN, A. A., EFRON, D. H. and HARRIS, S. R. (1971) Appearance of Monohydroxylated Chlorpromazine Metabolites in the Central Nervous System. Life Sci. 10, 679, Part I.
23. NYBÄCK, H. and SEDVALL, G. (1970) Further Studies on the Accumulation and Disappearance of Catecholamines Formed from Tyrosine-^{14}C in Mouse Brain. Effects of Some Phenothiazine Analogues. Europ. J. Pharmacol. 10, 193.
24. NYBÄCK, H. and SEDVALL, G. (1972) Effect of Chlorpromazine and Some of its Metabolites on Synthesis and Turnover of Catecholamines Formed from ^{14}C-Tyrosine in Mouse Brain. Psychopharmacologia, 26, 155.
25. PETKE, J. D., Work in progress.
26. PRESTON, H. J. T. and KAUFMAN, JOYCE, J., Work in progress.
27. Stedman's Medical Dictionary (1966) 21st Edition. Williams and Wilkins. Baltimore, Maryland.

28. USDIN, E. and EFRON, D. H. (1967) Psychotropic Drugs and Related Compounds, U. S. Public Health Service, Department of Health, Education and Welfare.
29. USDIN, E. (September 1971) Private communication.
30. WAY, E. L., LOH, H. H. and SHEN, F. (1968) Morphine Tolerance, Physical Dependence and Synthesis of Brain 5-Hydroxytrytamine. Science, **162**, 1290.
31. WILSON, K. (Spring 1963) The 4π photocomparator — a photo-optical aid useful for a study of molecular models. Abstract 144th ACS National Meeting, Division of Chem. Education #23.

J. J. K., Division of Anesthesiology, the Johns Hopkins University School of Medicine, Baltimore, Md. 21205, U.S.A.

LES ÉCHANGES DU PHARMACOLOGUE ET DU PSYCHIATRE

P. DENIKER et J. R. BOISSIER

Département de Psychiatrie, Faculté de Médecine de Paris (Cochin) et Département de Pharmacologie, Unité de Neuropsychopharmacologie de l'INSERM, Paris

Les échanges réciproques entre pharmacologues et cliniciens sont à l'origine des principales avances de la psychopharmacologie pour ce qui touche à la découverte de nouveaux types d'agents médicamenteux.

RAPPEL HISTORIQUE

La chlorpromazine, synthétisée dès 1950, ne fut introduite en clinique que deux ans plus tard. Le laboratoire fabricant était en possession d'une définition pharmacologique suffisante pour répondre à la demande des cliniciens en choisissant la phénothiazine possédant le plus d'effets centraux parmi d'autres composés anti-histaminiques ou anti-parkinsoniens. Toutefois on sait que les caractéristiques du nouveau groupe des neuroleptiques ne furent véritablement établies qu'en associant les données expérimentales et cliniques et en se basant sur les caractéristiques communes de la chlorpromazine et de la réserpine dont la structure et les modes d'action étaient pourtant éloignés.

Entre temps, la recherche pharmaceutique s'était intéressée aux agents psycho-sédatifs non-hypnotiques que sont les tranquillisants. Mais il fallut une longue suite d'échanges critiques pour établir une claire distinction entre les tranquillisants majeurs – ou neuroleptiques – et les tranquillisants mineurs. Actuellement, il existe un ensemble de tests de pharmacologie prévisionnelle de ces deux types de médicaments.

La découverte des médications antidépressives fournit deux exemples opposés des échanges réciproques pharmaco-cliniques. L'introduction de l'iproniazide, prototype des inhibiteurs de la M.A.O., est la conséquence directe d'un feed-back du laboratoire vers la clinique qui a essayé de reproduire approximativement l'antagonisme de l'iproniazide vis à vis de l'action réserpinique par des applications au traitement de l'inertie schizophrénique et des dépressions endogènes. L'imipramine et les composés tricycliques sont issus d'une démarche inverse: sélectionnée au laboratoire comme un possible tranquillisant, c'est l'expérimentation clinique systématique qui a montré les véritables propriétés de l'imipramine, à la suite de quoi se développèrent les recherches sur les tests pharmacologiques de sélection des propriétés antidépressives, recherches qui ne sont pas encore achevées. Cet inachèvement de la pharmacologie des anti-dépresseurs et le peu de rigueur de ses corrélations avec les constatations cliniques explique sans doute le flou qui persiste dans ce secteur de la psychopharmacologie.

D'autres divergences ont été notées avec l'introduction des neuroleptiques qui ont suivi les deux prototypes. La sélection des phénothiazines pipérazinées et la découverte du groupe des butyrophénones a tenu compte des corrélations entre la production d'effets extra-pyramidaux chez l'homme et celle de la catatonie ou de certains mouvements anormaux chez l'animal. Au contraire, l'utilisation des benzamides comme neuroleptiques ne repose sur aucune propriété psychotrope expérimentale à l'exception de l'action anti-émétique. Ainsi se trouva de nouveau posé le problème des tests pharmacologiques les plus caractéristiques de l'activité des neuroleptiques, les uns assimilant la catalepsie expérimentale aux effets neurologiques, et les autres tenant l'action anti-apomorphine comme reflétant mieux les actions psychothérapeutiques. Quoi qu'il en soit, ceci souligne la nécessité d'employer des batteries de tests pharmacologiques suffisamment étendues et en même temps de tenir compte d'actions isolées si elles peuvent être regardées comme spécifiques.

La pause qu'on a pu constater ces dernières années en matière de découverte de médicaments psychotropes peut tenir à la fois à une certaine saturation des secteurs suffisamment connus grâce aux corrélations pharmaco-cliniques, et surtout à l'insuffisance des tests existants pour caractériser des actions psychopharmacologiques nouvelles.

En général, on ne pourra trouver que ce qu'on cherche, et le laboratoire ne pourra mettre au point que des tests correspondant à des activités thérapeutiques déjà définies.

PRINCIPAUX TYPES D'ÉCHANGES PHARMACO-CLINIQUES

Les modalités de cette coopération sont essentiellement différentes selon le degré de précision et de fiabilité des faits expérimentaux et cliniques à mettre en corrélation. On peut ainsi avoir affaire, schématiquement, à quatre types de situations dans la recherche.

1. Il s'agit de composés appartenant à des types psychopharmacologiques aussi bien définis du point de vue pharmacologique que clinique, comme c'est le cas pour les exemples que nous avons cités en débutant. Il ne s'agit alors que d'obtenir une simple confirmation réciproque des données expérimentales et cliniques, qui est évidemment nécessaire mais dont la valeur euristique reste forcément limitée.

2. Plus intéressant est le cas où apparaissent des contradictions ou des divergences entre les données pharmacologiques et cliniques mais alors qu'il s'agit encore de types psychopharmacologiques suffisamment définis, comme les neuroleptiques, les antidépresseurs, etc. L'examen en feed-back des faits de non-concordance revêt alors tout son intérêt, surtout si l'on dispose d'observations suffisamment nombreuses et probantes au laboratoire comme dans les applications cliniques. On pourra ainsi être amené à établir des corrélations entre des faits apparemment contradictoires ou, au contraire, à les expliquer par des différences de métabolisme.

3. Une troisième éventualité est réalisée lorsque les données principales relatives à un nouveau composé sont fournies de façon unilatérale soit par le laboratoire soit, éventuellement, par les observations cliniques. Le problème est alors d'imaginer les correspondances à trouver dans le domaine expérimental ou clinique. Naturellement c'est dans ce type de situation que l'inventivité doit se montrer la plus active. Bornons-nous à souligner que la psychopharmacologie a beaucoup à faire pour créer et développer des modèles expérimentaux capables de refléter chez l'animal les troubles psychiatriques proprement dits, et que les cliniciens de leur côté ont une tâche considérable pour préciser et clarifier les cibles des actions thérapeutiques.

4. Une dernière éventualité est représentée par les cas où les données existantes sur un nouveau type de composé sont fragmentaires, par exemple d'ordre purement bio-

chimique, et obtenues *in vitro* ou à l'échelon du neurone. Dans ce cas il semble indispensable de réaliser un „screening" pharmacologique complet avant de passer aux applications cliniques, car rien n'est plus hasardeux que d'associer une propriété fondamentale et des constatations cliniques sans passer par l'étape des tests proprement pharmacologiques.

Problèmes méthodologiques

Avant d'envisager la question des principes propres à favoriser la dialectique pharmaco-clinique, il est bon de remarquer que la recherche en psychopharmacologie comporte au moins trois niveaux ou trois ordres de données relatives au mode d'action des substances psychotropes.

a) *Le niveau chimique* concerne d'abord la composition des agents eux-mêmes, puis leur métabolisme depuis leur introduction dans l'organisme, et enfin les processus neuro-chimiques qui se passent au niveau des récepteurs intéressés.

b) *Le niveau physiologique* concerne les fonctions neuro-psychologiques et les structures plus ou moins complexes qui les sous-tendent; parmi ces fonctions, quelques-unes sont assez bien définies comme les mécanismes de la vigilance, du sommeil ou du rêve, ou comme ceux de la mémoire; d'autres ne font qu'émerger parmi nos connaissances, telles la régulation de l'humeur ou la production des hallucinations.

c) *Le niveau psychologique* concerne les structures mentales proprement dites et leur fonctionnement normal ou pathologique.

Rarement les données dont nous disposons couvrent les différents étages de la connaissance. Aussi faut-il faire les plus expresses réserves sur les soi-disant observations qui sautent les étapes et vont directement d'une réaction bio-chimique à une indication psychiatrique.

Nous pouvons maintenant envisager les règles communes qui devraient régir les échanges réciproques entre pharmacologue et clinicien.

a) *Multiplication des donnés à comparer.* Il importe, en premier lieu, de multiplier les investigations tant expérimentales que thérapeutiques, de manière à obtenir une somme suffisante de données à mettre en présence. Rien n'est plus vain que les soi-disant recherches entreprises à propos d'un corps dont on suppose – à partir de quelques tests hétérogènes – qu'il pourrait avoir des actions psychotropes, après quoi le clinicien pourra répondre qu'il a obtenu certains effets favorables sur un lot de malades plus ou moins défini : cela peut suffire à lancer un nouveau médicament, mais non à réaliser une avance dans le domaine de nos connaissances.

Afin d'augmenter le nombre de données utilisables, il faut certainement multiplier les modèles expérimentaux, et, à cet égard, le feed-back du clinicien vers le pharmacologue est déterminant. Dans le passé en effet, les batteries de tests pharmacologiques n'ont pu être développées qu'à partir d'observations cliniques précises concernant par exemple l'activité thérapeutique des neuroleptiques, des tranquillisants ou des antidépresseurs. Nous y reviendrons à propos des lacunes actuelles de la pharmacothérapie. Il est sûr que les constatations négatives ont souvent autant d'importance que les données positives, et l'absence confirmée de tel effet chez l'animal ou chez l'homme contribue efficacement à l'évaluation des propriétés d'un composé nouveau. Encore faut-il préciser la signification des faits constatés.

b) *Spécificité des données à comparer.* L'essentiel du dialogue pharmaco-clinique réside probablement dans l'explicitation par chaque spécialiste de la valeur significative des faits qu'il rapporte, autrement dit dans l'interprétation de la spécificité de tel test ou groupe de tests de laboratoire, et dans celle de la valeur pathognomonique ou non des modifications sémiologiques observées en clinique. Suivant son expérience personnelle et ses vues critiques, chaque expérimentateur est conduit à affecter – de façon explicite ou non – un *coefficient de signification* aux faits qu'il observe. Ceci serait vrai pour l'évaluation de certains items d'échelles de comportement aussi bien que pour l'interprétation du screening de laboratoire. Aussi est-on amené à penser que, dans l'avenir, plus d'études devront être consacrées à la détermination scientifique de la signification des faits observés.

c) *Flexibilité dans l'établissement des corrélations*. Autant la rigueur est nécessaire dans l'établissement des données à comparer, autant il convient de garder de la souplesse d'esprit et de la prudence dans l'étude des corrélations pharmaco-cliniques. La démonstration de propriétés sédatives au laboratoire n'implique pas obligatoirement des effets similaires chez l'homme, surtout s'il s'agit d'un composé de type nouveau dont le spectre d'activité pharmacologique n'a pas été entièrement exploré. Le rappel d'un exemple peut illustrer ce point de vue. Depuis longtemps on recherche des antidépresseurs tricycliques plus puissants que l'imipramine introduite voici quinze ans. Or les cliniciens avaient observé que le dérivé chloré, la clomipramine, se montrait souvent plus actif en thérapeutique, mais leurs rapports se heurtèrent à un certain scepticisme du fait que la fiche pharmacologique du médicament comportait des résultats inférieurs à ceux de l'imipramine dans les tests réputés représentatifs de l'activité antidépressive. Actuellement, l'efficacité de la clomipramine en clinique est bien établie, et l'on est obligé d'admettre qu'au laboratoire sa supériorité sur l'imipramine se manifeste surtout pour des tests mesurant l'action sédative. Depuis on a appris au plan biochimique qu'il était possible de classer les antidépresseurs tricycliques suivant leur capacité à inhiber le re-captage de la 5-HT, qui serait parallèle à leur activité thérapeutique. Il y aurait donc intérêt à conserver une certaine flexibilité dans la confrontation initiale des résultats de la clinique et du laboratoire. Il est possible qu'en reprenant l'étude de certaines discordances pharmaco-cliniques on puisse aboutir à nouvelles avances, même pour des composés déjà connus.

Règles particulières à l'expérimentation clinique

L'application des principes envisagés plus haut comporte, dans le domaine clinique, des difficultés particulières tenant principalement au caractère „immatériel" des troubles et des modifications psychiques. Si les données sémiologiques représentent un ensemble sommairement utilisable pour la communication on doit reconnaître que la systématisation nosographique varie suivant les pays et suivant les Ecoles. L'interprétation pathogénique est encore plus contradictoire. On peut comprendre que, dans ces conditions, ceux qui ne sont pas initiés à la psychiatrie aient eu besoin de données objectives et si possible mesurables; c'est certainement une des raisons du développement des échelles d'évaluation du comportement. Celles-ci ont l'avantage de rendre compte de la mosaïque sémiologique souvent différente d'un cas à l'autre. Mais ce que l'on semble gagner en objectivité, on le perd en spécificité: en effet on peut rendre compte de l'action du médicament sur la mosaïque des items sémiologiques, mais sans savoir au juste vis à vis de quelle „maladie", de quelle entité, ou de quel processus, la thérapeutique peut être efficace.

On est ainsi conduit, dans la perspective de recherche qui nous intéresse, à pratiquer certaines options.

a) *Expérimentation intensive et expérimentation extensive*. Pour le clinicien, il est peu discutable que le matériel clinique est d'autant plus utilisable qu'il est mieux connu dans sa signification pathologique, ce qui naturellement est en faveur d'une étude intensive des cas. Se contenter d'un profil résultant de l'application d'une échelle de comportement sans référence à une qualification diagnostique précise expose aux objections indiquées ci-dessus. D'autre part le type évolutif des troubles morbides dans le temps a souvent une grande importance, si bien que les études longitudinales (follow-up studies) peuvent être d'un grand intérêt. On est ainsi conduit à préférer l'étude d'un nombre de cas limités mais bien connus à des études extensives dont les bases restent floues. Toutefois l'application des méthodes statistiques peut exiger la constitution de groupes cliniques d'une certaine ampleur, aussi la connaissance exacte de chaque cas de cet ensemble représente-t-il une tâche assez lourde.

b) *Importance de la qualification diagnostique.* Dans la perspective de la recherche thérapeutique, certaines qualifications diagnostiques précises ont une valeur particulière dans la mesure où elles désignent des états morbides peu susceptibles d'être modifiés par des placebo ou par une évolution imprévisible. Ainsi la réduction des états d'excitation maniaque typiques représente-t-elle un véritable test pharmacodynamique de l'activité des neuroleptiques et il reste valable pour la sélection des tranquillisants majeurs.

De même on pourrait dire que le meilleur critère de sélection des antidépresseurs est le traitement des cas de dépression endogène véritables: dans une étude-pilote quelques dizaines de patients convenablement sélectionnés fournissent des résultats plus valables que le traitement d'un grand nombre de dépressions simples ou névrotiques, ou encore de „dépressions" schizophréniques qui encombrent inutilement les statistiques.

Pour évaluer les activités „anti-psychotiques", on pourrait dire que la mise en évidence des hallucinations et de leur réduction a une certaine valeur probante. De même la qualité de la critique du délire par le malade serait à différencier du simple désintérêt ou de la réticence qui ne saurait être confondue avec une véritable amélioration.

c) *Articulation avec les explorations paracliniques.* Dès 1959 nous avions insisté sur l'intérêt qu'il y a à associer l'examen neuro-psychiatrique avec des techniques paracliniques telles que la polygraphie pour l'étude de drogues psycho-actives. Cette technique permet de mettre en évidence des effets qui ne seraient pas objectivés par la clinique ou par l'enregistrement pratiqués séparément. L'utilisation des ordinateurs apporte naturellement une contribution de grande valeur à la recherche de pointe. Mais on sait qu'en cette matière la qualité des données à exploiter se montre déterminante, et l'on distingue parmi elles les données „soft" et „hard". Parmi ces dernières, il convient sans doute de retenir les variables utilisées par l'électroencéphalographie quantitative (spectres de fréquences et de puissances, etc...). Ici encore, l'intégration des modifications E.E.G. et des observations cliniques concomittantes a probablement plus de valeur que des constatations séparées.

Pour remédier à la soi-disant subjectivité des observations psychiatriques dont les meilleures sont fondées sur l'expérience de l'observateur et sur sa capacité à grouper et à interpréter les nuances sémiologiques, ITIL (5) a proposé pour l'évaluation des médications antidépressives de comparer des enregistrements magnétoscopiques d'entretiens avec les malades avant et après thérapeutique. Cette méthode paraît d'un intérêt certain pour faciliter la communication entre psychiatres et non psychiatres, et éventuellement pour valider les résultats des échelles de comportement.

PERSPECTIVES DE RECHERCHE PROVENANT DES LACUNES ET BESOINS DE LA THÉRAPEUTIQUE

On peut considérer le problème du point de vue pratique des avances qui seraient nécessaires pour remédier aux lacunes et besoins de la thérapeutique psychiatrique qui avaient fait l'objet d'un bilan lors de notre VIème Congrès (4).

Un premier type de progrès serait représenté par une amélioration des moyens de traitement de l'excitation et de l'agitation, car en dépit de la transformation de l'atmosphère des services spécialisés, le contrôle de différents types d'agitation est encore insuffisant. Aussi serait-il logique d'étudier les correspondances pharmaco-cliniques pour réaliser les screening d'agents plus puissants ou plus spécifiques.

On sait que quinze ans après l'introduction des médicaments antidépresseurs, ces chimiothérapies n'ont pas toujours égalé l'électro-choc qui demeure dans certains cas irremplaçable. Il y a là une voie de recherche directement ouverte à la recherche pharmaceutique. Nous avons indiqué plus haut en quoi une corrélation plus souple et réaliste entre les propriétés pharmacologiques et les effets cliniques pourrait permettre de nouvelles avances.

Un autre exemple est fourni par la sémiologie hallucinatoire qui représente un processus psychotique assez facile à discerner et dont le traitement efficace influe souvent de façon déterminante sur l'évolution du délire. De plus l'activité hallucinatoire se rencontre fréquemment dans les psychoses rebelles et dans le „noyau" persistant des délires chroniques. Or, parmi les neuroleptiques, les butyrophénones – et tout spécialement l'halopéridol – semblent douées d'activités anti-hallucinatoires plus marquées. Mais, à notre connaissance, aucune étude systématique n'a été entreprise pour essayer de définir au laboratoire de semblables propriétés.

On pourrait encore citer les psychoses déficitaires pour lesquelles les recherches thérapeutiques sont abandonnées aux aléas des essais de médicaments censés améliorer la circulation ou le métabolisme cérébral.

On doit enfin mentionner le domaine des névroses, du déséquilibre psychopathique et des toxicomanies, où les possibilités offertes par les chimiothérapies demeurent très insuffisantes. Pourtant les progrès apportés par les thymoanaleptiques autant que par les tranquillisants ouvrent certaines perspectives de recherche.

Pour conclure, on peut dire que, mis à part les cadeaux que le hasard pourrait faire, l'avenir de la recherche psychopharmacologique en matière de médicaments repose essentiellement sur un dialogue ouvert et précis entre pharmacologues et cliniciens.

BIBLIOGRAPHIE

1. AYD F. J. et BLACKWELL B. (1970) Discoveries in Biological Psychiatry. Lippincott, Philadelphie.
2. BOISSIER J. R. et SIMON P. (1966) Pharmacologie prévisionnelle d'une substance psychotrope. Thérapie, **21**, 799.
3. FINK M. (1969) E. E. G. and human psychopharmacology. Pharmacol. Rev. **9**, 241.
4. DELAY J., DENIKER P., TEDESCHI D. H., GIURGEA C., LEHMANN H. E., HIPPIUS H., SIMON P. et LWOFF J. M. (1969) Insufficiencies and needs in psychopharmacology — Criteria of drug selection. In: The Present Status of Psychotropic Drugs, p. 139. Excerpta Med. Found., Amsterdam.
5. ITIL T. M. (1968) Electroencephalography and Pharmacopsychiatry. Modern Problems of Pharmacopsychiatry. Vol 1, p. 163, Karger, Basel.
6. JANSSEN P. A. (1970) Chemical and pharmacological classification of neuroleptics. In Modern Problems of Pharmacopsychiatry: 5. The neuroleptics. p. 33. Karger, Basel.

P. D., Département de Psychiatrie, Faculté de Médecine de Paris (Cochin), 100—102, rue de la Santé, Paris 14e, France

QUANTITATIVE AND COMPUTER EEG ANALYSIS IN ANIMAL NEUROPHARMACOLOGY

P. ETEVENON and J. R. BOISSIER

Research Unit of Neuropsychopharmacology, INSERM, Paris

Before considering the usefulness of EEG analysis in animal neuropharmacology, we describe briefly the principal methods of EEG analysis used by many workers in human pharmacology. Spontaneous activity of one-EEG channel may be analysed and quantitized by four different methods (Figs. 1 and 2).

METHODS OF ANALYSIS

First, histograms of instantaneous voltage amplitudes may be computed over a specific period of time (3, 4).

Second, the EEG signal may be rectified and integrated continuously over a period of integration T, providing mean values of quantitized integrated EEG. Time-course histograms, cumulative frequency curves and statistical analysis of distributions of integrated EEG data provide: means ± standard-deviations, coefficients of variability, modes of distribution, and chi-squared values of fitness to gaussian curves (5, 7). This method of quantitative electroencephalography, developed by DROHOCKI (3), since 1937 has been applied successfully in human subjects and in animal neuropharmacology by GOLDSTEIN and BECK (13).

The third method, the mean-frequency analysis or period analysis of BURCH and SALTZBERG, computes the major period, the mobility N of the EEG signal over the epoch T, by the averaged number of baseline zero-crossings divided by two. Similarly, the averaged number of maxima divided by two provides the intermediate period, the mobility of the first derivate of the signal (2, 11, 16, 19) (Fig. 1).

The last method applied by D. O. WALTER to EEG data is the power density spectrum analysis (20). The auto-spectrogram is the distribution of the EEG intensity (proportional to the squared amplitude) along the frequency axis. Statistical spectral analysis (9, 12, 14) computes mean power spectra between successive EEG epochs and provides statistical spectral characteristics relating all the three preceding methods to the mean power spectrum (Fig. 2). In fact, these four methods are related (1, 12), for example the voltage amplitude decreases linearly as the mean-frequency increases (Fig. 3).

When 2-EEG channels are simultaneously analysed, statistical regression or variance analysis may be computed from 1 channel-analysis data or spectral analysis may be applied

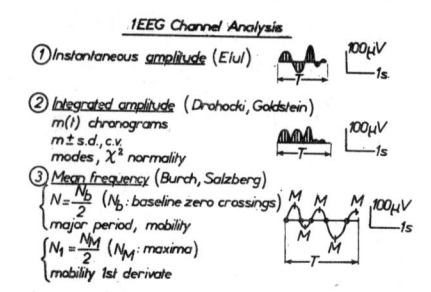

Fig. 1. First three methods of analysis of 1 EEG channel.

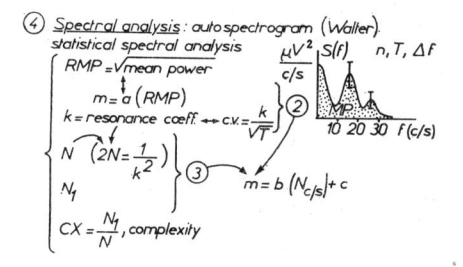

Fig. 2. Spectral analysis of 1 EEG channel. This fourth method of analysis is related to the second and the third one, by simple mathematical relations. The Mean Power value (MP) is the area under the mean power density curve. The mean integrated amplitude value is linearly proportional to the mean frequency value.

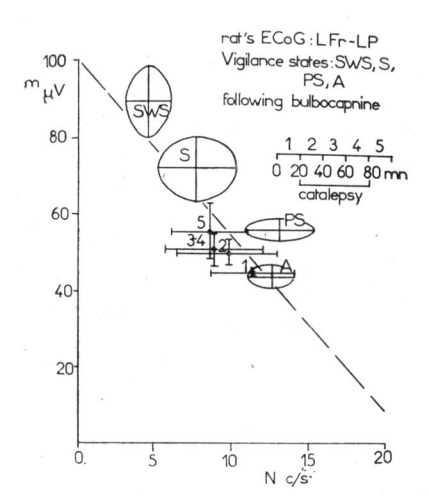

Fig. 3. Mean integrated amplitude linearly related to the mean frequency. For 8 seconds epochs of rat's left frontal-left parietal electrocorticograms. Statistical spectral analysis on PDP-10 computer, during different states of vigilance: slow wave sleep (SWS), sedation (S), paradoxical sleep (PS), arousal (A) and following bulbocapnine administration (50 mg/kg, i. p.).

providing cross-power spectrum, coherence function, transfer function or phase analysis (20, 21).

Computer analysis is needed for multiple EEG-analysis. Discriminant analysis has been used to discriminate between different states of vigilance. Factorial, multivariate analysis has been used from 1-channel EEG data to find the principal factors involved in psychotropic actions in time and for different neural structures (10).

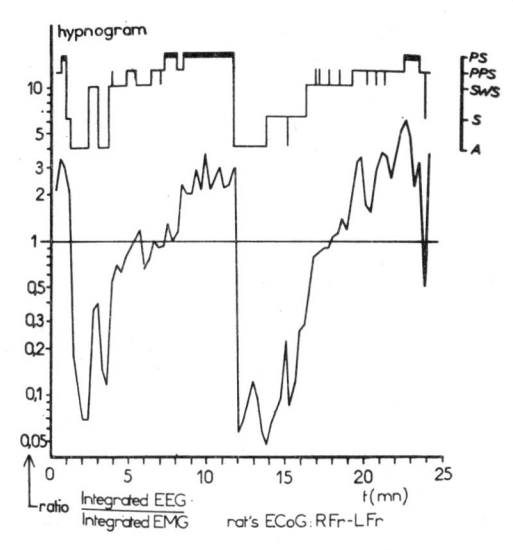

Fig. 4. Ratio of "integrated EEG vs. integrated EMG" and hypnogram. On the upper part: hypnogram or step-like curve of the time-course of vigilance changes of the rat from arousal (A), to sedation (S), slow wave sleep (SWS), phasic paradoxical sleep (PPS) and tonic paradoxical sleep (PS). On the lower part, the ratio of "integrated EEG vs. integrated EMG" computed from 20 seconds successive epochs of rat's left frontal-right frontal integrated electrocorticogram and integrated neck-muscles EMG.

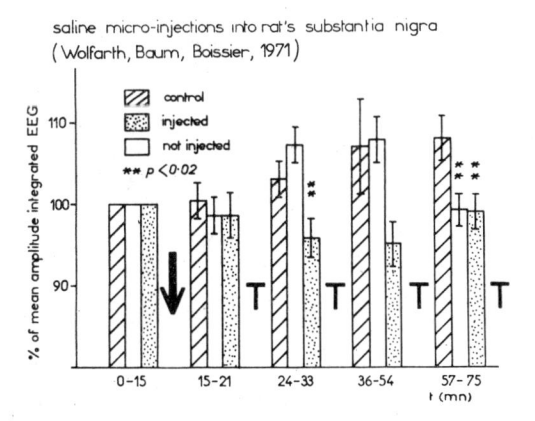

Fig. 5. Mean integrated amplitude values of rat's right and left substantia nigra EEG's, related to 100 % of control recordings. When one substantia nigra received saline microinjection (0.4 microliter), indicated by the arrow, this structure was desynchronized for 33 minutes prior to the contralateral non-injected other structure. Tests of catalepsy between EEG runs are labelled T.

Quantification of EEG

Used as a complement of visual analysis of recordings, together with psychopharmacological testing and neurophysiological techniques of lesions, stimulations or conditioning, EEG analysis provides an objective quantification of EEG data. In the rat, the ratio of "integrated EEG versus integrated EMG", is an index changing in time similar to the hypnogram describing normal vigilance fluctuations (Fig. 4).

A discriminating program based on the ratios of integrated EEG vs. integrated EMG values, has recently been developed, providing an automatic rat hypnogram plot (8), similar to the human "sleep-prints" obtained by Itil.

Wolfarth, Baum and Boissier have found that a microinjection of saline into the substantia nigra, produced an arousal which was well quantified by integrated amplitude values (Fig. 5) (22).

Display of unseen EEG changes

EEG analysis may also reveal new features undetected by visual inspection of recordings. Using quantitative electroencephalography, Goldstein and Beck were able to discriminate psychotropic agents in animals from mean and coefficient of variability changes. Whereas hypnotics increase mean and coefficient of variability, analeptics decrease these parameters (13). We found that neuroleptics increase the mean and decrease the coefficient of variability in the rat (5).

Beck found that when a chronically implanted rabbit is pre-treated by 5 mg/kg of pentobarbital inducing a sedated state, reversal towards arousal produced by psychostimulants is well measured by integrated amplitude data. The slope of dose-reversal lines may be related to the mechanism of action as in pharmacokinetics (13).

The effects of psychotropic agents on associative cortical response to reticular formation stimulation in cats, may be seen clearly after spectral analysis. Hugelin has observed a specific response after pentobarbital, masked on the tracé by the low frequency-high amplitude waves, and no response at all after atropine administration (15).

The hypovariability after psychotropic agents also appears to be an important factor,

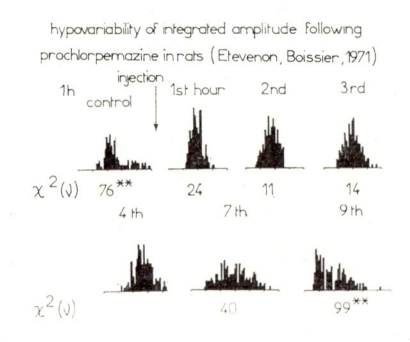

Fig. 6. Sequential distributions of 1-hour successive integrated amplitude values (20 seconds epochs). The first hour control period presents a non-gaussian distribution (chi-square value of 76), such as the 9th hour following prochlorpemazine treatment (12,5 mg/kg, i.p.). The first three hours following neuroleptic administration present gaussian distributions of integrated amplitude values, indicating the amplitude hypovariability during the neuroleptic induced cataleptic state.

well displayed by EEG analysis. NAQUET and coworkers have shown cortical hypovariability between 5 to 7 cycles/s in *Papio papio* after droperidol (18).

This dominant frequency band (5—7 c/s) corresponds to a dominant integrated amplitude peak in gaussian histograms taken after prochlorpemazine administration in rats (Fig. 6). One hour successive histograms of integrated EEG data show this cortical hypovariability (5) (Fig. 6).

By using quantitative electroencephalography with differential photic stimulation in rabbits, we have found a lateralisation of the visual cortex in control animals. The lateralisation and signal-to-noise ratio are increased following LSD treatment (6).

DIRECTIONS OF RESEARCH

Computer analysis between multiple structure previously quantitized and analysed by 1-channel or 2-channel techniques, may be a useful tool in research into mechanisms of action and cortical-subcortical relationships (13, 21).

FAIRCHILD and coworkers have recently used canonical multivariate analysis between long time frequency analysis in cats submitted to different treatments and have described specific relations between canonical variables (10).

Despite this and other interesting approaches, it does not seem that causality and interrelations between cortical and subcortical structures and their changes following psychotropic treatments, have yet been completely described, by this sophisticated computer EEG analysis (21).

Nevertheless, this avenue of research is still open and the difficulties increase from practical problem of the proper analysis of data so as to extract the highest amount of information from an experiment, to models simulating the neurophysiological processes and towards a model of mechanisms of psychotropic action. Such models have been developed in neuronal unitary neurophysiology and worked out by PERKEL, GERSTEIN and MOORE (17). We hope it will soon be possible to apply such models in experimental neuropharmacology.

CONCLUSION

If we consider the tremendous growth of the space-sciences today, it is due in great part to new instruments, new programs and technological improvements involved in space-missions as well as to the discovery of new theoretical models in cosmology. Along these lines, EEG analysis has been developed recently for astronauts health and vigilance checking (20, 21).

We believe that animal neuropharmacology will benefit from these new methods of EEG analysis and from the growing modelling of CNS functional activities. Animal neuropharmacology will then appear to be in a closed feedback loop with clinical neuropharmacology and pharmaco-electroencephalography; the former being complementary of the latter in a generalized set of neuropharmacological knowledge.

REFERENCES

1. BARBEYRAC, J. de and ETEVENON, P. (1969) On the relationships between two methods of EEG signals analysis: the integrative method and power spectrum analysis. L'analyse automatique du signal électrobiologique. Agressologie, **10** (numéro spécial), 573.

2. BURCH N. R. (1959) Automatic analysis of the electroencephalogram: a review and classification of systems. EEG clin. Neurophysiol. **11**, 827.
3. DROHOCKI Z. A. (1971) Les trois aspects du spectre d'amplitude de l'électroencéphalogramme. C. R. Acad. Sci. (Paris), **273**, 504.
4. ELUL R. (1969) Gaussian behavior of the electroencephalogram: changes during performance of mental task. Science, **164**, 328.
5. ETEVENON P. and BOISSIER J. R. (1971) Statistical amplitude analysis of the integrated electrocorticogram of unrestrained rats, before and after prochlorpemazine. Neuropharmacology, **10**, 161.
6. ETEVENON P. and BOISSIER J. R. (1972) LSD effects on signal-to-noise ratio and lateralisation of visual cortex and lateral geniculate during photic stimulation. Experientia, **29**, 1100.
7. ETEVENON P., GUILLON G. and BOISSIER J. R. (1969) Statistical analysis of the distributions of integrated EEG in psychopharmacology. Agressologie, **10** (numéro spécial) 641.
8. ETEVENON P., GUILLON G. and BOISSIER J. R. (1972) Sleep-prints automatic analysis and histamine changes in chronic unrestrained rats. Fifth International Congress on Pharmacology, Abst. 387, San Francisco, USA.
9. ETEVENON P., KITTEN G., BARBEYRAC J. de and GOLDBERG P. (1970) Analyse spectrale de l'EEG du rat. J. Pharmacol. (Paris), **1**, 383.
10. FAIRCHILD M. D., JENDEN D. J. and MICKEY M. R. (1971) Quantitative analysis of some drug effects on the EEG by long-term frequency analysis. Proc. West. Pharmacol. Soc., **14**, 135.
11. FINK M., SHAPIRO D. M., HICKMAN C. and ITIL T. (1968) Digital computer EEG analysis in psychopharmacology. p. 109. In: Computers and electronic. Devices in Psychiatry, KLINE and LASKA, Ed., Grune and Statton, N. Y.
12. GOLDBERG P. and ETEVENON P. (1973) Analyse spectrale statistique du signal EEG. Calcul de nouvelles données spectrales caractéristiques. Revue d'Informatique Médicale, Paris **4**.
13. GOLDSTEIN L. and BECK R. (1965) Amplitude analysis of the electroencephalogram: review of the information obtained with the integrative method. Int. Rev. Neurobiol. **8**, 265.
14. HORD D. J., JOHNSON L. C., LUBIN A. and AUSTIN M. T. (1965) Resolution and stability in the autospectra of EEG. EEG clin. Neurophysiol. **19**, 305.
15. HUGELIN A. (1968) Mise en évidence par analyse spectrale de trois bandes critiques de l'électrocorticogramme du Chat. J. Physiol. **60**, suppl. 2, 465.
16. ITIL T., SHAPIRO D. and FINK M. (1968) Differentiation of psychotropic drugs by quantitative EEG analysis. Agressologie, **9**, 267.
17. PERKEL D. H., GERSTEIN G. L. and MOORE G. P. (1967) Neuronal spike trains and stochastic point processes. II. Simultaneous spike trains. Biophys. J. **7**, 419.
18. RENN C., VUILLON-CACCIUTTOLO G., JUTIER M., BIMAR J. and NAQUET R. (1970) Contribution de l'analyse spectrale à l'évaluation électroencéphalographique de l'action des drogues anesthésiques. Ann. Anesth. Franç. **11**, 357.
19. SALTZBERG B., EDWARDS R. J., HEATH R. G. and BURCH N. R. (1968) Synoptic analysis of EEG signals. p. 267. In: Data acquisition and processing in biology and medicine, Vol. 5, Pergamon Press, Oxford.
20. WALTER D. O. (1963) Spectral analysis for electroencephalograms: mathematical determination of neurophysiological relationships from records of limited duration. Exp. Neurol. **8**, 155.
21. WALTER D. O. (1972) Digital processing of bioelectrical phenomena. Part B, Volume 4. In: Handbook of electroencephalography and clinical neurophysiology, Ed.-in chief ANTOINE RÉMOND, Elsevier, Amsterdam.
22. WOLFARTH S., BAUM E. and BOISSIER J. R. (1971) The effects of uni-and bilateral micro-injections of saline solutions into substantia nigra of conscious rat. III. Congress of the Polish Pharmacological Society, Wroclaw, Abstracts, p. 113.

P. E., Unité de Recherches de Neuropsychopharmacologie,
INSERM, 2, rue d'Alésia, Paris 14e, France

BEITRÄGE DER PHARMAKOPSYCHIATRIE ZUR ENTWICKLUNG NOSOLOGISCHER MODELLE

H. RENNERT und G.-E. KÜHNE

Universitäts-Nervenklinik, Halle (Saale)

Die bisherigen nosologischen Modellvorstellungen in der Psychiatrie hatten in der Regel betont systematisierenden Charakter; bei der Rubrifizierung stand der symptomatologisch-phänomenologische Aspekt im Vordergrund. Ätiopathogenetische Interpretationen der endogenen Psychosen werden zwar weiterhin angestrebt, kommen aber meist nur in genetischen und verlaufstypologischen Teilaspekten zur Geltung. Obwohl die Therapie der Psychosen in den letzten Jahrzehnten einen enormen Aufschwung genommen hat, sind in den meisten nosologischen Vorstellungen therapeutische Bezüge noch nicht enthalten. Die psychiatrische Therapie wird auch heute von vielen ausschließlich als Korrektiv betrachtet, um pathoplastische Faktoren zu eliminieren, Entgleisungen zu korrigieren, Schäden zu kompensieren und Restfunktionen rehabilitativ nutzbar zu machen.

Die heute wieder stärker aufkommenden, mehr oder weniger konsequent einheitspsychotisch bzw. unitarisch ausgerichteten pathogenetischen Konzeptionen tragen einen flexibleren Charakter, streben universell gültige Aspekte an und verbessern — zunächst quasi als Nebenergebnis — die Kongruenz nosologischer und klinisch-therapeutischer Probleme. Bei Annahme eines multifaktoriellen Entstehungsgefüges — etwa im Sinne der von uns vertretenen „Universalgenese der Psychosen" — ist eine als partiell-kausal aufzufassende Psychosentherapie diskutabel.

Wir meinen, daß das bisherige Fehlen einer durch die moderne Psychosentherapie wesentlich mitbestimmten psychiatrischen Nosologie Hemmnisse für Forschung und Praxis und damit auch für die Therapie selbst bewirkt. Die Erfahrungen der Psychopharmakologie der letzten 10 Jahre haben es ermöglicht, auf empirischer, massenexperimenteller, naturwissenschaftlich bestimmter Basis wichtige Rückschlüsse auf die Pathogenese zu ziehen. Wir konnten dabei sichtbar machen, daß ein multifaktorielles Konzept am besten mit den gewonnenen Ergebnissen vereinbar ist, und zwar nicht allein für die sog. endogenen Psychosen, sondern bis zu einem gewissen Grade auch für die symptomatischen und reaktiven Psychosen. Ein im jeweiligen Krankheitsfall unterschiedliches Schwergewicht einzelner pathogenetischer Faktoren und symptomatologischer Momente spricht nach unserer Auffassung keineswegs gegen ein multifaktorielles, multikonditionales Zusammenwirken grundsätzlich einheitlicher Kräfte bzw. gegen die Gültigkeit universeller Entstehungsbedingungen, und das sowohl bei den vorwiegend affektiven, als auch bei den vorwiegend schizophrenen Psychosen.

Unsere Erfahrungen haben uns also veranlaßt, die Nosologie der Psychosen nicht zuletzt aus der Sicht der Wirkungsweise therapeutischer Maßnahmen, und zwar sowohl erfolgreicher als auch nicht erfolgreicher, zu beleuchten. Beim Studium psychopharmakologischer Wirkungen sieht man, daß mit großer Regelhaftigkeit das Vorliegen bestimmter psychopathologischer Grundbefindlichkeiten und Konstellationen eine entscheidende Rolle spielt. Das gilt insbesondere für die Psychopharmaka-Wirkung im Antriebs-Stimmungsbereich; hier kommt es vorrangig auf das jeweilige Überwiegen von psychomotorischer und affektiver Erregung oder Hemmung bzw. auf gewisse quantitative oder qualitative Varianten und Kombinationen an. Wir erfassen damit die „Antriebs-Stimmungsrelation" im Sinne von PETRILOWITSCH differenzierter. Ähnliches gilt für die „dynamischen Grundkonstellationen" von JANZARIK und die „psychischen Zentralfunktionen" von ENGELMEIER. Diesen Autoren verdanken wir jedoch wertvolle Anregungen. Die Beachtung der Grundbefindlichkeiten und ihrer Beeinflußbarkeit erleichtert nicht nur wesentlich das Verständnis der Psychopharmakawirkung und die Indikationsstellung, sondern schafft auch neue pathogenetische Einsichten und kann nebenbei helfen, internationale nomenklatorische Schwierigkeiten zu überwinden und die statistische Erfassung und Aussagekraft zu verbessern.

Unsere klinischen Erfahrungen haben bestätigt, daß die bei den meisten Psychiatern noch als entscheidend geltende vordergründige „klassische" Psychosensymptomatik für die therapeutische Indikationsstellung und statistische Auswertbarkeit nur einen begrenzten, wahrscheinlich sogar fragwürdigen Wert besitzt. Psychomotorisch-affektive Grundbefindlichkeiten stellen in den von uns in verschiedenen Veröffentlichungen herausgestellten typischen Konstellationen, die wir als „Basissyndrome" bezeichnen, eine gute Grundlage dar. Hyper- und Hypomotorik, Para- und Dysmotorik in unterschiedlicher Kombination mit den entsperchenden Differentialen auf affektivem Gebiet ergeben charakteristische psychotische Reaktionstypen und erlauben eine bessere grundlagen- und therapiegerechte Rubrifizierung. Diese Basissyndrome, die über die „Zielsymptome" von FREYHAN wesentlich hinausgehen, können weitgehend unabhängig von der sonstigen phänomenologischen und verlaufsmäßigen Zugehörigkeit zu den sog. manisch-depressiven und schizophrenen Formenkreisen diagnostiziert und therapiert werden und öffnen den Weg zu einer nosologisch-therapeutischen Kongruenz. Ähnliches meinte auch VINAŘ, wenn er kürzlich bei uns in Berlin etwa von Chlorpromazin- oder Amitriptylintypen unter den Psychosen sprach. Nach ähnlichen Ordnungsprinzipien können übrigens auch in anderen Bereichen der pathologisch veränderten Persönlichkeit, also außerhalb von Antrieb und Stimmung, weitere Differentiale herausgearbeitet werden, wenn diese auch therapeutisch weniger bedeutungsvoll sind.

Eine derartige Korrelation therapeutischer Erkenntnisse und nosologischer Fragestellungen eröffnet die Möglichkeit, die Psychosenlehre strukturell klarer zu verstehen und eine engere Verbindung mit dem pragmatisch-kurativen Anliegen herzustellen. Auf diesem Wege einer „Nosogenese" wird die Weiterentwicklung therapeutischer Verfahren zwangsläufig allmählich auch eine neue problemoffene, dynamische psychiatrische Nosologie schaffen, die das internationale psychopharmakologische und pharmakopsychiatrische Verständnis erleichtern, Dokumentations- und Auswertungsverfahren vereinfachen und das humanistische Anliegen des heilenden Arztes auf eine neue wissenschaftliche Stufe heben kann.

H. R., Universitäts-Nervenklinik, Halle (Saale), D.D.R.

SOCIAL IMPLICATIONS OF PSYCHOPHARMACOLOGY

Chairmen: H. E. Lehmann and P. Kielholz

Associate chairman: S. Rasmussen

ZUKÜNFTIGE GESICHTSPUNKTE ÜBER DIE MÖGLICHE SOZIALE VERWENDBARKEIT DER PSYCHOPHARMAKOLOGIE

R. JUNGK

Technische Universität, West-Berlin

In ihrer jetzigen, selbstkritischen zweiten Phase löst sich die Zukunftsforschung mehr und mehr von jenen prophetischen, normativen oder deterministischen Bemühungen, die meinen Aussagen mit einem hohen Grad von Sicherheit über die Welt von morgen machen zu können und exakte Zielvorstellungen, sowie detaillierte Programme für die Gestaltung des Kommenden formulieren zu können. Immer mehr spricht man im Plural von möglichen „Zukünften", statt von „*der* Zukunft", immer stärker wird der spekulative heuristische Charakter aller Aussagen betont, die wir über das noch nicht Geschehene machen können.

In diesem Sinne sollten auch die nachfolgenden Überlegungen aufgefasst werden. Sie maßen sich nicht an zu wissen, was sein *wird*, sie entwickeln nur Gedanken über das, was sein *könnte*. Diese Vermutungen, obwohl gestützt durch Daten und Fakten, werden, wie alle je versuchten Prognosen, unvermeidlich von gegenwärtigen Sorgen und Hoffnungen beeinflusst. Die Abhängigkeit jeder Vorausschau von den Denkweisen, ja den Denkmoden der Epoche, in der sie erstellt wurden, und von den spezifischen Vorurteilen derjenigen, die sie machen (oder in Auftrag geben), darf niemals übersehen werden.

Ein in der westlichen Welt lebender, seine eigenen Bedingtheiten und Gebundenheiten mitreflektierender Zukunftsbetrachter wird gedrängt sein, die Krise, die der Menschheit in den nächsten Jahrzehnten droht, zum Ausgangspunkt seiner Betrachtungen zu machen.

Der amerikanische Biophysiker und Futurologe JOHN PLATT hat unlängst hervorgehoben, daß bis zur Jahrtausendwende und vermutlich auch noch darüber hinaus, eine Turbulenzzone der Menschheitsgeschichte erwartet werden müsse, die durch das fast gleichzeitige — und durch diese Gleichzeitigkeit verwirrende — Auftreten mehrerer schwerer Krisen besonders gefährlich sei. An erster Stelle ist da, trotz seines augenblicklichen Zurückweichens aus dem Zentrum der öffentlichen Aufmerksamkeit, der *Rüstungswettlauf* zu nennen. Durch die immer noch zunehmende Anhäufung von Vernichtungswaffen und deren Verteilung auf immer mehr Gefahrenzonen, bleiben die Überlebenschancen der Erdbewohner permanent bedroht. Dazu kommt erschwerend die Tatsache, daß durch die Erhaltung und permanente Modernisierung dieser hochtechnisierten Vernichtungssysteme enorme geistige und materielle Mittel, die zur Bekämpfung der anderen Krisen dringender denn je gebraucht würden, verschwendet werden.

Diese anderen Krisen sollen hier nur kurz erwähnt werden. Es ist die Umweltkrise, die Bevölkerungskrise, die Krise zwischen dem verschwenderischen hochindustrialisierten Norden und dem immer mehr verarmenden Süden der Erdhalbkugel, es ist das Wuchern der Städte, die Verknappung sowohl der Rohstoffe wie der Nahrungsmittel, die falsch verteilt und Spekulationsobjekt geworden, mit der sprunghaften Vermehrung der Menschheit und ihrem Bedarf bald nicht mehr schritthalten dürften. Aber neben diesen uns allen bekannten und zwar kaum gelösten, aber fast bis zum Überdruss diskutierten Problemen, erwähnt JOHN PLATT ein nur selten derart hervorgehobenes, das im Zusammenhang mit der Frage nach dem mir hier gestellten Thema, von besonderer Wichtigkeit ist. Er spricht nämlich von der "crisis of participation", von der Mitbeteiligungs,- von der Mitbestimmungskrise.

Was hat Partizipation mit den „möglichen künftigen sozialen Implikationen der Psychopharmakologie" zu tun? Lassen Sie mich darauf zuerst mit einer Hypothese antworten. Sie lautet: In dem Maße, wie die Partizipation der Bürger, speziell der jungen und der arbeitenden Menschen, an der Gestaltung ihres Schicksals in den kommenden Jahren weiterhin abnimmt, wird der Gebrauch von Psychopharmaka zunehmen.

Aber diese These lässt sich natürlich auch umkehren: In dem Maße, wie die aktive Partizipation der heute noch „Abhängigen" zunimmt, wird der Gebrauch von Psychopharmaka abnehmen.

Kielholz hat gezeigt, daß Drogenabhängigkeit besonders bei solchen Jugendlichen auftritt, die aus gestörten Familienverhältnissen stammen. Ähnlich gestört ist heute schon das Verhältnis von Millionen Menschen zur "family of man", zu menschlichen Gemeinschaften auf allen anderen Ebenen: In der Berufsgruppe, in der Gemeinde, im Staat. Der durchschnittliche Mensch unserer Tage fühlt sich, wie unlängst durch eine holländische Studie über Zukunftserwartungen auch quantitativ belegt wurde, nicht imstande, die komplizierte, in ihren wichtigsten Verknüpfungen ihm nicht zugängliche gesellschaftliche Wirklichkeit, zu erfassen oder gar zu beeinflussen.

Diese Unmündigkeit wird ihm zudem von den Fachleuten ständig vorgehalten. Selbst in den sozialistischen Staaten, in denen die Mitbeteiligung der Bürger nicht nur bei unmittelbar anstehenden Entscheidungen, sondern bereits in den Vorstadien der Prognose und der Planung prinzipiell ermöglicht werden soll, wird dann in der Praxis ein Maß von „Qualifikation" verlangt, das der Laie — und das ist fast jeder, ausser auf seinem speziellen Berufsgebiet — nicht besitzt und auch kaum schnell genug erwerben kann (5).

Dazu kommt, daß der schon von MARX beschriebene Prozess der „Entfremdung" weitergeht durch zunehmende Arbeitsteiligkeit, Rationalisierung und immer weiter eingeschränkte Möglichkeit zu eigener schöpferischer Initiative. Zwar ist vorläufig noch in den meisten hochindustrialisierten Ländern die berufliche Vollbeschäftigung gesichert, zugleich aber nimmt die „seelische Arbeitslosigkeit" zu.

Diese besondere und für den „homo consumens" typische Form der inneren Beschäftigungslosigkeit trägt noch mehr dazu bei, ihn abhängig und passiv zu machen. RASOR hat in seiner Studie über junge, drogenabhängige Amerikaner kritisiert, daß sie „nicht interessiert seien irgendjemandem etwas zu geben. Sie sind nur interessiert, etwas zu empfangen". Aber ist das nicht eben die Rolle, zu der man sie verurteilt? Und ist nicht gerade der Drogengebrauch ein allerdings völlig untauglicher Versuch ihr zu entfliehen? Denn die Droge entführt ihren Benutzer in eine andere „Realität", die er meint durchschauen zu können, die seine im Alltagsleben zur Untätigkeit verurteilte seelische Energie, Sensibilität und Kreativität für wenige Stunden anregt. Er wird innerlich aktiv und kann dabei doch körperlich und gesellschaftlich passiv bleiben.

Charakteristisch für den Zustand der „seelischen Arbeitslosigkeit" ist das Absterben der für den Menschen — besonders für den westlichen Menschen — so wichtigen Zukunftserwartungen. ERICKSON, FRANK, KENNISTON, KLUCKHOHN und SAUNDERS haben auf die wichtige Rolle der „Zeitperspektive" und „Zeitorientierung" in der Dynamik des psychisch aktiven Menschen hingewiesen, der bereit ist, die sofortige Erfüllung seiner auf Zukunftsgestaltung zielenden Wünsche vorübergehend aufzuschieben. Wenn aber dieser Aufschub zur permanenten Frustrationsquelle wird, stirbt schließlich die Fähigkeit zur Hoffnung ab. Die Zukunft hat dann aufgehört. Nur die *sofortige*, augenblickliche Befriedigung wird noch angestrebt. Ihr zuliebe ist man auch bereit, mögliche Gefährdungen der persönlichen Zukunft, die aus gesundheitlichen Schädigungen beim Drogengebrauch entstehen können, in Kauf zu nehmen.

Es lassen sich heute, politisch vor allem, zwei entgegengesetzte Entwicklungstendenzen prognostizieren:

1. die weiter oben skizzierten Krisen verstärken die heute bereits wahrnehmbaren technokratischen, elitären und autoritären Tendenzen;
2. die immer dringender werdenden Wünsche nach Partizipation und Erweiterung der Demokratie im Staat wie im Berufsleben setzen sich allmählich durch.

Für die erste Alternative spricht beim heutigen Stand der Dinge mehr als für die zweite. Da ist zunächst einmal das immer häufiger zu hörende Argument des Zeitdrucks. Typisch dafür ist die von führenden Managern gegründete Studie des „Klubs von Rom" über „Die Grenzen des Wachstums"(3). Sie plädiert dafür, in spätestens zehn Jahren jene Wachstumsprozesse zu stoppen, die nach den Computerberechnungen dieser internationalen Gruppe zu einer Katastrophe führen müssen. Unter Berufung auf die Notlage der Menschheit könnte es dann der Ruf nach „starken Männern" — diesmal wird man die „starken Fachmänner" verlangen — immer lauter ertönen. Sie sollen dann imstande sein, ohne viel Diskussion und Widerspruch das zu verordnen, was sie für „vernünftig" halten. Für solch ein "Krisenmanagement" von oben würden die von Untergangsangst gequälten Menschen der achtziger Jahre vielleicht von sich aus auf ihre ohnehin nicht sehr effektiven demokratischen Rechte ganz verzichten (2). Die Folge wäre eine weitere Konzentration der Planungss - und Entscheidungsgewalt, weiterer Abbau der als "hemmend" und "zu langsam" verketzerten Partizipation. Und vermutlich auch weiteres Ansteigen des möglicherweise sogar staatlich geförderten Drogenkonsums.

Die zweite Alternative ist nicht ganz chancenlos. Es nehmen zur Zeit nicht nur die Passiven, die „seelisch Arbeitslosen" zu, sondern auf der anderen Seite des Spektrums auch die kritischen, auf erweiterte Information und Mitgestaltung drängenden Kräfte. Soziale Experimente, Bürgerbewegungen, Initiativen im Schulwesen und im Wohnungsbau, die auf Aufbau von „Aussenlenkung" und Autorität drängen, treten in wachsender Zahl und Intensität auf. Nicht zufällig stellen sich diese, auf die Reaktivierung der Menschen zielenden Bewegungen gegen die Drogenbenutzung. Allerdings nicht durch den Ruf nach Verboten und polizeilichem Eingreifen, sondern indem sie versuchen, die gestörte "family of man" wenigstens partiell wieder herzustellen durch Bildung von Gruppen, von Gemeinschaften und Kommunen, in denen auch Drogenabhängige Aufnahme finden.

Theoretisch vorwärtsgetrieben und überspitzt wird diese Position durch die „radikalen Therapeuten" in den USA (7). Ihre Formel für die Beseitigung der Entfremdung, die sie als die Grundursache aller psychischen Störungen ansehen, lautet:

"Liberation equals awareness plus contact". Also: Befreiung (auch Befreiung von der Sucht) ist gleich Bewußtwerden plus Zusammenschluß. Dabei soll der Patient, der nun nicht mehr als Sonderfall angesehen wird, sondern als der Normale, durch die gesellschaftlichen Verhältnisse Beschädigte, einmal die Kräfte und Mechanismen der Unterdrückung und Verhinderung kennenlernen und weiterhin sich mit den Menschen verbinden, die gegen diese Bedingungen kämpfen.

Zu kritisieren ist an dieser Auffassung, daß sie zwar eine — und vermutlich sogar die wichtigste Wurzel — der „seelischen Arbeitslosigkeit" und der aus ihr entstehenden Drogensucht erkennt, aber annimmt, daß eine Veränderung der bestehenden gesellschaftlichen Machtverhältnisse schon ausreichen würde, um mit dem Problem fertig zu werden. Vermutlich würde aber eine politische und wirtschaftliche Strukturveränderung der Art, wie sie die sozialistischen Länder versucht haben, noch nicht jene „Selbst-Verwirklichung" der Einzelpersönlichkeiten erreichen, die imstande wäre die Partizipations krise und Identitätskrise der Menschen in dieser Epoche der Geschichte aufzuheben. Denkbar und nach Ansicht des Verfassers wünschbar wäre eine viel tiefer gehende Wende, eine „neue Richtung des Fortschritts", die sich andere Ziele setzt: Nicht mehr die Entwicklung und Herstellung von materiellen Erzeugnissen wäre ihr verpflichtendstes Ziel, sondern die Erhöhung der menschlichen Sensibilität, die Erweiterungen der menschlichen Fähigkeiten durch Förderung der Phantasie, die heute noch meist in den ersten Schuljahren abgetötet wird, die Weckung und Befriedigung des Schönheitssinns, die Entwicklung von Liebesfähigkeit, von kooperativem Verhalten an Stelle von Konkurrenz und von Freude am Spiel.

Lewis Mumford (4) hat darauf hingewiesen, daß eine grundlegende Bekämpfung der Krisen, in die uns die wissenschaftlich-technische Revolution hineingeführt hat, nur durch eine Wendung von aussen nach innen, von der Erforschung der Natur und der Materie zur Erforschung des Menschen gelingen könne.

Es ist als Zukunftsvision denkbar und möglich, daß durch eine unvermeidlich gewordenes Abbremsen des materiellen Wachstums nun ein anderes Wachstum des Menschen in den kommenden Jahren zum zentralen Gegenstand der Forschung wird. Es würden dann "mind laboratories" (Geisteslaboratorien), in den Anthropologen, Neurophysiologen, Biologen, Soziologen, Ethiologen, Ethnologen und "last but not least" auch Psychopharmakologen interdisziplinär zusammenarbeiten sollten, jene Pionierrolle übernehmen, die bisher den Laboratorien der Chemie und Physik zukam.

In solchen Versuchsstätten wäre dann z.B. herauszufinden, in welcher Weise „altered states of consciousness" zu einer Bereicherung der menschlichen Möglichkeiten beitragen könnten. Hier würden nicht nur meditative Techniken objektiv untersucht und entwickelt werden, wie es Kamiya heute schon in San Francisco versucht, sondern auch die Drogen — nun nicht mehr als Mittel der Scheinaktivierung sondern der kontrollierten Steigerung, Erweiterung und Vertiefung des „inneren Menschen" eine eminent positive Rolle spielen (1).

Psychodrogen haben—ich zitiere Günter Ammon — „bei stabiler psychischer Konstitution und in gesicherter sozialer Position" bewußtseinserweiternde Qualität. Das wissen die sogenannten „Unterentwickelten" seit langem, die diese den Gesetzen des Ritus und und der Heiligkeit unterstellen. Die „dritte Welt" könnte dann auf diesem und nicht nur auf diesem Gebiet dem westlichen Menschen vermutlich als Entwicklungshelfer wichtige Dienste leisten.

Einer der interessantesten und heute bereits effektiven Zweige der Zukunftsforschung ist das sogenannte "technology assessment". Im Rahmen dieser Bemühungen versucht man die künftigen schädlichen und nützlichen Folgen neuer technologischer Erfindungen für die Gesellschaft zu prognostizieren *bevor* diese Innovationen eingeführt werden (Beispiel Auto, SST).

Ähnlich wird eine Zukunftsforschung, welche die Bedeutung des Faktors Mensch erkannt hat, ein "psychology assessment" ausprobieren müssen, in dem die seelischen Folgen von Innovationen nicht für Einzelne sondern für die Gesellschaft vorherbedacht werden. Die Überprüfung der negativen und positiven Einflüsse der Psychopharmaka für die Weiterentwicklung der Geschichte sollte dann zu den zentralen Aufgaben eines solchen nie aufhörenden Studiums seelischer Entwicklungen gehören. Die Psychopharmakologen sollten bei solchen prognostischen Bemühungen mitarbeiten, um Schaden zu vermeiden und den Nutzen ihrer Arbeit zu erhöhen.

LITERATURVERZEICHNIS

1. AGEL, J. (1971) The Radical Therapist, New York.
2. JUNGK, R. (1972) Politik und Technokratie, IG Metall Kongress Oberhausen.
3. MEADOWS, D. et al. (1972) Die Grenzen des Wachstums, Stuttgart.
4. MUMFORD, L. (1970) The Pentagon of Power, New York.
5. MÜLLER, N. Mündliche Mitteilung (TU Berlin) auf Grund seiner Vorarbeiten zur Dissertation „Prognose und Partizipation in der DDR".
6. PLATT, J. (1969) What we must do. Mental Health Institute University of Illinois.
7. TART, CH. U. (Ed.) (1969) Altered States of Consciousness, New York.

R. J. Technische Universität, Fachbereich Planungswissenschaften, West-Berlin

PERSONAL AND SOCIAL IMPLICATIONS OF LITHIUM MAINTENANCE TREATMENT

M. SCHOU and P. C. BAASTRUP

Psychopharmacology Research Unit, Aarhus University Psychiatric Institute, Risskov, and Glostrup Psychiatric Hospital, Glostrup

The prophylactic efficacy of lithium in recurrent endogenous affective disorders has by now been proven beyond any reasonable doubt. Non-blind and double-blind studies have shown that when lithium is given as a maintenance treatment in proper dosage it effectively prevents or attenuates further manic and depressive episodes without interfering with normal mental functions. That is of course not so in all cases, but in most. This provides us with a unique opportunity to study what happens when a life that was previously dominated by frequent and severe manias or depressions is changed to one that is stable month after month and year after year. As anybody will know who is at all familiar with recurrent manic-depressive disorder, such a change is a major event, and it has far-reaching consequences not only for the patient himself but also for his family and acquaintances.

Around patients with frequent and severe affective episodes there often develops a peculiar psycho-social pattern in which patient, spouse, children, friends and associates all play special roles in a combined effort to mitigate the consequences of the patient's incessant mood changes. In protracted cases the family hardly knows an existance that is not dominated by fear of imminent disaster: depressive suicidal attempts or manic deeds of misjudgement. The atmosphere becomes one of constant vigilance, plans can be only tentative, and activities are curbed by the necessity of subordinating everything to the caprices of the patient's recurrent disorder.

All this is altered by successful lithium maintenance treatment. Recurrences become few and mild and eventually disappear completely. The patient, or rather ex-patient, once more becomes the person he or she was before the disease first started. Fear is eventually replaced by confidence in the future, and everybody can breathe a sigh of relief. It is among the psychiatrist's most gratifying experiences to hear descriptions of how the patient is now "on an even keel", "in much better shape than he has been for years", "is now able to cope with difficult situations much more adequately", "is now his old self again as he was when we married", etc., etc. The list could be continued almost *ad infinitum*.

However, not in every instance is all bliss. Patients who before lithium treatment profited personally or professionally from frequent and long periods of hypomania may dislike the effects of the treatment and even reject it (3, 5, 6, 15, 17, 21). Some businessmen and executives claim that the hypomanic impetus and energy is necessary for their work and that lithium makes them less capable. Some artists claim that the hypomanic inspiration and indefatigability are essential for both the quality and the quantity of their work and that lithium treatment inhibits their creativity. These claims are, however, strictly subjective and have not been substantiated by systematic studies. In fact, the patients' families and associates often explain that the work which is carried out by the patients during hypomanic periods is not nearly as valuable as the patients themselves think at the time. In our experience, most of the patients who initially miss their hypomanias eventually get accustomed to the new and stable life course and discover with pleased astonishment that their productivity and creativeness are then as good as or better than before lithium treatment started. The suggestion occasionally made that lithium treatment is contraindicated in artists because lithium interferes with creative ability, finds no support in our observations.

It is not always the elation that is missed. An undertaker's customers, mistaking depressive sadness for compassion, complained about his appearance of indifference when he was in lithium treatment (6). Another patient regretted that in discussions he was unable to attain the level of excitement he considered necessary: "Doctor, I am a communist and I *must* get excited when I discuss " (4). There are also patients who feel that lithium treatment makes life "flat" and less colourful, "curbs" their activity, and prevents them from going as fast as they would like (3, 9, 20, 21, 25, 27, 28). In most cases these complaints disappear when the patients become used to the stable life course.

For the patient's family and friends a feeling of immense relief is in almost all cases the dominant reaction to the result of successful lithium treatment. But the surroundings may sometimes need time to adjust to the new situation, which often creates difficult inter-personal conflicts. This is best illustrated by the effect of lithium treatment on marital relations (7, 9, 16). In most cases the marital climate is much improved during lithium maintenance treatment. The spouse notes a reduction of undesirable attributes in the ex-patient, who is found more reasonable and who shows more participation in family activities. But occasionally the spouse complains of a reduction in sexual responsiveness and enthusiastic behaviour, and in a few instances the spouse becomes anxious or severely depressed as a reaction to the unfamiliar normality of the patient on lithium. Suicide attempts by the spouse have in fact been seen in this situation (12).

Successful lithium maintenance treatment leads to a radical reshuffling of roles and responsibilities in the family. The main sufferer under this is the spouse, whose central role as heroic upholder of home and family is endangered by the patient's recovery and who therefore may sabotage the treatment secretly or openly. It is our experience that unless the cooperation and support of the family is secured from the very beginning, lithium treatment is almost doomed to fail.

A spouse may also for other reasons greet the patient's recovery with less than enthusiasm. We know of a case where the girl had fallen in love with and married a charming hypomanic person with occasional depressions; she found the lithium-treated normothymic spouse much less attractive and eventually left him. In another case the husband had during his wife's prolonged manic-depressive disorder with frequent hospital admissions arranged himself comfortably with a mistress, and he now found his wife's re-emergence as a normal person highly inconvenient.

Lithium-produced prevention or attenuation of manic-depressive recurrences may occasionally lead to the complete disappearance of what was previously considered neurotic features (4, 26). Obsessive-compulsive personality traits are sometimes secondary to or part of manic-depressive disorder and hence disappear when this is brought under control by lithium. This change in the patient's personality does not always please the family. Husbands have described how much they suffered when lithium treatment produced a more relaxed attitude in wives who previously with energy and conscientiousness managed a well-paid job and at the same time kept home, children, and husband scrupulously clean (4).

The removal of manic-depressive symptoms by lithium leads in some patients to the appearance of paranoid traits which previously had been hidden behind the affective psychosis (3, 10). The family may then claim that lithium treatment makes the patient "crazy" and should be stopped. Under these circumstances it is advisable to supplement lithium with a neuroleptic drug and to institute appropriate individual and family psychotherapy.

I have dealt so far only with the classical endogenous affective disorders: manic-depressive disorder and periodic endogenous depressions, because these are the illnesses for which a prophylactic effect of lithium has been definitely established. It is worth noting that further uses of lithium may be found. There is for example evidence that lithium may be used for the treatment or emotional stabilization of children suffering from infantile affective psychosis (1, 2, 11, 22), certain atypical mental disorders dominated by periodic aggressions (8, 13, 23, 24), and a group of young sociopaths described as suffering from emotionally unstable character disorder (18). It is tempting to see this as an indication that lithium may come to play a role also in the combat of violence and drug abuse, but clearly the observations must be tested in further studies.

In this presentation I have drawn attention to some of the negative effects which lithium treatment may have on the patients' surroundings — at least initially. When known in advance, the difficulties may be more efficiently handled if and as they arise. But in order to avoid misunderstandings I must stress again that in the large majority of cases the effects of successful lithium treatment are positive and of great benefit to the patients and to their family, friends, and associates.

Let me end on a sordid note: money. The cost of outpatient lithium maintenance treatment for one year is the same as the cost of 3 or 4 days spent in a psychiatric hospital (14, 19). Add to this the preservation of the patient's working capacity — and sometimes also that of his family —, and you will understand that money used to buy a flame photometer for serum lithium determinations is indeed well spent by hospitals and society.

REFERENCES

1. ANNELL, A.-L. (1969) Lithium in the treatment of children and adolescents. Acta psychiat scand., suppl. **207**, 19.
2. ANNELL, A.-L. (1969) Manic-depressive illness in children and effect of treatment with lithium carbonate. Acta paedopsychiat. **36**, 292.
3. BAASTRUP, P. C. and SCHOU, M. (1967) Lithium as a prophylactic agent. Its effect against recurrent depressions and manic-depressive psychosis. Arch. gen. Psychiat. **16**, 162.
4. BAASTRUP, P. C. (1969) Practical clinical viewpoints regarding treatment with lithium. Acta psychiat. scand., suppl. **207**, 12.
5. BERTAGNA, L., PEYROUZET, J.-M., QUÉTIN, A.-M. and DALLE, B. (1971) Lithium et affections psychiatriques cycliques. Action prophylactique et thérapeutique. Rev. Prat. (Paris) **21**, 1743.
6. BÖSZÖRMÉNYI, Z. (1970) Ueber einige psychische Nebenwirkungen der Lithiumtherapie. Int. Pharmacopsychiat. **4**, 204.
7. DEMERS, R. G. and DAVIS, L. S. (1971) The influence of prophylactic lithium treatment on the marital adjustment of manic-depressives and their spouses. Comprehens. Psychiat. **12**, 348.
8. DOSTÁL, T. and ZVOLSKÝ, P. (1970) Antiagressive effect of lithium salts in severe mentally retarded adolescents. Int. Pharmacopsychiat. **5**, 203.
9. DYSON W. L. and MENDELSON M. (1968) Recurrent depressions and the lithium ion. Amer. J. Psychiat. **125**, 544.
10. FANN, W. E., ASHER, H. and LUTON, F. H. (1969) Use of lithium in mania. (With comment on underlying personality types.) Dis. nerv. Syst. **30**, 605.

11. FEINSTEIN, S. C. and WOLPERT, E. A. (1973) Juvenile manic-depressive illness: Clinical and therapeutic considerations. J. Amer. Acad. Child Psychiat. **12**, 123.
12. FITZGERALD, R. G. (1972) Mania as message: Treatment of mania with family therapy and lithium. Amer. J. Psychoter. **26**, 547.
13. FORSSMAN, H. and WÅLINDER J. (1969) Lithium treatment on atypical indication. Acta psychiat. scand., suppl. **207**, 34.
14. GROSSER, H. H. (1968) Kurzer Erfahrungsbericht über die Lithiumtherapie. Gütersloher Fortbildungswoche, p. 101.
15. MARSHALL, M. H., NEUMANN, C. P. and ROBINSON, M. (1970) Lithium, creativity, and manic-depressive illness: Review and prospectus. Psychosomatics, **11**, 406.
16. MAYO, J. A. (1970) Psychosocial profiles of patients on lithium treatment. Int. Pharmacopsychiat. **5**, 190.
17. POLATIN, P. and FIEVE, R. R. (1971) Patient rejection of lithium carbonate prophylaxis. J. Amer. med. Ass. **218**, 864.
18. RIFKIN, A., QUITKIN, F., CARRILLO, C., BLUMBERG, A. G. and KLEIN, D. F. (1972) Lithium in emotionally unstable character disorder. Arch. gen. Psychiat. **27**, 519.
19. ROSSNER, M., KÖNIG, L. and LANGE, E. (1971) Oekonomische und soziale Aspekte im Zusammenhang mit der rezidiv-prophylaktischen Langzeitbehandlung manisch-depressiver Erkrankungen mit Lithiumsalzen. Psychiat. Neurol. med. Psychol. (Lpz.) **23**, 17.
20. SCHLAGENHAUF, G., TUPIN, J. and WHITE, R. B. (1966) The use of lithium carbonate in the treatment of manic psychoses. Amer. J. Psychiat. **123**, 201.
21. SCHOU, M. (1968) Lithium in psychiatric therapy and prophylaxis. J. psychiat. Res. **6**, 67.
22. SCHOU, M. (1972) Lithium in psychiatric therapy and prophylaxis. A review with special regard to its use in children, p. 479. In: ANNELL, A.-L. (ED.): Depressive States in Childhood and Adolescence. Almqvist and Wiksell, Stockholm.
23. SHEARD, M. H. (1971) Effect of lithium on human aggression. Nature, **230**, 113.
24. TUPIN, J. (1972) Lithium use in nonmanic depressive conditions. Comprehens. Psychiat. **13**, 209.
25. VAADAL, J. M. and ROBAK O. H. (1968) Litium-behandling av affektive sinnslidelser. T. norske Lægeforen. **88**, 1578.
26. VILLENEUVE, A., LANGLOIS, M., CHABOT, C. DOGAN, K., LACHANCE, R. and, LAURENT C. S. (1971) Lithium therapy in recurrent manic-depressive psychosis, p. 55. In: VINAŘ, O., VOTAVA, Z. and BRADLEY, P. B. (Eds.): Advances in Neuro-Psychopharmacology. North-Holland Publ. Co., Amsterdam.
27. WARICK, L. H. (1970) Lithium carbonate in the treatment and prophylaxis of recurrent affective disorders: Long-term follow-up. Bull. Los Angeles neurol. Soc. **35**, 169.
28. WITTRIG, J. J. and COOPWOOD, W. E. (1970) Lithium versus chlorpromazine for manics. Initiative and productivity versus tranquilization and hospitalization. Dis. nerv. Syst. **31**, 486.

M. S., Statshospitalet, 8240 Risskov, Denmark

VERÄNDERUNGEN DES DEPRESSIVEN ERLEBENS UNTER LITHIUM-DAUERTHERAPIE

O. H. ARNOLD

Psychiatrische Universitäts Klinik, Wien

Der langzeitige Gebrauch wirksamer Substanzen in der Therapie endogener Psychosen ließ die Frage auftauchen, wie weit damit spontane Längsschnittverläufe beeinflußt, bzw. in qualitativ neuartiger Weise variiert würden. Die Behandlung depressiver Manifestationen aus dem manisch-depressiven Krankheitsgeschehen (MDK) mit trizyklischen Antidepressiva führte zu den ersten Beobachtungen solcher Abänderungen des Längsschnittverlaufes (1—3). Die folgenden Beobachtungen unter Lithium-Dauertherapie wurden an einem Material von 24 ausgelesenen Fällen recidivierender Verläufe des MDK gemacht. Diese Fälle waren ursprünglich alle klinisch behandelt worden und wurden sodann ambulant-fallweise auch kurzfristig wieder klinisch weiterbehandelt. Sie stellen insofern eine Auslese dar, als sie Privatpatienten wurden und damit sowohl eine enge Bindung an den Therapeuten eintrat als andererseits auch eine besonders eingehende Kenntnis der Psychopathologie und vegetativ-somatischen Symptomatik der Längsschnitte gegeben war. Zudem liegen in diesen Fällen sehr eingehende Daten über Persönlichkeitsstrukturen, Familie und soziale Verhältnisse vor.

In allen Fällen wurde vor Beginn der Lithiumtherapie eine oder mehrere depressive Phasen mit trizyklischen Antidepressiva behandelt. Die folgende Tabelle 1 zeigt eine Übersicht über die wesentlichsten Daten jener 12 Fälle, bei denen letztlich Abänderungen der psychopathologischen Syndrome, bzw. des Eigenerlebens unter Lithium-Dauertherapie beobachtet worden sind.

TABELLE 1
Übersicht über die wesentlichen Daten der 12 Fällen unter Lithium-Dauertherapie

Typ	Fall	Geschlecht	Alter	Krankheitsdauer in Jahren	Verlaufstyp	Zahl der Phasen vor Beginn der Lithium-Dauertherapie
A	G.K.	m.	45	4	bipolar	2
	A.H.	m.	65	43	bipolar	ca 15
	J.T.	m.	45	9	bipolar	3

Typ	Fall	Geschlecht	Alter	Krankheits-dauer in Jahren	Verlaufstyp	Zahl der Phasen vor Beginn der Lithium-Dauertherapie
A	C.B.	w.	21	4	bipolar	2
	E.Z.	w.	52	12	bipolar	7
	E.P.	m.	35	5	bipolar	5
B	R.G.	m.	41	11	bipolar	6
	G.B.	m.	47	4	unipolar depressiv	3
	F.B.	w.	56	8	bipolar	4
C	E.Sch.	m.	64	41	bipolar	ca 12
	A.P.	w.	56	5	unipolar depressiv	3
	E.T.	m.	47	7	bipolar	5

Das Material ist bezüglich seiner meisten Daten inkongruent, die Gemeinsamkeiten liegen in den oben erwähnten Auslesefaktoren. Wenn dennoch der Versuch gemacht wird, die beobachteten Abänderungen in eine vorläufige Typisierung zu bringen, so vor allem deshalb, um das beobachtende Interesse anderer Therapeuten in eine bestimmte Richtung zu lenken und für die gemachten Erfahrungen einen gemeinsamen Nenner im Sprachgebrauch zu entwerfen.

Tabelle 2 zeigt einen solchen Entwurf der drei Abänderungstypen.

TABELLE 2

Entwurf der drei Abänderungstypen

A
Mischzustände an Stelle depressiver Phasen

Auftreten von missmutig-gereizten Mischzuständen mit durchschnittlich 6-wöchiger Dauer zu Zeitpunkten, an denen vor Li-Therapie depressive Phasen bestanden. Bei gedrückter Stimmung und gestörten Körper- und Vitalgefühlen rasche Denkabläufe, Plänemachen, Konflikte. Keine Tagesschwankung, Schlafstörung, ängstliche Träume.

B
Dysphorie, Sensitivität, Beziehungsideen

Langsam fortschreitende Dysphorie mit raschem Pendeln, Tagesschwankung, Wetterfühligkeit, zunehmende Sensitivität, Neigung zu Beziehungsideen und paranoider Verarbeitung als sich etablierender Dauerzustand. Vor Li-Therapie keine solchen Persönlichkeitsreaktionen.

C
Lebensverarmung „Automatendasein"

Nach dem 2. Therapiejahr Einsetzen eines stabilen Zustands mit Gleichgültigkeit, Entemotionalisierung, Zurückgezogenheit, Initiativverlust, Stereotypisierung der Tagesabläufe, jedoch nicht depressiv, familiär und sozial sehr gut angepaßt. Im Eigenerleben Gefühl des Automatenhaften.

Tabelle 3 gibt einige weitere Daten im Zusammenhang mit diesen beobachteten Veränderungen an.

TABELLE 3

Weitere Daten im Zusammenhang mit beobachteten Veränderungen

Abänderung	Fälle ♂ ♀	Li-Dosis	mVal	Dauer (Monate) der Li-Therapie	Durchschnittswerte nach Therapiebeginn Auftreten (Monate)	Anmerkungen
A: Mischzustände an Stelle depressiver Phasen	4 2	1,050 g	0,77	18	8	fallweise Zusatz-Medikation mit Diazepam/Lorazepam überlappende Einstellung nach trizyklischen Antidepressiva
B: Dysphorie Sensitivität Beziehungsideen	2 1	1,2 g	0,88	21	16	1 Fall mehrfach Zusatzmedikation mit 0,240 g Noveril
C: Lebensverarmung „Automatendasein"	2 1	1,050 g	0,85	35	25	1 Fall anfangs durch 18 Monate gleichzeitig 0,360 g Noveril

DISKUSSION

Depressive Manifestationen unter Lithium-Dauertherapie sind zur Genüge beschrieben (7, u. a.). Ihre Abschwächung bis zu subklinischer Ausprägung bzw. ihre successive Reduzierung stellt ein häufiges Übergansstadium bis zur völligen Unterdrückung der Manifestationen dar. Über zeitliche Kopplungen solcher reduzierter Manifestationen im Sinne der Beibehaltung eines vorher bestandenen Rhythmus bei Recidivverläufen unter Lithiumtherapie ist noch wenig bekannt. Unter Dauertherapie mit trizyklischen Antidepressiva sahen wir gelegentlich ein gegenteiliges Phänomen, das wir als Phasenentkoppelung bezeichnet haben (3). Auch bei dieser Behandlung fanden wir anstelle depressiver Manifestationen das Auftreten von missmutig-gereizten Mischzuständen. Die unter Lithium-Dauertherapie beobachteten Mischzustände unterscheiden sich nicht von jenen sowohl spontan als auch unter anderen Therapien gelegentlich sichtbaren, es sei denn, daß sie unter Lithium-Therapie vielleicht eine längere Dauer aufweisen. Keinesfalls sollte man sie vorerst als gleichsam spezifische Antworten auf die Lithiumtherapie interpretieren. Wir haben in keinem der 6 Fälle abgesetzt, jedoch zu zusätzlicher Medikation greifen müssen, insbesondere zur Zugabe von Tranquilizern der Diazepamgruppe. Weitere Schlußfolgerungen können wir zum gegenwärtigen Zeitpunkt noch nicht ableiten.

Die langsam fortschreitende Dysphorie als solche ist unter Therapie mit trizyklischen Antidepressiva gelegentlich beobachtet worden, im besonderen, wenn man zur Langzeittherapie mit kleinen Erhaltungsdosen gezwungen war (z. B. 2). Die hier beobachteten 3 Fälle zeigten aber doch ein zusätzliches Phänomenbild. Auffallend war eine zunehmende Empfindlichkeit, Abwendung vom eigenen Körper, Neigung zur Außenprojektion und zu Beziehungsideen, wobei letztlich das Pendeln der dysphorischen Verstimmtheit etwa gleichzeitig mit der Verminderung der anfänglichen Wetterfühligkeit und vegetativen Labilität zurücktrat und sich ein stabiler Gleichgewichtszustand dysphorischer Gestimmtheit mit paranoider Einstellung zur engen Umgebung, im besonderen zum Familien- und Berufsmilieu einpendelte. Um dies anders auszudrücken, hätten wir hier eine paranoide Milieueinbindung gegen die vorher bestandene depressive oder dysphorische Periodik gleichsam als Dauerzustand und unter Weiterbestehen dysphorischer Gestimmtheit eingetauscht. Natürlich taucht hier sofort die Frage auf, wieweit die vorher bestehende Persönlichkeitsstruktur zu solchen Reaktionen prädestinierte. Im Falle der F. B. fanden sich in einem Lebensabschnitt nach dem 24. Jahr (Zeitpunkt der Verheiratung) fallweise Eifersuchtsideen, in der Aszendenz keine Psychose. Während der depressiven Phasen verschwanden diese Eifersuchtsideen völlig, während schlecht abgrenzbarer hypomanischer Wellen traten sie vielleicht etwas in den Vordergrund. Nunmehr stellen sie nur ein Phänomen dar, Beeinträchtigungsideen durch andere Familienmitglieder, insbesondere aber auch durch den Freundeskreis, in den letzten Monaten auch Hinweise auf eine Ausweitung auf die gesamte Umgebung stellen doch eine veränderte Gesamtreaktion dar.

In den beiden anderen Fällen (R. G., G. B.) waren vor dem erstmaligen Auftreten einer dysphorischen Verstimmung jeweils nach vielmonatiger Lithiumtherapie mit Sicherheit keine sensitiven oder paranoiden Persönlichkeitstendenzen auffindbar. Bei beiden Fällen besteht neben der dysphorischen Gestimmtheit mit noch gewisser Neigung zum Pendeln der Intensität bei voller sozialer Angepaßtheit eine deutliche Tendenz, Reaktionen der familiären und beruflichen Umgebung mit großer Sensitivität zu beobachten und mit eigenbezüglichen Vermutungen zu interpretieren. Hierbei wird nicht eine Außenursache etwa im Sinne einer systematischen Organisiertheit angenommen, wohl aber, daß eben der eigene Zustand derartige Reaktionen der Umgebung ja begreiflicherweise hervorrufen müsse. Die wiederholte Besprechung mit den Familien beider Fälle ergab eine deutliche Verzerrung in der Erlebnisweise der Realität entsprechend der erhöhten Sensibilität und Eigenbezüglichkeit. Alle drei Fälle würden wir im Sinne der Untersuchungen von BERNER (4) unter Berücksichtigung ihrer Struktur und Aufbauelemente noch als paranoische Syndrome einordnen. Ihre Beziehungen zur chronischen Dysphorie hat ebenfalls BERNER (5, 6) ausführlich analysiert.

Das Auftreten eines Zustandes mit deutlicher Einengung der emotionalen Reaktionsbreite, absoluter Stimmungsstabilität, aber andererseits deutlichem Verlust an Initiative und persönlichem Engagement stellt trotz der sich nunmehr einstellenden völligen familiären und sozialen Angepaßtheit und durchaus auch beruflichem Erfolg doch ein bedenkliches Ergebnis dar: Schöpferische Qualitäten gehen verloren und alle drei Patienten berichteten übereinstimmend, daß sie zufrieden seien, aber doch nicht mehr eigentlich *sie selbst*. Sie bezeichneten ihre Lebensweise als automatenhaft, den Verlust an Gefühlserlebnissen sie irgendwie nicht tangierend, aber rein rational doch feststellbar.

Dieses automatenhafte Dasein haben wir vor der Lithium-Dauertherapie nicht beobachtet. Es unterscheidet sich doch deutlich vom Erleben der chronischen Depressivität mit Resignation und Lebensverarmung (3, 8). Diesen Menschen wurde gleichsam ein Teil ihrer Personalität entzogen. Man könnte formulieren, daß manische und depressive Manifestationen das Ausleben sonst tabuisierter und unterdrückter Erlebnisbereiche gestatten (tiefenpsychologisch betrachtet), oder die Selbstverwirklichung im Sinne der progressiven Personalisation in weiteren Bereichen erlauben (anthropologisch betrachtet). Dann würde in einigen Fällen eine Lithium-Dauertherapie neben Stabilisierung und sozialer Anpassung mit der Einengung und Automatisierung des Daseins doch eine wesentliche Beschneidung der Persönlichkeitsentfaltung und der personalen Selbstverwirklichung mit sich bringen.

Literaturverzeichnis

1. Arnold, O. H. (1965) Zur Frage der Beeinflussung des Verlaufes endogener Psychosen durch Psychopharmaka. D. Bente u. P. B. Brandley Eds.: Neuro-Psychopharmacology, 4, Elsevier, Amsterdam, p. 255.
2. Arnold, O. H. (1968) Das chronisch-depressive Syndrom in anthropologischer Sicht. Baudiš, Peterová u. Šedivec Eds.: De psychiatria progrediente, 216. Pilsen.
3. Arnold, O. H. (1969) Zur Frage der Abwandlung depressiver Verläufe nach Antidepressiva-Therapie. H. Hippius u. H. Selbach Ed.: Das depressive Syndrom, Urban und Schwarzenberg, München, p. 575.
4. Berner, P. (1965) Das paranoische Syndrom, Springer, Berlin.
5. Berner, C., Berner, P., Gabriel, E., Küfferle, B., Mader, R., Müller, E. und Saleu, B. (1971) Aktuelle Probleme der Wahnforschung, Nervenarzt, 42, 511.
6. Berner, P. (1972) Paranoide Syndrome, Psychiatrie d. Gegenwart, Bd II/1. 2. Auflg. Springer, Berlin, p. 154.
7. Schou, M. (1971) Die Lithium-Therapie bei manisch-depressiven Psychosen. Nervenarzt, 1, 1.
8. Tellenbach, H. (1961) Melancholie, Springer, Berlin.

O. H. A., Psychiatrische Universitäts Klinik, Wien, Austria

SOCIAL ASPECTS OF PSYCHOPHARMACOLOGY

N. BOHAČEK

Department of Psychiatry, University of Zagreb

In assessing the social aspects and factors of modern psychiatry it is rather difficult to limit oneself to the field of psychopharmacology only. The social significance of psychopharmacology is deeply and closely connected with a variety of other treatments in psychiatry. Social psychiatry is not to be credited alone with special treatments in rehabilitation, and psychopharmacology must also be taken into account because it makes such treatments possible. Many of the various types of socio-therapeutical measures were not even possible earlier because of poor co-operation on the part of the patient due to less satisfactory therapeutical results.

It must also be borne in mind that the attitudes towards the mental patient, both of the psychiatrist and the lay public, have essentially changed. It is difficult to say whether the attitudes changed first or pharmacotherapy prompted the change of attitudes, or whether perhaps both factors matured and were at work at the same time.

The social repercussions of psychopharmacology are extraordinarily great, and it was certainly psychopharmacology that has greatly contributed to the development and impact of current socio-psychiatric trends and orientations on psychiatry.

If we only remember what psychiatric wards and hospitals were like before the era of psychopharmacology, the change as the first social merit of psychopharmacology will become evident. The new, altered, serene atmosphere under the influence of psychotropic drugs made all other procedures possible in the treatment of mental patients, ranging from individual and group psychotherapy to occupational, work and recreation therapy, and to all other measures that can be undertaken in a therapeutic community. The global therapeutical effect was undoubtedly of prime social significance, leading to numerous other social repercussions.

A phenomenon, diametrically opposite to previous experience, began to be noticed in the United Kingdom after 1954, in the USA after 1955 and in other parts of the world even later: admission of psychiatric patients to hospitals was diminishing. The percentage of admitted patients in France in these years did not actually fall, but it did not increase at the rate of 7% but only 1.5%. BRILL'S first report in 1957 (4) hinted at the decrease and in 1958 (3) connected it directly and beyond a shade of doubt with intensive use of psychotropic drugs. DELAY in 1958 (5) reported 3 significant findings in respect of the number of admissions to and discharges from psychiatric wards:

1. a decrease of the yearly rate of admissions,
2. an increase in discharges and a rise in the discharge rate over the admission rate, and
3. a correlation between the discharge rate and consumption of neuroleptics.

It was obvious that the drop of psychiatric patients admitted for psychiatric treatment was caused by the use and increasing popularity of therapy with psychotropic drugs, whether the opponents of pharmacotherapy admitted it or not. It is a fact that hospitalization leads to a number of psychological and social repercussions. The possibility of avoiding hospital treatment and the possibility of out-patient therapy is a great, new asset of pharmacotherapy in the broadest social perspective.

Not long afterwards, with the spreading of psychopharmacs all over the world, with an ever larger gamut of psychotropic drugs, there came voices, individual at first and more numerous later, claiming that although pharmacotherapy did help patients to remit quickly, they soon returned back to hospitals and continued to commute between admissions and discharges. This is known in psychiatry as "Drehtürpsychiatrie" (revolving-door psychiatry).

Our numerous investigations have proved beyond doubt that psychopharmacotherapy applied in cases of schizophrenic psychosis, together with well organized and supervised long-term treatment, eliminates the patient's commuting, so that I consider the "revolving-door psychiatry" only an expression of "vitium artis" and not an inevitable necessity (1). Our observations on 114 schizophrenic female patients who were discharged from the University hospital in Zagreb in 1965, and were given constant out-patient therapy with psychotropic drugs in long-term treatment, showed 5 years later — in 1970 — that of 32 patients who were regularly treated and supervised, only 4 (12.5%) were rehospitalized, and of 82 irregularly treated there were 62 (75.5%) such cases (10). These figures need no comment; they indicate the social significance of a well organized psychopharmacotherapy in long-term treatment. It seems to me that the question today is not so much whether we shall be able to achieve remission in the patient by psychotropic drugs in the majority of cases, but whether we shall be able to sustain the patient in remission and for how long. It is my opinion that in most cases, with few exceptions, the remission can be maintained providing the required conditions are satisfied: trained staff (doctors, nurses, social workers) familiar with the effects and side-effects of psychotropic drugs; a well organized home-visiting service (nurses, social workers); good regional distribution of service — the same doctor should preferably take care of the patient in hospital and in out-patient treatment (2).

A lowered admission rate naturally diminishes the demand for psychiatric beds*) which brings us to the crucial socio-economic question of how many beds are needed today and how many should be planned for the future. There are various ways of assessing psychiatric bed needs, but the various studies do not agree with the required ratio. It is known that 4 beds per thousand inhabitants was considered the optimal number for psychiatric purposes before the era of psychopharmacology. Current estimations are much lower. Thus e.g. some Britisch studies (8, 9, 12) foresee between 1 and 2 classical psychiatric beds per thousand inhabitants in the future. But all these estimates divide the system into classical psychiatric beds and a number of other purposes. Some consider geriatric or gerontopsychiatric beds separately, others count out beds intended for the mentally retarded; but all agree that a great number of beds and a lot of space is necessary for

---

*) Owing to misunderstanding, or rather, terminological differences in the meaning of „psychiatric bed", it is often quite impossible to compare numbers of beds and the ratio in various countries and sometimes even between data of authors from the same country.

the so-called day and night hospitals which could be more successful in solving numerous socio-psychiatric problems than the traditional type of hospitals. (One should not forget that undesirable hospitalism is in this way avoided, but that a new form of hospitalism is possible even in these modern type institutions.)

If we consider the position in Yugoslavia, which had 0.78 beds per thousand inhabitants in 1969, and the oscillations within the country among the republics (of which Croatia ranged first with 1.29 and Bosnia-and-Herzegovina last with 0.33 per thousand inhabitants) it becomes obvious that the introduction and application of psychotropic drugs saved this country from continuous and unbearable pressure of mental patients on inadequate facilities which it would be difficult to build up in time (7). We see and feel in Yugoslavia today that on the whole we are in a position to accomodate the present number of patients who need hospitalization because a great many of them can be treated with psychotropic drugs as out-patients.

The ways and methods of psychopharmacological treatment have significant social implications. Taking tablets and drops, or getting shots — all these are ways of treatment identical to the treatments of any somatic patient, and the mentally ill person is not discriminated. Gradual development of psychotropic drugs in various forms, especially in long-term therapy, is of greatest significance. There has been great progress from the original daily use of drugs taken orally 2 to 4 times a day, through retard and slow-released forms to depot-preparations which are taken once in 1 to 4 weeks. Taking of drugs has been made easy and with it the attitudes of both the patient and his family have changed in a positive sense towards this kind of treatment.

Consumption of psychotropic drugs is increasing immensely all over the world. (We have heard more about it in J. Levine's paper.) The use of psychotropic drugs in Yugoslavia went up over four times in only six years, between 1963 and 1969, but the increase is not equal for the various groups of drugs. Neuroleptics went up a little less than 4 times, antidepressants and tranquillizers 7 times, psychostimulants as much as 20 times. (Consumption of antiparkinsonic drugs also rose 20 times.) Expressed in absolute amounts, expenditure on neuroleptics and tranquillizers was approximately equal, expenditure on antidepressants represented half the expenses on neuroleptics and expenditure on psychostimulants was only 1/4 of that on neuroleptics.

However, if we compare the cost of one psychiatric bed (fully equipped) which amounts to at least 30,000 Dinars, with the expenses on psychotropic drugs for the whole of Yugoslavia (amounting to 42 million Dinars in 1969), we shall see that this money would cover only 1400 new psychiatric beds. This would raise the absolute number of beds to 17,400, i.e. 0.87 per thousand inhabitants. Although, expenditure on psychotropic treatment goes up several times every year (regardless of the increased prices of drugs), these amounts would cover only an insignificant number of psychiatric beds, in fact only 9 beds per 100,000 inhabitants.

Having lowered the need for new beds, pharmacotherapy has proved to be an extraordinarily economical method of treatment in psychiatry. It has been particularly helpful in developing and in underdeveloped countries, since it has allowed them to skip the stage of building large, even too large, hospital facilities, as was the case in developed countries. The problem, however, is not as simple as that. It appears that each country must have a certain, though a minimal number of standard beds, before it can dispose of the surplus beds or use them for other purposes. If this minimal number does not exist, other psychiatric efforts and other forms of psychiatric protection are not fully effective. The calculation of the optimal number of necessary beds could be done on the basis of Mezey's proposal (9). It is of course necessary to delimit purposes for which beds are intended.

The savings achieved on traditional beds can and must be used for the "superstructure" in modern psychiatry, for day and night hospitals, for hostels, for special rehabilitation workshops and centres etc. (6). The enormous social significance of psychopharmacology lies in the fact that the mental patient can be treated in out-patient departments with modern psychotropic drugs. The savings on traditional beds were reflected in all the modern trends in psychiatry, i.e. the means can now be used for subtler differentiation of rehabilitation and resocialization of the mental patient.

The goal of all treatment is complete cure of the patients. If this is impossible to achieve in mental patients, the goal is to sustain them in good remission and without symptoms, which usually means out of hospital, for as long a period of time as possible. This goal has been achieved in a great number of psychiatric patients by means of pharmacotherapy. In a previous study (10) we found that in 59 cases of regularly treated schizophrenias the psychotic symptoms lasted for 7 weeks on an average in the course of a year while the rest of the period was without symptoms, in contrast to irregularly treated patients whose symptoms were manifested for 25 weeks, with the rest of the year without symptoms.

There are other social factors of significance in pharmacotherapy: regularity of treatment does not greatly depend on the distance between the patient and the doctor, but rather on motivation; it has been noticed that patients who are employed or attending school are more motivated and appear to be more strict in taking psychotropic drugs as shown in the mentioned study (10).

Recovery of working capacity, in which pharmacotherapy has been more successful than previous methods of treatment, is directly related to the national economy. This has been recently shown in a study by Shain (11) of the University of Michigan. He claims that the costs of mental diseases in Croatia (Yugoslavia) amount to 0.46% of the national income of this Republic, which means that 46 Dinars out of each 10.000 go for mental diseases. The loss of working capacity during illness has two major economic consequences: the loss of wages and the allotment of sickness allowance. These two factors alone make up for a ten times higher amount in the total price of costs of the mental disease than is the expenditure on the whole medical treatment and therapy. If we manage to return the patient back to work faster by means of continuous, consistent, well organized pharmacotherapy, if we can help recover his working capacity by differentiated measures of rehabilitation, we shall have achieved considerable savings for the national health and the national economy. Working capacity depends mainly on the regularity of treatment. It is considerably better established by patients who are treated regularly, as our experience has proved (10).

If, in the end, we try to calculate the economic costs of treatment of mental diseases, with a well organized pharmacotherapy taken for granted, where considerably fewer psychiatric beds in the traditional sense are necessary, we shall have to conclude that pharmacotherapy by itself is a considerably cheaper method of treatment than any formerly used methods have been, because it offers a series of possible savings. If, however, we consider all the new impacts that pharmacotherapy has offered with the whole gamut of socio-psychiatric institutions and treatments, our conclusion will be that it is not a cheaper method but one greatly superior and more efficient in fully rehabilitating and resocializing the mental patient today.

References

1. Bohaček, N. (1969) Probleme und Organisation der psychopharmakologischen Dauerbehandlung, Arzneim.-Forsch. **19**, 529.
2. Bohaček, N. (1971) Socialno značenje psihijatrijske farmakoterapie (Social aspects of psychopharmacotherapy). In: Socijalna psihijatrija, p. 494, Pliva, Zagreb.
3. Brill, H. (1959) The impact of psychotropic drugs on the structure, function and future of psychiatric services in hospitals. In: Neuropsychopharmacology, Vol. 1, p. 189, Elsevier, Amsterdam.
4. Brill, H. and Patton, R. E. (1957) Analysis of 1955—1956 population fall in New York State mental hospitals in first year of largescale use of tranquillizing drugs. Amer. J. Psychiat. **114**, 509.
5. Delay, J. (1959) Discussion. In: Neuropsychopharmacology, Vol. 1, p. 196, Elsevier, Amsterdam.
6. Heinrich, K. (1967) Der entlassene Anstaltspatient in der psychiatrischen Rehabilitation, Alma-Mater, Konstanz.
7. Kilibarda, M. (1971) Pregled razvitka psihijatrijske službe u socijalističkim republikama Jugoslavije (Development of the psychiatric services in Yugoslavia and her socialist republics). In: Socijalna psihijatrija, p. 685, Pliva, Zagreb.
8. Mezey, A. G. and Eileen Evans (1971) Psychiatric in-patients and out-patients in a London borough. Brit. J. Psychiat. **118**, 609.
9. Mezey, A. G. and Syed, I. A. (1972) Forecasting psychiatric bed needs. Lancet (1) 7744, 251.
10. Palmović, R. and Bohaček, N. (1970) Preliminarna analiza otpuštenih shizofrenih bolesnika liječenih psihofarmacima (Preliminary analysis of a discharged group of schizophrenic treated with psychotropic drugs), Psihofarmakologija, Vol. 2, p. 145, Medicinska naklada, Zagreb.
11. Shain, M. (1972) Ekonomska cijena mentalnih oboljenja, II. dio: u Hrvatskoj (Economic costs of psychotic illness, II. part: in Croatia). (In press).
12. Editorial (Wing, J. K.) (1971) How many psychiatric beds? Psychol. Med. **1**, 188.
13. Statistics of the Drug Research Centre, Zagreb (1963—1969).

N. B., Department of Psychiatry, University of Zagreb,
41000 Zagreb, Rebro, Yugoslavia

TRANQUILLITY DENIED

A. HORDERN

King's College Hospital, London

The psychotropic drugs introduced in the last two decades have demonstrated their effectiveness — as well as perhaps the need for their existence — in an epoch unique in its appreciation of the widespread prevalence of psychiatric illness, its scientific and technical mastery and its concern for the individual (4). The cynical may correlate the synthetic nature of the majority of modern psychotropics — and their increasing use — with the synthetic nature of many aspects of Western civilisation and the problems this has engendered. The historically minded, however, will like ALTSCHULE (1), recognize in the present age of anxiety no fundamentally new phenomenon but merely an intense 20th century preoccupation with this emotion, with a corresponding yearning for tranquillity which the tranquillizing drugs, like their older counterparts, purport to provide.

Excessive anxiety results from uncertainty which may be engendered in the environment, in the individual or in the interaction between the two. There are many potent causes of anxiety in the environment today, and the changes that progress in technology have produced in the social fabric are exerting pressures on individuals in every age group.

ENVIRONMENTAL CAUSES OF ANXIETY

The last twenty five years have been characterized by an increasing penetrance of science into every aspect of life (9). As a result of advances in technology a continuous and all-pervasive process of change has taken place, with loss of the stable society and all that this implies. As SHON (10) has emphasized, men and women now have to cope with transformations that formerly were handled by the replacement of one generation by another. The present situation was accurately presaged nearly forty years ago by the slogan of the 1933 Chicago World Fair: "Science proposes, technology executes, man conforms."

Amongst the technological advances that have transformed Western Society are the improvements that have been made in food manufacture, in power supplies, in methods of transportation and in automated, continuous-flow, production techniques. With industrialization has come urbanization, the growth of huge business corporations, the elaboration of expanding networks of communication — military, commercial, mass and industrial — the development of computors and microelectronics, the synthesis of new materials and the conquest of infectious diseases. The arrival of death control without birth restriction, especially in the developing countries of Asia, Africa and Latin America, has produced a colossal problem of explosive population growth with expanding needs and dwindling world resources.

The affluent society which these advances have made possible is largely dependent on advertising and near-universal credit linked with deceptively convenient hire purchase agreements: is has brought technological and social problems on a massive scale. High-energy, high-profit technology, catering for the consumer, has resulted in overproduction, waste and depletion of resources on one hand, and pollution on the other (12). Social problems include poverty which, despite the ambience of affluence, persists in the old, in the disadvantaged and in minority groups, and a steady increase in crime and violence. Loss of respect for law and order has reflected the declining status of patristic institutions such as the Church, the Crown and the Armed Forces. Due to taxation and more universal education, class barriers have been lowered: the upper and the middle classes have had to relinquish much of their power and, as management has lost its nerve, an embourgoisement of workers, organized through their highly-efficient unions, has taken place. This and the shorter working week facilitated by modern machinery has enabled the "Protestant ethic" to be replaced by the "Leisure ethic". *Pari passu* with these changes "permissive" attitudes have emerged, symbolized in the 1960s in Britain by the enactment of increasingly liberal laws dealing with capital offences, censorship, homosexuality, abortion and divorce. The "permissive" society, characterised by the success of the 20th century "sexual revolution" with its less inhibited patterns of behaviour and dress, has been associated especially, but not exclusively, with the young (5).

Anxiety in the individual

As a result of these changes, marriage as an institution is less stable than formerly. In the Western World the extended family — grandparents, aunts, cousins and so forth — has been replaced by the nuclear unit: father, mother and two or three children. The elderly have become increasingly isolated — impoverished materially and emotionally — and, unable to keep abreast of current trends, have become lonely and dispirited. Middle aged men, both workers and executives, sensing the uncertainty that pervades industry, have become prone to anxiety and loss of confidence. The mindless technology of the industrial state condemns the majority to lives of boredom and anonymity; its affluence has brought insecurity and tension with illnesses such as obesity, alcoholism, bronchial carcinoma and diverse psychosomatic ailments. It is noteworthy that the forms of oral overindulgence — in food, in alcohol, in nicotine — that lead to these diseases, are identifiable as methods by which individuals seek to free themselves from tension and ennui, and that the increase in these and in psychosomatic ailments has been paralleled by a widespread increase in the consumption of tranquillisers. Women too have become affected; well on the way to securing a "liberated" status, in many cases they have not found the satisfaction they expected in abrogating their domestic roles. For infants and children the impermanence of many marriages and the risk of separation from their mothers in the first few vital years of life constitute a threat to their future emotional stability (2).

The elderly and the middle aged would probably agree on the importance for tranquillity of privacy and, in particular, of freedom from noise, whether their comfortable 80 decibel limit is exceeded by machinery, aircraft, vehicles, singing or musical instruments. In regard to the latter, they are at odds with the young, who in the main, favour a continuous cacophony created by cars, crowds and electronically amplified pop music. The youth of the world, united in their contempt for the materialism, impersonality, hypocrisy and pollution they perceive in Western civilisation, have collectively organized protests and have individually striven to discover a meaning in life, seeking to achieve fulfillment through transcendental experiences obtained via music, sexuality and drugs.

Tranquillisers old and new

The remedies resorted to for relief of anxiety can be divided into those which are procured from non-medical sources, and those which are prescribed by physicians. The psychotropic drugs, with the exception of a few synthetic dysleptics like LSD, fall into the latter category.

Amongst substances obtained from non-medical sources, alcohol and nicotine have long held pride of place. Alcohol intake continues to rise globally — it was estimated in 1967 that 1 per cent of the adult population of the world might be alcoholic (14) — whilst in the last thirty years the mass manufacture and skilful promotion of sought-after images spuriously associated with cigarette smoking has ensured that, despite adverse medical publicity, cigarette consumption has become the norm in men and women in every social stratum (13). In addition, the popularity of cannabis is very striking. Probably about 300 million people — almost 10 per cent of the world's population — employ it, whilst in the United States it is estimated that about 30 million have tried it and that 8.3 million are regular users. In Western Europe the magnitude of the figure is proportional to the intensity with which the situation is investigated (11). Of non-pharmaceutical tranquillisers, television is now the most popular. An anodyne for boredom it feeds perhaps 500 million people, young and old alike, with a constant diet of violence, generating anxiety as it entertains and blunting an individual's tolerance to aggressive actions. In North America, television watching often begins at two years old and three hours daily are customarily devoted to it; by the time he is 14 the average child has seen 16,000 murders on the television screen and at this rate, when he reaches 65, will have spent 9 years of his life watching it (7).

Trends in psychotropic drug use are particularly easy to study in the United Kingdom where 95 per cent of all drugs are prescribed under the National Health Service. The total expenditure on drugs (£ 184 million in 1968), which includes manufacturers', wholesalers' and chemists' margins, has remained fairly constant at about 10 per cent of Health Service costs. The cost of drugs, though substantial, should be kept in perspective: thus whilst the daily amount spent on N.H.S. drugs for each person is one new penny, his daily expenditure on alcohol is 8 new pence, on smoking is 8 new pence and on food is over 31 new pence (3). In 1970, total N.H.S. expenditure on psychotropic drugs — stimulants and appetite suppressants, barbiturates, non barbiturate hypnotics, tranquillisers and antidepressants — amounted to £ 21.5 million. Since 1965 the number of scripts for these drugs, most of which were prescribed under their trade names, had risen steadily by about 4 per cent per annum to a total of 47.2 million prescriptions in 1970. In that year 43 per cent of prescriptions were for hypnotics, 36 per cent were for tranquillisers, 14 per cent were for antidepressants and 7 per cent were for stimulants and anorexogenics.

It is noteworthy that whilst between 1965 and 1970 there was a 24 per cent decrease in prescriptions for barbiturates and a 36 per cent fall in scripts for stimulants and anorexogenics, over the same six year period there took place a 145 per cent increase in non-barbiturate prescriptions (mainly due to scripts for Mandrax and for Mogadon), an 83 per cent increase in prescriptions for antidepressants (mainly Tryptizol and Tofranil) and a 59 per cent increase in scripts for tranquillisers (this being due to an 110 per cent rise in scripts for Librium and Valium, rather than to a concurrent 49 per cent increase in prescriptions for Largactil and similar neuroleptics). Commenting on these trends, PARISH (8) observes that most of the recent increase in the use of psychotropic drugs in the United Kingdom has been due to the increased prescribing of six compounds: Mandrax, Mogadon, Librium, Valium, Tryptizol and Tofranil. In 1970, for example, 2.3 million prescriptions were dispensed for Mandrax, 2.5 million for Mogadon, 4.8 million for Librium and 4.3 million for Valium. These figures show that patients obtain prescriptions to help them to sleep and to allay anxiety; in other words, that doctors are prescribing vast quantities of drugs which, they feel, can induce tranquillity.

In seeking to provide this, British doctors have gradually become aware of the hazards of the barbiturates and of the addiction potential of the amphetamines and of similar appetite suppressants. They are prescribing more non barbiturate hypnotics, though unfortunately they have not as yet fully recognized the dangers of Mandrax. They are well aware of the value of the neuroleptics in the management of the psychoses, and they know that, skilfully used, the minor tranquillisers can relieve the anxiety of many patients with neuroses and psychosomatic disorders. Yet it is becoming increasingly apparent that insomnia and anxiety are frequently symptoms of depressive illnesses and that such illnesses, for a variety of reasons, often fail to be recognized, whether they occur atypically as phobic anxiety states or more characteristically as endogenous depressions. the presentation of which, especially in good personalities, may be muted or masked (6). When such illnesses are diagnosed, ineffective, even deleterious, treatment with tranquillisers and psychotherapy is often given. For many deserving individuals, therefore, tranquillity is denied, not only by the pressures of "civilized" living, but also by the failure of their doctors to recognize endogenous depressions and other affective illnesses and to treat them effectively with adequate doses of suitable antidepressants. The most appropriate remedy is to educate family doctors, hospital physicians and medical students — as well as perhaps chemists and clergymen — in the diagnosis and treatment of depression.

REFERENCES

1. ALTSCHULE, M. D. (1957) Roots of Modern Psychiatry, p. 1. New York: Greene and Stratton.
2. BOWLBY, J. (1953) Child Care and the Growth of Love. Harmondsworth: Penguin.
3. BRECKON, W. (1972) The Drug Makers, p. 93. London: Eyre Methuen.
4. HORDERN, A. (1961) Psychiatry and the tranquillisers. New Eng. J. Med. **265**, 584 and 634.
5. HORDERN, A. (1971) The permissive society: some psychological aspects. Proc. roy. Soc. Med. **64**, 1112.
6. HORDERN, A. and WHEATLEY, D. (1972) The Black Cloud: The recognition and treatment of depression in general practice. Med. J. Aust. **1**, 637.
7. JOHNSON, N. (1968) Evidence given to the President's Committee on Violence. Washington D.C.
8. PARISH, P. A. (1971) The prescribing of psychotropic drugs in general practice. J. Coll. gen. Practic. **21**, (supp. 4).
9. ROSE, R. and ROSE, S. (1970) Science and Society. Harmondsworth: Penguin.
10. SHON, D. (1970) The B.B.C. Reith Lectures for 1970.
11. VOSSENAAR, T. (1972) Psychotropic drugs in the world today. Wld. med. J. **19**, 3.
12. WARD, B. and DUBOS, R. (1972) Only One Earth. Harmondsworth: Penguin.
13. Addiction to tobacco. (1971) Documenta Geigy.
14. Alcohol abuse. (1970) London: Office of Health Economics.

A. H., Department of Psychological Medicine, King's College Hospital, London S.E.5, England

EGO-STRENGTH CHANGES DURING PHARMACOTHERAPY

Z. BÖSZÖRMÉNYI

National Institute for Nervous and Mental Diseases, Budapest

The side effects of minor tranquillizers have often been mentioned, but only rather briefly, and not much importance was attributed to the subjects. The psychic side effects of these drugs were not a favourite topic, either. Some authors, however, observed that when using this type of anxiolytic drugs, such as meprobamate, or earlier, a small amount of barbiturates, then a new trend of drug addiction, the so-called tranquillomania may occur, which drug dependence seems to be connected with the chronic consumption of these day-time sedatives. This type of addict is not craving for euphoria, overzealousness or hyperactivity, but aims rather at obtaining an increased level of tolerance towards every-day nuisances, tensions, frustrations or stress situations, by reducing the possibilities of reactive anxiety conditions. Therefore, the tranquillomanic wishes to remain a conformist and an active working member of his community, in the majority of cases sticking to a moderate daily dosage. Still, it appeared that this seemingly harmless attitude can be dangerous to the persons involved: it occurred, for example, that a neurotic patient tranquillized himself so thoroughly that he failed to be present at the hearing of his own law-suit, whereby he lost a substantial sum of money.

LEHMANN (4) also emphasized that "anxiolytic sedatives, in contrast to neuroleptics, tend to be ego-weakening with chronic usage. "He supposed this effect to be due to "their capacity of disinhibiting the individual and increasing conflict behaviour, thereby weakening the persons judgement and selfcontrol which are indispensable components of an ego structure capable of coping successfully with the reality principle..."

In Hungary, luckily, we have only this type of drug addiction problem — thus far. Therefore, we looked for an opportunity to investigate the supposed ego-weakening effect of some anxiolytic drugs in a hospital setting, where the ingestion of the prescribed medication had been assured and the periodical checking of the psychic state through standardized interviews, symptom check lists etc., had been guaranteed. For "measuring" the ego-strength, we utilized the Barron ego-strength scale (2) which was made up from the 550 items of MMPI, containing 68 items, originally selected to be able to predict the response of psycho-neurotic patients to psychotherapy. BARRON thought to measure the various aspects of effective personal functioning that are usually subsumed under the term "ego-strength". Since his first publication, this scale has been used by him and many others for the same or for some similar purposes, e.g. for measuring the capacity of mastering agressive impulses among army officers, for the prediction of success in antialcoholic treatment (6—8).

The concept of ego-strength itself is somewhat vague for a pharmacopsychiatrist, and even I am using it "faute de mieux", not, however, referring thereby to the same definition as BARRON. I think that this scale can help us to assess someone's capacity to realize what are the role expectancies or obligations directed towards him by his environment, and how he feels about his ability to cope with them. One can expect a variety of answers

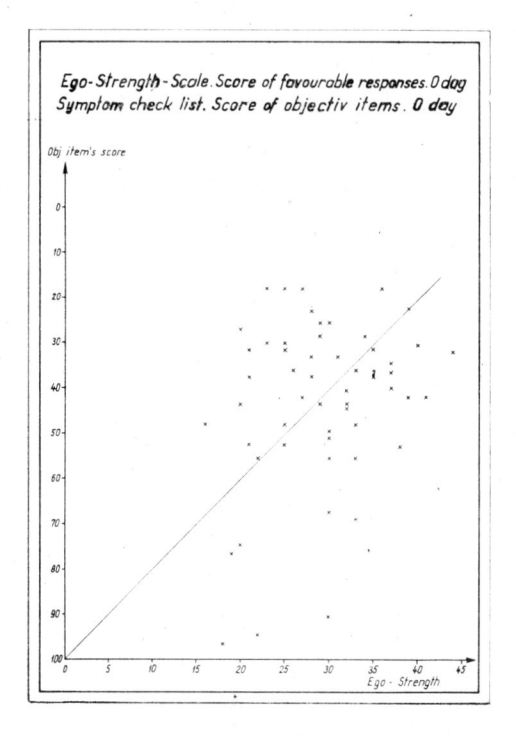

Fig. 1. Ego-Strength-Scale. Score of favourable responses. 0 day. Symptom check list. Score of objective items. 0 day.

depending upon the personality structure, as well as age and somatic condition, still, the scale was thought by us to be usable for our purposes as part of a test-battery employed on the same patient before and after pharmacotherapy.

We accepted the task of investigating the clinical efficacy of a new brand of anxiolytic drug which is a 1-(3,4-dimethoxy-phenyl)-4-methyl-5-ethyl-7,8-dimethoxy-5H-2,3-benzdiazepine, named Tofizopam. This experiment was already the second, following a former "pilot" study with this drug, directed chiefly at clinical toxicity and at the delimitation of symptomatic indication. On this occasion we do not want to go into detail of our findings, but summarily it may be stated that this drug is a good anxiolytic and reduces psychic tension with a slight euphorizing effect. Therefore, we applied this drug on 56 hospitalized female and 9 non-hospitalized male patients, chiefly on the grounds of the predominant target syndrome composed of the symptoms of minor anxiety, dysphoria and stressfulness, independently of nosological categories. The dosage, on the average, was between 75—150 mg/day. Nosologically, the majority of our patients were neurotics, psychopaths or persons with pathological personality reactions, but only 5 of them were psychotic, these five patients had endogenic depression.

On the first 10th and 22nd day we registered the psychic changes with the help of a self-composed symptom check list that contained subjective, as well as objective items, with the Taylor-manifest anxiety scale, with the Brengelman-Eysenck questionnaire and

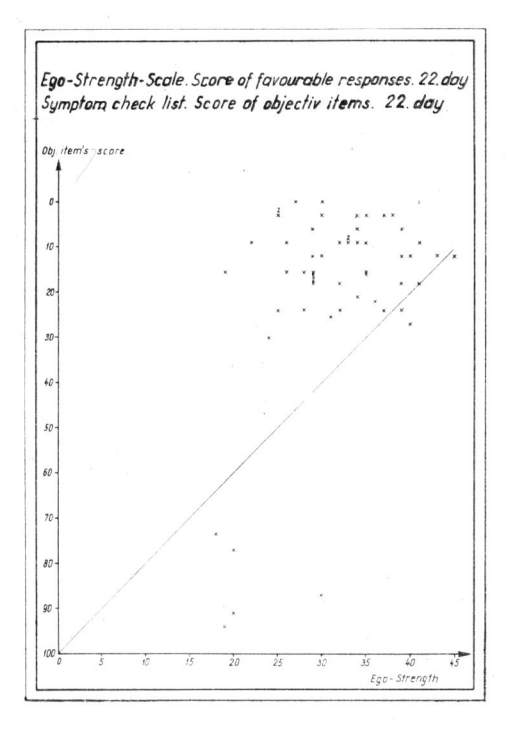

Fig. 2. Ego-Strength-Scale. Score of favourable responses. 22nd day. Symptom check list. Score of objective items. 22nd day.

with the modified Barron ego-strength scale. The gist of the modification was that we omitted the 6 items concerning attitudes towards religion. Three other items were partly changed, too.

With 20 female patients we organized a double blind experiment after matching them syndromatically, anamnestically, as well as according to age and educational level. In the two groups, consisting of ten patients each, we gave either 75 mg/day Tofizopam or 15 mg/day diazepam. These patients too, were examined, as detailed above. The results for the 56 not-blind treated patients were statistically evaluated, especially concerning the correlation between the change of favourable answers according to the Barron ego-strength scale and that of the objective items on our symptom check list before treatment and after a 21 day's therapeutical trial, utilizing the Student's paired t-test. The following table and scatter-diagrams will demonstrate the results, which are significant on a 1% level concerning the favourable changes of the ego-strength scale (Table 1 and Figs. 1—3).

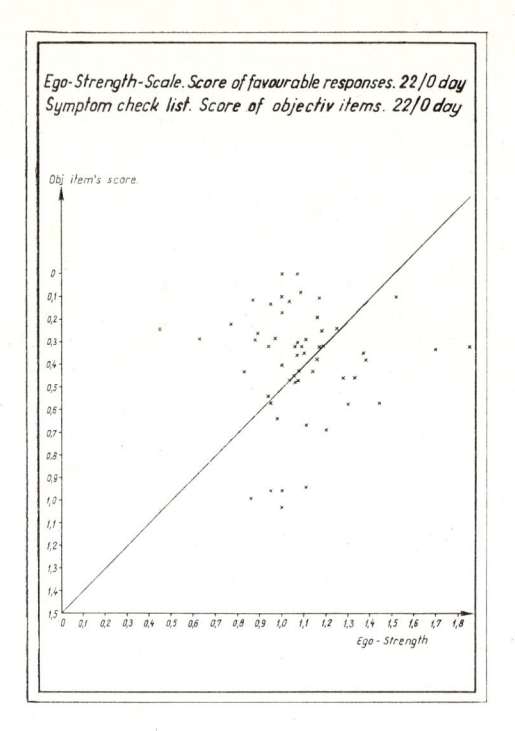

Fig. 3. Ego-Strength-Scale. Score of favourable responses. 22nd/0 day. Symptom check list. Score of objective items. 22nd/0 day.

TABLE 1

Barron, ego strength scale

	22nd day/0 day	
	Favourable responses	Unfavourable responses
n	56	56
$\bar{x}$	1,036—1,149 1,093 9,3 %	0,8993—0,997 0.948 (—) 5,2 %
var.	0,0449	0,0359
S.D	0,212	0,189
$t = \dfrac{S.D}{\sqrt{n}}$	3,117	2,110
p	< 1 %	< 5 %

There were some other noticable changes too, which, however, were not significant, that is to say, the so-called neuroticism showed a diminishing tendency after treatment, according to the Brengelman-Eysenck questionnaire. The increase in the ego-strength seemed to be smaller after the diazepam treatment, but the difference was not statistically significant. One can only surmise such a tendency at this stage of our investigations which are still in progress. We have to agree with BAN (1) who mentioned that "the sample size requirements for a controlled clinical study cannot be fulfilled within the frame of reference of the traditional approach."

After three week's treatment with Tofizopam, we obtained just the opposite of the anticipated results: In the majority of the patients an ego-strengthening and not an ego-weakening effect could be observed. We are well aware of the fact that three weeks is not a long enough span of time to label this as chronic usage, and in hospitalized patients there are a lot of other non-pharmacologically induced effects which play a part as well, such as the unintentional or indirect psychotherapy, the avoidance of some conflict-situations in the family setting, the encounter with other patients in a less favourable psychic condition or with a worse family etc. background as their own. Our follow-up study comprises till now only 19 patients who are taking the new drug at least 6 months at home. This number is not yet large enough for a statistical evaluation.

Nevertheless, we believe that if we can later prove a difference between two anxiolytic drug effects on a greater number of patients under similar circumstances and reveal simultaneously, with the help of the Barron scale, some relevant components of the ego-structure, this would be of great help in planning the most appropriate drug therapy for those who have to use anxiolytic sedatives chronically.

It seems to us that we have already demonstrated the utilizability of the Barron ego-strength scale for the purpose mentioned. It goes without saying that research must go on, extending the investigations to non-hospitalized, mental health center patients living at home, and even working at the same time (naturalistic clinical research, OVERALL — 5). Then it may be possible to achieve some statistically important results showing: a) whether there is a possibility to predict the types of personalities that have an inclination to become tranquillomanic, b) whether there is a difference between the anxiolytics currently used concerning future addiction and/or ego-weakening effect.

Of course, it still remains unanswered, whether some patients who chronically use anxiolytics are going through an ego-weakening process because of the taking of these drugs, or inspite of their steady consumption. Some neurotics have the tendency to an ego-deterioration anyway; they are trying eventually to cope with their difficulties through the anxiolytics — mostly unsuccessfully. But theoretically there also exists the possibility that the steady "drug-eating" causes a feeling of inferiority reducing self-respect and thus creating a vicious circle through minority feelings which might facilitate a further deterioriation in the condition of the patient. In view of all these considerations, it is suggested that one must be cautious when prescribing mild anxiolytics for a longer time, even though they be labelled as "not habit forming" and non-euphorizing drugs.

ACKNOWLEDGEMENTS

The author wishes to thank for their help Dr. I. Juvancz, Dr. G. Solti and V. Venter, who made the psychological and statistical evaluation of this study possible.

REFERENCES

1. BAN, T. A. (1971) In: Advances in Neuropsychopharmacology. Eds.: P. B. BRADLEY, O. VINAŘ, Z. VOTAVA, North Holland Publ. Comp. Amsterdam and Avicenum, Prague
2. BARRON, F. (1953) J. consult. Psychol. **17**, 737
3. BÖSZÖRMÉNYI, Z. (1960) Therap. Hung. **8**, 1.

4. LEHMANN, H. E. (1969). In: The Present Status of Psychotropic Drugs. Eds.: A. CERLETTI and F. J. BOVÉ, Excerpta Medica Foundation, Amsterdam.
5. OVERALL, J. E. (1969) Presented at the Interdisciplinary Week on Neuroleptics, Liège.
6. SILVERMANN, J. (1963) J. consult. Psychol. **27**, 532.
7. TAFT, R. (1957) J. consult. Psychol. **21**, 247.
8. VERHELST, E. (1969) Presented at the Antialcoholic Congress, Budapest.

Z. B.: *National Institute for Nervous and Mental Diseases, Vöröshadsereg u. 116, Budapest 1021, Hungary.*

CERTAINS ASPECTS SOCIAUX DE L'EMPLOI DES NEUROLEPTIQUES À ACTION PROLONGÉE: À PROPOS D'UNE ENQUÊTE AUPRÈS DES PSYCHIATRES FRANÇAIS SUR L'INTRODUCTION DE CES MÉDICAMENTS

R. ROPERT

Hôpital psychiatrique de Perray-Vaucluse, Epinay-sur-Orge

Dès l'introduction des neuroleptiques dans la thérapeutique psychiatrique, il y a plus de 15 ans, on a souligné l'importance et le nombre des problèmes que soulevait, au point de vue social, ce nouveau mode de traitement des maladies mentales. Les effets en apparaissaient immédiatement sur la structure des hôpitaux psychiatriques, sur l'encombrement de ceux-ci, sur la nécessité du développement des institutions extra-hospitalières.

En 1955, lors du premier colloque consacré, à Paris, à la thérapeutique par la chlorpromazine, le psychiatre américain OVERHOLSER soulignait, à propos du traitement des psychoses par les neuroleptiques, „le retour à la médecine des médecins psychiâtres et des infirmiers psychiatriques". Il indiquait également que les nouvelles thérapeutiques neuroleptiques, loin de réduire le nombre de problèmes qui se posent à une équipe psychiatrique vis-à-vis du malade et de sa famille, ne faisaient que les modifier.

Avec l'introduction des neuroleptiques à action prolongée (N.A.P.), il nous est apparu que ces problèmes sociaux et relationnels subissaient une nouvelle modification et prenaient une nouvelle importance. Nous l'avions déjà souligné, en 1969, à propos de l'œnanthate de fluphénazine, dans une communication au Congrès de Psychiatrie de Langue Française de Bruxelles. Nous l'avons confirmé, en 1971, au Congrès Mondial de Psychiatrie de México, dans un travail consacré aux dérivés neuroleptiques-retard de la pipothiazine.

Il semble en effet qu'à la trilogie classique „médecin-malade-maladie", il faille substituer un système relationnel „médecin-malade-médicament-maladie", dans lequel la forme très particulière d'administration des neuroleptiques à action prolongée introduit une dimension nouvelle et originale du système relationnel global.

EXPÉRIENCES

— *Nos premières recherches* (1969) avaient porté sur un groupe de 42 malades traités par l'œnanthate de fluphénazine. Chez ces malades, on avait étudié le mode de perception du traitement par le malade lui-même et par son entourage familial et professionnel.

— *Ultérieurement*, nous nous sommes interrogés sur l'incidence du traitement par les neuroleptiques à action prolongée sur l'attitude des médecins (médecins psychiatres et médecins généralistes) et sur l'attitude des infirmiers psychiatriques. Plusieurs colloques qui se sont tenus en France en 1970 nous ont montré l'importance de cette technique nouvelle sur la pratique du „secteur" psychiatrique. Cela nous a montré également que le rôle des neuroleptiques-retard dans certaines relations „soignants-soignés", en particulier au niveau extra-hospitalier, pouvait être très variable selon le type de pratique psychiatrique en cause: milieu urbain, ou milieu rural à habitat dispersé, par exemple.

— *Enfin, récemment, nous avons effectué une large enquête auprès de nos collègues psychiatres français*, en nous adressant aussi bien à ceux qui travaillent dans le secteur public que dans le secteur privé. Dans cette enquête nous avons inclus un certain nombre de questions concernant les implications sociales et relationnelles des traitements par les N.A.P. Nous avons reçu à ce jour 400 réponses, chiffre fort important qui témoigne à lui seul de l'intérêt suscité par ces problèmes dans le milieu psychiatrique français. Nous présenterons quelques-uns des résultats concernant les réponses qui ont été analysées à ce jour, soit 342 réponses, qui se décomposent ainsi:

— 200 psychiatres travaillant en pratique publique
— 74 psychiatres travaillant en pratique strictement privée
— 68 psychiatres travaillant en pratique mixte.

Parmi ces 342 psychiatres:

— 283 ont indiqué qu'ils avaient la pratique courante des neuroleptiques à action prolongée.
— 15 ont précisé qu'ils en avaient une pratique insuffisante à leur avis.
— 44 ont répondu qu'ils ne les utilisaient jamais.

Les produits utilisés sont:

— l'œnanthate de fluphénazine (273 réponses)
— le décanoate de fluphénazine (170 réponses)
— les dérivés-retard de la pipothiazine (51 réponses)
— divers autres neuroleptiques à action prolongée (10 réponses)

De ces différentes recherches nous pouvons tirer les conclusions suivantes, concernant les implications sociales et relationnelles des neuroleptiques à action retardée:

1. — *Dans tous les cas il se produit une modification de la relation*„*médecin-malade*" *et* „*équipe soignante-malade*", et ceci est surtout sensible lors des traitements ambulatoires, dans le secteur extra-hospitalier.

2. — *Attitude du malade vis-à-vis du traitement neuroleptique-retard:* le problème posé est celui de savoir si les neuroleptiques à action prolongée représentent pour le malade mental une contrainte moins importante que la poursuite quotidienne d'un traitement neuroleptique oral. Voici, à ce propos, les réponses fournies par les 342 psychiâtres de notre enquête:

— 189 estiment que les N.A.P. représentent une diminution de la contrainte imposée au malade.
— 90 estiment que les N.A.P. ne diminuent pas la contrainte.
— 63 estiment que le malade risque d'être trop contraint par l'emploi des N.A.P.

Parmi les malades eux-mêmes, nous notons deux types de réponses:

1. — *Les réponses positives des malades*

Les réponses positives au traitement par les N.A.P. apparaissent le fait:

— Des malades qui préfèrent une injection tous les 15 jours ou 3 semaines plutôt qu'une astreinte quotidienne régulière de la prise d'un médicament.

— D'autre part, de ceux pour qui l'emploi des N.A.P. en pratique ambulatoire représente une „médicalisation" du traitement en même temps qu'un rythme naturel de la relation avec l'équipe soignante.

2. — *Les réponses négatives des malades*

Au contraire, les réactions négatives des malades sont le fait dans notre expérience actuelle:

— Soit des malades qui supportent mal le recours aux injections, celles-ci étant vécues comme des agressions dans un contexte sadomasochiste.
— Soit des malades qui supportent mal la notion de „l'inclusion" et de la persistance d'action du produit au niveau du corps. (Cette réaction est aussi bien le fait de certains psychotiques que de certaines personnalités psychopathiques.)
— Soit enfin des malades pour lesquels l'abandon du traitement neuroleptique quotidien représente une sorte de frustration orale.

3. — *Attitude du médecin vis-à-vis des N.A.P.*

Seules les attitudes du médecin psychiâtre sont possibles à analyser; d'ailleurs notre enquête ne s'adressait qu'à des psychiatres. Les attitudes des médecins généralistes sont: soit marquées par une méconnaissance totale des N.A.P.; soit entachées à leur égard d'enthousiasme ou, au contraire, de réactions très négatives; — l'un comme les autres étant souvent directement proportionnels à la qualité, bonne ou mauvaise, de la relation qui existe entre le médecin généraliste et l'équipe soignante psychiatrique.

Les résultats de notre enquête concernant l'attitude des médecins psychiatres vis-à-vis des N.A.P. donnent les résultats suivants, sur 342 réponses:

a) *Intérêt des N.A.P.*

— 263 considèrent les N.A.P. comme un progrès thérapeutique incontestable;
— 245 insistent surtout sur l'intérêt lié au fait qu'avec les N.A.P. ils ont la certitude que le traitement est effectivement absorbé par le malade;
— 204 insistent (toujours en parallèle avec la reponse précédente) sur la simplicité de la technique.

b) *Objections à l'égard des N.A.P.*

— 76 sur 342 considèrent que la simplicité apparente du traitement N.A.P. risque de masquer d'autres problèmes thérapeutiques;
— ces réponses sont impossibles à analyser dans le détail, mais la crainte la plus fréquemment exprimée est celle que l'emploi des N.A.P. puisse diminuer ou supprimer la relation *médecin-malade* ainsi que l'écoute du malade. En fait les réticences à ce propos apparaissent plus grandes chez les médecins qui ont une activité purement ambulatoire que chez les médecins ayant une activité hospitalière ou une activité mixte.

Deux types d'attitude se dégagent d'ailleurs à ce sujet parmi les psychiatres ayant la pratique du travail „de secteur", notamment ambulatoire:

— *les uns admettent de revoir seulement le malade à intervalles très éloignés* (plusieurs mois), l'essentiel de la relation étant alors confié à des infirmiers ambulatoires chargés de pratiquer les injections de N.A.P., tous les 15 jours à trois semaines;

— *d'autres, s'élèvent au contraire contre le „danger" de l'attitude précédente* et estiment que l'emploi des N.A.P. en pratique ambulatoire les amène à revoir plus fréquemment leurs malades et à faire des N.A.P. la base d'une nouvelle relation médecin-malade.

c) *Rôle des N.A.P. par rapport à la famille du malade.*

Dans notre enquête, *ce rôle est apprécié de façon concordante:*
— 186 réponses estiment que les N.A.P. provoquent une plus grande confiance de la famille vis-à-vis du traitement;
— 190 estiment que les N.A.P. provoquent une meilleure tolérance de la famille vis-à-vis du malade psychotique;
— 33 relèvent au contraire des réactions d'inquiétude de la famille par rapport à l'emploi des N.A.P.

4. — *Attitude de l'équipe soignante*

Le traitement par les N.A.P. a sans doute modifié très profondément la relation des infirmiers avec les malades, comme l'avait déjà fait à partir de 1952 l'introduction des neuroleptiques à l'hôpital psychiatrique. Il est inutile de revenir ici sur le fait que de semblables progrès thérapeutiques ne „simplifient" pas le rôle du personnel infirmier, mais rendent celui-ci disponible pour de nouvelles tâches qui font apparaître d'autres problèmes: notamment la possibilité d'une plus grande relation psychothérapique. Mais il faut souligner que l'emploi des N.A.P. modifie surtout la tâche et la position de l'équipe *extra-hospitalière.*

Voyons, là encore, quelles sont les réponses obtenues dans notre enquête auprès des médecins psychiatres français:

a) *Estimation globale:*
— 136 psychiâtres estiment que l'opinion de leurs infirmiers à l'égard des N.A.P. est „globalement favorable";
— 109 estiment l'opinion de leurs infirmiers „plutôt favorable",
— 5 seulement l'estiment „franchement défavorable".

b) *Réponses motivées:*
— 116 psychiatres estiment que leurs infirmiers sont *rassurés*, par cette technique;
— 112 considèrent que les N.A.P. *libèrent* leurs infirmiers au profit d'autres tâches (relationnelles, ergothérapie, etc.);
— 72 déclarent que le travail de leurs infirmiers subit du fait des N.A.P., *une modification et une valorisation* nouvelles.

Ce dernier point est souligné notamment par ceux de nos confrères psychiatres qui desservent un secteur rural, et qui disposent d'équipes d'infirmiers-visiteurs se rendant régulièrement au domicile du malade à l'occasion de l'injection du neuroleptique-retard. Ceci répond également au fait général suivant, — que nous observons aussi bien en pratique urbaine qu'en pratique rurale: plus un malade psychotique acquiert de possibilités de s'autonomiser, plus ses liens avec le psychiatre ont tendance à se distendre. De ce fait, il devient très important qu'une technique telle que l'emploi des N.A.P. entraîne le malade à conserver un „point d'ancrage", de liaison, régulier avec le reste de l'équipe psychiatrique (infirmiers, assistantes sociales), même si cela risque d'entraîner une inversion de l'importance relative des rapports entre médecin-malade et équipe soignante-malade.

CONCLUSION

Il nous faudrait évoquer également un dernier aspect social et socio-psychiatrique de l'emploi des neuroleptiques à action prolongée: celui de l'importance d'une méthode thérapeutique de cet ordre par rapport au développement futur de l'assistance psychiatrique.

Des calculs précis, concernant notamment le coût de l'emploi des N.A.P. par rapport aux autres méthodes de traitement des malades psychotiques (et notamment par rapport à l'hospitalisation de ces malades) ont déjà été faits, en particulier en Grande-Bretagne. Certaines estimations de cet ordre ont été rapportées en 1971 au Congrès Mondial de Psychiatrie de México. On peut également se poser la question de savoir si les N.A.P. sont susceptibles de modifier profondément les projets ultérieurs d'extension de l'assistance psychiatrique, — notamment dans les pays en voie de développement, où cette assistance psychiatrique est actuellement en cours d'implantation. Faut-il, dans de tels cas, renoncer totalement à la construction de nouveaux établissements psychiatriques et traiter les malades mentaux psychotiques exclusivement par les N.A.P., et uniquement en thérapeutique ambulatoire? Y-a-t-il au contraire un danger que, par le biais des N.A.P., la thérapeutique psychiatrique puisse „se mécaniser", aux dépens d'une approche en profondeur des problèmes en cause et aux dépens de la relation médecin-malade?

Ces questions sont importantes à soulever et à débattre. Elles montrent en tout cas à quel point une nouvelle technique thérapeutique de cet ordre peut engendrer des problèmes qui dépassent rapidement le simple plan des effets pharmacologiques et impliquent une réflexion d'ordre relationnel et sociothérapique.

R.P., Hôpital Psychiatrique de Perray-Vaucluse, 91, Epinay-sur-Orge, France

TRAINING MODELS IN PSYCHOPHARMACOLOGY

Chairmen: T. A. BAN and F. A. FREYHAN

Associate chairman: B. CHRISTENSEN

PSYCHOPHARMACOLOGY IN THE TEACHING OF PSYCHIATRY

T. A. BAN

Division of Psychopharmacology of the Department of Psychiatry, McGill University, Montreal, Quebec

INTRODUCTION

With the rapidly increasing number of new drugs with possible psychoactive properties there has developed a growing sophistication in the methodology of clinical investigation. The recognition, however, that controlled experiments are essential for meaningful clinical, psychopharmacological research has led to double standards in psychiatry, one standard in the evaluation of changes induced by psychological and another standard in the evaluation of changes induced by biological means. Of course, the fact that psychiatry today is taught, and consequently practiced, on the basis of knowledge derived from clinical impressions and on the basis of findings verified in clinical testings, i.e. on the basis of two different standards, does not mean that there are two psychiatries now, nor does it suggest that there are two psychiatries in the making. On the contrary, it implies, that psychiatry, in spite of all the retarding and dividing forces at work, is progressing from a descriptive into an experimental discipline.

At present there are indications that the scope of psychiatry is changing, that a new structure of psychiatric organization is in the making and that a new content is gradually replacing the old in psychiatric teachings.

SCOPE AND STRUCTURE OF PSYCHIATRY

The re-evaluation of traditional psychiatric concepts and thought, however, is only one of the manifestations of the "psychopharmacological era". Concurrently, drugs in general are becoming a part of everyday living, and new psychopathologies related to these new pharmacological contingencies are in the making.

To update the training program in psychiatry with the psychopharmacological contributions, the Division of Psychopharmacology of the Department of Psychiatry, McGill University, was established. The aims of the Division are to improve the teaching and practice of psychiatry, and to encourage research in psychopharmacology.

Adult psychiatric facilities affiliated with McGill University comprise seven psychiatric units — 6 to 100 beds each — in general hospitals and a large psychiatric hospital with approximately 1500 beds. In this system, the purpose of the general hospital psychiatric units is to serve as primary diagnostic and therapeutic screens, and the purpose of the psychiatric hospital is to provide services for patients who remain refractory to traditional methods of treatment within a limited period of time.

A special monitoring technique was devised to study the operating system of psychiatric services. This system consists of a set of forms, which are completed at regular intervals in four general hospital psychiatric units (GH) and in one of the admission units of the psychiatric hospital (PH).

Comparative data between two representative monitored units — over a three month period — revealed that the number of patients admitted to the GH is only 70 percent of those admitted to the PH; and that the average weekly turnover is less at the GH than at the PH. In addition to the greater patient load, in the PH there was also a significantly ($P < 0.001$) greater number of patients with previous psychiatric hospitalization and with the psychopathological symptoms of thought disorders, delusions and memory disturbances. Nevertheless, the total number of staff was larger at the GH (total of 32) than at the PH (27); and the staff-patient ratio, with the exception of nursing assistants, was only one fourth that of the GH in the PH.

The operating system unveiled by the monitored data was quite obviously inadequate to deal with the most severely sick patients. It was based on a psychiatric education which was strongly skewed in favor of psychotherapies, in which psychopathology was almost entirely substituted by psychodynamics, and in which training in psychoanalysis outweighed the training in pharmacotherapies. Furthermore, it was based on a psychiatry which was characterized by an almost complete separation of psychiatric practice from psychiatric research.

To prevent the one-way road to chronicity and imbalance in training and treatment priorities, a new, planned, continuous and accountable, structural organization of psychiatric services was suggested. "Planning" implies that the extent of psychiatric services is based on the prevalence of mental disorder and the availability of professional manpower. Or, in other terms, "planned" means that the extent of psychiatric services is not based on meaningless polemics on what psychiatry is or what psychiatry should offer, but on the concrete definition of what psychiatry can offer with the available manpower and what psychiatry should provide for the community. While "planning" defines the scope of psychiatry, "continuity" refers to the structure of psychiatric organization. Accordingly, "continuity" implies that there is a structure in the organization of psychiatric services which enables all psychiatrists, operating in the system, to exercise full responsibility towards their patients in the different stages of their illnesses, from the beginning to the end. It also implies the coordination of teaching, practice and research. Finally, "accountability" means a system with built-in controls in which changes are recommended on the basis of needs — and not personal biases — brought to light by data analysis.

In the proposed structural organization, psychiatric services are provided on five levels, i.e. (1) Primary Hospitalization Service, (2) Central Consultation Service, (3) Continuing Treatment Service, (4) Specialized Treatment Service, and (5) Rehabilitational Facilities. The Primary Hospitalization Service (PHS) has been designed to provide for a psychiatric inpatient facility which covers a well delineated geographical area, while the Central Consultation Service (CCS) has been designed for patients who remain diagnostic and/or therapeutic problems after an 8 to 12 weeks period at the PHS. In contrast to the PHS, where both diagnosis and therapy are primarily based on clinical judgement, at the CCS laboratory — behavioral, neurophysiological and biochemical — findings play a role equal to clinical judgement in diagnostic and therapeutic decisions. Similarly, while at the PHS, treatments are primarily based on the application of well established techniques and procedures, at the CCS, careful testing of new therapeutic approaches, based on rational hypotheses, plays, at least, an equally important role. The primary aim of the Continuing Treatment Service (CTS) is to establish optimal maintenance treatment as well as to reveal the potential for social rehabilitation of patients who are in need of longer than 12 to 16 weeks of hospitalization; and the Specialized Treatment Service (STS) has been designed to provide for a service for patients who remain resistant to treatment after 18 to 24 months of hospitalization at the CTS, by utilizing specialized, but not fully evaluated, methods of treatment in the therapy of chronic psychiatric patients. Finally, the establishment of Rehabilitational Facilities (RF) takes into consideration the limits of psychiatry as a medical discipline.

In the proposed structural organization clinical operations are extended and supplemented with adequate facilities for applied research, i.e. (1) Behavioral Analysis Service, (2) Neurophysiological Analysis Service, (3) Biochemical Analysis Service, (4) Clinical Investigational Service, and (5) Specialized Investigational Service. The primary aims of the laboratory services are to establish standardized objective measurements based on behavioral, neurophysiological and biochemical procedures; to supplement and correlate the data obtained by the application of these procedures by the data obtained in clinical assessments; and to conduct research in the experimental analysis of behavior, psychopathology, psychiatric diagnosis and behavioral pharmacology.

While the role of clinical and research services is to secure "continuity" within the system, the role of the educational services — General Monitoring Service (GMS), Adverse Reaction Monitoring Service (ARMS) and Psychopharmacological Consultation Service (PCS) — is to render the various operations accountable and to provide the necessary information for appropriately planned developments. Accordingly, it is essential that all of these services, i.e. GMS, ARMS and PCS, utilize the obtained information in the continuous education of professional personnel via regularly submitted and discussed reports. Beyond these seminars, the educational services offer formal training courses in Biological Psychiatry (75 hours), Practical Psychopharmacology (10 hours), Systematic Psychopharmacology (10 hours), Applied Psychopharmacology (10 hours) and in Research Design (6 hours).

CONTENT OF PSYCHIATRY

If it is true that structure defines content, the new structural organization of psychiatry should bring about fundamental changes in psychiatric practice and psychiatric teachings. There is no doubt that extension of psychiatric care from a particular social strata to society as a whole, without a considerable increase in psychiatric manpower, can only be achieved if family doctors and/or general practitioners are trained in the use of the new psychoactive drugs, if paramedical professionals are prepared to undertake the educational role of psychiatrists in the community, and if psychiatry becomes a consulting medical specialty. Similarly, there is no doubt that extension of optimal psychiatric care from a selected group of psychiatric conditions, usually referred to as psychoneuroses, to all psychiatric diseases, can only be achieved if the emphasis in psychiatric education shifts from psychodynamics to psychopathology and from an intensive training in the psychotherapies to an extensive training in the application of physical, especially pharmacological, therapies. As the new structure of psychiatry extends the provision of psychiatric care from a limited period of time to care covering the whole long duration of psychiatric disease, optimal utilization of these new facilities can only be achieved if psychiatric education includes training in biochemistry, neurophysiology, psychophysiology and behavioral pharmacology as well as in the methodological principles of contemporary research.

It is still too early to evaluate the actual changes in the context of psychiatric education which were brought about by the introduction of the new therapeutically effective psychoactive drugs. Nevertheless, there is sufficient evidence to believe that in contrast to the traditional approach in psychiatry, which is based on a descriptive analysis of psychopathological signs and symptoms, the psychopharmacological approach is based on the description of those interactions between drugs and biochemical structures which trigger off neurophysiological mechanisms with measurable behavioral effects.

With the advent of psychopharmacology many psychoactive drugs with distinctly different pharmacodynamic properties were synthetized. These new drugs with increasingly better defined behavioral, neurophysiological and biochemical actions, have provided new means for therapeutically influencing and systematically studying clinical psychopathological conditions. As a result, a clinical psychopharmacological approach is slowly developing and attempts are made to group psychiatric patients on the basis of their response patterns to various psychoactive drugs. This psychopharmacological approach has already contributed observations pertinent to the analysis of clinical syndromes, to the elucidation of psychopathological mechanisms and theories, and to the delineation of concepts and nosological entities. The newly accumulated information supports the hypothesis of a true psychopathological diversity, confirms the nosological concepts of schizophrenia and of manic-depressive psychosis and supports the view that contemporary pharmacotherapy does not act merely by modifying the symptoms of these disorders, but may also modify the clinical course and evolution of these conditions (1). Other findings which have accumulated during the psychopharmacological era strongly suggest that the classical nosological groups are only in part homogeneous entities. What is becoming obvious is the heterogeneity within these various groups. This corresponds with the clinical observation that any particular patient may be unaffected by a specific neuroleptic/antidepressant agent, yet the same patient may respond to another neuroleptic/antidepressant drug.

Pharmacological and clinical investigations with the rapidly growing number of new psychoactive substances revealed many drugs with common pharmacological characteristics and similar clinical effects. These common pharmacological characteristics were found to be useful in the prediction of the clinical indications for newly developed drugs. On the other hand, in the absence of any fundamental knowledge of either the structural or the functional basis of most of the clinical psychopathological conditions, the co-called "rational approach" has still very limited application in the search for new psychotherapeutic drugs. This implies, that no fundamental changes occurred in our concepts of mental illness which could be directly attributed to the introduction of the numerous psychotherapeutic drugs.

Summary

The effect of psychopharmacology on the teaching of psychiatry has been discussed. It was suggested that as a result of the introduction of effective psychotherapeutic drugs, the scope of psychiatry is changing, that a new structure of psychiatric organization is in the making, and that a new content is gradually replacing the old in psychiatric teachings.

As far as the scope of psychiatry is concerned, psychopharmacology provides a means which redefines the field of psychiatry as a medical discipline. On the other hand, by creating a planned, continuous and accountable structural organization of psychiatric services, it leads to an extension of optimal psychiatric care throughout the long duration of psychiatric disease.

The newly accumulated information in the psychopharmacological era focused attention on the fact that classical nosological groups are only in part homogeneous entities. In spite of all this, no fundamental theoretical change has occurred in psychiatry, which could be directly attributed to the introduction of the numerous new psychotherapeutic drugs.

Probably the most important contribution of the psychopharmacological era to date, is the fact that the increasing sophistication in the methodology of clinical investigations has forced a re-examination of traditional concepts in psychiatry — an essential prerequisite for the transformation of psychiatry from a descriptive into an experimental discipline.

REFERENCES

1. WHO SCIENTIFIC GROUP ON PSYCHOPHARMACOLOGY: Research in Psychopharmacology. World Health Organization Technical Report Series No. 371, Geneva 1967.

T.A.B., Division of Psychopharmacology, Department of Psychiatry, McGill University, Montreal, Quebec, Canada

POSTGRADUATE TRAINING IN PSYCHOPHARMACOLOGY

B. MÜLLER-OERLINGHAUSEN and H. HELMCHEN

Department of Psychiatry of the Free University, West Berlin

WHAT IS CLINICAL PSYCHOPHARMACOLOGY

Most professional pharmacologists might feel slightly embarrassed when asked for a definition of the term "clinical psychopharmacology". Some certainly would suggest that this notion is identical with clinical screening of psychotropic drugs or pharmacotherapy of mental diseases or maybe with both. However, it should be emphasized that such definitions are by far too narrow. In fact, drug screening can be considered as part of (psycho)pharmacology, and pharmacotherapy may be occasionally the result of pharmacological arguments.

In order to promote a definition which describes just what a clinical psychopharmacologist actually does or is expected to do we suggest two different operational meanings of the term which should not exclude but rather complete each other:

a) Elaboration of a theoretical concept about the mechanisms of clinical action of psychotropic drugs, — which would lead then to a rational pharmacotherapy based on scientific facts and hypotheses.

b) Investigations of the actions of psychotropic drugs in man, — implying among other things drug screening in volunteers and patients.

WHY DO WE NEED TRAINING IN PSYCHOPHARMACOLOGY

The issue of improved psychopharmacological training of resident psychiatrists seemingly has not raised much interest hitherto in discussions about postgraduate psychiatric education (1, 2). So it may be worthwhile to spend some time on the question: why is a postgraduate training in psychopharmacology necessary at all? At present the undergraduate training in basic and clinical psychopharmacology is still not satisfactory, at least as regarding the situation in our country. Most students of clinical psychiatry do not know what special kind of drugs are used in the treatment of mental diseases, and which are their assumed mechanisms of action or their most common side effects. This is in line with the fact that even a decade ago teaching in psychiatry focussed mainly on diagnostic-nosological problems whereas very little attention was paid to details of therapeutic measures. A deeper understanding of basic psychopharmacological facts seems to be essential for the resident psychiatrist for the following reasons:

a) It is getting more and more difficult to fulfill the requirements of the FDA, WHO and other national or international institutions concerning drug studies in man, and this will be even more so in the near future. There is a strong trend developing to make the clinician who is in charge of a drug trial *fully responsible* for that part of the study which is actually performed by himself, and for any complication resulting from an investigation not properly done. Therefore, the clinician must study and must be able to understand the experimental data of a substance *before* starting a study in patients. Only his own knowledge in psychopharmacology or the assistance of a pharmacologist will prevent him from overlooking important details of the foregoing animal experiments. The physician should be able to evaluate himself the quality of screening instructions and the necessity of e.g. FDA-restrictions referring to his own activities. He should be trained in psychopharmacology so that he can make suggestions to the authorities how to improve the reliability and safety of drug trials.

b) We shall discuss now what will be the consequence if basic psychopharmacological knowledge will not be increased among the clinicians performing drug trials which the pharmaceutical manufacturers are forced to do by law. Up to now the cooperation between clinicians and the pharmacologists working in the pharmaceutical companies was rather poor. Those who are responsible for clinical research in the pharmaceutical companies often do not have much clinical competence; so they have to accept clinical results though being informed about faults and negligence in the performance of certain drug trials. Moreover, the pharmacologists of the companies often do not participate in planning the details of a drug study because this is considered belonging to the competence of the clinician. Efficient feedback is also often missing between clinicians and pharmacologists during the period of a drug trial. Sometimes the manufacturer may have an ideal concept how to perform a clinical study, but this concept might turn out quite unrealistic in view of organisational difficulties on the wards where the study is to be done. It can be expected that the pharmacologists of the manufacturers, as far as they are aware of this situation will try in the future to take a more active part in the planning and performing of drug trials. This obviously implies the danger that finally the clinician himself is no longer planning a drug study but is only fulfilling the detailed requests of the clinical pharmacologists in the pharmaceutical company. Such a development can only be counteracted if the clinician acquires enough knowledge in psychopharmacology himself or if he is helped by a clinical pharmacologist in his department on whose advice he can rely upon.

c) The therapeutic success of modern psychotropic drugs has deeply influenced the theories and speculations about the biochemical processes correlated with specific psychopathological symptoms or certain nosological entities. It has also stimulated efforts to discuss the problem again whether the conventional classifications of mental diseases are justified, i.e. whether they make any sense for a differential pharmacotherapy ("the right drug for the right patient"). Above all, the discussion about the nature of affective disorders has received many impulses from experimental and clinical psychopharmacology. On the other side, only clinicians who are well informed about the pharmacology and biochemistry of psychotropic drugs might draw any scientific or practical benefit from these discussions of highly sophisticated arguments.

In other words, advanced psychopharmacological training should not be confined to those physicians who are to take part in clinical drug trials but it should constitute a general background for discussions about the nature and origin of psychotic and other mental disorders.

d) Finally, it may seem trivial to repeat what most clinicians have already agreed upon, namely that continous postgraduate training in pharmacology is essential for every physician in order to be on the safe side when it comes to the use of drug combinations. Seldom psychiatric in- or out-patients will be treated exclusively with psychotropic drugs. Instead they may have been prescribed antidiabetics, laxatives, analgetics, hormones, antihypertensive drugs etc. at the same time. General pharmacological knowledge is required to foresee and evaluate critically side effects and hazards resulting from the use of drug combinations, especially since the clinical effects of many combinations — even very common ones — have never been closely scrutinized.

Which are the aims of postgraduate psychopharmacological training

From what has been mentioned above three practical aims for postgraduate training in psychopharmacology might be set up:

a) To make the resident psychiatrist more familiar with the results of experimental psychopharmacology thereby providing him with a deeper understanding of clinical drug effect and possible side effects. Basic knowledge about the chemical structure and the general pharmacological properties of centrally acting and other drugs should enable the clinician to foresee side effects of allegedly "new" drugs or drug combinations.

b) To advise and support the clinician in the effective performance of controlled pharmacological studies in man.

c) To increase critical-methodological thinking in order to sensitize the physician against the existence of e.g. hidden placebo effects, of bias, and of the many unexpected pitfalls in the final evaluation of so-called "controlled" drug trials.

Thus, summarizing, it may be stated that "clinical psychopharmacology" signifies investigations in man concerning the action of psychotropic drugs. Active postgraduate training consists in:

a) Conveying the results of experimental investigations to the residents.
b) Giving advice how to perform experimental and clinical investigations.

It should be the aim of such efforts to integrate the results of experimental psychopharmacology into the everyday routine work of the psychiatrist.

How can training in clinical psychopharmacology be realized

Instead of presenting a fully elaborated concept we would rather like to give some idea of how we try to increase the level of psychopharmacological knowledge among the resident psychiatrists at our department in Berlin.

First of all, we are fortunate to have an experimental unit for animal studies under the direction of Prof. Coper which is attached to the clinic but works independently. The frequent and informal discussions between members of this section and clinicians provide various opportunities to increase the knowledge about experimental methods. Sometimes residents may feel stimulated to investigate a clinical observation more intensively by means of animal experiments.

One pharmacologist is working fulltime within the hospital in order to enforce and improve cooperation with the experimental unit. It is essential that the clinical pharmacologist is actually working *within* the hospital and that he has sufficient clinical experience and training so that he can take care of patients whom he is especially interested in. He keeps intensive contact with every ward and pays special attention to drug side effects, unexpected outcomes of therapy, "poor responders" etc. He will discuss therapeutic problems with the physicians on the ward and during the weekly conferences. For metabolic and pharmacokinetic studies in man, special laboratory facilities are at his disposal and some standard methods are kept ready for determination of certain psychotropic drugs in body fluids. Thus, residents on the ward may also feel motivated to check more frequently serum concentrations of drugs. Constant feedback from the laboratory to the resident and *vice versa* is very important, — and this communication should be steadily reinforced by the clinical pharmacologist who will discuss pharmacological problems with his colleagues much more effectively (from a didactic point of view) on the ground of single case observations.

The easiest and most promising way to get in touch with the practical problems of psychopharmacology is the planning, performing, and evaluating of controlled drug trials in which as many residents as possible should take part at least once during their training period (3). The controlled drug trial is a special case where often very intriguing and sophisticated questions have to be dealt with; they may sometimes also constitute a starting point from where special methodological problems can be discussed and elucidated (e.g. "placebo effects" or the difficult criteria of "improvement"). In our opinion a more positive attitude towards methodological problems would be the most valuable tool for the physician in order to be able to evaluate the results of pharmacotherapeutic measures in his patients and to compare critically the benefits of different kinds of treatment, they may be called "biological", "psychological" or "social" therapy.

References

1. G. F. M. Russell and H. J. Walton, Eds.: The training of psychiatrists. Proceed. of the conference on postgraduate psychiatric education. Headley Brothers Ltd., Ashford/Kent 1970.
2. "Residency Training." In: Amer. J. Psychiat. **128**, 1097—1131 (1972).
3. M. Hamilton: The teaching of psycho-pharmacology. Paper pres. at the 2. Zentraleurop. Symp. Neuropsychopharmakologie und Pharmakopsychiatrie in Split, 1971.

B.M.-O., Department of Psychiatry of the Free University, West Berlin

TRAINING MODELS IN PSYCHOPHARMACOLOGY

P. KIELHOLZ

Psychiatric Clinic, University of Basel

Research programmes in the U.S.A. — especially those executed by M. B. BALTER, J. LEVINE and I. RUBINSTEIN — and in various countries of Europe have demonstrated that psychotropic drugs, especially minor tranquilizers and anti-depressants, are prescribed, for the most part, by specialists for internal medicine, by doctors in general practice, and by gynaecologists, the psychiatrist following in the fourth place. The most important target groups for training in psychopharmacology are, therefore, primarily doctors who will later enter practice as specialists for internal medicine, general medicine, gynaecology and psychiatry. As in many other fields of medicine this training in psychopharmacology, which has an immense practical importance, receives too little attention during medical studies and in postgraduate training.

Preconditions for the successful use of psychotropic drugs are knowledge of psychopathology, uniform nomenclature and uniform classification. There are, however, great differences not only from language to language, not only from one psychiatric school to another, but even in the same clinic among the doctors. Differences exist not only in nomenclature but also in diagnostic definition. It is therefore necessary that all the different university clinics, in which students and post-graduates are trained, should aspire to an uniform interpretation of symptoms, syndromes, diagnostic criteria and indications for psychopharmacotherapy.

Training in psychopathology during the bedside dialogue between the patient and the doctor under the supervision of an experienced psychiatrist is too time-consuming for each training centre to undertake. Therefore we use, as a training model, television, teletape and films. Audiovision has the advantage that each rater can judge the same interview and has the same degree of visible and audible information and also that this information can be repeated at any suitable time. The doctors must fill in a questionnaire, quantifying all the symptoms and syndromes they observe in the patient and finally recording the indication for therapy. The results of the assessments are continuously statistically evaluated and then discussed critically and objectively until a good Interrater-Reliability is achieved.

Such a training programme, using a new method, was carried out by FISCHER-CORNELSSEN, HOLE and ABT with the medical staff of our clinic and was reported recently at the V. World Congress of Psychiatry in Mexico-City. In contrast to all reliability tests published previously, in this study the raters neither saw the new rating scale in advance nor had they received previous training with it. Although all doctors worked in the same clinic, in interrater reliability there were significant differences in 3 out of 14 symptom-groups, but none in total score. Correlation in interrater reliability was good. In view of the rigid conditions and a weak definition of two symptoms in the rating scale used, these results demonstrated a good level of education which nevertheless could be improved.

Moreover, it was seen that the more years of experience and training in psychiatry a rater had, the more cautious he became in rating the value of symptoms. This difference was statistically significant.

It could also be seen that students and doctors participated in the training model with enthusiasm, since each one took an active part. In the subsequent discussion over the differences in the rating of symptoms, diagnostic criteria and indications for therapy the practical application of psychopharmacology in the example of the patients interviewed can be demonstrated.

The same training model is to be used for students and in further education for doctors in practice.

A similar study was made at a WHO meeting in Basel with international participation. It was shown that there is a very great agreement between countries in the registration of the psychopathological symptoms and syndromes, but that there are great differences in diagnostic criteria and indications for pharmacotherapy. In a symposium for joint international research in depression which was organised by the WHO in Basel the investigators were able to establish within 10 days on an international basis uniformity in the registration and classification of symptoms, and a close agreement on indications for pharmacotherapy.

For many years we have used, for large educational programmes, the Eidophor system to allow the discussion of psychopharmacological problems by a scattered audience. First, we show the patient and his symptoms and discuss the differential diagnosis. Next, we answer questions posed by doctors in the assembly-room and finally we discuss in detail the indications for psychopharmacotherapy.

A precondition for the successful use of psychotropic drugs is a knowledge of the effects and side-effects of the drug, which should be demonstrated as clearly as possible. Audiovisual methods are of proven value as they allow the doctors participating to see the patient and the related problems in a situation identical to that of the consulting room.

Summary

1. The basis for successful use of psychotropic drugs is a good knowledge of psychopathology and diagnostic factors as well as uniform terminology and classification.

2. Exact diagnostic criteria and indications can be best achieved through the help of audiovisual methods. The aim of the training is a close agreement in the assessment of the symptoms, syndromes and classification which is statistically checked and corrected continuously until good interrater reliability is achieved.

3. The choice of drug will be decided on the basis of the patient's symptoms and signs and presupposes a good knowledge of the effects and of the side-effects of the drug.

4. Before each joint research project, the participating doctors should achieve uniformity of diagnostics and a good interrater reliability, as otherwise the research results cannot be compared.

5. The present standard of training in psychopharmacology is insufficient. The training should as rapidly as possible be intensified and improved in view of the world-wide importance of psychotropic drugs.

For reading list, please contact the author.

P.K., Psychiatric Clinic of the University, Wilhelm Klein-Strasse 27, CH-4000 Basel, Switzerland

WHO TRAINING COURSE IN PSYCHOPHARMACOLOGY FOR TEACHERS IN MEDICAL SCHOOLS

O. J. RAFAELSEN

Psychochemistry Institute, University of Copenhagen School of Medicine, Copenhagen

This Course was initiated by DR. B. A. LEBEDEV, former Chief of Mental Health, WHO, Geneva. In his outline the Course would include lectures, practical studies in various psychiatric institutions, and round table discussions.

The proposed subjects were:

1. Psychotropic drugs and their classifications.
2. Clinical effectiveness of the main groups of psychotropic drugs: neuroleptics, anxiolytic sedatives, antidepressants, psychostimulants and psychodysleptics (hallucinogens).
3. Adverse clinical effects. Prevention and treatment.
4. Biochemical and neurophysiological mechanisms of action of psychotropic drugs.
5. Psychotropic drugs in treatment of mental disorders: schizophrenic, depressive, manic, organic, neurotic, and personality disorders, delusional states.
6. Psychotropic drugs in combination with other forms of somatic therapy: electroconvulsive therapy, insulin coma therapy, sub-coma insulin, etc.
7. Psychotropic drugs in comprehensive therapy: in combination with psychotherapy (individual, group or family, work therapy, rehabilitation).
8. Psychotropic drugs in out-patient practice, supportive therapy and follow-up of patients discharged from mental hospitals.
9. Organisation of training and supervision of auxiliary personnel (e.g. in basic health services) distributing psychotropic drugs to mental patients.
10. Psychopharmacological training in medical schools.
11. Research in clinical psychopharmacology; comparative studies on drug effectiveness.

The financial costs of the course were covered by Danish Government Authorities (DANIDA).

The duration of the course was 3 weeks: 2 weeks in Copenhagen and 1 week in Aarhus. The Course was planned and conducted by the author and Professor MOGENS SCHOU.

16 participants from as many developing countries were accepted as fellows, all being teachers of psychiatry in medical schools, preferably heads of departments of psychiatry or their associates, having continued clinical experience in the psychopharmacological treatment of mental disorders.

The programme consisted of:

1. Lectures and discussions.
2. Group sessions and discussions.
3. Visits to hospitals, research institutes, drug companies, including practical demonstrations.
4. Multiple choice tests.
5. Critique and evaluation of the course.

Most lectures were preprinted and distributed to the participants in advance to make it possible to study the text beforehand. Lecturers were then requested only to give a short introduction to the subject, leaving most of the time at session for discussion.

For group work the participants were divided in groups of 4 or 5, new group structures being formed on each group session.

The participants were encouraged to change group leaders and rapporteurs and all functioned on rotation as chairman.

Most lecturers were from Denmark, but foreign lecturers were invited from Canada, West Germany and Sweden.

Multiple Choice Tests were administered on 7 occasions during the Course. The purpose of this was threefold:

1. To acquaint the participants with this type of evaluation.
2. To give the Course Management some crude information at the onset on the participants' factual knowledge.
3. To activate the participants during the Course as the Multiple Choice questions used in most of the tests were constructed by one half of the participants for the others, and vice versa.

From the participants critique and evaluation of the Course, it became evident that the modern pedagogical principles involved and the group dynamics were felt as a worthwhile experience for most of the participants.

The participants showed maximum interest on principles and techniques for the practice of psychopharmacology. Half of the fellows suggested that new Courses take place in developing countries, the other half that as the present one it should take place in a developed country.

The participants gave high ratings for the Course relevance to their own clinical and teaching activities, lower ratings for research and administration.

The participants suggested that WHO should take a lead:

1. To extend the network for information on psychopharmaca, both on their beneficial action and on their adverse effect.
2. To stimulate and coordinate research in psychopharmacology and biological psychiatry.
3. To arrange training for young research workers in these fields.
4. To provide more travelling fellowships for these purposes.
5. To provide financial aid for collaborative research.

It has been agreed between WHO and the Danish teaching staff to repeat the Course in the spring of 1974, and in closing I can say on behalf of the Danish teaching staff that we, at least, learnt a lot from such a Course.

O.J.R., Psychochemistry Institute, Rigshospitalet, 9 Blegdamsvej, DK-2100 Copenhagen, Denmark

TRAINING MODELS IN PSYCHOPHARMACOLOGY

J. J. LOPEZ IBOR and J. J. LOPEZ-IBOR ALIÑO

Department of Psychiatry, University of Madrid

It is strange that the technical aspects of the teaching of psychopharmacology have until the present been neglected. We do not mean pharmacology or biochemistry, but rather clinical psychopharmacology.

Psychotherapeutic methods, starting with the attempts of systematization of psychoanalysis, have shown themselves to be eager to technify their activities, which has given rise to the birth of the various schools. Each one was born of a more or less explicit concept of man and the patient, from which therapeutic activity is deduced almost immediately. Each school has its methods and the teachings they propose are based on very simple postulates. The first is the acceptance of a model of the patient or disease to be treated; the second, to become acquainted with the techniques through *learning* and *training* (learning and training being the most important bases of every school). FREUD, in his early days, gave more importance to the former (learning), so much that according to ZUTT, in 1905 he refused to accept one of BONHOEFFER's students on the excuse that his methods, as all technology, could be learned through his publications. Later on, it is well known that training became the axis of psychoanalysis, and, therefore, of psychotherapy. Training is what endows psychotherapeutic schools with their raison d'être, converting their members into students.

Psychopharmacotherapy has a different background. Starting with more empirical origins, it has been expanding, but not without strong resistance and inspite of many misunderstandings. One of these tends to minimize the influence it has had in the psychiatric revolution of the last few decades. It is obvious that the progress of a science such as psychiatry and more so that of its clinical problems, cannot be carried out exclusively along one line. Occupational therapies, group or individual psychotherapy, and sociological and political influences have modified methods, but they would have all been insufficient without the new drugs. Occupational therapy has existed for many centuries, not just since TUKE's time. It is likely that it was higly developed in Spanish insane asylums during the 18th century, according to PINEL himself. Psychotherapy is as old as humanity itself, and is perhaps the foremost and most-often used therapeutic weapon up until a few centuries ago. Social and political factors were not as ominous as FOUCAULT has suggested, who was barely aware of the situation outside France and Germany. Suffice is to read the founding proceedings of the first insane asylum of the Western world in Valencia in 1452 and compare it to the WHO declaration; or to the Mental Health Act regarding the mentally ill.

On the other hand, psychopharmacology has had an extraordinary success, to the point that any illness, syndrome or symptom is a candidate for it, at times with little discrimination. Its evolution has been analogous to that of psychoanalytic psychotherapy, but with a fundamental difference. Freud began with hysteria and ended by applying psychoanalysis to all human affairs — pathological, those that were less so, private and social affairs. Chlorpromazine was first applied to a group of schizophrenics and today practically any situation or conflict would seem to offer possibilities for psychotropic drugs. Psychopharmacology and psychotherapy are applied in each case in a prolonged and lasting manner. We know when both begin, but many volumes have been written on how to end them, and often this fundamental decision is left up to the patient (lithium therapy is an exception; according to our present knowledge, it should last indefinitely).

However, there is a great difference between pharmacotherapy and psychotherapy in this aspect to which we refer, and which has been wisely pointed out by Szasz in the case of psychoanalysis. This is a technique equally applied to all types of patients. The question arises only whether the client is or is not susceptible to analysis, not even if he is ill or what his distrubances might be. And even more, Szasz even said that the first question should not even arise.

Psychopharmacotherapy, inspite of its enormous field of action and diffusion, none of which is limited inspite of our efforts, requires a much finer discrimination than psychoanalysis.

Thus we can understand how psychopharmacological training imposes new demands on the teaching of psychiatry. The difficulties are even greater in schools (such as the American ones) which have formerly followed a fundamentally psychotherapeutically oriented course.

The new psychopharmacological demands first arise in the problems of *differential diagnoses*.

At the beginning of this period, Freyhan saw this when he postulated the existence of some "target symptoms". Although today it is difficult to maintain this concept within the limited context suggested by the author, it did serve to point out the need for a precise differential diagnosis before beginning psychopharmacological treatment. This is one of the paths that has had most success in recent investigation from the most simple symptom scales to multinational studies with standardized rating scales. The problem of the disparity of diagnostic criteria and the studies originated are fundamentally influenced by the impact of psychopharmacology on the practice of psychiatry. On the other hand there is no doubt, that certain psychological and psychopathological studies (Beck, Hamilton, etc.) have been motivated by the consequences of the action of some psychotropic drugs. And we could add that the evolution of manic depressive psychoses is better understood today precisely because lithium has a favorable effect on its course, and because of the need for a more precise evaluation.

But we feel that this path is today followed with inadequate instruments. The majority of symptom rating scales are based on an insufficient psychopathological analysis and a merely statistical evaluation criteria. Thus Hamilton states that the most characteristic symptom of depression (as it is the most frequent) according to his studies, is lack of appetite. The differential diagnosis in psychiatry must be taken into a broader perspective than the merely syndromatic or that of classification. Therapeutic directions are not only based on the diagnosis of a disease, syndrome or symptom; but rather on a more holistic evaluation using a widely-spread expression. Tellenbach says that in depressions one cannot describe symptoms but rather "phenomena", all of which are derived from a disturbed totality. Lopez-Ibor points out that the so-called primary symptoms of schizophrenia are all somewhat primary — that is, we can see in all of them a common disturbance which is a reflection of the break-down of psychic life, which is characteristic of what we call schizophrenia. That is to say, it is not enough to point out the existence of an hallucination and propose the method of treatment with hallucinolytic drugs, since such abstractions, as much as they are dressed up in the magic of figures and statistical analyses, only remove us from clinical reality. The problem of the classification of depressions has not found in these approaches a satisfactory solution since the problem is not properly put. Nor is there a place in them for the new aspects of masked depressions, or affective equivalents which, according to our experience and that of others, constitute the majority of depressions.

C. A. H. WATTS, a British general practitioner, has shown how only a minimal part of depressions are treated by psychiatrists and calls this the "iceberg" phenomenon. We then must ask ourselves seriously if the "symptoms" we find in our patients are truly characteristic of the disease or if in the course of the years we will not have to broaden our perspectives. Something similar occurs with schizophrenia, although here, for reasons too complex to go into here, some aspects are accentuated. This is fundamental in the relationship between psychopharmacology and other therapeutic methods, especially rehabilitation. Here, too, the new drugs oblige us to modify certain points of view. For example, we have used long acting neuroleptics in chronic residual patients and have observed more beneficial effects than in similar patients only treated with ergotherapeutic methods. This makes us ask ourselves if the residual states are not so different from the more "active" psychopathological states; that is, if in them there is not also a form of activity. Thus we find it more important to study in our patients those factors which contribute to their chronic state and the means of intercepting this evolution, even by using psychotropic drugs.

In the field of neuroses, the problems are even greater. By now no one dares to doubt the influence of drugs in their evolution inspite of what is considered their psychodynamic origin. At times it is said, though not in a convincing way, that medicines hide or mask symptoms (this is also said of schizophrenia), thus impeding a true cure.

Without denying that one form of abusing psychopharmacology is precisely that of placing a "chemical straight jacket" on patients and avoiding reflection and taking care of them, this type of criticism is diminishing. In the so-called neurotic or reactive depressions the problem arises in a very clear way before our eyes. Years ago our clinical experience led us to conclude that monoamine oxidase inhibitors were quite effective and that precisely against their supposed thymeretic effect, they were powerful anxiolytics. The passing years have confirmed our viewpoints, which we have published many times. In the United States, in recent times, there has been a new wave of usage of this type of drugs, which has freed itself of its bad reputation of the past, perhaps due to satisfactory results achieved in other branches of medicine. We should ask ourselves why some medicines that have a well-known pharmacological effect on the physiopathology of depressions as we understand it today, are more effective in those forms of depressions in which the majority of psychiatrists deny their physiological basis.

These considerations help us to understand how to approach our teaching of psychopharmacology and above all how a psychiatric and medical preparation is an indispensable requisite, and maintains a highly critical spirit in its use and in the evaluation of our results.

In the Institute of Neuropsychiatric Research, first, and later at the Clinical University Hospital of Madrid, we have placed great insistence on therapeutics for mentally-ill patients through chemotropic treatments that have given extraordinary results. The doctors' direct clinical experience is the basic requisite for the formation and evaluation of results.

We place great stress on the need for seeing the patients at least twice a day, once in the morning and again in the afternoon, and exchanging opinions in a daily meeting with the rest of the team members (other doctors, nurses, assistants, psychologists, occupational therapists) and even with the patient's family. The exchange of opinions in these institutions takes place every day, and any discrepancy must be studied, evaluated and adequately cleared up. In some cases the study is completed with the use of rating scales, not because we consider them indispensable, but rather because they are tacitly required in all scientific publications and we would be shirking our duty if we did not use them. In this way we have tested active treatments intravenously of tricyclic antidepressives and also monoamine oxidase inhibitors and neuroleptics with surprising results and a great margin of safety as well as with great benefit for training doctors. Psychopharmacological therapy has reached such a point in our services that we have hired nurses from surgical teams, with no psychiatric training, to work with us on a daily basis. We have had one great surprise which we had almost expected: the patients feel cared for as patients and not guinea pigs, always with analogous ideas, in their own psychological intimacy, by nurses, social workers, etc., who possess a superficial training in these problems. The psychotherapeutic action is always added to the psychiatric action, and in our case it can be used in a more liberated and serene form. Another advantage we have had is a greater understanding on the part of the patients' families and freedom of action and trust on their part. We thus see that psychopharmacological training amongst us has all but a unilateral character.

Naturally enough, the instruction of clinical psychopharmacology is completed by theoretical courses in biochemistry and pharmacology which help us to understand, although only on a partial basis, the mechanisms of action.

The results are so clear and obvious that we have initiated a third phase in the training of psychopharmacologial treatment, which consists in extending their use to other hospital departments which are themselves full of patients who should be psychiatrically treated, and created mobile psychiatric and psychosomatic units at the Clinical Hospital of the University of Madrid. This allows the doctors and also future general practitioners to understand therapeutic possibilities of which they were ignorant in the past.

There are not yet enough psychiatrists in those countries in which their number is greater to treat patients who should really be considered psychiatric cases. In such cases, general practitioners should be able to handle minor psychopharmacological problems and be adequately prepared to do so.

The same thing will occur to another degree with clinics for internal medicine, surgery and other specialties. This experience has not occurred only in our country; working with a large group of well-prepared psychiatrists and psychiatric collaborators, we have had the opportunity of observing this at the same time in other countries, not only in Europe, but also in South America.

J.J.L.I., Department of Psychiatry, University of Madrid, Avenida Nueva Zelanda No. 78, Madrid 35, Spain

A COMPUTER PROGRAM TO ASSIST INDEPENDENT STUDY OF THE CLINICAL USE OF PSYCHOTROPIC DRUGS

D. J. SMELTZER, W. KNOPP, D. L. HUNTER, R. MAKO and F. M. SMELTZER

*Department of Psychiatry of the Ohio State University, Columbus, Ohio,
University of Minnesota and University of Missouri*

THE COMPUTER AS A "MEDICAL EDUCATOR"

Modern electronic digital computers are rapidly finding application in both clinical medicine and medical education. In 1970, the Ohio State University College of Medicine offered entering medical students the option of obtaining their pre-clinical medical education through an Individual Study Program (ISP). One of the novel features in this approach is that the computer does the routine chore of guiding each student's studies, freeing faculty time for individual student needs and enhancing faculty effectiveness by providing updated feedback on individual student performance. Despite the relatively smaller number of faculty involved, the students in the ISP were found to learn the required material as effectively and as quickly as the students in the traditional curriculum.

Encouraged by the success of the ISP, we decided to experiment with computer-assisted study methods to teach the increasing number of students requiring clinical training in psychiatry without increasing the number of faculty members involved. However, our proposal introduced several problems not encountered by the ISP. For one, the nature of the student-computer interaction would have to be considerably different. The ISP used the computer to help *assess* the student's knowledge and understanding, while we hoped to use it to *increase* student knowledge directly. Moreover, the ISP material was basically *objective* and *factual*, though highly complicated; our material included a *subjective* goal, namely development of sound clinical judgment. A second concern was the heterogeneity of our student population, requiring computer programs that could adjust to the level of clinical experiences of the individual student.

After consideration of the difficulties involved, we decided that we would attempt our own innovation in medical education, namely *computer-assisted clinical training*. We decided to limit the material to "what every physician ought to know about psychotropic drugs," and that our primary audience should be medical students and non-psychiatric physicians.

---

*) The authors gratefully acknowledge the assistance of The Ohio State University Computer Assisted Instruction Center, and partial financial support from the Samuel J. Roessler Memorial Medical Scholarship Fund and the Psychiatric Research Foundation of Columbus.

The Computer as a "Tutor" in Clinical Psychopharmacology

The student-computer interaction resembles closely the interaction that would occur between the student and a human tutor. The student is instructed to read two brief papers, which are simply introductions to psychopharmacotherapy in outline form. After reading the assignments, the student makes an appointment to meet his "tutor".

To the student, his "tutor" looks like an electric typewriter. These terminals are quite inexpensive, and since standard telephone lines are used to connect them to the computer memory, they can be located in places readily accessible to the students. After making the telephone connection with the computer, the student identifies himself and requests the program on psychopharmacology. The computer then initiates a conversation with the student by operating the typewriter. Once he has begun, the student is free to stop whenever he wishes, and each time he returns the instruction is resumed at the point at which the previous session ended.

The tutor begins his instruction by asking a simple introductory question which the student should be able to answer from his reading. Following the student's response, the tutor reinforces a correct answer or patiently explains the error in an incorrect answer. He then begins presenting new material to the student. Interspersed through this material are various questions — some are easy, some are fairly difficult, and some will usually require the student to guess. After each question, the student is congratulated for a correct answer or provided explanation about an incorrect one. Just as a human tutor would do, the computer is able to take into account all of the student's previous answers and such other variables as the amount of hesitation before replying. The tutoring thus quickly becomes individualized to the student, so that experienced students spend a minimal amount of time on familiar topics, and inexperienced students are given much more detailed information.

TABLE 1

Only one category of neuroleptic side effects appears to be unequivocally "dose-dependent", namely the extrapyramidal reactions. The frequency and severity of these side effects is directly related to the relative antipsychotic potency of the drugs *and* to the actual dosage of whichever drug is used. The remaining categories of side effects are more or less *"dose-independent."* Just as the term implies, the likelihood of occurrence of these complications is generally not related closely to the actual dosage of the neuroleptic drug. These side effects occur with *decreasing* frequency relative to the antipsychotic potency of the drugs. In other words, they are relatively *most* likely to occur with a *low* potency neuroleptic, *less* likely with an *intermediate* potency drug, and *least* likely with a *high* potency drug. We will be discussing each group of these side effects in detail later. Here is a list of the general categories:

1. cardiovascular complications
2. peripheral autonomic side effects
3. "endocrine-like" effects
4. potentiation of epileptic seizures
5. hypersensitivity reactions
6. sedation

Since the cardiovascular complications may be life-threatening to some patients, we ought to discuss them first. Often you will want to select an intermediate or high potency neuroleptic in order to avoid these problems for a high-risk patient. There are three of these conditions which occur often enough to warrant remembering.

Please try to name one of the three. A good guess is appropriate.

*****

Table 1 shows part of the discussion on neuroleptic drugs. The student has by now learned the names of all the drugs and the concept of "relative antipsychotic potency." The tutor is explaining that this concept provides a convenient method for classifying the drugs according to effects and side effects. The student has learned, for example, that sedation is characteristic of the low potency neuroleptics, and that extrapyramidal reactions are more likely to occur with the high potency ones.

The row of five asterisks after the second paragraph indicates that the student in now expected to respond to the question asked — in this case, to make a guess about the principal cardiovascular effects of neuroleptics. The computer, being much more patient than a human tutor, will wait as long as necessary for the student to read the material and make his response. When he is ready, the student types his response on the line next to the five asterisks. As you see in Table 2, the first guess of the student was incorrect. The tutor comments that it was incorrect and gives a subtle hint (the word "paradoxical"), then waits for another guess from the student.

TABLE 2

***** they elevate blood pressure
Incorrect.
Although a few cases of paradoxical hypertension have been reported, these are extremely rare. Please try again.
*****

The next response of this student (Table 3) indicates that he missed the hint, and demonstrates one of the ways he is able to ask for assistance. After receiving a clearly labelled hint, the student is now able to state one of the three correct answers to the question asked. Following this (Table 4), the tutor discusses the answer proposed by the student in some detail, emphasizing the clinically relevant considerations about neuroleptic-induced hypotension. The discussion then continues so that the other correct answers, electrocardiographic changes and ventricular arrhythmias, are presented to the student.

TABLE 3

***** Please give me a hint.
HINT: One of these problems is often manifested by dizziness or "light-headedness."
*****

TABLE 4

***** hypotension
Correct!
Hypotension is a fairly common side effect of especially the low potency neuroleptics, and can be a concern if the patient has cardiovascular disease. It is especially common following parenteral administration of the drug. For example, intramuscular injection of 25 milligrams of chlorpromazine may cause a decrease of 15% in systolic blood pressure, often with compensatory tachycardia.
Postural or orthostatic hypotension, usually with reflex tachycardia, is a very common side effect, especially if antidepressant medication is being given simultaneously. While it is seldom serious or life-threatening in itself, the faintness or light-headedness experienced by the patient when he rises suddenly from a sitting or lying position may cause him to fall and injure himself. Some patients are sufficiently disturbed by this to become resistive to taking the medication.
Some degree of tolerance to the hypotensive effect of the drug usually develops after several weeks, but orthostatic hypotension may persist indefinitely.

Table 5 shows another form of assistance the student can request any time he wishes. The student needed and requested a definition of an unfamiliar term, "akathisia," and was immediately given a concise definition which emphasizes the importance of the term in relation to the subject being studied.

TABLE 5

***** define akathisia

DEFINITION: *akathisia:*
An uncontrollable restlessness, often manifested by continual shuffling of feet or pacing up and down. A common *extrapyramidal* side effect of certain psychotropic drugs. It may be mis-diagnosed as a hyperactive exacerbation of the psychosis or as some other form of anxiety, and the medication erroneously raised.

A final section of the course has been partially implemented, and Table 6 shows part of a typical problem. The tutor has "assigned a patient" to the student for treatment. Of course, the variety of possible responses from the student is immense, and the tutor must be able to make intelligent, instructive comments about virtually any possibility. There are many acceptable answers to these problems, and after the student has proposed one the tutor discusses it and contrasts it with various other possibilities. The student is then presented with subsequent information about his patient — for example, the patient may develop a side effect to the treatment, or might not respond to what appears to be a reasonable treatment. The student thus "follows his patient" just as a real clinician would do, and hopefully acquires something similar to "clinical experience" by this method. These problems have elicited enthusiastic responses from our students, many of whom have commented that "I feel almost as if I'm treating a real patient."

TABLE 6

Your patient is a 53-year-old white married woman. Her problems apparently began two years ago when the last of her children moved out of town, and have become progressively more serious. Her husband describes her as being "very nervous" and says she spends most of the day pacing, fidgeting, and getting little done. She has come to you only because of the gentle but firm insistence of her husband, and seems to be convinced that you can't help her because "nobody cares what happens to me." Her husband, however, seems to be a warm, loving person who really does care about her.
A complete medical workup reveals no obvious somatic difficulties, although the patient complains of constant fatigue, poor appetite, and unhappy dreams. Her speech is somewhat slow, and she frequently pauses for long intervals, especially while discussing her children. She seems to believe that her children have all moved away because "I wasn't a good enough mother to them." There is no evidence of hallucinations or suicidal ideation, although the patient admits that she sometimes feels that she wants to die.
A recent vacation in Puerto Rico with her husband did not seem to elevate her mood. She had tried working at a part-time job, but gave it up after several weeks because she was "too nervous." How will you treat this patient?
*****

A wide variety of persons have now taken this course — medical students, psychiatry residents, experienced psychiatrists, several nurses, and a class of pharmacy students. Despite the diversity of educational and clinical backgrounds of all these people, each has reported that his experience with the computer was at an appropriate level of instruction. Thus, we have apparently been successful in our goal of making the program modify itself to the level of experience of the student.

Validation Problems

Our attention is now devoted to several "validation problems," both short range and long range. One concerns the content and functioning of the computer program. We have approached this "short range content validation problem" pragmatically by asking for assistance from a number of experienced psychiatrists. Each of these clinicians took the entire computer course, and provided deliberately incorrect or ambiguous replies to many of the questions. This not only enabled us to locate and correct a number of minor errors and misleading statements, but it also identified those issues which are open to different points of view among clinicians.

The "long range content validation problem" is being approached differently. We recognize that this course will require frequent up-dating, just as a good professor will continually update his lectures. Both literature review and monitoring of student performance are constantly underway; the computer assists us by routinely providing detailed analysis of student responses and performance, so that we can identify and correct sections whose educational value change or which cause misunderstanding or confusion.

The more crucial type of validation problem, however, concerns the value of this course as an adjunct to clinical training. We are now designing research to answer such questions as these: Do students perform better as clinicians after taking our course than they would otherwise have done? Does their attitude toward psychotropic drugs and toward psychiatric problems change? Is there in fact any measurable advantage to the use of this program as far as the students are concerned? (We feel there certainly is an advantage to the faculty.)

Some Comments About Development of the Program and Future Plans

This program described above was designed and implemented by a team consisting of a psychiatrist experienced in psychopharmacologic research, a computer scientist, and a number of medical students. Although the entire team planned the overall strategy, the medical students actually composed most of the content. We feel that this is a significant advantage, since these students may be better able than the professors to perceive the educational status and needs of other medical students. In the course of their work, these students had access to a number of basic scientists and clinicians, and consequently benefited directly by acquiring an extensive knowledge of practical psychopharmacology.

We have already begun developing similar programs on psychosomatic medicine and human sexuality, and are also adapting the psychopharmacology program for nurses' training, so optimistic do we feel about the potential uses of the computer in clinical training and continuing medical education.

Summary

Modern computers are producing innovations in medical education. The authors have developed a computer program to teach applied psychopharmacology to medical students, non-psychiatric physicians, and others. The program first simulates a human tutor conversing with a single student about psychotropic drugs, covering such topics as drug selection, effects, and side effects. After the student has learned the basic principles, he is then presented with hypothetical patients, and the program simulates an experienced psychiatrist supervising the student.

The program is now being used as a regular part of the clinical training curriculum in psychiatry with apparently good success. A strategy has been implemented to assure ongoing verification of its correctness, completeness, and educational validity in relation to changes in medical education and in the science of psychopharmacology. Research is also in progress to study changes in student performace and attitudes resulting from this novel form of teaching.

D.J.S., Department of Psychiatry, Ohio State University, Columbus, Ohio, U.S.A.

DRUG EFFECTS IN NORMALS: CORRELATIONS WITH PHARMACOLOGICAL AND CLINICAL EFFECTS

Chairmen: H. Heimann and F. Hoffmeister

Associate chairman: E. Bechgaard

METHODOLOGICAL PRINCIPLES FOR PSYCHOBIOLOGICAL COMPARISON OF THE EFFECTS OF PSYCHOTROPIC DRUGS

H. HEIMANN

Department of Research in Psychopathology, The Psychiatric Clinic, University of Lausanne

Psychotropic drugs have an influence on animal and human behavior that is both temporary and dosage-dependent. Their effects can, therefore, be demonstrated in principle at several psychobiological levels of organization: from influencing molecular-biological processes at the cell membrane, down to the modification of specific inter-actions between living organisms. For this reason, the investigation of the effects of psychotropic drugs is necessarily inter-disciplinary — in a far more comprehensive sense than, for example, the pharmacology of specific organ functions. A pharmacology of behavior, therefore, encounters special difficulties resulting from the necessary specialization of research, and the differing degrees of complexity of the phenomena under investigation.

Indeed, the first step in an investigation using scientific methodology, i.e., valid evidence of qualitative and quantitative differences, in effect, confronts us with a multiplicity of findings that are difficult to compare. The pharmacologist derives this evidence from animal experimental models of isolated behavior, the pharmacopsychologist, from a number of experimental psychological parameters; the clinician, from therapeutic intervention in more or less sharply delineated psychopathological symptoms and syndromes. For the therapeutic management of syndromes of psychic disturbance, the relevance of an effect observed in isolated behavior-models in animal experimentation, is controversial — for the majority of these models — and is repeatedly challenged by more recent findings. Recall, for example, the case of Clozapine (2) which discredits the animal experimental models of anti-psychotic effects, which had, prior to that time, been accepted as valid.

The pharmacopsychologist occupies a middle position between the two exponents, the pharmacologist and the clinician — because he investigates, in the healthy human individual, the effects of psychotropic drugs, using experimental methods, i.e., to a certain extent isolated — *but human behavioral models*. As a result, he is in a position to demonstrate factors that influence the psychopharmacological effect on human behavior, for example, those of the setting and of the personality. One could ascribe to him, therefore, a mediating role and he might, perhaps, be in a position to develop in close cooperation with the clinician and the pharmacologist, the theoretical models of the psychopharmacological effect on the road toward a *general theory* of the psychopharmacology of behavior. Some steps in this direction were already taken with EYSENCK's drug-postulate. It was, perhaps, only because of certain theoretical weaknesses (as analyzed, e.g., by LEGEWIE —8) that the EYSENCK postulate has not found a corresponding response in the other disciplines.

In the hope of promoting the inter-disciplinary cooperation sketched here, we have in this symposium placed in the forefront the effects of psychotropic drugs on the healthy human individual, as point of reference of pharmacological and clinical modes of approach. In successive order, the neurophysiologist, the neuropharmacologist, the pharmacopsychologist and the clinician will discuss from their viewpoints, the problems of the effect of psychotropic drugs. We invite an inter-disciplinary discussion which, hopefully, clarifies certain theoretical and practical research problems that would have to be attacked in a common effort. By way of introduction, I trust you will allow me to make a few preliminary remarks concerning methodology. Following that, on the basis of an example, a brief analysis of the various levels of complexity encountered at the interface between physiological and psychological measuring techniques. Using this example, it is, in my opinion, possible to show how — from a theoretical point of departure, we can come to grips with — and bring into relationship, phenomena of different complexity.

PRELIMINARY COMMENTS ON METHODOLOGY

In the theme of our symposium, mention is made of "correlations" between pharmacological, pharmacopsychological and clinical effects. Here, one can only understand "correlations" in the sense of an analogous relationship between changes in different reference-systems which, additionally, becomes even more complicated by the different complexity of these reference-systems. When, for example, the pharmacologist influences "anxiety" in an isolated animal-behavior model, then he exposes himself to anthropomorphism because he uses for animal behavior the same terminology which, in the case of human behavior, is replete with very specific, many-faceted meanings — from a clinical point of view. When one regards only the purely *physiological* aspect, then in both animal and human behavior a general activation can be demonstrated in neurophysiological, vegetative and endocrine systems. By contrast, when we shift our focus of attention to the *behavioral* level, it is merely by analogy — and this, on the basis of human understanding of self — that we can interpret a particular behavioral pattern as "anxiety". This state of affairs is the basis for the great interest that physiological parameters have for the clinician. Holding forth the promise of a direct comparison with pharmacological data, these parameters can be related to general, theoretical models which, in turn, have a bearing on the prediction of clinical outcomes.

Taking refuge in such general and fundamental relationships of physiological functional-systems abstracts from the differentiated clinical-psychopathological experience wherein the psychiatrist in the "doctor-patient" relationship, encounters the phenomenon of "anxiety." For the clinical experience, "anxiety" is essentially bound up with the subjective aspect related to a situation with specific meaning-content. According to our own investigations, an evaluation based on purely *external* criteria of behavior and expression is quite uncertain: the criteria for a common observation-language are still, for the most part, non-existent (4).

Let us pursue this problem on the basis of another well-known example, i.e., *sedation* by means of a sedative drug. In the clinical reference-system we first encounter verbalizations of the patient that are *individually* colored. One reports that he cannot concentrate under the effect of sedative drug; another, that he feels fatigued and knocked-out;

a third, that he experiences his body as heavy and burdensome. From a psychodynamic viewpoint, this individual expression can contain essential information. For in all likelihood, it is not accidental when one experiences sedation as a bodily event or as decrease of one's mental performance. The clinician is accustomed to integrate this subjective multiplicity of possible modes of experiencing, and to categorize it within the observable decrease of psychomotor activity. At the same time, a reduction in complexity as well as loss of information takes place, leading from the individual — to a more *general* viewpoint. A reduction of psychomotor activity induced by a sedative drug is recognized by both the clinician as well as the pharmacologist as characterizing sedation.

From a pharmacopsychological standpoint, i.e., from the differentiating investigation of sedatives using quantitative methods, the individual, subjective aspect is too special and accidental. On the other hand, the *global* behavior-description is too general. For human application, a differentiation of sedatives cannot be determined with reliability in either this way, or that way. By contrast, the pharmacopsychologist using quantitative methods that encompass subjective changes and parameters of performance, tries to show differential profiles of sedation. He disregards individual assertions by forcing the test-persons to project their own subjectively experienced changes onto — for example — lists of adjectives or the semantic differential. On the other hand, he is able to assess directly the effect of a sedative on performance parameters. I refer, for example, to the work of KORNETSKY (6) on the differentiation of barbiturates and chlorpromazine, and to our own investigations (5) with different types of psychotropic drugs. Pharmacopsychologically, the salient aspects of this procedure emerge, as follows:

1. One can limit the personality-specific variance by selection of a homogeneous sample. For example, after testing with the Maudsley Medical Questionnaire (MMQ) limiting the choice of test-persons to a central group that exhibits neither extremely stable nor unstable personality-traits. Similarly, the effect of situationally-related variance can be reduced by standardization of the test-situation. Thus, under such conditions a comparable differentiation of sedatives by means of several psychological tests becomes possible. In this experimental setting, the pharmacopsychologist plays an analogous role to that of the pharmacologist. By limiting himself to certain animal species of a certain age, and by rigorous standardization, the pharmacologist creates experimental conditions that permit comparison between drugs.

2. It is possible to demonstrate a personality-specific component in the sense of a differential effect of sedatives by comparison of the unstable with the stable groups of test-persons. We are especially indebted to the work-group of JANKE (7) for such investigations.

3. One can also determine the *situationally-related portion* of the variance by systematic variation of the experimental condition, e.g., through an increase in the noise level. One can even combine with the personality-specific factor, in order to assess the interactions of both components with the drug. Here, the drug and its action-profile are no longer in the foreground, but rather, specific factors of the psychopharmacological effect on behavior as determined by the substrate and the setting.

The relationship of personality dimensions, especially of neuroticism, with the level of arousal as measured by the EEG — and with their effects on mental performance has only recently been demonstrated in a most impressive manner by BECKER-CARUS (3). These investigations show that probably, essential differences in personality-dimensions (assessable by means of corresponding questionnaires) determine differences in performance-behavior. Moreover, that the level of activation which varies in a personality-specific way is an indicator of performance results to be expected.

All of these pharmacopsychological and psychobiological findings underscore the importance of the level of activation for the effect of psychotropic drugs. In my opinion these findings have the potential of bridging the findings of the pharmacologist and the clinician. LEGEWIE, (8) modifying EYSENCK's "drug-postulate" has correctly emphasized the importance of activation and its relationship to performance and subjective changes. Because the pharmacologist "homogenizes" the level of activation of his experimental animals in a specific and verifiable manner — by a certain standardization of his experimental conditions — he obtains relatively uniform findings compared with clinical data. Clinically, however, we are probably dealing with an abundance of different levels of activation which we can define only by approximation, by means of psychopathological description. It is possible that precisely these differences between patients provide an explanation of paradox-effects and therapeutic failures.

PSYCHOBIOLOGICAL MODEL OF SEDATION

A pharmacopsychological experiment conducted with 20 normal testpersons, using a sedative, should exemplify the importance of the level of activation for influencing the subjective appraisal of one's own well-being and mental performance. Our test-persons belonged to the middle group on the neuroticism-dimension of the MMQ. They were tested individually on several mornings: prior to, and 2 hours following administration of placebo, 20 mg, and 60 mg of a sedative. The dosage of 60 mg was repeated to verify consistency of the findings. On every occasion before psychological testing, 2 electroencephalograms were made under resting-conditions: with open-eyes, and with closed-eyes — each recording, of 4 min duration (Mingograph Elema-Schönander. F_3—C_z, F_4—C_z, O_1—P_z, O_2—P_z).

Fig. 1 shows means and standard deviations in the two factors, "energetic" and "tired"-"inactive"-"indifferent", from Lorr's "List of Adjectives." Under 20 mg, no significant *subjective* changes are found. Under the two 60 mg dosages, however, they occur consistently.

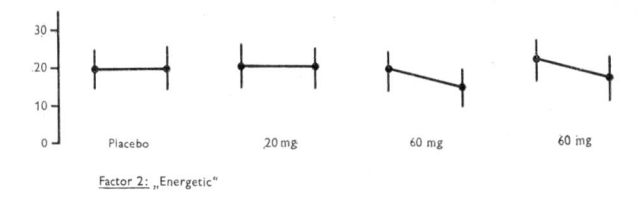

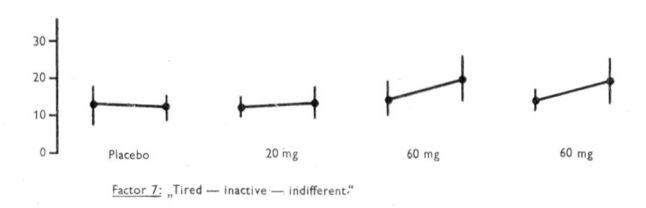

Fig. 1. List of adjectives from LORR-DASTON-SMITH effect of a sedative drug.

In the performance tests (Meili's Test of Concentration; Two-Plates-Tapping, and the Minnesota Rate of Manipulation), the results are analogous: with 20 mg of the sedative, no significant changes; with 60 mg, significant reductions which are, however, less consistent than in the subjective area.

Evaluation of the electroencephalograms was done on a semi-quantitative basis. Under blind-conditions, the first and last 30 seconds of each recording were studied with regard to the presence or absence of the following four signs of psychic relaxation: 1. increase in alpha-waves per unit of time, 2. greater regularity in alpha-rhythm, 3. increased amplitude of alpha-waves, 4. shift of alpha-waves into the frontal region. Additionally, three signs of the transition into the first stage of sleep: 1. disappearance of the alpha-rhythm, 2. appearance of theta-waves, 3. appearance of beta-spindles.

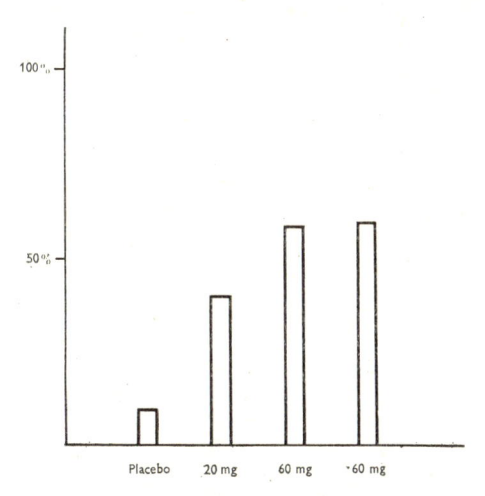

Fig. 2. EEG "eyes-open." 4 min. recording, the first and last 30 seconds positive signs of relaxation in %.

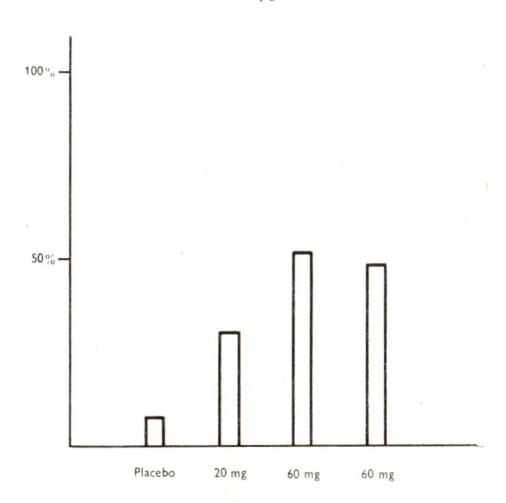

Fig. 3. EEG "eyes-closed." Only subjects with positive alpha rhythm in basal EEG 4 min. recording, the first and last 30 seconds, positive signs of transition into the first stage of sleep in %.

Fig. 2 shows the results for the recording condition, "eyes-open": both under 20 mg as well as under 60 mg, signs of relaxation are found, significantly, more often ($2\alpha \leq .01$). In the EEG, placebo differs from 20 mg, and 20 mg differs from 60 mg. In the case of the 60 mg application on successive days, no difference was observed.

Fig. 3 shows the situation for the recording procedure, "eyes-closed": here the frequency of signs of the transition into the first stage of sleep, differ significantly between placebo, 20 mg and 60 mg ($2\alpha \leq .01$).

One might well argue that the electroencephalogram is intrinsically a more sensitive

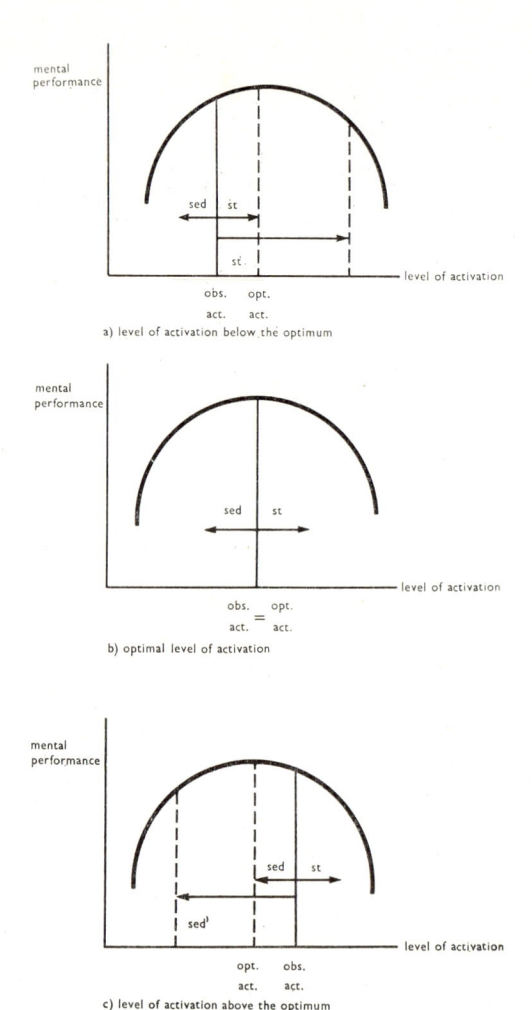

Fig. 4. Performance and activation inverted U-chaped relationship according to the principle of YERKES and DODSON. Effects of a psychostimulant and a sedative drug. Relationship between initial level of activation and effects of various dosages. opt. act. — optimal level of activation; obs. act. — observed level of activation; st. — stimulant drug; sed. — sedative drug; st'—stimulant drug in overdose; sed' — sedative drug in overdose.

method of demonstrating the sedative effect of a given preparation than the method of psychological testing. In my opinion, however, this would be a premature conclusion, for according to the law of YERKES and DODSON (10) on the relationship between the level of activation and mental performance we must consider the level of activation of the test-person *before* the administration of the sedative.

Fig. 4 illustrates the "picture" which can be inferred from the law of YERKES and DODSON for the action of sedatives and stimulants. Between level of activation, and mental performance, there exists a curvilinear, i.e., an inverted U-shaped relationship and we may assume that our test-persons are distributed around the optimal level of activation. The *small* sedative-action of 20 mg, which, in the EEG is uniformly reflected in an increase in relaxation and transition into the first stage of sleep, leads in overactivated test-persons to improved performance. In test-persons who are below the optimum, it leads to worsened performance. Thus, in the psychological procedures, these two effects, i.e., improved performance in overactivation and worsened performance in underactivation, cancel each other out within the group. However, 60 mg which induce a stronger shift in the level of activation lead, in the majority of test-persons, to reduced performance.

The greater complexity on the *psychological level* can, in this case, be reconciled with the aid of the principle of YERKES and DODSON and by taking into account the initial situation. The inverted U-shaped relationship between level of activation and psychic performance has been demonstrated in numerous studies. Moreover, according to MURRAY (9), it also applies to the relationship between speech-rate and anxiety. Beyond that, however, it is also an inherent *neuro-physiological* factor as shown by ANDERSEN and ANDERSSON (1) in the genesis of spindle-activity in the EEG. These authors postulate variable thalamic generators which, in the presence of a certain amount of input in the cortex, lead to rhythmic activity. Both a decrease, as well as an increase in input, lead to de-synchronization. Thus, we have here a common principle of regulation built upon the organization of central nervous structures and functional-systems. This principle is operant on different levels of the biological organization. It could also take on meaning for pharmacotherapy in the clinic, because — for therapeutic purposes — the clinician has, so far, paid too little attention to the *level of activation* of the individual patient. We must make the reservation, however, that while the EEG is an essential measure for the level of activation, it is not the only measure; and, furthermore, that "activation", according to more recent psychobiological investigations, is not a uniform measure. Nevertheless, it appears to me that a theoretical platform is provided here which satisfies not only the theoretical interest of the pharmacopsychologist but, might well serve as the basis for an understanding and cooperation between our various disciplines.

REFERENCES

1. ANDERSEN, P. and ANDERSSON, S. (1968) Physiological Basis of the Alpha Rhythm. Appleton-Century-Crofts, New York.
2. ANGST, J. et al. (1971) Das klinische Wirkungsbild von Clozapin (Untersuchung mit dem AMP-System). Pharmakopsychiat. **4**, 201.
3. BECKER-CARUS, Ch. (1971) Relationships between EEG, Personality and Vigilance. Electroenceph. clin. Neurophysiol. **30**, 519.
4. HEIMANN, H. (1972) Grundsätzliche Überlegungen zur erfahrungswissenschaftlichen Methodik in der Psychiatrie. Nervenarzt, **43**, 345.
5. HEIMANN, H. (1971) Wirkungsvergleich von Psychopharmaka am menschlichen Verhalten. Beitr. zur Gerichtl. Medizin, Band 28, 155.
6. KORNETSKY, C. and MIRSKY, A. F. (1965) On Certain Psychopharmacological and Physiological Differences between Schizophrenic and Normal Persons. Psychopharmacologia, **8**, 309.
7. JANKE, W. and DEBUS, G. (1968) Experimental Studies on Antianxiety Agents with Normal Subjects: Methodological Considerations and Review of the Main Effects. In: Psychopharma-

cology. A Review of Progress 1957 to 1967. Ed. by EFRON, D. H., Publ. Health Service Publication No. 1836, 205.
8. LEGEWIE, H. (1968) Persönlichkeitstheorie und Psychopharmaka. Kritische Untersuchung zu Eysencks Drogenpostulat. A. Hain, Meisenheim am Glan.
9. MURRAY, D. C. (1971) Talk, Silence, and Anxiety. Psychol. Bull. **75**, 244.
10. YERKES, R. M. and DODSON, J. D. (1908) The Relation of Strength of Stimulus to Rapidity of Habit-Formation. J. comp. Neurol. Psychol. **18**, 459.

H.H., Department of Research in Psychopathology, The Psychiatric Clinic, University of Lausanne, Switzerland

NEUROPHYSIOLOGICAL FOUNDATION OF BEHAVIOUR

W. P. KOELLA

Biological Research Laboratories, Pharmaceutical Division, CIBA-GEIGY Ltd. Basel

It is generally accepted that pharmacological substances act on specific receptors which, serving as transducers, bring about a reaction in a particular effector organ. Extending this concept to psychopharmacology, one has to postulate that drugs which affect behaviour also act through specific receptors to induce in an *organized reactive substrate* a change in activity which is the immediate cause for the change in behaviour. If this reactive substrate is the nervous system*), we implicitly acknowledge the concept of brain-mind-unity and have to accept — as a good many neurophysiologists already do (see 8) — that every pattern of behaviour, including non-overt mental aspects such as thinking, feeling, remembering, will, love, hate, gratitude, etc., is the manifestation of a particular time-space-intensity-dispositive of activity of all neurons constituting the nervous system. For the sake of identity of dimensions one may view any behavioural pattern as a composite of vectors, each of particular direction and time-dependent length (i.e. intensity), and equally view nervous activity as a composite of vectors, each one representing one neuron of particular direction (meaning a particular set of functional connections in the NS) and time-dependent length (i.e. activity of the unit). Seen in this fashion, one could state that a particular set of time-dependent behavioural vectors is the topological representation of a particular set of time-dependent neuronal vectors. To illustrate this concept while still staying within a more or less theoretical framework, one could consider first a single motor act, viz. the lifting a forepaw by a cat, or the turning of eyes to the side by a human subject. In either case movement means mobilization of muscular forces, i.e. a time-dependent activity of several muscles each representing a particular (though not necessarily constant) direction. Motor behaviour can be viewed as a particular time-dependent vector bundle of muscular forces.

As muscles do depend in their activity upon information originating in motoneurons, the above mentioned movement or time-dependent pattern of muscular vectors is the manifestation of a topologically identical time-dependent pattern of neuronal vectors in the motoneuron pool supplying the muscles involved.

Concerning the causal relations between these two sets, one could, at first, visualize

---

*) Although being aware that the "long-distance" humoral information channels, i.e. the hormonal system, is involved in behaviour regulation and modification it will not — to avoid undue complication of a story already complicated enough — be mentioned here anymore.

a unidirectional, open-loop arrangement in the sense that the neuronal activity dispositive always and exclusively *controls* behaviour. This certainly is not so, as is well demonstrated by even the simplest fragments of motor behaviour: Feedback information arising from the behaving effector organ, the muscle, itself and from other parts of the moving organism is apt to modulate the activity in the neuronal pool. Evidently, the muscular activity, i.e. behaviour, influences the activity in the neuronal pool, and one is forced to accept the fact that the set of neuronal vectors only initially, i.e. for a very small fraction of a second, is intrinsically determined and thus only initially controls behaviour. In later phases of the motor behaviour it manifests the combined influence of intrinsically and extrinsically (i.e. peripheral) originating information.

It can be assumed that the mutual relation between, or the respective weight of, the intrinsic and the extrinsic components changes in time, that it depends upon the type of behaviour and that it is subject to the additional external influences.

It appears not too far fetched to extend these same concepts to motor activities originating in, and organized in part by, the motor cortex. Again one could postulate that a particular movement seen as discrete vector bundle of muscular activities is related in its time-intensity-space structure to the vector bundle represented by the cell pool in the motor cortex. At this point it is tempting to speculate a little bit further and visualize the situation that such a "cortical" movement is planned, but that its execution is prevented either by willful suppression or say, by paralyzing the muscles. Evidently under such conditions the "thought" or plan "movement" is still present in the cortex, that is to say, the neural pattern ordinarily attending, and in its time-space pattern representing, the movement, still occurs although, due to the lack of feedback information, its actual form may deviate from the one occurring in the course of an executed movement.

If one transfers this concept to the motor activity forming speech, one could imagine that one "talks" to one-self only without uttering actual words. Thus one could hypothesize that in the Broca-Cortex there exists a neural pattern representing words which could indeed be parts of abstract thoughts, or, if one likes, some fragments of thought processes. An explanation for the fact that we can in a conscious manner observe our thought processes, that we are conscious of what we are thinking, still escapes our imagination. Still, starting out with some principles of motor activity it has been possible to develop, in a highly theoretical, speculative, and certainly most crude fashion, some lines of thought which may prove to be fruitful for later and possibly better based inquiries.

Presently, an important aspect of our speculations depends heavily on the necessity that we somehow are able to determine the neuronal activity pattern, the neuronal vector set. If we try to approach supraspinal levels of highly developed species, a solution of this problem appears impossible. In man, we have to reckon with roughly 10^{10} to 10^{12} elements, and a considerably large fraction of these would participate to constitute the vector bundles discussed above. At best we could take recordings from a few only, if we could record at all in this species. A detailed analysis of the neuronal activity pattern attending overt and/or mental behaviour is out of question.

Furthermore, our knowledge about the functional connections and thus the relations between these units is still very scarse or almost non-existent; consequently little if anything is known about the "direction" of the vectors.

Finally, if it comes to the relation between neurophysiological activity and entirely subjective aspects of behaviour like feeling, thinking, re-living through past experiences, etc., one depends for these "vectors" entirely upon verbal communications which are very unrealiable indeed and force the subject to live through again, and thus to modulate the experience. Still, in spite of these at first gaze, unsurmountable obstacles, one should not be too much discouraged from attempting to get at least some insight into behaviour-neuronal relations.

Firstly, recordings with macro-electrodes of EEG patterns, evoked potentials, and DC drifts give already a certain, though crude indication of neuronal activities.

Secondly, it is always possible to use organisms with relatively simple networks and it appears not unlikely that knowledge about the relation between behaviour and certain neuronal patterns gained from studies in such primitive subjects may serve as guide lines and models to understand and direct new investigations about such relations in more complex organisms.

Thirdly, it appears feasible to break down complex behaviours in higher organisms into simpler fragments (for instance some simple spinally organized movements such as we dealt with on the outset) and to study the neuronal-behaviour relations in such components only to try to integrate the information thus gained for more complex patterns of behaviour.

Fourthly, though one is not able to investigate with to-day's micro-electrophysiological means more than a few of a large number of neurons, it is not unlikely that some approximative conclusions about the activity pattern of the large population are possible through the employment of computer techniques for spatial and temporal inter- and extrapolation.

The extensive work in the field of the last 10 to 20 years had proven indeed that this "modest" approach with "reduced" goals is quite apt to yield important information and that we are well justified in saying that we are well on the way toward a considerably better understanding of neuronal-behavioural relations or — in short — of neuropsychology.

In the remaining parts of this chapter we shall mention and discuss a number of such observations picked almost at random to illustrate that indeed we have made some inroads.

In the preceeding part we have used the model of motor activity to develop some ideas about neuro-behavioural relations. In this connection one should mention just shortly EVARTS' older (10) and newer work (11—15) in which he describes particular neuronal activities in the motor as well as a sensory cortex attending spontaneous and learned movements of the limbs in the monkey. DE LONG (5) has succeeded in finding particular relations between unit discharge in the basal ganglia and learned movements of the limbs. His data provided "strong evidence for a role of the basal ganglia in voluntary movements". KLEMM (29) recorded the EEG and — using macroelectrodes — multiple-unit activity during movements and immobility in the rabbit. He found that hippocampal theta rhythms were triggered during movements. Coinciding with the hippocampal activity or slightly earlier there occurred phasic increases in multi-unit activity in the brain stem reticular formation.

The study of vigilance and related problems also offers some interesting aspects of neuronal-behavioural relations. It is by now very well established that for a good many types of activity, be it viz. overt (i.e. actually: motor) behavioral activity in sub-human species or be it mental activity (i.e. viz. thinking, re-experiencing past events, dreaming) in man the cerebral neo-cortex, as well as some subcortical areas and parts of the limbic system have to be in a state of activity. This active state is signalled in the first two areas by an irregular rather fast and low-amplitude pattern in the electroencephalogram. In the hippocampus the aroused state is manifested by a rather highly synchronized theta-wave pattern (19). JOUVET and JOUVET (25) have shown that the same holds true for the "dreaming" state in cats.

Although little is known yet about details of neuronal activity attending these arousal patterns, some general aspects have become clearer through the work of EVARTS (9, 10, see also 31). This author has shown that the discharge frequencies of various classes of neurons are quite different during the aroused state but that they approach each other with the transition from waking to sleep. According to EVARTS this "de-differentiation" manifests a reduction of "gradients" between the various units; thus a reduction in "information content"; a shift which indeed is compatible with the loss of consciousness. With such observation one evidently does not learn much as yet about the neuronal vectors representing particular "thought vectors" but one certainly becomes aware that "temporal collimation" of vectors is incompatible with consciousness.

Another interesting finding has recently been reported by KAMP et al. (27) who noted "beta bursts" in the EEG of the inferior frontal cortex in a psychiatric patient related probably to brief and sudden release of mental tension. The EEG of various areas of the brain seems to be an indicator of learning abilities. In two genetically different strains of rats, i.e. one the good and the other the bad learners, DOLCE et al. (6) found differences in the EEG power spectra between the two strains in the EEG's from the right sensory motor cortex. After the learning procedure, there appeared also significant differences in the EEG of the left cortex and of the dorsal hippocampus.

In connection with the EEG one should mention the sensory evoked potential which — though little is known yet about their relation to unit activity — somehow represent one aspect of cerebral activity modified by incoming information. Here it is of interest to learn about the inherent possibility for focussing one modality while the electrophysiological manifestations of other modalities are suppressed (21). Some years ago we have proposed and experimentally demonstrated a cortico-subcortico-cortical feedback system which could very well represent the mechanism responsible for this focussing phenomenon (30).

Recently VELASCO and VELASCO (41) have demonstrated a positive correlation between "significance" of sensory stimuli and amplitude of late components of sensory evoked potentials. According to DUSTMAN and BECK (7) evoked potential amplitude in man is related to intelligence although the relationship is small.

Turning now to the question of feelings, mood, and drives, one may mention first the wellknown "centers" of hunger (or better drive for eating) and satiation in the lateral and ventromedial areas respectively of the hypothalamus. Microelectrode experiments have revealed that the cells in the lateral "hunger" area are more active in the fasting animal and react with reduced firing in response to glucose (1). Quite probably the activity of this cell pool is at least in part the neurophysiological correlate of subjective hunger. It is of interest to note here that the hypothalamic areas are controlled by limbic structures (34).

From HESS' classical work (22) we know that electrical stimulation of the perifornical hypothalamic area of the cats elicits a "package-deal" of behavioural changes such as hissing, growling, snarling, piloerection, flattening of the pinnae and extreme mydriasis, as one usually sees if the feline encounters a dog. Again there can be little doubt that activation of a relatively small cell pool is in first place responsible for this behavioural change. In turn one may conclude that under natural conditions, activity of this cell pool brought about by complex afferent information, "dog", is the, or, more probably, one of the, neurophysiological correlates of rage, possibly leading to attack or flight.

SAWYER (37) noted a particular electrographic pattern in the septal area attending the terminal stages of co-habitation in rabbits. Again one can see a relation between a — as yet unknown — neuronal discharge pattern (responsible for the local EEG pattern) and sexual excitement.

In this connection one could mention also OLDS and MILNER's classical work (32) which demonstrated on the basis of self-stimulation experiments a relation between (induced) activity in certain limbic structures and pleasure.

Memory including many fringe phenomena offers further evidence of behavioural — neurophysiological correlations. Although the work of the last 15 or so years has revealed that in all probability consolidation of memory material is based on biochemical processes one cannot fail to see that at least at the "beginning" and the "end" of memory, i.e. during incorporation of fresh information and during read-out, nervous activity must play a pertinent role if what we mentioned at the out-set of this chapter — the neuronal vector bundle or spatio-temporal patterns as the basis of thought and mental process in general — should hold true.

In more general terms, it is by now well known that during the initial phases of learning there occurs a generalized activation of the cerebral cortex possibly as a generalized reaction to the "training" stimuli. In the mere advanced stages of learning the evoked activity is more and more restricted to the cortical primary projection area of the modality stimulated and the part of the motor cortex somatotopically related to the body area moving in (learned) response to the stimulus (see viz. the review of Thompson et al., 40). Halas et al. (20) have shown that preceeding the development of the localized cortical activities there appears increased unit activity in the subcortical unspecific systems. De long's work (5) could be mentioned again here which has revealed activity in the basal ganglia preceeding learned leg movements in monkeys.

Olds (33) has demonstrated that pontine and hippocampal units can be conditioned to discharge more frequently by rewarding the animal and, moreover, that this discharge can be controlled by discriminative stimuli.

While mentioning changes in activity of single neurons attending the process of "general" conditioning one should also refer to experimental evidence which indicates that even single cells may be subject to plasticity. For instance, Bureš and Burešová (3) have shown that cells of the inferior colliculus can be "conditioned" to acoustic stimuli. Ban-Ari (2) noted "spontaneous" discharges of amygdala units representing possibly traces of latent conditioned responses, as well as associations of discharge to paired stimuli. For a more detailed account the reader is referred to the review of Thompson et al. (40).

A considerable number of data obtained from man (see viz. 38, 36, 4) and animals (see viz. 35, 17, 26, 24) strongly suggest that the hippocampus (and the temporal lobe) plays a key role in the organization of engram consolidation and read-out although it probably would be wrong to state that memory has its seat in this structure. Still, during the process of training, the hippocampus reveals patterns of electrical activity — both on the macro- and micro-level — which underline the notion of the key role just mentioned. These observations are also additional examples for the general theme of this chapter. Thus, Grastyan et al. (18) found 4 to 7/sec hippocampal waves to be most pronounced in the early stages of learning whereas desynchronized patterns were characteristic later in the process of training cats. Walter and Adey (42) described in the same species maximal synchronization in the theta band during approach performance in the course of learned behaviour. Segal and co-workers (39) observed in the dentate gyrus an increase of the discharge rate of single cells in response to rewarding conditioned stimuli and a rate decrease in response to punishing stimuli. In contrast, cells of the hippocampus reacted to both types of stimuli with an increase. Although for obvious reasons only very few cells can be observed in such experiments, the data point toward characteristic patterns of activity and thus allow at least some "advanced guess" as to the "activity vectors" in these structures attending the "recall" of past experience.

Especially in the area of learning and memory, experimental data from small and relatively simple networks may prove to be invaluable for a better understanding the activity patterns paralleling behavioural patterns usually studied in larger subjects. In this connection mention should be made of the probing and excellent work of Kandel and his co-workers in Aplysia (see viz. 28) and of the beautiful experiments of Horridge (23) on "leg-position-learning" in decapitated insects.

These are just a few examples only of neurophysiological correlates of behaviour. Certainly, the observations mentioned and many others are but a beginning in our endeavour to understand the relation between behaviour and neural activity, yet a beginning which already offers some insight at least into some principles of these relations. It seems that with the presently available knowledge future research can move along in better defined directions.

May be, one reason for the still somewhat slow progress in the field can be seen in the fact that most of the investigators have been satisfied with the parallel study of behavioural and neuronal pattern. Yet, to-day the biologist should make more use of some of the modern methods of information theory, systems analysis, the mathemathics of stationary and non-stationary time series and computer techniques, just to name a few, to extract from their observations as much information as possible. As a matter of fact, entirely artificial models may prove quite helpful in furthering our understanding in this field. It has indeed been possible to construct from computer components networks of artificial neurons which behave quite similarly to neuronal networks in producing wave patterns looking strikingly akin to the alpha waves picked up from the skalp of a resting human subject (FARLEY — 16).

A better understanding of the *neurophysiology of behaviour* would at the same time further our insight into the abnormal neural patterns attending, or, in part causative to, abnormal behaviour; i.e. the pathoneurophysiology of those mental aberrations which we still must refer to as "functional psychoses". Finally, knowing at least some of the functional relations between neuronal activity and behaviour we shall stand on firmer ground if we assume — as we said at the beginning of this chapter — that psychoactive drugs must act on an organized reactive substrate, the neuronal networks. At that time, we shall be able to talk about a *neuropharmacology of behaviour* and this accomplishment would be instrumental to develop a new and better pharmacotherapy of mental disease with compounds of well defined mode and locus of action.

REFERENCES

1. ANAND, B. K., CHHINA, G. S., SHARMA, K. N., DUA, S. and SINGH, B. (1964) Activity of Single Neurons in the Hypothalamic Feeding Centers: Effect of Glucose. Amer. J. Physiol. **207**, 1146.
2. BEN-ARI, Y. and LE GAL LA SALLE, G. (1972) Plasticity at Unitary Level II. Modifications during Sensory-sensory Association Procedures. Electroenceph. clin. Neurophysiol. **32**, 667.
3. BUREŠ, J. and BUREŠOVÁ, O. (1967) Plastic Changes of Unit Activity Based of Reinforcing Properties of Extracellular Stimulation of Single Neurons. J. Neurophysiol. **30**, 98.
4. DE JONG, R. N., ITABASHI, H. H. and OLSON, J. R. (1969) Memory Loss Due to Hippocampal Lesions. Arch. Neurol. **20**, 339.
5. DE LONG, M. R. (1972) Activity of Basal Ganglia Neurons During Movement. Brain Res. **40**, 127.
6. DOLCE, G., OFFENLOCH, K., SANNILA, W., MÜLLER-CALGAN, H. and DECKER, H. (1972) Spectral EEG Analysis in Two Strains of Rats with Genetically Determined Different Conditioned Behaviour. 40. Tagung der Deutschen Physiol. Ges. (September 1972) R 77.
7. DUSTMAN, R. E. and BECK, E. C. (1972) Relationship of Intelligence to Visually Evoked Responses. Electroenceph. clin. Neurophysiol. **33**, 254.
8. ECCLES, J. C. (1953) The Neurophysiological Basis of Mind. Oxford University Press, London.
9. EVARTS, E. V. (1963) Photically Evoked Responses in Visual Cortex Units During Sleep and Waking J. Neurophysiol. **26**, 229.
10. EVARTS, E. V. (1964) Temporal Patterns of Discharge of the Pyramidal Tract Neurons during Sleep and Waking in the Monkey. J. Neurophysiol. **27**, 152.
11. EVARTS, E. V. (1966) Pyramidal Tract Activity Associated with a Conditioned Hand Movement in the Monkey. J. Neurophysiol. **29**, 1011.

12. EVARTS, E. V. (1968) Relation of Pyramidal Tract Activity to Force Exerted during Voluntary Movement. J. Neurophysiol. **31**. 14.
13. EVARTS, E. V. (1969) Activity of Pyramidal Tract Neurons during Postural Fixation. J. Neurophysiol. **32**, 375.
14. EVARTS, E. V. (1972) Activity of Motor Cortex Neurons in Association with Learned Movement. Internat. J. Neurosci. **3**, 113.
15. EVARTS, E. V. (1972) Contrasts between Activity of Precentral and Postcentral Neurons of Cerebral Cortex during Movement in the Monkey. Brain Res. **40**, 25.
16. FARLEY, B. G. (1963) A Model of the Brain. Discovery.
17. GRASTYÁN, E. and KARMOS, G. (1961) The Influence of Hippocampal Lesions on Simple and Delayed Instrumental Conditioned Reflexes. In: Physiologie de l'Hippocampe. Ed. J. CADILLAC, CNRS, Montpellier.
18. GRASTYÁN, E., LISSAK, K. MADARASZ, I. and DONHOFFER, H. (1959) Hippocampal Electrical Activity during the Development of Conditioned Reflexes. Electroenceph. clin. Neurophysiol. **11**, 409.
19. GREEN, J. D. and ARDUINI, A. (1954) Hippocampal Electrical Activity in Arousal. J. Neurophysiol. **17**, 533.
20. HALAS, E. S., BEARDSLEY, J. V. and SANDLIE, M. E. (1970) Conditioned Neuronal Responses at Various Levels in Conditioning Paradigms. Electroenceph. clin. Neurophysiol. **28**, 468.
21. HERNÁNDEZ-PÉON, R., SCHERRER, H. and JOUVET, M. (1956) Modification of Electrical Activity in Cochlear Nucleus during "Attention" in Unanesthetized Cat. Science, **123**, 331.
22. HESS, W. R. (1948) Die funktionelle Organisation des vegetativen Nervensystems. Benno Schwabe, Basel.
23. HORRIDGE, G. A. (1962) Learning of Leg Position by the Ventral Nerve Cord of Headless Insects. Proc. roy. Soc. B **157**, 33.
24. HUGHES, R. A. (1972) Retrograde Amnesia Produced by Hippocampal Injections of Potassium Chloride: Gradient of Effect and Recovery. J. comp. Physiol. Psychol. in press.
25. JOUVET, M. and JOUVET, D. (1963) A Study of the Neurophysiological Mechanisms of Dreaming. Electroenceph. clin. Neurophysiol. Suppl. **24**, 133.
26. KAADA, B. R., RASMUSSEN, E. W. and KVEIM, O. (1961) Effects of Hippocampal Lesions on Maze Learning and Retention in Rats. Exp. Neurol. **3**, 333.
27. KAMP, A., SCHRIJER, C. F. M. and STORM VAN LEEUWEN, W. (1972) Occurrence of "Beta Bursts" in Human Frontal Cortex Related to Psychological Parameters. Electroenceph. clin. Neurophysiol. **33**, 257.
28. KANDEL, E. R. and SPENCER, W. A. (1968) Cellular Neurophysiological Approaches in the Study of Learning. Physiol. Rev. **48**, 65.
29. KLEMM, W. R. (1971) EEG and Multiple-Unit Activity in Limbic and Motor Systems during Movement and Immobility. Psychology and Behavior **7**, 337.
30. KOELLA, W. P. and FERRY, A. (1963) Cortico-Subcortical Homeostasis in the Cat's Brain. Science, **142**, 586.
31. NAUTA, W. J. H. and KOELLA, W. P. (1966) Sleep, Wakefulness, Dreams and Memory. Neurosci. Res. Program. Bull. **4**, No. 1.
32. OLDS, J. and MILNER, P. (1954) Positive Reinforcement Produced by Electrical Stimulation of Septal Areas and Other Regions of the Rat Brain. J. comp. Physiol. **47**, 419.
33. OLDS, J. (1967) The Limbic System and Behavioral Reinforcement. In: Structure and Function of the Limbic System. Eds. R. W. ADEY and T. TOKIZANE, Elsevier, Amsterdam, London, New York.
34. OOMURA, Y., OOYAMA, H., YAMAMOTO, T., NAKA, F., KOBAYASHI, N. and ONO, T. (1967) Neural Mechanism of Feeding. In: Structure and Function of the Limbic System. Eds. R. W. ADEY and T. TOKIZANE. Elsevier, Amsterdam, London, New York.
35. ORBACH, J., MILNER, B. and RASMUSSEN, T. (1960) Learning and Retention in Monkeys after Amygdala-Hippocampus Resection. Arch. Neurol. **3**, 230.
36. PENFIELD, W. (1958) The Excitable Cortex in Conscious Man. C. C. Thomas, Springfield.
37. SAWYER, C. H. (1962) Triggering of the Pituitary by the Central Nervous System. In: Physiological Triggers. Ed. T. H. BULLOCK, Wawerly Press, Baltimore.
38. SCOVILLE, W. B. and MILNER, B. (1957) Loss of Recent Memory after Bilateral Hippocampal Lesions J. Neurol. Neurosurg. Psychiat. **20**, 11.
39. SEGAL, M., DISTERHOFT, J. F. and OLDS, J. (1972) Hippocampal Unit Activity during Classical Aversive and Appetitive Conditioning. Science, **175**, 797.
40. THOMPSON, R. F., PATTERSON, M. M. and TEYLER, T. J. (1972) The Neurophysiology of Learning. Ann. Rev. Psychology **23**, 73.
40. VELASCO, M. and VELASCO, F. (1972) Correlation between the Psychological Significance of

Stimuli and the Amplitude of the Cortical Somatic Evoked Potential in Man. Electroenceph. clin. Neurophysiol. **33**, 239.
42. WALTER, D. O. and ADEY, W. R. (1963) Spectral Analysis of Electroencephalograms Recorded during Learning in the Cat, before and after Subthalamic Lesions. Exp. Neurol. **7**, 481.

W.P.K., Biological Research Laboratories, Pharmaceutical Division, Ciba-Geigy Ltd., Basel, Switzerland

KORRELATION PHARMAKODYNAMISCHER EFFEKTE IN VERSCHIEDENEN HÖHEN BIOLOGISCHER ORGANISATION

G. STILLE und K. DIXON

Forschungsinstitut Wander, Einheit der Sandozforschung, Bern

Wenn der Pharmakologe über die Korrelation psychopharmakologischer Befunde am Tier mit Beobachtungen an gesunden Versuchspersonen berichten soll, kommt er unweigerlich in Schwierigkeiten. Das verwendbare Material zu diesem Thema ist so unzulänglich, daß kaum jemand über ausreichende Unterlagen verfügen kann.

In den folgenden Ausführungen soll daher nur versucht werden, einige grundsätzliche Probleme beim Vergleich der Ergebnisse an Tier und Mensch aufzuzeigen, soweit sie die Arbeit mit Psychopharmaka betreffen.

Jeder Versuch, zwischen Mensch und Tier Beziehungen darzustellen, setzt zwei Annahmen voraus:

1. Die phylogenetische Gemeinsamkeit, auch für die Verhaltensparameter,
2. das Nervensystem als Organisator des Verhaltens.

Die Untersuchung von Psychopharmaka kann nun beim Tier, aber auch beim Menschen, auf verschiedenen Organisationshöhen, also bei unterschiedlicher Komplexität des Substrates erfolgen:

1. Die niedrigste Stufe der Komplexität biologischer Organisation stellen die *Zellorganellen* dar, bei der Arbeit mit Psychopharmaka in erster Linie die der Zellen des Nervensystems. Wir erschließen ihre Funktion beim Tier durch enzymologische, biochemische und elektronenmikroskopische Befunde. Beim Menschen sind entsprechende Untersuchungen nur *post mortem*, also nicht an frischem Material möglich.

2. Die nächst höhere Stufe der Komplexität stellt die Zelle, also in unserem Fall die *Ganglienzelle oder auch die vernachlässigte Gliazelle,* dar. Zugänglich ist das funktionierende Neuron beim Tier durch die Mikroelektrodentechnik und die Mikroelektrophorese. Beim Menschen kann man vergleichbare Untersuchungen gegenwärtig nur an Gewebsexplantaten durchführen.

3. Die nächste Stufe sind die *zerebralen und spinalen Systeme.* Methodisch sind diese beim Tier durch verschiedene elektrophysiologische, histochemische und biochemische Methoden zugänglich. Beim Menschen gibt es hier nur Einzelbefunde während stereotaktischer Operation.

Besonders erwähnt sei hier das *autonome System,* bei dem sich Vergleichsuntersuchungen zwischen Tier und Mensch anbieten, die ja auch mit Erfolg durchgeführt werden.

4. Als nächste Stufe biologischer Integration folgt das *Gesamtgehirn*. Hier zeichnet sich, wie wir noch sehen werden, die Möglichkeit einer engen Zusammenarbeit zwischen Pharmakologen und Klinikern ab, wenn man z.B. das EEG, besonders auch das Schlaf-EEG und evozierte Antworten im Kortex als Kriterien verwendet.

Steigen wir noch weiter in der Komplexität, so kommt es zu einem Sprung, der den Naturwissenschaften immer Schwierigkeiten bereiten wird, zum Sprung zwischen Hirnphysiologie und Verhalten, als Sublimation zerebraler Funktionen.

5. Wir möchten die nächste Stufe das *Elementarverhalten* nennen. Es ist bei Mensch und Tier an der Gesamtaktivität, am Schlaf-Wach-Rhythmus, an der Schmerzreaktion u.a. zu erfassen.

6. Erwähnt sei ferner das *Dressur- oder Lernverhalten*. Hierher gehören die Vielzahl beschriebener operanter Methoden. Besonders Untersuchungen am konditionierten Verhalten sind beliebt, da

— Lernen eine Eigentümlichkeit aller Lebewesen ist,
— bei allen Species vergleichbare Techniken durchgeführt werden können,
— die Ergebnisse gut reproduzierbar sind.

Die Brauchbarkeit dieser Methoden für psychopharmakologische Vergleiche ist jedoch dadurch stark beeinträchtigt, daß in der phylogenetischen Reihe die Flexibilität des Verhaltens stark zunimmt. Lernen führt, soweit es das Verhalten betrifft, zu einer Rigidität, die in einer definierten Situation von Vorteil sein kann, in der Mehrzahl anderer eine Fehlanpassung bedeutet. Es ist gerade die flexible Komponente des Verhaltens, nicht die rigide, die unsere Aufmerksamkeit verdient.

Die Interpretation konditionierten Verhaltens erfordert die Einführung von Begriffen als mitbestimmende Variable, die wie „Angst", „Wut" u.a. für das Tier nicht ausreichend definierbar sind. Diese Feststellungen entsprechen der Erfahrung, daß uns bisher die umfangreichen Arbeiten über konditioniertes Verhalten, was den Vergleich von Tier und Mensch anbelangt, nicht wesentlich weiter gebracht haben.

7. Mit der bereits oben erwähnten flexiblen Komponente des Verhaltens kommen wir zu den *differenzierten angeborenen und phylogenetisch festgelegten Verhaltensweisen* dem Forschungsgebiet der Ethologie. Die Ethologie verzichtet auf alle vorgefaßten Begriffe und versucht, die Bedeutung von Verhaltensbildern vergleichend bei den einzelnen Species zu erfassen. Hier zeichnen sich für den Pharmakologen eine Fülle unausgeschöpfter Möglichkeiten ab, und entsprechende klinische Untersuchungen sind noch ganz in den Anfängen. Psychopharmakologische Befunde oder sogar Vergleiche zwischen den Species dürften kaum vorliegen.

8. Als letzte Möglichkeit ergibt sich, die *durch psychologisierende Termini charakterisierten Verhaltensweisen* beim Tier wie „Angst", „Aggression", „Spannung" usw., mit den Ergebnissen psychologischer Tests am Menschen zu vergleichen.

Beginnen wir mit der Diskussion dieses letzten Punktes, also der Verhaltenspharmakologie unter Verwendung unreflektierter anthropomorpher Termini und untersuchen wir den Begriff der „Aggression" und der „Aggressionshemmung" im Tierversuch.

Die Werte in Tabelle 1 wurden aus einer Arbeit von Sofia (6) errechnet. Es wurde in diesen Untersuchungen mit vier Aggressionstests gearbeitet: die Aggression der für längere Zeit isolierten Maus, die Kampfaktivität bei elektrischem Fußschock, die Aggression bei Septumläsion und das muricide Verhalten von Ratten nach Isolation. Die für die einzelnen Pharmaka angegebenen Werte sind der Quotient aus der mittleren Wirkdosis zur mittleren neurotoxischen Dosis. Liegt der Wert also über 1,0 so ist die antiaggressive Dosis größer als die neurotoxische. Dies trifft in den meisten Fällen zu und nur wenige Werte sind kleiner als 1. Zudem schwanken die Werte von Modell zu Modell erheblich.

Tabelle 1

Wirkung von Psychopharmaka in 4 „Aggressions"-Tests. In der Tabelle dargestellt wurde der Quotient aus mittlerer effektiver Dosis und mittlerer neurotoxischer Dosis (Die Werte wurden einer Arbeit von Sofia entnommen.)

	Quotient der mittleren effektiven Dosis: mittleren neurotoxischen Dosis			
	Agression der isolierten Maus	Kampfaktivität bei elektrischem Fusschock	Agression bei Septumläsion an Ratten	Muricides Verhalten von Ratten
Chlorpromazin	2,3	4,9	7,1	5,3
Methotrimeprazin	1,3	1,1	6,1	16,5
Thioridazin	0,6	0,6	2,3	15,9
Thiothixen	1,1	0,7	3,5	8,0
Clomacran	0,7	0,3	4,4	18,9
Chlordiazepoxid	2,6	0,5	2,7	2,3
Diazepam	1,6	0,1	4,3	54,8
Tetrabenazin	1,1	0,7	32,4	41,3
Benzquinamid	0,9	1,9	3,9	8,5
Meprobamat	1,1	0,9	1,8	3,5
Trifluperidol	2,5	1,2	5,0	2,0
Pentobarbital	1,9	0,7	1,7	2,4
Imipramin	1,0	1,0	2,3	0,4
Desimipramin	0,6	1,6	1,3	0,3
Thiazesim	0,5		0,8	1,1

Die Mehrzahl solcher Modelle versagt bei der Korrelation der aus ihr gewonnenen Ergebnisse mit der Beobachtung am Menschen, weil ihnen keine exakten Kenntnisse des Verhaltensrepertoires der einzelnen Species zugrunde liegen. Die „muricidal rat" ist das beste Beispiel für ein unangemessenes Vorgehen. Es ist in der freien Natur höchst ungewöhnlich, daß Ratten Mäuse töten: es gehört nicht zum normalen Verhaltensrepertoire der Ratte. Der Test ergibt zwar eine sauber erfassbare ED 50, ihm fehlt jedoch jede ethologische Basis, die einen Vergleich mit der Reaktion beim Menschen gestatten würde.

Das gleiche gilt für das durch elektrische Fußschocks ausgelöste Kampfverhalten von Mäusen. Das normale Verhaltensbild der Maus bei Applikation elektrischer Schläge durch den Boden des Käfigs besteht zunächst in Erstarren („freezing"), Zusammenkauern („crouching") oder defensivem Aufrichten. Aggressives Verhalten gehört nicht zum typischen Verhalten unter diesen Bedingungen. Die Mäuse sind in dieser Situation in erster Linie fluchtmotiviert. Nur wenn die Flucht blockiert ist wie im Käfig, kommt es zu dem, was zu Unrecht als „Aggressivität" bezeichnet wird. Ähnliche Einwände gibt es auch bei anderen tierexperimentellen Kriterien und Meßgrößen, denen ein emotives Verhalten zugrunde liegt. Erwähnt sei nur die Bedeutung des Urinierens bei der Ratte, das gelegentlich, wie die Defäkation, als Symptom der „Angst" von Pharmakologen verwendet wurde.

Urinieren bedeutet für die Ratte nicht Angst, sondern

— Abgrenzung des Territoriums,
— Soziale Aktivität vor allem im Hinblick auf das Geschlechtsverhalten, und schließlich,
— die Ausscheidung von Endprodukten des Stoffwechsels (2).

Der Pharmakologe muß sich bei tierischem Verhalten vor oberflächlicher Ähnlichkeit mit menschlichen Eigenschaften schützen, vor allem aber vor der Eigengesetzlichkeit bei der Verwendung von Begriffen wie „Angst", „Aggression" usw.

Mit dem Vorangehenden haben wir bereits die Ethologie berührt, das Bemühen um die Erfassung des Darstellungswertes bestimmter Verhaltensweisen in der Phylogenese. Das folgende Beispiel soll zeigen, wie die ethologische Methodik und Betrachtungsweise dem Pharmakologen zu helfen vermag, Brücken zur Beobachtung am Menschen zu bauen.

Wir wissen, daß nach allen Halluzinogenen bei Mäusen regelmässig ein intensives Kopfschütteln auftritt. CORNE und PICKERING (3) haben die für Mäuse notwendigen Dosen mit den halluzinogenen Dosen beim Menschen korreliert. Abb. 1 zeigt diese Korrelation und man sieht, daß offensichtlich eine Beziehung zwischen beiden Wirkungen besteht, soweit man die Dosen vergleicht. Die ethologische Frage müßte nun lauten: Was bedeutet im Verhaltensrepertoire der Maus das Kopfschütteln? TOLSCVAI-NAGY (7) ist in unserem Laboratorium dieser Frage nachgegangen und hat festgestellt, daß das

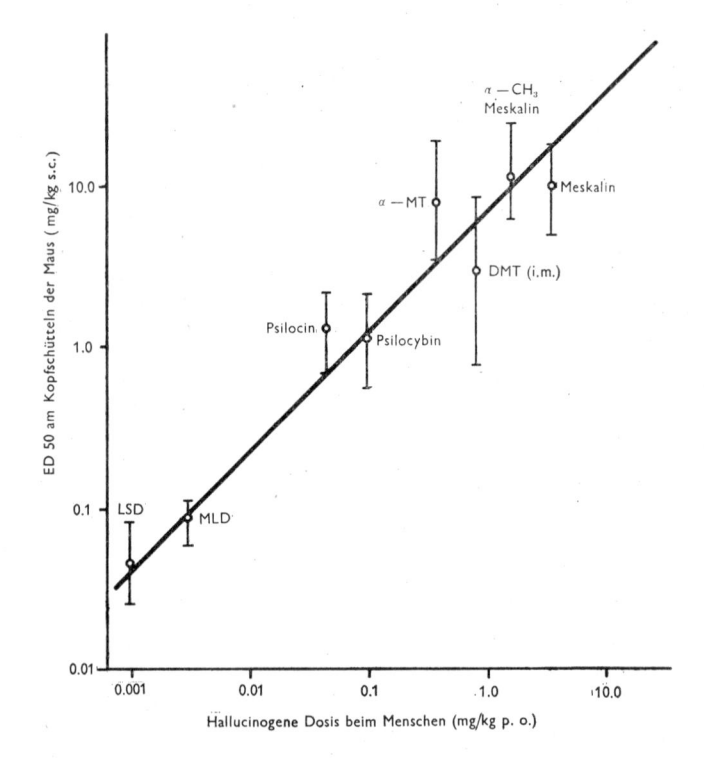

Abb. 1. Beziehung zwischen der halluzinogenen Dosis beim Menschen (Abszisse) und der mittleren effektiven Dosis (ED 50) am Kopfschütteln der Maus (Ordinate) unter der Wirkung von Halluzinogenen des LSD-Typs. (Modifizierte Darstellung nach CORNE und PICKERING—3)

Kopfschütteln bevorzugt beim Wechsel von einer Verhaltensweise in eine andere auftritt. Besonders auffällig war Kopfschütteln bei unbehandelten Mäusen nach Unterbruch eines Handlungsablaufes. Man könnte in ihm also eine Art Übersprungsbewegung sehen. Was dieses Verhalten für die Wirkung von Halluzinogenen an Mäusen ausdrückt, kann man im Augenblick noch nicht sagen. Hier müssen weitere Untersuchungen ansetzen.

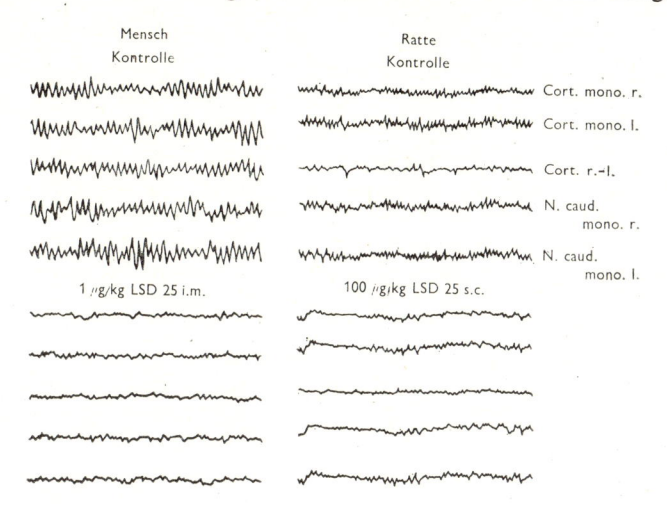

Abb. 2. EEG beim Menschen und bei der Ratte, oben vor und unten nach Behandlung mit LSD (BACHINI et al. — 1).

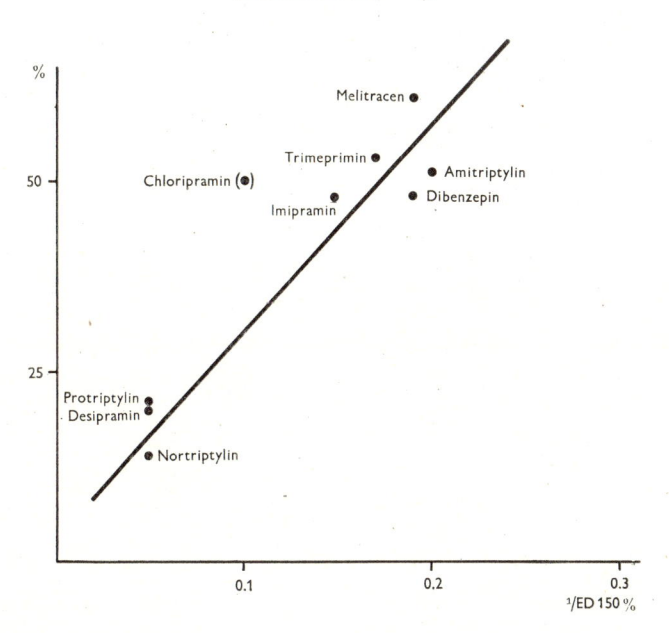

Abb. 3. Korrelation zwischen der Wirkung von Antidepressiva auf die elektrische Arousalschwelle beim Kaninchen (Abszisse) und der Hemmung der Agitation beim Menschen (Ordinate). Spearman'scher Rangkorrelationskoeffizient $r_s = +0.813$; $p \sim 0.0025$.

Das letzte Beispiel sollte nur zeigen, wie Verhaltensforschung ethologischen Ansatzes verwendet werden und darüber hinaus dazu beitragen kann, Beziehungen zwischen tierischem Verhalten und menschlichem Erleben (Halluzinationen) zu erhellen.

Sicher einfacher als beim Verhalten ist die Möglichkeit einer Korrelation physiologischer Parameter. So bietet unter anderem das EEG mit allen seinen durch die Computertechnik erweiterten Möglichkeiten ein ideales Feld des Vergleiches. Ein Beispiel in Abb. 2 zeigt dies. Links ist die Wirkung von LSD auf das menschliche EEG (1), rechts auf das einer Ratte, dargestellt. In beiden Fällen steht Abnahme von Rhythmizität und Spannung im Vordergrund der LSD-Wirkung. Hier, wo wir auf dem gleichen Niveau der Integration arbeiten können, sollten vermehrt Bemühungen um eine Korrelation psychopharmakologischer Werte zwischen Mensch und Tier einsetzen.

Das letzte Beispiel zeigt, daß ein Vergleich aber auch dann möglich ist, wenn man unterschiedliche Organisationsstufen bei Tier und Mensch verwendet. Abb. 3 stellt ein Korrelationsdiagramm dar, bei dem die Abszisse, die Wirksamkeit auf die elektrische Weckschwelle beim Kaninchen ausdrückt, die Ordinate die Agitationshemmung beim Menschen (5). Wir korrelieren also hier einen elektrophysiologischen Parameter beim Tier mit einer klinischen Beobachtung, und zwar der psychomotorischen Aktivität der Versuchspersonen (rating scale). Es ergibt sich eine statistisch gesicherte positive Korrelation zwischen der Wirkung der Antidepressiva auf die Arousalschwelle beim Kaninchen und der Dämpfung der Agitation beim Menschen (Rangkorrelation nach Spearman $r_s = + 0,813$; $p \sim 0,0025$).

Die Bemühungen, Beziehungen herzustellen zwischen den Beobachtungen im Tierexperiment und der Wirkung von Psychopharmaka beim Menschen, stehen erst im Anfang. Die grundsätzlichen Schwierigkeiten sind nicht gering und wir haben versucht, hier einige zu beschreiben. Eines wird uns immer verschlossen bleiben, das Erleben des Tieres. Die Beobachtung des Verhaltens, wie es die Ethologie übt, kann dafür immer nur eine Approximation sein. Hier ist eine Kluft zwischen Tierexperiment und Untersuchung am Menschen, die man nie schliessen wird.

LITERATURVERZEICHNIS

1. BACHINI, O., et al. (1965) Acta neurol. lat.-amer. **11**, 383.
2. CHANCE, M. R. A. (1957) Lancet II, 687.
3. CORNE, S. J. und PICKERING, R. W. (1967) Psychopharmacologia, **11**, 65.
4. GRANT, E. C. und MACKINTOSH, J. H. (1963) Behaviour, **21**, 246.
5. POELDINGER, W. und STILLE, G. (1968) VI. Internat. Congress des CINP in Tarragona. Excerpta Medica Int. Congr. Series No. 180, 529.
6. SOFIA, R. D. (1969) Life Sci. 8, 705.
7. TOLSCVAI-NAGY, unveröffentlichte Ergebnisse.

G. S., Forschungsinstitut Wander, Einheit der Sandozforschung, Bern, Switzerland

DIFFERENTIELLE UND GENERELLE WIRKUNGEN PSYCHOTROPER PHARMAKA AUF DAS MENSCHLICHE EEG

Nervenklinik der Universität Erlangen — Nürnberg, Forschungseinheit für Psychophysiologie

D. BENTE

Quantitative EEG-Untersuchungen mit der Frequenzintegrationsanalyse (1, 2, 3) haben gezeigt, daß sich im Verlauf einer standardisierten neuroleptischen Medikation nicht nur generelle, sondern auch differentielle Effekte manifestieren, die sich in dem von uns untersuchten Fall als populationsabhängige Unterschiede der medikamentösen Reaktivität erwiesen und mit im einzelnen noch ungeklärten Faktoren biologischer, öko- oder soziophysiologischer Art in Zusammenhang stehen dürften. Unter den hier verwendeten Begriff der differentiellen EEG-Effekte fallen demnach alle von dispositionalen individualen oder kollektiven Momenten und Einflußgrößen abhängigen Formen der hirnelektrischen Reaktivität, während als generell die dem Pharmakon konstant zugeordneten EEG-Veränderungen bezeichnet werden. Da eine methodisch fundierte, pharmakologisch relevante Klassifikation pharmakogener EEG-Veränderungen letztlich nur auf der Basis scharf umrissener genereller Effekte möglich ist, andererseits aber über die Rolle und das wahre Ausmaß differentieller Wirkungen bisher noch nichts Genaueres bekannt ist, kommt der systematischen Klärung dieser Verhältnisse, die bei der Untersuchung gut definierter Normalgruppen beginnen muß, eine große theoretische und praktische Bedeutung bei.

Was für Fragen sich diesbezüglich ergeben und welche Aussagen hier zu gewinnen sind, soll an Hand von zwei elektroencephalographischen Arzneimittelstudien erörtert werden. Beide Untersuchungen wurden an Gruppen gesunder, nach gleichen Kriterien ausgewählter Probanden unter identischen Bedingungen und mit derselben Analysetechnik durchgeführt, wobei als Analyseverfahren die auf der Theorie der Zufallsprozesse beruhende Korrelations- und Spektralanalyse benutzt worden ist.

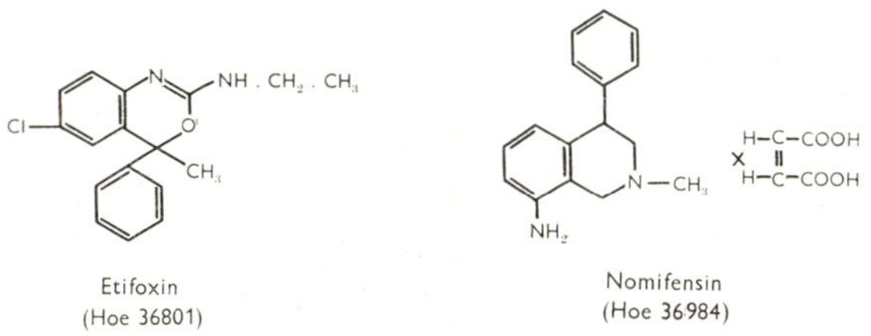

Abb. 1. Chemische Strukturen der geprüften Arzneimittel.

Als Testsubstanzen wurden Etifoxin und Nomifensin geprüft (Abb. 1). Etifoxin ist eine Benzoxazinverbindung, die anxiolytische, antikonvulsive, spasmolytische sowie peripher und zentral anticholinerge Wirkungen hat. Bei Nomifensin handelt es sich um ein Tetrahydroisochinolinderivat, eine Stoffklasse, die bisher in der Psychopharmakologie noch keine Verwendung fand. Pharmakologisch weist die Substanz antikataleptische, antiaggressive und noradrenalinverstärkende, aber keine anticholinergen Effekte auf.

Zur Versuchsanordnung und Aufbereitung der gewonnenen Kenngrößen ist folgendes auszuführen: Um elektroencephalographisch eindeutig definierte und möglichst homogene Versuchsgruppen zu erhalten, wurden in entsprechenden Voruntersuchungen aus jeweils ca.50 Studenten 11 bzw. 10 Probanden ausgewählt, deren Ruhe-EEG bei visuell-morphologischer Beurteilung folgenden Kriterien genügte: Gut ausgeprägter, weitgehend kontinuierlicher Alpharhythmus mit konstantem occipitalem Ausprägungs- und Amplitudenmaximum ohne nennenswerte Einstreuung von Beta- oder Thetawellen.

Placebo und Wirkstoff wurden jeweils in zwei in einem Abstand von 7 Tagen aufeinanderfolgenden Versuchen peroral appliziert, wobei die Sequenz Placebo-Verum in jeder Probandenreihe systematisch alternierte. Placebo und Wirkstoffgabe erfolgten jeweils um 15 Uhr. 140 Minuten später im erwarteten Wirkungsmaximum des Pharmakons begann die Aufzeichnung der in sitzender Haltung bei geschlossenen Augen registrierten Ruheaktivität, die mit Mayo-Klebeelektroden von der rechten Occipitalregion zu einer Referenzelektrode am Vertex abgeleitet wurde.

Die Auswertung der EEG-Daten wurde off line an Hand der auf Analogband gespeicherten Aufzeichnungen vorgenommen (Abb. 2). Für die Berechnung und Schätzung des empirischen Autospektrums wurde das indirekte Verfahren gewählt, da es eine optimale Nutzung der in unserem Labor vorhandenen Möglichkeiten gestattete und sich arbeitstechnisch als eine sehr maniable Lösung für solche Aufgaben erwies. Wie das Blockdiagramm zeigt, wurde zunächst mit dem an die CAT 400 angeschlossenen Korrelator COR 256 die Autokovarianzfunktion bestimmt, während deren Normierung und Fouriertransformation nach entsprechender Umcodierung der auf Lochsterifen ausgegebenen Daten dann im Digitalrechner erfolgte.

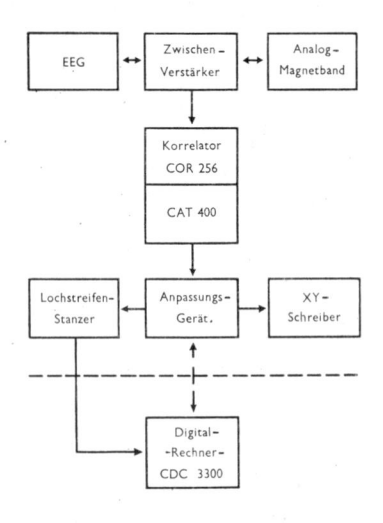

Abb. 2. Schematische Darstellung der Auswertung der EEG-Daten.

Bestimmt wurde das mit einem Hammimg-Fenster geglättete Autospektrum der rechten Occipitalregion, wobei sich die der Schätzung zugrundeliegende Stichprobenfunktion auf jeweils 3 Minuten Ableitedauer erstreckte. Nachdem die Autokovarianzfunktion für 256 Punkte mit tau = 20 msec und tau(max) = 5120 msec berechnet wurde, ergibt sich bei der Fouriertransformation eine Frequenzauflösung von 0,19 Hz. Da bei dieser Parameterwahl die im Falle eines Gaussprozesses einer Chi^2-Verteilung folgende Stichprobenverteilung der spektralen Schätzwerte etwa 70 freiheitsgrade aufweist, ist die Stabilität der resultierenden Kenngrößen als genügend groß zu betrachten.

Für die weitere Verarbeitung der extrahierten Spektralparameter kommen verschiedene Methoden in Betracht. Da es im Rahmen solcher Studien auf eine möglichst prägnante Darstellung des elektroencephalographischen Wirkungsbildes der untersuchten Pharmaka ankommt, nehmen wir eine an Frequenzbereichen orientierte Auswertung vor, wobei wir die auf die Gesamtleistung normierten Spektralwerte in entsprechenden Grenzen summieren und damit ein Maß für den relativen Leistungsinhalt der verschiedenen Bereiche gewinnen. Diese Kenngrößen werden durch Angaben über die Lage des Leistungsmaximums oder der dominanten Frequenz und ein Alpha-Bandbreitenmaß ergänzt, das aus dem Quotienten von Leistungsinhalt und Leistungsmaximum gebildet wird und damit die Leistungskonzentration bzw. Synchronisation im Alphabereich erfaßt.

Nach diesen methodischen Anmerkungen möchte ich mich nun den Ergebnissen der Etifoxin-Studie zuwenden. Wie die in Tabelle 1 Mittelwerte der auf den Subdelta-, Theta-, Alpha- und Betabereich entfallenden Leistungsanteile sowie die der dominanten Frequenz und der Alphabandbreite zeigen, finden sich zwischen Placebo und Wirkstoff nur unbedeutende Differenzen. Ebenso sind auch keine statistisch bedeutsamen Unterschiede in den Streuungsmassen festzustellen, sodaß, zunächst die Nullhypothese eines fehlenden Medikationseffektes beibehalten werden muß.

TABELLE 1

Mittelwerte Placebo-Etifoxin
(n = 11)

	0,19–0,97 Hz	1,17–3,90 Hz	4,10–7,81 Hz	8,00–12,89 Hz	13,08–22,85 Hz	$f_{\alpha max}$	B_α
Placebo	4,09 %	8,47 %	11,68 %	46,69 %	25,15 %	10,30 Hz	9,12 Hz
Etifoxin	3,86 %	7,98 %	11,25 %	47,41 %	24,89 %	10,30 Hz	8,68 Hz

Ordnet man jedoch die Probanden nach der Größe ihres im Placeboversuch auf den Alphabereich entfallenden Leistungsanteils und berücksichtigt man die jeweilige Richtung der unter Wirkstoff auftretenden Verschiebungen, so ergibt sich ein bemerkenswerter Befund. Wie Tabelle 2 zeigt, tritt unter Etifoxin eine systematisch gerichtete, von der Größe des Alphaausgangswertes abhängige Veränderung verschiedener Kenngrößen auf. Während unter Medikation bei den über dem Placebo-Gruppenmittelwert liegenden Probanden die Leistung im Alphabereich sinkt, dagegen im Theta- und Betabereich steigt, zeigen alle Probanden unterhalb des Mittelwertes eine inverse Reaktion. Die sich bei dieser Dichotomie am Gruppenmittelwert ergebende Verteilung-differenz der Vorzeichen ist für die genannten Variablen auf dem 2% bzw. 5% Niveau signifikant. Ebenso läßt sich auch die bei geringeren Alpha-Ausgangswerten auftretende Beschleunigung der dominanten Frequenz nach dem exakten Test von R. A. FISHER auf dem 5% Niveau sichern.

TABELLE 2

Vergleich Placebo-Etifoxin

Vp.	0,19—0,97 Hz	1,17—3,90 Hz	4,10—7,81 Hz	8,00—12,89 Hz	13,08—22,85 Hz	$f_{\alpha max}$	B_α
WI	—	—	+	—	+		+
HE	—	—	+	—	+		+
NA	+	+	+	—	+		—
KN	—	—	+	—	—		—
LI	+	—	+	—	+		—
ED	+	+	+	—	+		+
KA	—	—	—	+	—	+	—
ME	—	—	—	+	—	+	+
EI	+	+	—	+	—	+	+
ET	+	—	—	+	—		—
FR	—	—	—	+	—	+	—

+ Zunahme nach Etifoxin
— Abnahme nach Etifoxin

Etifoxin übt demnach keine generelle Wirkung auf die untersuchten spektralen Kenngrößen aus. Vielmehr tritt ein differentieller Effekt auf, der von der Größe des Alphaleistungsanteils im medikamentös unbeeinflußten EEG abhängig ist. Dabei tendieren Probanden mit hoher Alphaleistung zu einem polyrhythmischen Zerfall der Ruheaktivität mit Anstieg der Theta- und Beta-Aktivität, während solche mit geringere Alphaleistung einen Alphaanstieg zeigen, der mit einer spektralen Harmonisierung und einer Beschleunigung der dominanten Frequenz gekoppelt ist. Abb. 3, in der links die Placebo- und rechts die Etifoxinspektren eines Probanden aus der oberen und unteren Halbgruppe gegenübergestellt sind, verdeutlicht diese Aussage. Während bei dem oberen Probanden der spektrale Gipfel absinkt, sich im Alphabereich aufsplittert und sich stärkere Nebenmaxima im Theta- und Beta-Bereich ausbilden, kommt es bei dem unteren Probanden zu einer deutlichen Glättung und Harmonisierung der Spektralfigur.

Unter morphologischen Gesichtspunkten betrachtet läßt sich dieses differentielle Verhalten dahingehend interpretieren, daß Etifoxin in beiden Fällen zu einer leichten Vigilanzverschiebung und -minderung führt, die sich jedoch in Abhängigkeit von individualen Strukturmerkmalen der hirnelektrischen Organisation in unterschiedlicher Weise manifestiert. Während Probanden mit akzentuierter Alphaausprägung und -synchronisation in einen dem Stadium B1 vergleichbaren Alphazerfall übergehen, tendieren Probanden mit geringerer Alphaleistung zu einer dem A-Stadium entsprechenden Änderung ihres hirnelektrischen Musters, zeigen aber gleichzeitig eine Beschleunigung ihrer dominanten Frequenz.

Nachdem die Ergebnisse dieser Untersuchung zeigten, dass der im Zuge einer pharmakogenen Vigilanzminderung auftretende Strukturwandel der hirnelektrischen Aktivität offenbar in Zusammenhang mit der Alphaorganisation des medikamentös unbeeinflussten Ruhe-Elektroencephalogramms steht, wurde bei der Nomifensin-Studie die Analyse auf einen zweiten 3-Minutenabschnitt ausgedehnt, um damit auch Aufschlüsse über die Verlaufsdynamik zu erhalten. Beide Abschnitte werden im folgenden mit I und II bezeichnet.

Bei der Analyse der Nomifensindaten ergibt sich zunächst, daß die in den beiden Abschnitten der Wirkstoffableitung erreichten Maxima der Betaleistung signifikant höher liegen als unter Placebo, wie der Wilcoxon-Test für Paardifferenzen zeigt (Tabelle 3). Es handelt sich demnach um einen generellen Effekt, der in einer pharmakogenen Anregung der Betaaktivität besteht und sich besonders im Abschnitt II entfaltet.

Teilt man nun wieder die nach der Größe der Alphaleistung geordneten Probanden in zwei Halbgruppen auf, so werden auch in diesem Fall ausgeprägte differentielle Effekte

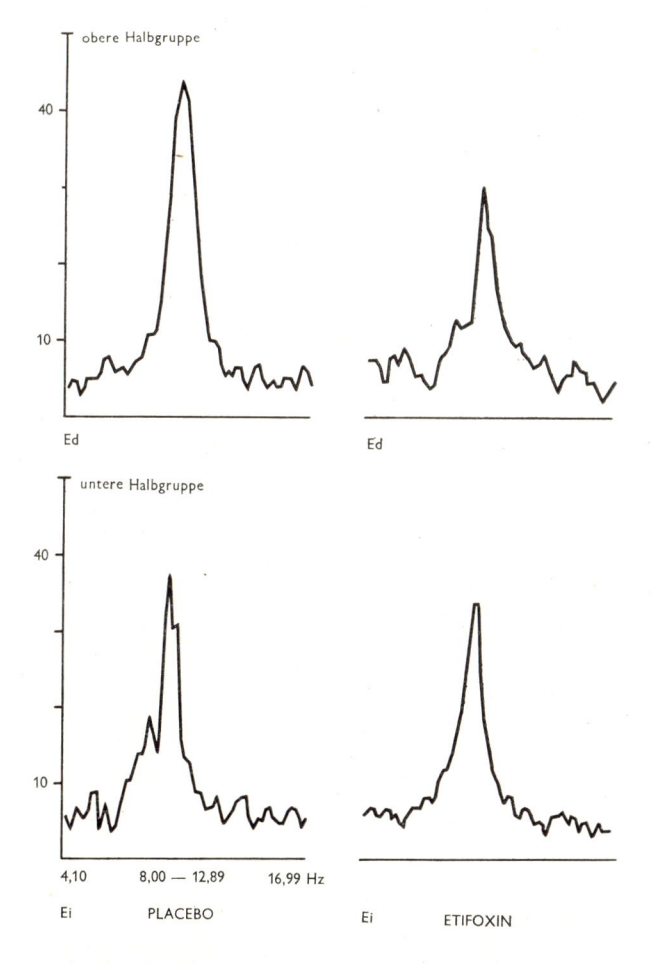

Abb. 3. Frequenzspektralanalyse der zwei Probanden (Ed - obere Halbgruppe, Ei - untere Halbgruppe) nach der Placebo (links) und Etifoxinverabreichung.

sichtbar. Tabelle 4, in der die unter Wirkstoff auftretenden Verschiebungen in den Abschnitten I und II für beide Halbgruppen dargestellt sind, macht diese Tendenzen deutlich. Während die obere Halbgruppe unter Nomifensin mit einem fortschreitenden Leistungsabfall im Alphabereich und einem gleichzeitigen Anstieg der langsamen und schnellen Aktivität reagiert, zeigt die untere Halbgruppe ein zweiphasiges Verhalten, wobei einem anfänglichen Alphaanstieg und Delta-Thetaabfall eine inverse Verschiebung miz weiten Abschnitt folgt.

TABELLE 3

Maxima der Betaaktivität

Placebo	Nomifensin	Differenz	Rangplatz
21,73	27,11	+ 5,38	9
21,51	24,19	+ 2,68	7
24,49	26,65	+ 2,16	4
26,18	26,78	+ 0,60	1
24,14	29,58	+ 5,44	10
25,83	28,00	+ 2,17	5
27,92	31,32	+ 3,40	8
22,83	25,39	+ 2,56	6
29,13	28,09	— 1,04	2
29,58	30,86	+ 1,28	3

Irrtumswahrscheinlichkeit nach Wilcoxon: **0,01**

TABELLE 4

Veränderung der normierten Spektralanteile unter Nomifensin

	Delta u. Theta	Alpha	Beta
I	+ 13,13	— 16,03	+ 4,08
II	+ 2,43	— 23,07	+ 16,42

obere Halbgruppe

	Delta u. Theta	Alpha	Beta
I	— 12,54	+ 14,53	+ 1,68
II	+ 16,42	— 11,14	+ 9,45

untere Halbgruppe

Wie sich dem Verhalten der Bandbreitenmasse entnehmen läßt, wird der Alphaabfall in der oberen Halbgruppe von einer Synchronisationszunahme begleitet, während die untere Halbgruppe nach verstärkter Synchronisation im Abschnitt I mit einer erheblichen Zunahme der Alphabandbreite im zweiten Abschnitt reagiert. Abb. 4, in dem die Alphaspektren der Abschnitte I und II für Placebo und Wirkstoff gegenübergestellt sind (Proband Ed), demonstriert diesen für die untere Halbgruppe typischen inversen Verlauf: Alphazunahme und verstärkte Synchronisation im Abschnitt I, Alphareduktion und Synchronisationsabnahme im Abschnitt II.

Zugleich wird damit auch die morphologische Bedeutung dieser differentiellen Wirkung erkennbar. Während Probanden mit hoher Alphaleistung unter Nomifensin zu einer den späten Phasen des A-Stadiums entsprechenden Musterbildung tendieren, gehen solche mit geringer Alphaleistung nach vorübergehender Alphazunahme und Synchronisation, was dem Durchlaufen eines A-Stadiums entspricht, in ein B-Stadium über.

Immer ist jedoch diese Vigilanzminderung mit einer Zunahme der Betaaktivität verknüpft. Da, wie wir annehmen, der Anteil schneller Aktivitätsformen ein Indikator für das Maß an erregenden Funktionstendenzen ist — die diesbezüglichen Befunde und Hypothesen habe ich 1964 ausführlich dargestellt —, sprechen diese Befunde dafür, daß gleichzeitig mit der Vigilanzminderung ein Erregungsanstieg erfolgt. Dieses Verhalten, das dem Typus einer dissoziativen Vigilanzverschiebung entspricht, findet sich nach unserer Erfahrung bei einer Reihe durch antidepressive Wirkungsqualitäten ausgezeichneter Substanzen. Es ist daher bemerkenswert, daß auch Nomifensin, wie ECKMANN (5) bei der klinischen Prüfung fand, ausgeprägte antidepressive Effekte entfaltet.

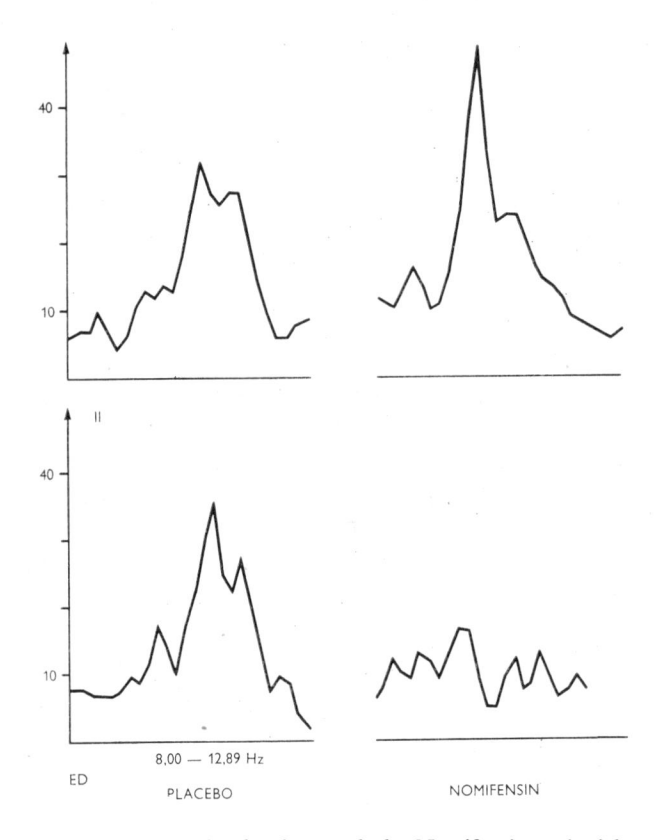

Abb. 4. Frequenzspektralanalyse nach der Nomifensinverabreichung.

Aus den Ergebnissen dieser quantitativ-elektroencephalographischen Arzneimittelstudien sind folgende Schlüsse abzuleiten: Außer generellen Effekten wird das hirnelektrische Wirkungsbild psychotroper Pharmaka in nicht unerheblichem Maße durch differentielle Effekte geprägt. Wie sich in beiden Untersuchungen zeigte, werden hierdurch Form, Ausmaß und Verlauf der durch das Pharmakon hervorgerufenen Vigilanzverschiebung bestimmt, wobei ein deutlicher Zusammenhang mit der individualen Alphaorganisation besteht. Methodisch setzt die Erfassung und Klärung solcher Effekte 1. ein genügend trennscharfes quantitatives Analyseverfahren voraus. 2. ist eine theoretisch angemessene Strukturierung, Verarbeitung und Interpretation der resultierenden Kenngrößen erforderlich. Da die jeweils gewonnenen Maßzahlen nicht alle Merkmale der das Phänomen EEG konstituierenden Strukturen abbilden, sondern nur bestimmte Dimensionen des zugrundeliegenden Prozesses widerspiegeln, ist bei dem heutigen Stande unseres Wissens eine sinnvolle Einordnung quantitativer Befunde und deren Deutung nur unter ständiger Bezugnahme auf die Ebene der morphologischen Betrachtungsweise möglich.

ZUSAMMENFASSUNG

Spektralanalytische Untersuchungen zur elektroencephalographischen Wirkung psychotroper Pharmaka — Etifoxin und Nomifensin — zeigen, daß außer generellen Wirkungen, die sich beispielsweise beim Nomifensin in einer Anregung der Betaaktivität äußern, auch beträchtliche differentielle Effekte vorkommen. Sie stehen in Abhängigkeit von der individualen Organisation der Alphaaktivität und manifestieren sich in einem unterschiedlichen Verlauf des im Rahmen der pharmakogenen Vigilanzverschiebung auftretenden Strukturwandels der hirnelektrischen Aktivität.

LITERATURVERZEICHNIS

1. BENTE, D. (1964) Die Insuffizienz des Vigilitätstonus. Habilitationsschrift Erlangen.
2. BENTE, D., DENBER, H. C. B., HARTUNG, M. L. und RANNEBERG, K. M. (1968) Extrapyramidalmotorische und elektroencephalographische Reaktivität unter neuroleptischer Medikation. Pharmakopsychiatrie-Neuropsychopharmakologie, **1**, 27.
3. BENTE, D. M., MATEJCIK, J., PENNING und SCHENK, G. Spektralanalytische Untersuchungen zur Wirkung von Etifoxin auf das menschliche EEG. Arzneimittel-Forsch. (im Druck).
4. BOHAČEK, N. (1969) Populationsabhängige Unterschiede der zentralnervösen Reaktivität auf Neuroleptika. Psihofarmakologija 2 (Zagreb), 95.
5. ECKMANN, F. Klinische Untersuchungen mit dem Antidepressivum Nomifensin. Arzneimittel-Forsch. (im Druck).
6. KRANZ, H. und HEINRICH, K. (1964) Vigilanz, dissoziative Vigilanzverschiebung und Insuffizienz des Vigilitätstonus, Begleitwirkungen und Misserfolge der psychiatrischen Pharmakotherapie (Stuttgart) 13.

D. B., Forschungseinheit für Psychophysiologie, Nervenklinik der Universität Erlangen — Nürnberg, B.R.D.

METHODOLOGISCHE ASPEKTE ZUR RELEVANZ VON PSYCHOPHARMAKA-UNTERSUCHUNGEN AN GESUNDEN FÜR DIE PHARMAKOTHERAPIE

W. JANKE

Psychologisches Institut der Universität Düsseldorf

Die Verabreichung psychotroper Substanzen an gesunden Personen vollzieht sich zu einem beträchtlichen Teil als Vorstufe zu klinischen Untersuchungen und als Nachstufe zu tierexperimentellen pharmakologischen Prüfungen.

Pharmakopsychiatrie wie auch Pharmakologie scheinen die Brauchbarkeit der pharmakopsychologischen Befunde an Gesunden daran zu bemessen, in welchem Maße sie sich mit den von ihnen erhobenen Befunden zur Deckung bringen lassen. Dabei wird oft übersehen, daß Verhaltensuntersuchungen an Gesunden vom Psychologen meist mit Blick auf Fragestellungen der psychologischen Grundlagenforschung durchgeführt werden. Wenn aber Psychopharmaka-Untersuchungen zur Klärung grundlagenpsychologischer Fragestellungen konzipiert werden, so sollten sie natürlicherweise nicht mit der Frage belastet werden, welche Relevanz sie für klinische Prüfungen haben. Es sollte vielmehr konzidiert werden, daß Pharmaka als unabhängige oder als intervenierende Variablen ausgezeichnete Forschungsinstrumente zur Manipulation des „inneren Milieus" darstellen und damit pharmakopsychologische Untersuchungen im Rahmen der wissenschaftlichen Psychologie ihren Selbstzweck finden.

Mit diesen Bemerkungen soll die Hoffnung ausgedrückt werden, daß klinische Pharmakologie oder Pharmakopsychiatrie gerechterweise keine Forderungen an die Pharmakopsychologie hinsichtlich der Übertragbarkeit von Befunden stellen sollten. Trotzdem glaube ich, daß eine so verstandene Pharmakopsychologie durchaus unentbehrlich im Rahmen der Entwicklung eines neuen Präparates ist und einige Ergebnisse aufzuweisen hat, die von Interesse für die klinische Pharmakologie sein sollten. Die Bemerkungen, die ich machen will, sollen sich auf die Ebene des Verhaltens beschränken.

Es scheint zweckmäßig, die Relevanz pharmakopsychologischer Untersuchungen für die Pharmakotherapie nicht global zu betrachten, sondern aufzudifferenzieren in eine Relevanz der Methoden, der Wirkungen und der Methodik bzw. Untersuchungsstrategien. Im Folgenden sollen diese drei Relevanzaspekte kurz an Hand einiger Beispiele besprochen werden.

Relevanz der Methoden

Die in der Pharmakopsychologie benutzten abhängigen Variablen sind zum überwiegenden Teil im Prinzip auf die pharmakotherapeutische Untersuchung übertragbar, wenn auch bestimmte Techniken, etwa bestimmte Selbstbeobachtungsskalen oder komplexe Leistungstests vor Anwendung auf Patienten oft gewisser Modifikationen bedürfen.

Allerdings scheint die Übertragbarkeit bestimmter Standardmethoden, z.B. der Selbstbeobachtung größer zu sein als angenommen. So ist etwa eine von Janke und Debus (10) in unserem Institut entwickelte mehrdimensionale Eigenschaftswörterliste zur Erfassung augenblicklicher Befindlichkeit, die sich bei gesunden Personen als äußerst pharmakonsensitiv erwies, nur mit geringen Modifikationen bei Pharmako-Therapiekontrollen von Depressiven, Parkinsonkranken und Schizophrenen verwendet worden. Die wesentlichen Ergebnisse, die sich in diesen Untersuchungen zeigten, waren: (1) Die inneren Konsistenzen bei Gesunden und Patienten sind nicht verschieden, (2) Die Therapieverläufe nach Selbstbeurteilung und Fremdbeurteilungen durch den Arzt sind vergleichbar, (3) Selbstbeurteilungen und globale Therapieerfolgsbeurteilungen korrelieren beträchtlich und (4) als besonders interessantes Ergebnis: Die faktorielle Struktur der Selbstbeurteilungen und Fremdbeurteilungen ist *vor* Therapiebeginn vergleichbar differenziert. Im Verlaufe der Therapie finden wir jedoch für die Arztbeurteilung eine beachtliche Entdifferenzierung der Faktorenstruktur (Reduktion der Faktoren von 6—8 auf 2—3), im Unterschied zur Selbstbeurteilung.

Aus derartigen Untersuchungen, die auch von anderen (etwa Park et al. — 14) bestätigt wurden, wird deutlich, daß eine in der Normal-Pharmakopsychologie sich an der Spitze pharmakosensitiver Methoden befindliche Testgruppe auch in der Pharmakotherapie sensitiv ist. In diesem Zusammenhang sei auch daran erinnert, daß Rashkin et al. (15) fanden, daß faktorenanalytisch gewonnene „Psychopathologie-Dimensionen" für Selbst und Fremdbeurteilungen bei Depressiven fast identisch waren.

Auf Grund der vorliegenden pharmakopsychologischen Literatur ist zu vermuten, daß die Pharmakonvaliditäten auch anderer Tests in Pharmakopsychologie und Pharmakopsychiatrie vergleichbar sind. So wird aus den Sammelreferaten von Berger und Potterfield (1) und Janke und Debus (11) deutlich, daß hinsichtlich der Diskriminierungsfähigkeit bei Tranquilizern und Neuroleptika grob gesehen eine Rangreihe derart besteht: Verbale Mitteilung der Befindlichkeit — Variablen des VNS — Psychomotorik — Variablen der Aufmerksamkeit — Wahrnehmungsprozesse — intellektuelle Prozesse.

Diese Rangreihe läßt sich im ganzen dem Aspekt der Beteiligung emotionaler und aktivatorischer Prozesse unterordnen. Wie wir wissen, sind dies auch diejenigen Befindlichkeitsdimensionen, die durch Tranquilizer und Neuroleptika sicher beeinflußt werden.

Auch in Pharmakotherapiekontrollen scheint eine ähnliche Rangreihe zu bestehen, wobei hier nur meist Selbst- in der Regel durch Fremdbeobachtungsdaten ersetzt sind.

Mit diesen Bemerkungen sollte angedeutet werden, daß psychopharmakologische Untersuchungen an Gesunden beitragen, auch für klinische Prüfungen potentiell sensitive Methoden zu entwickeln. Der Vorteil eines solchen Screening ist natürlich darin zu sehen, daß es einfacher ist, hinreichend große homogene Stichproben im normalpsychologischen Bereich zu finden als bei Patienten.

Relevanz der Wirkungen

Die Frage nach der Übertragbarkeit der bei Gesunden gewonnenen Befunde auf Kranke ist komplexer als es auf den ersten Eindruck erscheinen mag. Insbesondere sind 3 Komplexe auseinanderzuhalten: Einmal können wir uns fragen, ob die bei Kranken und Gesunden präparatalterierten psychophysischen Funktionen vergleichbar sind, m.a.W. ob vergleichbare Wirkungsprofile bei vergleichbaren Dosierungen und vergleichbaren Applikationszeiten bestehen, zum anderen ist die Frage zu stellen, ob bei einmaliger oder wiederholter Applikation ähnliche Veränderungen in den Zielsymptomen auftauchen und zum dritten können wir uns die Frage stellen, ob trotz etwaiger Ungleichheit der Wirkungsprofile, es die Ergebnisse bei gesunden Personen zulassen, Vorhersagen über therapeutische Effizienzen zu machen.

Keine der drei Fragen läßt sich bislang nur halbwegs gestützt auf empirisches Material beantworten, weil es einfach an exakten vergleichenden Untersuchungen mit der unabhängigen Variablen „gesund-krank" fehlt.

Betrachten wir kurz den ersten Komplex, den der Vergleichbarkeit der Wirkungsprofile von Kranken und Gesunden. Untersuchungen an Gesunden und Kranken *gleichermassen* mit vergleichbaren Dosierungen lassen sich an den Fingern einer Hand abzählen. Selbst indirekte Vergleiche verschiedener Untersuchungen sind kaum möglich, weil Prüfmethoden und Dosierungen bei Gesunden und Kranken in der Regel verschieden sind. Auch diejenigen klinischen Untersuchungen, die psychologische Prüfmethoden verwenden, sind für Vergleiche „gesund-krank" in der Regel nicht verwendbar, weil die Prüfanordnung lediglich darauf abzielt, Veränderungen vor Behandlung/nach Behandlung zu erfassen, nicht aber Querschnittsbeobachtungen des Verhaltens, wie es der pharmakopsychologischen Methodik entspräche, herauszuarbeiten.

Einige Hinweise ergeben sich lediglich aus dem Untersuchungskreis um SHAGASS und CLARIDGE zur „Sedierungsschwelle" bei Normalen einerseits und Dysthymen und Hysterikern sensu EYSENCK (7) andererseits. Diese allerdings nur eindimensionalen Untersuchungen zeigen, daß neurotische Patienten und „Normale" *qualitativ*, jedoch nicht *quantitativ* vergleichbar reagieren. Zugleich legen bestimmte Korrelationen der Sedierungsschwelle mit dem Therapieerfolg nahe, daß die akuten Präparatwirkungen prognostisch bedeutsam sein können, ein Grund mehr, die Vernachlässigung der Erstellung von akuten Wirkungsprofilen bei Patienten zu bedauern.

Der zweite Aspekt, der zur Wirkungsrelevanz erwähnt wurde, betrifft die Frage, inwieweit bei gesunden Pbn Wirkungen im Sinne der Zielsymptomatik zu beobachten sind. Konkreter: Läßt sich z.B. die anxiolytische Wirkung eines Tranquilizers, der stimmungsaufhellende Effekt eines Antidepressivums auch bei Gesunden nachweisen?

Wenn man die Literatur zu Untersuchungen mit Gesunden durchsieht für typische Vertreter typischer Präparatgruppen, etwa für Meprobamat, Chlorpromazin und Imipramin, so wird man feststellen, daß das nicht der Fall zu sein scheint. Bei allen Präparaten dominieren Leistungsbeeinträchtigungen und Müdigkeit, ohne daß der „emotionale Bereich" im Sinne der Erwartung verändert würde. Insofern wäre die Frage der Übertragbarkeit negativ zu beantworten. Trotzdem darf mit an Sicherheit grenzender Wahrscheinlichkeit festgestellt werden, daß mindestens für Tranquilizer und für Antidepressiva Veränderungen der Zielsymptomatik auch bei Gesunden nachweisbar sind, wenn man *ausgelesene* Stichproben verwendet, also Personen mit hohen Angst- bzw. Neurotizismus-Werten und hohen Punktwerten in Depressionsskalen. DIMASCIO (5) und JANKE (9) haben mehrfach gezeigt, daß bei Aufteilung von unausgelesenen Pbn entsprechend der Zielsymptomatik aus *negativen positive* Befunde gemacht werden können. Wieweit auch für Neuroleptika durch Verwendung umschriebener gesunder Pbn-Gruppen gewisse Wirkungseigentümlichkeiten dieser Substanzen bei Schizophrenen aufgezeigt werden können, ist allerdings fraglich, wenn auch noch nicht definitiv beantwortet.

Die Behauptung, daß pharma*kopsychologische* Untersuchungen vergleichbare Ergebnisse wie pharmakopsychiatrische bringen können, wird sicherlich von mancher Seite bestritten werden. Kritikern ist jedoch entgegenzuhalten, daß nicht behauptet wird, daß positive Befunde bei ausgelesenen Gesunden bereits eine hinreichende Bedingung für klinische Wirksamkeit sind. Allenfalls muß vermutet werden, daß ein Tranquilizer, der bei ausgelesenen ängstlich-neurotlischen Pbn unwirksam ist, wahrscheinlich auch klinisch nicht effektiv ist. Dieses Modell geht davon aus, daß fließende Übergänge von „normal" zu „krank" auf der Verhaltensebene bestehen. Im übrigen ist darauf aufmerksam zu machen, daß ein größerer Teil „gesunder" Pbn, wenn er nach bestimmten Kriterien ausgelesen wurde, mit Sicherheit sich von allen möglichen klinischen Gruppen (z.B. Neurosen, psychosomatische Störungen) kaum unterscheiden dürfte, einfach deshalb, weil solche Pbn häufig nur zufällig nicht in Behandlung sind.

Eine weitere Möglichkeit, die Prüfbedingungen für Kranke und Gesunde einander anzunähern, besteht darin, die Drogenwirkung bei Tranquilizern unter experimentellen Stress-Bedingungen zu prüfen. Eine große Anzahl von Experimenten zeigt, daß unter Lärm oder Erwartungsangst typische anxiolytische oder entspannende Wirkungen bei Tranquilizern zu beobachten sind. Auch diesem Ansatz wird der eingeschworene Kliniker kritisch beggnen und evtl. feststellen, daß die chronifizierte Angst eines Neurotikers prinzipiell etwas anderes sei als die experimentell induzierte eines Gesunden. In Übereinstimmung mit IRWIN (8) und anderen kann der Verhaltensforscher allerdings solchen Einwänden leicht begegnen. Der Erfolg der Pharmakotherapie besteht nicht darin, daß Psychopharmaka irgendetwas an von uns konstruierten nosologischen Einheiten verändern, deren empirisch-verhaltensmäßige und ätiologische Verankerung fragwürdig ist, sondern darin, daß bestimmte Verhaltensweisen wie die motorische und psychische Aktiviertheit oder die Reaktionsweise auf äußere Reize modifiziert werden. Auf der Ebene operational definierter Variablen (Verhalten, physiologische Variablen des ZNS und VNS) aber bestehen, so wie ich die Dinge sehe, keine qualitativen Unterschiede zwischen Patienten und Gesunden unter Stress. Selbst wenn sie *bestehen*, so sind sie *gerade* vom klinischen Pharmakologen nicht kritisch aufzugreifen, weil nach unserer Meinung praktisch alle Psycho-Pharmakotherapie (mit Einschränkungen bei Patienten des manischdepressiven und schizophrenen Formenkreises) darauf beruht, daß durch die wiederholte Präparatverabreichung bestimmte Verhaltens-Umwelt-Interaktionen induziert werden, die bei geeigneten Dosierungsschemata den Eindruck eines mehr oder weniger langdauernden Therapieerfolges vermitteln.

Mit dieser lerntheoretischen Akzentuierung der Pharmakotherapie wird die eingangsgestellte Frage, wieweit auch bei Gesunden Variationen der Zielsymptome nachweisbar sind, etwas anders gestellt: Wieweit lassen sich bei unausgelesenen, ausgelesenen oder unter bestimmten experimentellen Bedingungen stehenden gesunden Pbn im Verhalten und in damit korrelierenden Variablen des autonomen Nervensystems Psychopharmaka-Wirkungen nachweisen, die wir auch bei wiederholten Querschnittsstudien an Patienten finden? Ist dies der Fall, so ist zu klären, welche der Verhaltensalterationen der Patienten für den entgültigen Therapieerfolg relevant sind, d.h. mit dem Therapieerfolg korrelieren und welche der therapierelevanten Verhaltensänderungen auch bei den Gesunden auffindbar sind.

Nach diesen Ausführungen zum Punkt 2. der Wirkungsrelevanz kann der dritte sehr kurz gefaßt werden. Er besagte: Trotz nicht belegter oder gar widerlegter Gleichheit therapierelevanter Wirkungsprofile bei den hier diskutierten Vergleichsgruppen, erscheint es denkbar, daß Vorhersagen von „gesund" nach „krank" möglich sind.

So mögen etwa somatische Nebenwirkungen oder andere therapieirrelevante Effekte auf die potentielle therapeutische Effizienz hinweisen. Die Pharmakopsychologie würde hier in genau der gleichen Lage wie die animale Verhaltenspharmakologie sein. Beispielsweise ist es durchaus denkbar, daß Verhaltensänderungen Gesunder, die nichts mit den Zielsymptomen zu tun haben und die bei Patienten z.B. aus methodischen Gründen nicht nachweisbar sind, eine direkte Vorhersage der antipsychotischen Wirksamkeit eines Neuroleptikums ermöglichen. Um ein Beispiel zu konstruieren: Angenommen ein Neuroleptikum entfaltet bei Gesunden unter Aktivationsbedingungen Verminderung des physiologischen Arousals, Reduktion der Beachtung irrelevanter Stimuli in einem Wahrnehmungstest, Erhöhung der Habituationsrate bei emotionalen Stimuli und Dämpfung der psychomotorischen Aktivität. All das sind Symptome, die wir durchaus bei Normalen regelmäßig beobachten können. Zugleich aber haben sie direkt nichts mit bestimmten Zielsymptomen, etwa Halluzinationen, zu tun. Und doch sind es Merkmale, die indirekt mit den Zielsymptomen zu tun haben, indem sie wahrscheinlich in der Kausalkette der Genese von Halluzinationen involviert sind.

Natürlich könnte hier die Frage auftauchen, warum zu einer solchen indirekten Vorhersage Gesunde benutzt werden. Die Antwort hat sich einfach auf die Ökonomie der Versuchsdurchführung zu beziehen. Untersuchungen an Gesunden sind billiger als klinische Untersuchungen; zumindest dann, wenn von den letzteren eindeutige Ergebnisse erwartet werden.

Relevanz der Methodik bzw. der Untersuchungsstrategien

Auch wenn unterstellt wird, daß Methoden und Wirkungen, so wie sie die gegenwärtige Pharmakopsychologie benutzt oder erarbeitet hat, von geringer Bedeutung für die Pharmakotherapie sind, so wird kaum zu bezweifeln sein, daß bestimmte Forschungskomplexe, die die internationale Pharmakopsychologie gegenwärtig bearbeitet, von mittelbarer Bedeutung sind für klinische Prüfungen. Viele Untersuchungen haben Modellcharakter für die klinische Prüfung oder werfen Hypothesen für praktische oder theoretische Probleme der Pharmakotherapie auf. Zwei Beispiele, die willkürlich ausgewählt sind, sollen dies verdeutlichen. Als erstes Beispiel sei die differentielle Pharmakopsychologie berührt. Pharmakopsychologische Untersuchungen seit Mitte der 50iger Jahre haben wiederholt Korrelationen zwischen Pharmakawirkungen und Persönlichkeitsmerkmalen aufzuzeigen versucht (7, 9, 10). Korreliert wurden Eigenschaften auf dem Trait-level wie Suggestibilität, auf dem Type-level wie Neurotizismus und Extraversion und Merkmale auf dem Habit-level sowie Einstellungen und Werthaltungen. Ähnliches gilt für Untersuchungen aus dem Bereich der Pharmakotherapie (13). Es zeigt sich, daß Kombinationen von Persönlichkeitsprädiktoren hohe multiple Korrelationen mit Pharmakonreaktionen ergeben können (2).

Wenn wir die in der Literatur zu findenden Ergebnisse aber genauer betrachten, so fällt auf, daß Prädiktoren, die sich konsistent als gut erweisen, eine ausgesprochene Rarität sind. Lediglich der Neurotizismus scheint reproduzierbar in der Weise mit Tranquilizerreaktionen zusammenzuhängen, daß hoch neurotische Pbn Angst- und Erregungsreduktionen, nicht-neurotische Pbn dagegen oft paradoxe Erregungen nach Minor und Major Tranquilizers zeigen (6, 7).

Die Gründe für die Inkonsistenz der Persönlichkeits-Wirkungskorrelationen werden deutlich, wenn wir sowohl Persönlichkeitsmerkmale als auch Untersuchungssituationen in experimentellen Anordnungen variieren: So ergab sich beispielsweise in einer unserer Untersuchungen eine hohe positive Korrelation zwischen Neurotizismus und emotionaler Entspannung nach Promazin-Gaben unter einer Untersuchungsbedingung, die keine *mentale* Beanspruchung verlangte. Unter Bedingungen mit hoher mentaler Beanspruchung hingegen war die Korrelation hoch negativ (9). Dies bedeutet, daß Persönlichkeits-Wirkungskorrelationen nicht generalisierbar zu sein scheinen, sondern situationsspezifisch sind.

Solche Ergebnisse, die auch mit allen möglichen anderen Situationsvariationen gewonnen werden können, zeigen erstens, daß die Suche nach generell gültigen Präparatwirkungsprädiktoren wahrscheinlich verfehlt ist, zweitens, daß die Wirkung ein- und derselben Substanz experimentell weitgehend in quantitativer und qualitativer Hinsicht manipulierbar ist. Obzwar es sich hierbei um grundlagenpsychologische Untersuchungen handelt, ist ihr Modellcharakter für pharmakotherapeutische Prozesse unmittelbar evident: Erregende Wirkungen eines Tranquilizers unter mentaler Beanspruchung bei neurotischen Personen etwa bedeuten von vornherein geringe Wahrscheinlichkeiten für therapeutischen Erfolg.

Eine Abklärung, ob, wieweit und in welcher Weise eine Substanz ihre psychotrope Wirkung in verschiedenen situativen Kontexten variiert, bedeutet für die Pharmakotherapie fast mehr als einen Modellversuch, und zwar aus folgendem Grund. Unsere Untersuchungen legen nahe, daß Situationsvariabilität der Wirkungen präparatspezifisch ist. Da man annehmen kann, daß die bei Gesunden gefundene Situationsvariabilität auf Patientenkollektive übertragbar ist, würden differentiellpharmakopsychologische Untersuchungen mit Situationsvariationen Vorhersagen über die Indikationsgeneralität ermöglichen.

Als zweites Beispiel seien Untersuchungen und zur Dosierung erwähnt.

DiMascio (4) hat in einem Referat darauf aufmerksam gemacht, daß die üblicherweise in der Pharmakotherapie verwendeten kontinuierlichen Dosierungsschemata (z.B. 3×25 mg täglich) durch Untersuchungsergebnisse zum Therapieerfolg nicht zu begründen seien. Psychopharmakologische Untersuchungen können hierzu modellhaft bedeutsame Beiträge leisten.

Unter der Annahme, daß gewisse Erfolge der Neurosen-Pharmakotherapie darauf beruhen, daß der Patient lernt, daß bestimmte Situationen unter Tranquilizern mit geringen emotionalen und vegetativen Reaktionen verknüpft sind und er daraus etwa lernt, bestimmte soziale Interaktionen angepaßter zu vollziehen, werden Untersuchungen zum zustandsabhängigen Lernen pharmakotherapeutisch hoch bedeutsam. Das Phänomen des zustandsabhängigen Lernens ist bislang praktisch ausschließlich tierexperimentell untersucht. Es bedeutet, daß unter Präparateinfluß gelerntes Verhalten unter Placebo-Bedingungen schlechter reproduzierbar wird als unter Einfluß eben des Präparates, das während des Lernens verabreicht wurde. Untersuchungen an Gesunden, die bei uns durchgeführt werden, würden bei Übertragbarkeit der Tierbefunde auf den Menschen, zur Erklärung der fatal geringen mittelüberdauernden Heilungen bei Neurosen (12), vielleicht auch bei Schizophrenien beitragen, da nach der Theorie des zustandsabhängigen Lernens während der Pharmakotherapie erzielte Verhaltensänderungen nicht auf die präparatlose Nach-Therapie-Zeit übertragen werden muß. Für die Dosierung von psychotropen Substanzen folgt aus den bisher vorliegenden Befunden zum zustandsabhängigen Lernen nach unserer Meinung zweierlei: Einmal, daß mit möglichst geringen Dosierungen gearbeitet wird, und zum anderen, daß nicht kontinuierliche Dosierungsschemata angewandt werden. Das erste, weil die Übertragungseffekte mit steigender Dosis einer desaktivierenden Substanz geringer werden. Letzteres, weil durch intermittierende Präparatverabreichung mindestens in der letzten Therapiephase dem Patienten ermöglicht wird, Lernvorgänge *ohne* Präparateinfluß zu aktivieren. Pharmakopsychologische Untersuchungen zum Lernen bei intermittierenden Präparatverabreichungen stehen jedoch noch aus.

Die Beispiele pharmakopsychologischer Untersuchungen, die Modellcharakter für Fragen der Pharmakotherapie haben, könnten beliebig fortgesetzt werden. Die beiden dargestellten Beispiele sollten in diesem Zusammenhang lediglich zeigen, in welcher Weise eine „Methodik-Relevanz" zu verstanden werden kann.

Literaturverzeichnis

1. BERGER, F. M. und POTTERFIELD, J. (1969) The effect of Antianxiety Tranquillizers on the Behavior of normal Persons. In: The Psychopharmacology of the Normal Human, Springfield (Thomas), 38.
2. BOUCSEIN, W. (1971) Experimentelle Untersuchungen zum Problem interindividueller Reaktionsdifferenzen auf Psychopharmaka. Giessen, Math.-Nat. Diss.
3. DIMASCIO, A. (1968) Personality and variability of response to psychotropic drugs: relationship to „paradoxical" effects. In: RICKELS, K. (Ed.): Non-specific factors in drug therapy, Springfield (Thomas).
4. DIMASCIO, A. (1970) Dosing scheduling. In: DIMASCIO, A., SHADER, R. I.: Clinical Handbook of Psychopharmacology, New York (Science House).
5. DIMASCIO, A., MEYER, R. E. und STIFLER, L. (1968) Effects of imipramine on individuals varying in level of depression. Amer. J. Psychiat. 124, 55.
6. DIMASCIO, A. und SHADER, R. I. (1968) Behavioral Toxicity. In: EFRON, D. H. (Ed.): Psychopharmacology, Washington (U. S. Gov. Print. Off.).
7. EYSENCK, H. J. (Ed.) (1963) Experiments with drugs. Oxford (Pergamon).
8. IRWIN, S. (1966) Considerations for the pre-clinical evaluation of new psychiatric drugs: a case study with phenothiazine like tranquilizers. Psychopharmacologia (Berl.) 9, 259.
9. JANKE, W. (1964) Über die Abhängigkeit der Wirkungpsychotroper Substanzen von Persönlichkeitsmerkmalen. Ein Beitrag zur Begründung einer differentiellen Pharmakopsychologie. Frankfurt (Akad. Verlagsgesellsch.).
10. JANKE, W. und DEBUS, G. (1973) Die Eigenschaftswörterliste. Göttingen (Hogrefe).
11. JANKE, W. und DEBUS, G. (1968) Experimental Studies on Antianxiety Agents with Normal Subjects: Methodological Considerations and Review of the Main Effects. In: EFRON, D. H.; COLE, J. O.; LEVINE, J.; WITTENBORN, J. R. (Ed.): Psychopharmacology: A Review of Progress 1957—1967, Washington (U. S. Gov. Print. Off.).
12. KAMANO, D. K. (1966) Selective review of effects of discontinuation of drug treatment: Some implications and problems. Psychol. Rep. 19, 743.
13. KOEGLER, R. R. und BRILL, N. O. (1967) Treatment of Psychiatric Outpatients. New York (Appleton-Century-Crofts, Meredith Publishing Co.).
14. PARK, L. C., UHLENHUTH, E. H., LIPMAN, R. S., RICKELS, K. und FISCHER, S. (1965) A Comparison of Doctor and Patient Improvement Ratings in a Drug (Meprobamate) Trial. Brit. J. Psychiat. 111, 535.
15. RASKIN, A., SCHULTERBRANDT, J., REAKY, N. und McKEON, J. J. (1969) Replications of factors of psychopathology in interview, ward behavior and self-report ratings of hospitalized depressives. J. nerv. ment. Dis. 148, 87.

W. J., Psychologisches Institut II der Universität, 4 Düsseldorf, Moorenstrasse 5, B.R.D.

ZUR PERSÖNLICHKEITSSPEZIFISCHEN WIRKUNG PSYCHOTROPER SUBSTANZEN AUF DER NEUROTIZISMUSDIMENSION

H. P. HUBER

Abteilung für klinische Psychologie am Psychologischen Institut der Universität, Düsseldorf

Vorbemerkungen

Am Ende seines Übersichtsreferates kommt BAKER (1) zu der ernüchternden Feststellung, daß es nur wenige Untersuchungen gibt, in welchen es gelang, die generelle Wirkung psychotroper Substanzen mit Hilfe von psychologischen Tests zu objektivieren. Aufgrund einer kritischen Sichtung der einschlägigen Literatur zur allgemeinen Wirkung anxiolytischer Tranquilizer bei gesunden Normalpersonen gelangten BERGER und POTTERFIELD (2) zu einem ähnlichen Ergebnis. Die Verhältnisse liegen jedoch anders, wenn man sog. nicht-spezifische Faktoren im Sinne von RICKELS (26, 27) bei der Planung und Durchführung psychopharmakologischer Experimente berücksichtigt. Es handelt sich hierbei um nicht-pharmakologische Wirkungsgrößen (wie z.B. die äußeren Untersuchungsbedingungen, die Erwartungshaltungen des Experimentators oder die persönliche Ausgangslage der Probanden), die mit der Pharmakonwirkung interagieren können. Die Bedeutung, die solchen nichtspezifischen Größen in der psychiatrischen Pharmakotherapie zukommen kann, wurde bereits in den Beiträgen der Symposien IX und XI des fünften Kongresses 1966 in Washington betont.

Persönlichkeit und Pharmakonwirkung

Für die differentielle Psychologie sind vor allem jene nicht-spezifischen Faktoren von Interesse, die in der Intelligenz- oder Persönlichkeitsstruktur der Pbn begründet sind. Der erste Versuch, das Phänomen der differentiellen Drogeneffekte im Rahmen einer experimentell-orientierten Persönlichkeitstheorie darzustellen, wurde von EYSENCK (6—11) unternommen. Das im Jahre 1957 zum ersten Mal formulierte Drogenpostulat bezieht sich auf die Extraversions-Introversionsdimension, als deren konstitutionelle Grundlage EYSENCK in Überwiegen zentralnervöser Erregungsprozesse bei Introvertierten und ein Überwiegen von Hemmungsprozessen bei Extravertierten annimmt. Unter Bezug auf die Untersuchungen von MAGOUN (24) postuliert EYSENCK als neurophysiologisches Substrat dieser Verhaltensdimension die Formatio reticularis des Hirnstammes. Das Drogenpostulat besagt nun, daß zentraldämpfende Pharmaka das kortikale Erregungs-Hemmungsgleichgewicht in Richtung eines Überwiegens der Hemmungsprozesse verschieben und auf diese Weise extravertierte Verhaltensmuster induzieren. Im Gegensatz dazu bewirken zentralstimulierende Substanzen eine Verschiebung des kortikalen Erregungs-Hemmungsgleichgewichtes in Richtung eines Überwiegens der Erregungsprozesse und führen auf diese Weise zu introvertierten Verhaltensmustern.

Das EYSENCKsche Drogenpostulat wurde in jüngster Zeit vor allem von LEGEWIE (21) scharf kritisiert. Vor LEGEWIE hat jedoch bereits JANKE (17) u.a. darauf hingewiesen, daß die von EYSENCK vorgetragene neurophysiologische Theorie der kortikalen Erregung und Hemmung und deren Zusammenhang zur Extraversions- und Introversionsdimension zu eng sei.

In einem zweiten, bislang allerdings nur programmatisch formulierten Drogenpostulat vertreten EYSENCK (8) und TROUTON und EYSENCK (29) die Hypothese, daß Sympathomimetika auf der Neurotizismusdimension eine Verschiebung in Richtung psychische Labilität bewirken, während Parasympathomimetika zu einer Verlagerung in Richtung psychische Stabilität führen. Als hypothetische neurophysiologische Grundlage des Neurotizismus nimmt EYSENCK (10) eine unterschiedliche Labilität des autonomen Nervensystems an.

Der Neurotizismus kann als eine experimentell fundierte Verhaltensdimension gelten. Zur operationalen Definition dieses Merkmals konstruierte EYSENCK verschiedene Fragebogenskalen wie den MMQ, MPI und EPI (vgl. 8, 12). Daß die mit Hilfe von Fragebogen erfaßte Tendenz zu neurotischen Verhaltensweisen tatsächlich für die Wirkungsbeurteilung psychotroper Substanzen relevant sein kann, haben zahlreiche experimentelle Untersuchungen gezeigt. Als Beispiele seien aus dem deutschen Sprachraum die Arbeiten von FAHRENBERG und PRYSTAV (13), JANKE (17, 18), LIENERT und HUBER (22) sowie MUNKELT und LIENERT (25) genannt. Eine Übersicht über weitere einschlägige Arbeiten findet man bei BERGER und POTTERFIELD (2), JANKE und DEBUS (19) und LEGEWIE (21).

Man kann wohl sagen: Es ist bislang noch nicht gelungen aus der Vielzahl der z.T. kaum vergleichbaren Untersuchungsergebnisse Gesetzmäßigkeiten zu erkennen, die eine zuverlässige Vorhersage der Pharmakonwirkung gewährleisten. Allerdings lassen sich — vor allem was die Wirkung anxiolytischer Tranquilizer auf der Neurotizismusdimension anbelangt — bestimmte Hypothesen formulieren. So besteht Grund zur Annahme, daß Größen aus dem Bereich der Psychomotorik und des bewußten Erlebens besonders empfindliche Indikatoren für differentielle Effekte sein dürften. Insbesondere dürfte es sich hierbei um nicht unmittelbar intelligenzabhängige Variablen handeln, die im Sinne des Satzes 1 von FISHER (14) eine starke Bewußtseinsrepräsentanz besitzen, weil sie entweder konfliktbezogen sind oder aus anderen Gründen eine besondere Ichbeteiligung implizieren. Diese Hypothese soll im folgenden an einem Beispiel aus der Arzneimittelprüfung untersucht werden.

Die persönlichkeitsspezifische Wirkung der Benzoxazinverbindung Hoe 36 801 (Etifoxin)

Die Experimente, die nun berichtet werden sollen, sind Teil einer umfangreicheren Untersuchung, die an zwei Extremgruppen von je 16 Labilen (mit einem N-Score von 15 bis 20) und 16 Stabilen (mit einem N-Score von 0 bis 2) durchgeführt wurde. Die Pbn wurden aufgrund ihrer EPI-Werte aus einer Stichprobe von 327 männlichen Studenten ausgewählt. Die beiden Extremgruppen unterschieden sich jedoch nicht auf der Extraversions-Introversionsdimension des EPI.

Bei der Testsubstanz handelt es sich um die in den Laboratorien der Farbwerke Hoechst AG synthetisierte Benzoxazinverbindung Etifoxin (16). Nach den vorliegenden Tierexperimenten ist Hoe 36 801 ein Tranquilizer mit anxiolytischer, spasmoystischer und anticholinergischer Wirkung.

Um das differentielle Wirkungsspektrum des Testpräparates möglichst breit zu erfassen, wurden folgende Bereiche der Aktivierung untersucht: (a) Katecholaminausscheidung im Urin, (b) Kreislauf, (c) Muskelaktivität, (d) Wahrnehmung, (e) Psychomotorik, (f) Aufmerksamkeit und Konzentration, (g) Anspruchsniveau und (h) subjektive Befindlichkeit. Nach der oben genannten Hypothese ist insbesondere eine differentielle Beeinflussung der Psychomotorik, der Zeitwahrnehmung, des Anspruchsniveaus und der subjektiven Befindlichkeit durch das Testpräparat zu erwarten.

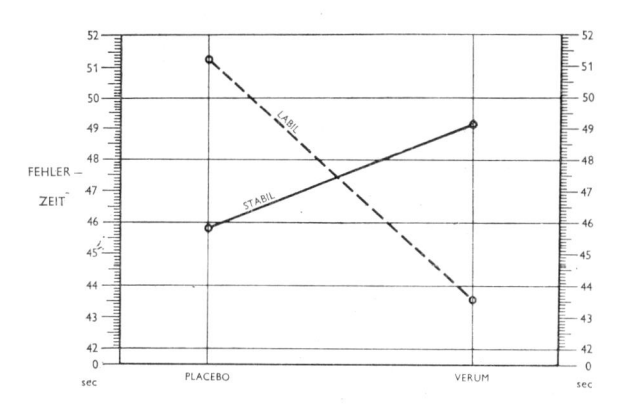

Abb. 1. Die durchschnittlichen Fehlerzeiten (aufsummiert über 5 Durchgänge) von 16 Labilen und 16 Stabilen beim Spiegelzeichnen unter den pharmakologischen Bedingungen A (= Placebo) und B (= Etifoxin)

Den Pbn der Versuchsgruppe wurden 6 Kapseln zu je 50 mg verabreicht. Die Experimente wurden unter rigorosen Doppelblindbedingungen durchgeführt. Die varianzanalytische Auswertung erbrachte u.a. folgende Resultate, die statistisch gesichert sind:

1. *Spiegelzeichnen:* Signifikante Ergebnisse in der Psychomotorik zeigten sich nur beim Spiegelzeichnen. Bei diesem Test muß der Pbn mit einem Kontaktstift eine mit unregelmäßigen Windungen versehene Metall-Leiste nachfahren, wobei er seine Tätigkeit nur über einen Spiegel kontrollieren kann. Hierbei erwies sich die *Fehlerzeit* (gemessen in sec.) als ein empfindliches Maß: Die Fehlerzeit stieg bei den Stabilen im Vergleich zur Placebobedingung unter Verum an; dagegen konnten die Labilen unter dem Einfluß des Testpräparates ihre Fehler schneller korrigieren, was bei gleichbleibender Fehlerzahl zu einer Abnahme der Fehlerzeiten führte (Abb. 1). Die Unterschiede sind auf dem 1 % Niveau gesichert.

2. *Zeitschätzung.* Durch das Herstellen von Zeitstrecken — die Pbn mußten ein Lämpchen in drei Durchgängen 45 Sekunden lang leuchten lassen — versuchten wir präparatebedingte Veränderungen in der Zeitwahrnehmung zu objektivieren. Die Zeitstrecken wurden mit einer Venner-Uhr (mit digitaler Zeitangabe) auf 1/100 Sekunden genau gemessen. Es zeigte sich, daß die Stabilen im Vergleich zu den Labilen unter Placebo kürzere Zeitintervalle produzierten, während sie im Gegensatz zu den Labilen unter Verum signifikant längere Zeitstrecken herstellten ($p < 0{,}10$).

3. *Anspruchsniveau und Ergebnisschätzung.* Beim *Stiftbrett* erwies sich die *Zieldiskrepanz* als ein empfindlicher Indikator für die Aufdeckung differentieller Pharmakoneffekte. Unter der Zieldiskrepanz versteht man die Differenz zwischen dem Anspruchsniveau (der Leistung also, die der Pb gerne erbringen möchte) und der tatsächlich erbrachten Leistung; beim verliegenden Test wurde die Zieldiskrepanz in 1/10 sec gemessen. Der

differentielle Effekt bestand darin, daß die positiven Zieldiskrepanzen der Stabilen unter der Verumbedingung größer wurden, während sie sich bei den Labilen verringerten (p < 0,10). Unter Placebo unterschieden sich die Labilen von den Stabilen nur unwesentlich.

Persönlichkeitsspezifische Effekte zeigten sich ferner in den sog. Erreichungsdiskrepanzen beim *Zieltippen*. Darunter versteht man die Differenz zwischen der geschätzten Leistung und der tatsächlich erbrachten, die bei diesem Test in der Anzahl der Treffer besteht. Während sich die Labilen gegenüber Placebo und Verum relativ indifferent verhielten, zeigten die Stabilen unter Verum eine Überschätzung und unter Placebo eine Unterschätzung ihrer Leistungen (p < 0,10).

4. *Subjektive Befindlichkeit*. Die Kontrolle der subjektiven Befindlichkeit erfolgte u.a. durch die Vorgabe von 23 7-stufigen Polaritätsskalen. Persönlichkeitsspezifische Befunde fanden sich auf den Dimensionen „mutig-ängstlich" (p < 0,05), „traurig-heiter", (p < 0,005) und „aufmerksam-unaufmerksam" (p < 0,10). Dabei erleben sich die Labilen unter Verum im Vergleich zu Placebo als weniger ängstlich, als heiterer und weniger unaufmerksam. Die Stabilen fühlen sich dagegen unter Verum „ängstlicher" und „unaufmerksamer" als unter Placebo.

Zur praktischen Bedeutung von differentiellen Pharmakoneffekten auf der Neurotizismusdimension

a) Die Bedeutung der Ängstlichkeit als klinische Entität und ihre Rolle in der klinischen Psychopharmakologie wurde von WITTENBORN (30) ausführlich diskutiert. Ferner sind sich COLE, BONATO und GOLDBERG (5), HAMILTON (15) und RICKELS (26) in der Auffassung einig, daß nicht-spezifische Faktoren für die pharmakotherapeutische Behandlung neurotischer Patienten eine größere Rolle spielen als für psychotisch Erkrankte.

b) Psychopharmakologische Neurotizismusstudien sind aus persönlichkeitstheoretischen Gründen für die differentielle Psychologie insoferne von besonderem Interesse, als es sich beim Neurotizismus entgegen einer weitverbreiteten Meinung nicht ausschließlich um ein umweltbedingtes Merkmal handeln dürfte. LIENERT und REISSE (23) haben mit Hilfe der BURTschen Kalküle gezeigt, daß der genetisch bedingte Anteil dieses Merkmals bei 50% anzusetzen ist.

c) Möglicherweise können psychopharmakologische Neurotizismusstudien Hinweise zum wissenschaftlichen Verständnis bestimmter Suchtformen geben. KLEIN und DAVIS (20) fanden, daß emotional labile Pbn häufig empfindlicher auf Rauschgifte reagierten als Stabile. Umgekehrt konnten TEASDALE, SEGRAVES und ZACUNE (28) nachweisen, daß von den vier von ihm untersuchten drogenkonsumierenden Versuchsgruppen drei gegenüber den Kontrollgruppen signifikant erhöhte Neurotizismuswerte aufwiesen.

d) Schließlich könnte unter Nutzbarmachung der differentiellen Wirkungskomponenten die Anwendung psychotroper Substanzen u.U. helfen, die Diagnostik des Neurotizismus zu verbessern. In einer eigenen Untersuchung (Symposium für medizinische Psychologie in Halle/S., 1971) konnte demonstriert werden, daß man mit einer linearen Diskriminanzfunktion, in welche die MV-Frequenz, die mittlere Intervall-Länge beim Zeitschätzen, die Fehlerzeit am Pursuit Rotor und beim Spiegelzeichnen sowie die Gesamtleistung im Test d-2 von BRICKENKAMP (3) eingehen, unter Etifoxin besser zwischen psychisch Labilen und Stabilen unterscheiden kann als unter Placebobedingungen. Die Diskriminationsschärfe dieser „Batterie" steigt unter Verum von 37% auf 48% an, wenn man den Prozentsatz der aufgeklärten Varianz über das ε^2 Maß von COHEN (4) schätzt.

Literaturverzeichnis

1. Baker, R. R. (1968) The effects of psychotropic drugs on psychological testing. Psychol. Bull. **69**, 377.
2. Berger, F. M. und Potterfield, J. (1969) The effect of antianxiety tranquilizers on the behavior of normal persons. In: W. O. Evans and N. S. Kline (Eds.), The psychopharmacology of the normal human. Charles C. Thomas. Springfield.
3. Brickenkamp, R. (1962) Test d 2. Aufmerksamkeits-Belastungs-Test, 2. Aufl. J. C. Hogrefe. Göttingen.
4. Cohen, J. (1965) Some statistical issues in psychological research. In: B. B. Wolman (Ed.) Handbook of clinical psychology. McGraw Hill, New York.
5. Cole, J. O., Bonato, R. und Goldberg, S. C. (1968) Non-specific factors in the drug therapy of schizophrenic patients. In: K. Rickels (Ed.) Non-specific factors in drug therapy. Charles C. Thomas. Springfield.
6. Eysenck, H. J. (1957) Drugs and personality. I. Theory and methodology. J. ment. Sci. **103**, 119.
7. Eysenck, H. J. (1959) Das „Maudsley Personality Inventory" (MPI). C. J. Hogrefe. Göttingen.
8. Eysenck, H. J. (1960) Objective psychological tests and the assessment of drug effects. Int. Rev. Neurobiol. **2**, 333.
9. Eysenck, H. J. (1963) Experiments with drugs. Pergamon Press, Oxford.
10. Eysenck, H. J. (1966) Neurose, Konstitution und Persönlichkeit. Z. Psychol. **172**, 145.
11. Eysenck, H. J. (1967) The biological basis of personality. Charles C. Thomas. Springfield.
12. Eysenck, H. J. und Eysenck, S. B. G. (1964) Manual of the Eysenck Personality Inventory. University Press. London.
13. Fahrenberg, J. und Prystav, G. (1966) Psychophysiologische Untersuchung eines Tranquilizers nach kovarianzanalytischem Plan zur Kontrolle von Ausgangswerten und Persönlichkeitsdimensionen. Arzneim.-Forsch. (Drug Res.) **16**, 754.
14. Fisher, S. (1970) Nonspecific factors as determinants of behavioral response to drugs. In: A. Dimascio and R. I. Shader (Eds.) Clinical handbook of psychopharmacology. Science House. New York.
15. Hamilton, M. (1968) Discussion of the meeting. In: K. Rickels (Ed.) Non-specific factors in drug therapy. Charles C. Thomas. Springfield.
16. Hoffmann, I., Kuch, H., Schmitt, K. und Seidl, G. (1970) 2-Äthylamino-6-chlor-4-methyl-4-phenyl-4H-3,1-benzoxazin. Arzneim.-Forsch. (Drug. Res.) **7**, 975.
17. Janke, W. (1964) Experimentelle Untersuchungen zur Abhängigkeit der Wirkung psychotroper Substanzen von Persönlichkeitsmerkmalen. Akademische Verlagsgesellschaft. Frankfurt am Main.
18. Janke, W. (1966) Über psychische Wirkungen verschiedener Tranquilizer bei gesunden, emotional labilen Personen. Psychopharmacologia, 8, 340.
19. Janke, W. und Debus, G. (1968) Experimental studies on antianxiety agents with normal subjects: Methodological considerations and review of the main effects. In: D. H. Efron (Ed.) Psychopharmacology. A review of progress 1957—1967. U.S.Government Printing Office. Washington.
20. Klein, D. F. und Davis, J. M. (1969) Diagnosis and drug treatment of psychiatric disorders. The Williams and Wilkins Company. Baltimore.
21. Legewie, H. (1968) Persönlichkeitstheorie und Psychopharmaka. Anton Hain. Meisenheim am Glan.
22. Lienert, G. A. und Huber, H. P. (1966) Strukturwandel der Intelligenzfaktoren unter der Wirkung von Amphetamin. Arzneim.-Forsch. (Drug Res.) **16**, 304.
23. Lienert, G. A. und Reisse, H. (1961) Ein korrelationsanalytischer Beitrag zur genetischen Determination des Neurotizismus. Psychol. Beitr. 7, 122.
24. Magoun, H. W. (1963) The waking brain, 2nd Edition, Charles C. Thomas. Springfield.
25. Munkelt, P. und Lienert, G. A. (1964) Blood alcohol level and psychophysical constitution. Arzneim.-Forsch. (Drug Res.) **6**, 573.
26. Rickels, K. (1968) Non-specific factors in drug therapy of neurotic patients. In: K. Rickels (Ed.) Non-specific factors in drug therapy. Charles C. Thomas. Springfield.
27. Rickels, K. (1968) Critique. In K. Rickels (Ed.) Non-specific factors in drug therapy. Charles C. Thomas. Springfield.
28. Teasdale, J. D., Segraves, R. T. und Zacune, J. (1971) "Psychoticism" in Drug-users. Brit. J. soc. clin. Psychol. **10**, 160.

29. TROUTON, D. und EYSENCK, H. J. (1960) The effects of drugs on behaviour. In: H. J. EYSENCK (Ed.) Handbook of abnormal psychology. Pitman Medical Publication Company, London.
30. WITTENBORN, J. R. (1966) The clinical psychopharmacology of anxiety. Charles C. Thomas. Springfield.

H.P.H., *Abteilung für klinische Psychologie am Psychologischen Institut der Universität, Himmelgeisterstr. 127, Düsseldorf, B.R.D.*

VERSUCH ZUR DARSTELLUNG EINER NEUROLEPTISCHEN BEHANDLUNG MIT EMD 16 139 AN GESUNDEN VERSUCHSPERSONEN

P. DIETSCH, F. ALBRECHT und H. J. MÖNIKES

Psychiatrische Klinik des Bürgerhospitals Stuttgart und Fachbereich Psychologie der Universität Giessen

Über den erfolgreichen Versuch, bei Ratten die dämpfende Wirkung von Benactyzin auf die Vermeidungsreaktion auf eine Medikation mit Kochsalzlösung zu übertragen, berichteten HECHT et al. (5). Die unter Placebo weiterhin gedämpfte Vermeidungsreaktion stieg aber auf ihr altes, d. h. nach dem Training bestehendes Niveau bei Änderung der äußeren Bedingungen von Dunkel auf Hell wieder an.

Ähnliche, allerdings einfachere Experimente wurden zuvor von MILLER (9) mit Chlorpromazin durchgeführt. Über gegenteilige Effekte, d. h. Fehlen Mittel-überdauernder Wirkungen im Tierversuch berichteten BARRY et al. (1).

Es erscheint möglich, daß eine psychotrope Wirkung erlernt werden kann und dann unter vergleichbaren Auslösebedingungen ohne Verabreichung des ursprünglichen chemischen Auslösers wieder hervorgerufen werden kann. Diese „erlernte" psychotrope Wirkung ist jedoch an bestimmte situative Auslösebedingungen gekoppelt. Dieser nach Tierversuchen aufgestellten Behauptung sollte an gesunden Versuchspersonen in unserer Untersuchung nachgegangen werden. Es wird versucht, einen experimentellen Beitrag gerade zur Frage der unzuverlässigen Mittel-überdauernden Wirkung von Neuroleptika in der Therapie zu leisten (8).

Ein weiterer Ansatzpunkt dieser Untersuchung war die Frage nach einer spezifischen Prüfung von Neuroleptika bei gesunden Versuchspersonen. Das Inventar der Untersuchungsmethoden ist charakterisiert durch die Prüfung von Tranquillizern, Schlafmitteln und Stimulantien. Die hier üblichen Instrumente zeigen auch bei Neuroleptika einen Ausschlag (3). Diese meist sedierende Wirkung kann aber nicht als spezifisch für Neuroleptika angesehen werden. Dagegen wurde von COOK (2) gezeigt, daß die Dämpfung der Vermeidungsreaktion zumindest durch Chlorpromazin, die eine entscheidende Bedingung für die Klassifikation eines Neuroleptikums im Tierversuch ist, auch beim Menschen spezifisch ist, d. h., daß sie bei Tranquillizern von COOK nicht festgestellt wurde. Für das hier untersuchte Präparat EMD 16 139 (MERCK) (Abb. 1), das nach Pharmakologie und klinischen Vorversuchen als Neuroleptikum klassifiziert wurde, hatten wir in Vorversuchen bei einmaliger Applikation vor allem deutlich dysphorische subjektive Wirkungen gefunden. Für das Präparat stellte sich die Frage, ob es das von COOK aufgestellte Kriterium der Dämpfung der Vermeidungsreaktion, das es im Tierversuch natürlich erfüllt, auch bei gesunden Versuchspersonen erfüllen würde.

Der Versuchsplan sieht eine Versuchszeit von insgesamt 18 Tagen, d. h. 3 × 6

Wochentagen ohne Sonntage vor. 7 Tage lang wurde die Vermeidungsreaktion eingeübt. Danach wurde 6 Tage lang die Mittel-gebundene Wirkung bei 48 Personen unter EMD 16 139 gegen Placebo bei 16 Personen geprüft. Gleichzeitig wurden die Versuchspersonen unter Medikament an die Wirkung gewöhnt. Um den Versuchspersonen nicht Medikamentwirkungen zu suggerieren, wurde schon in der Einübungszeit Placebo appliziert. Am 14. Versuchstag wurde das Medikament bei 16 Versuchspersonen ganz

Abb. 1. EMD 16 139 = 2-Hydroxy-2-äthyl-1,2,3,4,6,7-hexahydro-11bH-benzo[a]chinolizinmalonat

abgesetzt und bei 16 Versuchspersonen durch Placebo ersetzt. Bei den restlichen 16 Versuchspersonen wurde die Medikation mit EMD 16 139 fortgesetzt. Es ergeben sich so vom 14. bis 16. Versuchstag vier Gruppen: Placebo nach Medikament (A1), nichts nach Medikament (A2), Medikament (A3), Placebo nach Placebo (B). Am 17. und 18. Tag wurde jeweils die Hälfte der vier Gruppen zusätzlich während der Messung der Vermeidungsreaktion mit Lärm (70 db) beeinflußt.

Versuchspersonen waren 64 gesunde männliche Studenten verschiedener Fachrichtung.

Das Präparat wurde in der Dosis von 50 mg/Tag oral am täglichen Versuchsbeginn appliziert. Es handelt sich um eine nach pharmakologischen Gesichtspunkten sehr niedrige Dosis. Eine Kumulierung des Präparates, die eine Mittel-überdauernde oder sich mit der Zeit verstärkende Wirkung bedingen könnte, ist so nicht einzukalkulieren.

Die Versuchspersonen hatten keine Einsicht in die Änderung der Medikation. Die Versuchsleiter wußten, an welchen Tagen Änderungen stattfanden, aber nicht, bei welchen Personen.

Der tägliche Versuchsablauf ist Tabelle 1 zu entnehmen. Hier wird nur über die Ergebnisse im Schnell-Lese-Versuch berichtet.

TABELLE 1

Täglicher Versuchsablauf

Zeitpunkt	Vorgang
0— 5 min	Applikation des Präparates/Placebo/Nichts
5— 15 min	EWL, 1. Messung, Tagesausgangslage
15— 75 min	Pause, Zeitungslesen, Beurteilung des körperlichen Befindens in den letzten 24 Stunden
75— 80 min	Wechsel des Versuchsraumes
80— 90 min	EWL, 2. Messung
90—110 min	Schnell-Lese-Versuch
110—120 min	EWL, 3. Messung

Als Vermeidungsreaktion wurde von uns ein Schnell-Lese-Versuch verwendet, weil wir eine ausgesprochen humane Leistungsmodalität beeinflussen wollten. Zu lesen war täglich der gleich Text. Die Versuchspersonen hatten 12 × 30 Sekunden so schnell wie möglich zu lesen. Davor und dazwischen wurde jeweils 60 Sekunden in normalem Tempo gelesen. Die Versuchspersonen wurden vom 2. bis 6. Tag gestraft, wenn sie ihre Leistung in 30 Sekunden nicht gegenüber dem Vortag steigern konnten. Als Strafe hatte die Versuchsperson direkt im Anschluß an die ungenügende Leistung innerhalb von 30 Sekunden wiederum 30 Sekunden lang unter verzögerter Rückkoppelung zu lesen. Die Wirksamkeit von verzögerter Rückkoppelung als Strafe wurde u. a. von GOLD-DIAMOND (4) hervorgehoben. Ab 7. Tag wurde keine Strafe mehr appliziert, was aber für die Versuchspersonen aus der Anordnung nicht vorherzusehen war. Das Training vom 1. bis 7. Tag erbrachte eine Leistungssteigerung von durchschnittlich 2012 auf 2684 Silben in 12 × 30 Sekunden.

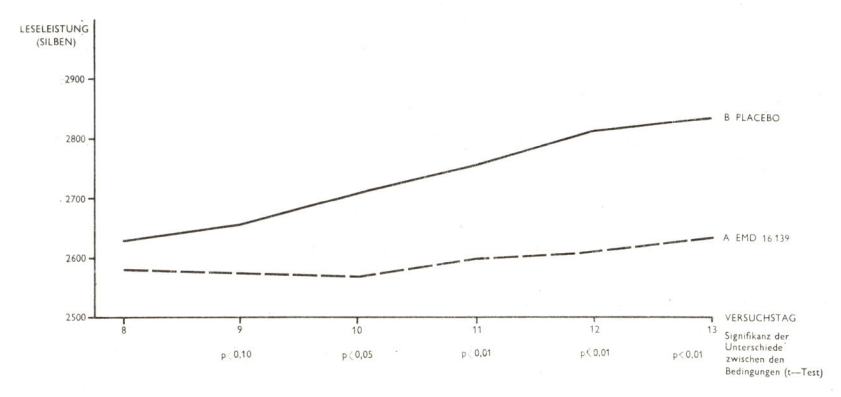

Abb. 2. Schnell-Lese-Versuch am 8. bis 13. Tag. Kovarianzanalytisch korrigierte Mittelwerte (Kovariable: Messwert am 6. Tag)

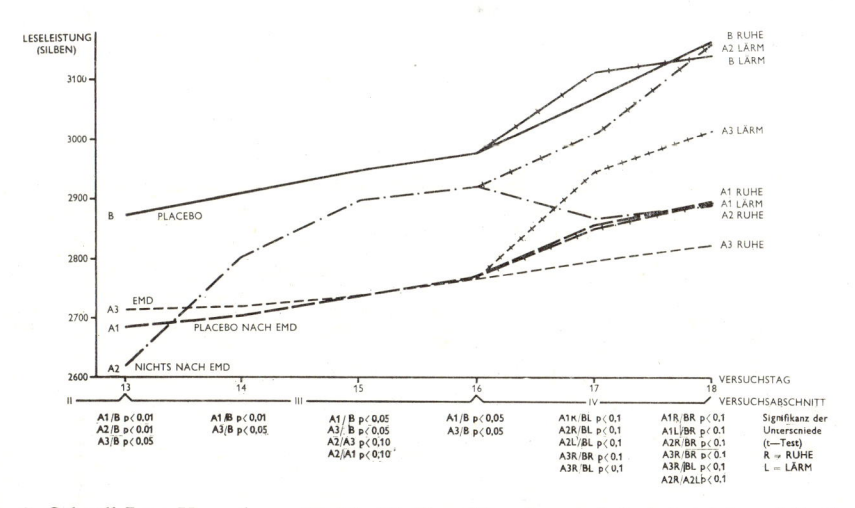

Abb. 3. Schnell-Lese-Versuch am 13. bis 18. Tag. Kovarianzanalytisch korrigierte Mittelwerte. (Kovariable: Meßwert am 6. Tag)

Zunächst ist ab 8. Versuchstag zu beobachten (Abb. 2), daß die Leistung in der Vermeidungsreaktion unter Placebo auch ohne Strafen weiter ansteigt. Vermutlich handelt es sich um Effekte eines fortgesetzten Trainings. Zu beachten ist, daß hier die Leistung in einer Vermeidungsreaktion gemessen wurde, nicht die Häufigkeit der Ausführung, wie dies in den meisten Tierversuchen üblich ist.

EMD 16 139 beeinflußt die Leistung in der Weise, daß im Mittel eine Stagnation eintritt (Abb. 2). Ab 10. Versuchstag ist die Medikamentwirkung statistisch signifikant von Placebo abgehoben. Die Signifikanz ergibt sich im t-Test nach kovarianzanalytischer Korrektur der Werte auf den Meßwert des sechsten Tages, d. h. die individuell optimale Ausprägung unserer Vermeidungsreaktion. Die Forderung, daß EMD die Vermeidungsreaktion bei der gesunden Versuchsperson dämpfen soll, kann also als erfüllt gelten.

Bei Veränderung der Medikationsbedingungen am 14. Tag unterscheidet sich entsprechen unseren Erwartungen die Gruppe A1 (Placebo nach Medikament) ebenso wie die Gruppe A3 (weiterhin Medikament) von Placebo, während der Unterschied gegen Placebo bei A2 (nichts nach Medikament) verschwindet (Abb. 3). Am 15. Tag ergibt sich ein fast signifikanter Unterschied zwischen A2 und A1 bzw. A3. Es kann also gefolgert werden, daß eine Mittel-überdauernde Wirkung, die nicht auf chemische Nachwirkungen bezogen werden kann, erzielt wird, wenn wir Placebo weiter applizieren.

Weniger klar sind die Ergebnisse, die bei der zusätzlichen Lärmbelastung bei jeweils der Hälfte der Gruppen erzielt wurden am 17. und 18. Tag. Dies ist in erster Linie durch die geringe Zahl von 8 Versuchspersonen pro Gruppe zu erklären. Der erwartete Abbruch der Mittel-überdauernden Wirkung unter Lärm (A1 Lärm) tritt, sofern man den statistisch schlecht gesicherten Unterschieden vertrauen will, nicht ein. Es ist aber auch unter Placebo keine Lärmwirkung auf die Leseleistung nachzuweisen. Die Tatsache, daß der erwartete Abbruch der Mittel-überdauernden Wirkung nicht einzutreten scheint, sollte zunächst so verstanden werden, daß es uns bisher nicht gelungen ist, den angemessenen Stressor zur Provokation dieses Effektes bei gesunden Versuchspersonen zu finden. Auch das absehbare Ende der Versuche könnte eine Alteration der Motivation der Probanden bedingt haben.

Über die subjektiven Wirkungen von EMD 16 139, gemessen mit der Eigenschaftwörter-Liste von Janke und Debus, (7) kann hier nur mitgeteilt werden, daß eine entsprechende Mittel-überdauernde Wirkung nicht festgestellt werden kann, weil schon während der Medikation die anfänglich starken sedierenden und stimmungsdämpfenden subjektiven Wirkungen zurückgehen. Störungen des körperlichen Befindens, gemessen mit der Liste körperlicher Symptome von Janke traten zu keinem Zeitpunkt unter EDM 16 139 gegenüber Placebo vermehrt auf.

Literaturverzeichnis

1. Barry, H., Etheredge, E. E. und Miller, N. E. (1965) Counterconditioning and extinction of fear fail to transfer from Amobarbital to nondrug state. Psychopharmacologia (Berl.) 8, 150.
2. Cook, L. (1964) Effects of drugs on operant conditioning. In: Steinberg, H., de Reuck, A. V. S., und Knight, J.: Ciba Foundation Symposium on Animal Behaviour and Drug Action. London, Churchill Ltd.
3. Debus, G. (1971) Neuroleptica. In: Arnold, W., Eysenck, H. J. und Meili, R.: Lexikon der Psychologie. Freiburg, Herder.
4. Golddiamond, I. (1965) Stuttering and fluency as manipulatable operant response classes. In: Krasner, L. und Ullmann, L. P.: Research in Behavior Modification. New York, Holt, Rinehart and Winston.
5. Hecht, K., Treptow, K., Hecht, T. und Poppei, M. (1969) Die Bedeutung der Organismus — Umwelt — Beziehung für die Neuro-Psychopharmakologie. Arzneim.-Forsch. (Drug Res.) 19, 417.

6. JANKE, W.: Liste körperlicher Symptome, LKS — V/1970 — 51i, 7s, unveröffentlicht.
7. JANKE, W. und DEBUS, G.: Eigenschaftswörterliste (E-W-L). Göttingen, Hogrefe, in Vorbereitung.
8. KAMANO, D. K. (1966) Selective review of effects of discontinuation of drug treatment: Some implications and problems. Psychol. Rep. **19**, 743.
9. MILLER, N. E. (1961) Some recent studies of conflict behaviour and drugs. Amer. Psychologist, **16**, 13.

P.D., Psychiatrische Klinik des Bürgerhospitals, Tunzhoferstr. 14—16, 7 Stuttgart 1, B.R.D.

EINE NEUE METHODE ZUR AUSWERTUNG DER PSYCHOTROPENWIRKUNG BEI NORMALEN VERSUCHSPERSONEN

Z. BÖSZÖRMÉNYI und GY. SOLTI

Staatliches Institut für Nerven- und Geisteskrankheiten, Budapest

Das Problem der Psychopharmaka-Wirkung bei normalen Versuchspersonen (nVp) wird immer schwieriger, da man immer kompliziertere Forschungspläne anwenden muß, um die verschiedenen wichtigen Parameter, sowie die Interaktionen einkalkulieren zu können. In mehreren Artikeln behandelt dasselbe Thema auch HEIMANN et al.(2, 3), neulich auch die Wichtigkeit bzw. Wechselwirkungen zwischen Gruppendynamik und Psychopharmaka bei Gruppenbeobachtungen betonend. Da wir schon früher Sozialpsychologische Untersuchungen bei mit Psychopharmaka behandelten Patienten im Gruppenrahmen durchführten (1), wollten wir die Gruppensituation gepaart mit Problemlösungsaufgaben ausnützen, um die Wirkung eines neuen Anxiolytikums bei nVpn zu studieren. Es handelte sich um ein neues Präparat der Benzdiazepinreihe, mit der Kurzbezeichnung Tofizopam. Während unserer Versuche erkannten wir, daß SPIEGEL et al. (4) schon ähnliche vergleichende Studien publizierten betr. Psychopharmaka-Wirkung auf die verbalen Interaktionen einiger Studenten, im Gruppenrahmen Desimipramin, Thioridazin bzw. Placebo verabreichend. Sie konnten keine nennenswerten Unterschiede bei ihren nVpn feststellen.

Unser Verfahren war jedoch vom Oberwähnten sehr verschieden: wir veranstalteten nähmlich mit unseren nVp-en sog. Brainstorming-Sitzungen vor und nach Medikamentengabe bzw. Placebo-Verabreichung. Dadurch wollten wir feststellen, ob manche Psychopharmaka die gezielten „ideenschöpfenden" Assoziationen quantitative und qualitative beeinflussen können und auf welche Weise. Deshalb formten wir 2 Gruppen mit je 10 Mitgliedern, eine von Universitätsstudenten, die englische und ungarische Literatur als Fach wählten, die andere Gruppe bestand aus Teilnehmern einer Krankenschwesternschule. Die Versuchsreihe war folgende: zuerst hielten wir eine Probesitzung mit beiden Gruppen als Übung, neutrale Denkaufgaben vorführend und die Mitglieder jeder Gruppe sollten entsprechende Vorschläge machen vor und nach einer Placebo-Verabreichung. Diese Übungssitzung wurde nicht gewertet. Nach diesem Vorversuch veranstalteten wir betr. Medikation die weiteren in folgender Reihe:

1. Placebo
2. Tofizopam (ein neues Derivat aus der Benzdiazepinreihe, 50 mg)
3. Placebo
4. Placebo
5. Amitriptylin (15 mg)
6. Placebo

Das Programm der Sitzungen war gleicherweise folgendes:

1. Bekanntgebung der Denkaufgabe mit der Aufforderung relevante, d. h. brauchbare Ideen zu äußern.
2. Einnahme der Tabletten.
3. 50—60 Minuten Pause.
4. Dasselbe wie in Punkt 1., mit anderer Aufgabe, d. h. Wiederholung des Brainstorming.

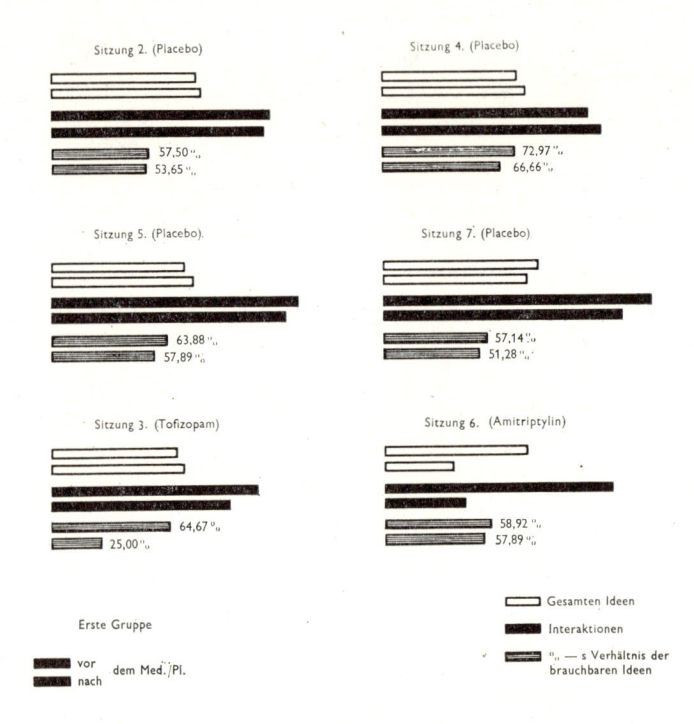

Abb. 1. Die Sitzungen mit den Philologiestudenten.

Die ideenprovozierenden Aufgaben waren — außer der oberwähnten Probesitzung — alle dem Fachgebiet der Beteiligten entsprechende, die gleichzeitig gewisse Fachkenntnisse voraussetzen. Als Beispiel möchten wir diejenigen Aufgaben, die in beiden Gruppen vor und nach der Tofizopam-Verabreichung vorgeschlagen wurden, erwähnen:

1a. Was würden sie tun um bessere Resultate zur Neuroformierung des Sprachunterrichts in der Schule zu erzielen?
2a. Wie könnten sie die alte ungarische Literatur bei ihren Studenten beliebter machen?
1b. Was halten sie für die schwierigste Aufgabe der Krankenpflege und wie könnten sie diese erleichtern?
2b. Falls sie Oberschwester bzw. Oberpfleger wären, welche Führungsmethoden würde Sie wählen und warum?

Die Latein-Quadrat-Methode konnten wir leider nicht anwenden, trotzdem glauben wir, da wir bei den ausgewerteten Sitzungen in gewisser Karakteristika keinen Unterschied feststellen konnten, daß die Übung die Ergebnisse wesentlicht nicht beeinflußte. Selbstverständlich wurden alle Sitzungen auf Tonband aufgenommen, daneben registrierten zwei Psychologen mit Aktogrammen neben verbalen auch die nichtverbalen Interaktionen.

Die Informationsströmung während der Problemlösung bei den Gruppen untersuchten wir durch Zählen der gesammten geäusserten Ideen bzw. Interaktionen und Ausrechnung der brauchbaren Ideen, auch ein prozentuales Vorkommen derselben

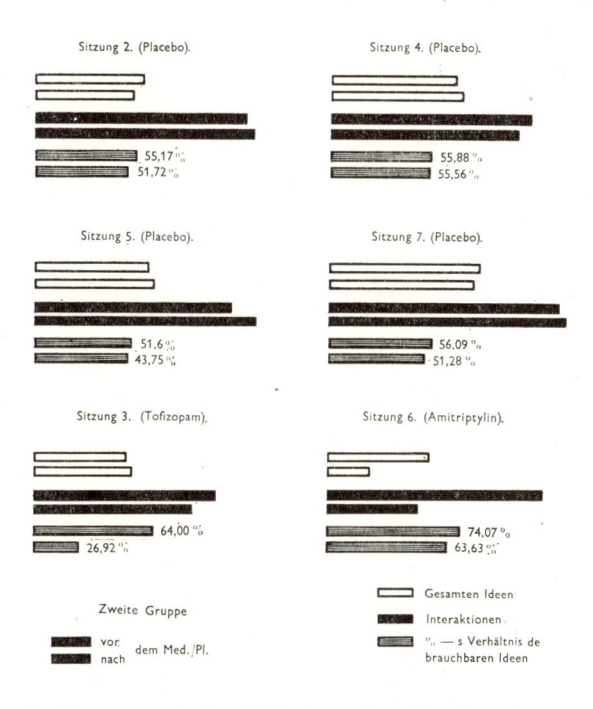

Abb. 2. Die Sitzungen mit den Teilnehmern der Krankenschwesterschule.

feststellend. Als brauchbar werteten wir alle diejenigen problemlösenden Vorschläge, die keine bizarren oder phantastische Elemente enthielten, unabhängig davon, ob diese verwirklichbar waren oder nicht. Als einer der Literaturstudenten z. B. die Planung eines Computersystems vorschlug, das für den Examenkandidaten Fragen stellen könne, die Antworten jedoch nur dann akzeptierend, wenn diese grammatisch und phonetisch fehlerfrei seien, bei einem Knopfdruck sogar die Fehler auch aufzählen könne, nahmen wir dies als brauchbar an, trotz des utopistischen Charakters.

Unsere Ergebnisse sind in der 1. und 2. Abbildung dargestellt.

Abb. 1. zeigt die Resultate der mit den Philologiestudenten organisierten Sitzungen.

Abb. 2. demonstriert die entsprechenden Daten der anderen Gruppe. Ergänzend zu den Abbildungen geben wir auch tabellarisch die exakten zahlenmässigen Daten an. (Siehe Abb. 1 und 2, sowie Tabelle 1)

TABELLE 1

No. der Sitzung		Gesamte Vorschläge G. I.	G. II.	Interaktionen G. I.	G. II.	%-der brauchbaren Einfälle G. I.	G. II.
2.	vor Pl.	40	29	62	57	57,50	55,17
	nach Pl.	41	26	58	59	53,65	51,72
3.	vor Tofizop.	34	25	56	49	64,70	64,00
	nach Tofizop.	36	26	53	43	25,00	26,92
4.	vor Pl.	37	34	56	54	72,97	55,88
	nach Pl.	39	36	60	51	66,66	55,55
5.	vor Pl.	36	31	67	53	63,88	51,61
	nach Pl.	38	32	64	60	57,89	43,75
6.	vor Amitr.	39	27	63	58	58,92	74,07
	nach Amitr.	19	11	22	24	57,89	63,63
7.	vor Pl.	42	41	73	62	57,14	56,09
	nach Pl.	39	39	65	64	51,28	51,28

Pl. — Placebo
Tofizop. — Tofizopam
Amitr. — Amitriptyline

Wie aus den Abbildungen zu ersehen ist, war in der Gruppe der Universitätsstudenten die Summe der geäußerten Ideen und Interaktionen vor und nach den Placeboversuchen, sowie vor den medikamentösen Versuchen gleicherweise hoch genug, die andere Gruppe war dagegen eher durch Reichtum der nichtverbalen Interaktionen charakterisiert. Durch die Wirkung des Tofizopams wurde die relative und absolute Menge der brauchbaren Ideen in beiden Gruppen wesentlich reduziert; gleichzeitig blieb die weitere Charakteristika der Gruppeninformationsströmung, d. h. die Anzahl die geäußerten Einfälle und die interaktionelle Tätigkeit im allgemeinen unverändert. Amitriptylin verursachte eine wesentliche Verminderung der gesamten Ideen und Interaktionen, auch der absoluten Anzahl der brauchbaren Vorschläge; diese Verminderung ging bis zu 35—50 % der Ausgangswerte. Nach Tofizopam-Verabreichung war die Reduktion der brauchbaren Ideen auch auffallend, zugleich statistisch signifikant, $p < 3\%$.

BESPRECHUNG

Obwohl wir die Methode der Lateinischen Quadrate nicht anwenden konnten, glauben wir, daß unsere Resultate trotzdem verwendbar sind. Wir konnten die Rolle der Übung bzw. Lernens bei beiden Gruppen für unwichtig halten, da bei allen Placebo-Versuchen, sowie vor der Medikamentverabreichung nur wenige Änderungen registriert wurden. Deshalb erwies es sich als zweckmäßig, daß für die Versuche schon präformierte, d. h. zusammengewöhnte Gruppen gewählt wurden, bei denen die gemeinsame Problemlösung eine alltägliche Situation bedeutete, weshalb die Arbeitsweisen der Informationsverwertung als Systemfunktionen schon vorhanden waren. Diese ermöglichte es, daß die Gruppe als selbständiges System funktionierte, derer Leistung die individuellen Schwankungen mit Hilfe ausgleichender-protektiver Mechanismen stabilisiert bleiben konnte.

Wir halten unsere Beobachtungen mit gewissen Beschränkungen für überzeugend, d. h. man kann annehmen, daß Tofizopam in problemlösenden Situationen mit Brainstorming-Charakter die Informationsströmung der Gruppen bizarrer oder phantastischer umgestalten kann, dadurch die prozentuale Häufigkeit der brauchbaren Ideen signifikanterweise senkend. Ähnlicherweise sinkt letztgenannte Häufigkeit auch durch die Amitriptylin-Wirkung, aber parallel mit der Zahl der gesamten geäußerten Einfälle und in Begeitung bedeutender Verminderung aller Interaktionen.

Wir nehmen an, daß obige Resultate karakteristisch für die beiden Medikamente, bzw. für jene Gruppe der Arzneimittel sind, denen diese angehörigen. Deshalb kann man wahrscheinlich oberwähnte Methode zum Testen neuer Psychopharmaka anwenden, wenn man einige typische Beeinflussungsmöglichkeiten betr. Informationsströmung und Aufarbeitung der Einfälle während Problemlösung im Gruppenrahmen mit bekannten encephalotropen Mitteln ausgesondert hat. Ähnliche retrospektive Folgerungen benützt man in der Biochemie schon seit langem, z. B. bei farbenphotometrischen Untersuchungen, deren Gültigkeit auch nur unter gewissen strikten Bedingungen gültig sind.

Die beschriebenen pharmakopsychologische Versuche sind nur als Erkundigungsexperiment zu betrachten. Die einfallprovozierende Methode im Gruppenversuch repräsentiert vielleicht einen Weg, welcher zu einer Differenzierung der Wirkung von Psychopharmaka in einer relativ praktischen Situation führen konnte.

LITERATURVERZEICHNIS

1. BÖSZÖRMÉNYI, Z. und SOLTI, GY. (1969) Sozialpsychologische Untersuchungen bei mit Psychopharmaka behandelten Psychotikern. Arzneim.-Forsch. (Drug Res.) 19, 446.
2. HEIMANN, H. (1971) Wirkungsvergleich von Psychopharmaka am menschlichen Verhalten. Beitr. z. gerichtl. Med. 28, 155.
3. HEIMANN, H. und EISERT, H. G. (1971) Emotionale Labilität bei gesunden Versuchspersonen und Ergebnisse in einigen Leistungstests. In: Advances in Neuropsychopharmacology, Eds: O. VINAR, Z. VOTAVA and P. B. BRADLEY, North Holland Publ. Co., Amsterdam; Avicenum, Prague, p. 389.
4. SPIEGEL, R., BATTEGAY, R. und ABT, K. (1971) Comparative study of the effect produced by psychotropic drugs on verbal interaction in a group of students. Ibidem, p. 353.

Z.B., Staatliches Institut für Nerven- und Geisteskrankheiten, Vöröshadsereg u. 116, Budapest 1021, Ungarn

BIOCHEMICAL FINDINGS IN MENTAL ILLNESS. SCHIZOPHRENIC DISORDERS

Chairmen: I. MUNKVAD, O. J. RAFAELSEN and D. RICHTER

Associate chairman: T. HALLAS-MØLLER

THE NATURE OF THE SCHIZOPHRENIC PSYCHOSES

D. RICHTER

Medical Research Council, Neuropsychiatry Unit, Carshalton and Epsom, Surrey

The clinical investigation of schizophrenia has been influenced in recent years by biochemical hypotheses which attribute the mental symptoms to a metabolic error involving the formation of an abnormal hallucinogenic or toxic metabolite (Table 1). One such hypothesis was that the oxidation of adrenaline by ceruloplasmin might lead to toxic levels of adrenochrome. Another suggestion was that abnormal transmethylation of dopamine might produce dimethoxyphenylalanine (DMPEA or "pink spot"). A more recent proposal is that a defect in the enzyme dopamine-ß-hydroxylase might lead to the formation of toxic quantities of 6-hydroxydopamine. The biochemical hypotheses have been amply reviewed elsewhere and will not be discussed in detail here (17).

TABLE 1

Biochemical hypotheses

Adrenochrome formation (HOFFER, 7)
Abnormal transmethylation (OSMOND and SMYTHIES, 11)
Abnormal plasma protein: "taraxein" (HEATH et al., 5)
Frohman plasma factor (FROHMAN et al., 4)
Autoimmune response (HEATH and KRUPP, 6)
Hydroxydopamine intoxication (STEIN, 16)

The general idea that schizophrenia might be due to a biochemical error, as in phenylketonuria or in diabetes, has led to many clinical investigations in which series of schizophrenic patients have been compared with series of matched controls to demonstrate a statistically significant difference: but these investigations, although informative in many cases, have failed so far to show any characteristic biochemical abnormality that can be accepted as a common cause. While clinical investigations of this type could show a uniform abnormality in a homogeneous group they are clearly inappropriate for studying the causal factors in a mixed population. It would therefore appear that before embarking on studies of this kind we should consider very carefully the evidence that schizophrenia is really a homogeneous condition. It is significant that the concept of "schizophrenia" has changed to a considerable extent since it was first proposed and many conditions previously included in "the schizophrenias" are now identified and diagnosed in other terms (12). This is true for example of the schizophrenia-like psychoses that occur from time to time in myxoedema, in toxic-infective states, in temporal lobe epilepsy, in pellagra and in many other conditions. Even the psychoses caused by the spirochaete include cases in which in the words of NOLAN LEWIS (9) "we have such a clear-cut dementia praecox symptomatology, even with outspoken catatonia, that if it were not for the accompanying neurologic symptoms and serologic findings these cases would be placed forthwith in the category of dementia praecox." Psychoses associated with temporal lobe epilepsy were described by SLATER, BEARD and GLITHERO (14) as "psychiatrically indistinguishable" from schizophrenia. The relatively frequent association of schizophrenia-like psychoses with these conditions differs from the relationship in other types of cerebral disorder such as multiple sclerosis, Parkinsonism and cerebro-vascular disease, in which the incidence of schizophrenia-like psychoses is no greater than the chance expectation (2). The evidence suggests that there are certain kinds of cerebral disorder which are specially prone to give rise to psychoses of the schizophrenic type. Some of these have only recently been recognized, and most of them were formerly included in "the schizophrenias". An important aspect of the history of schizophrenia has been the repeated recognition of sub-groups of this kind and it must therefore be questioned whether the remaining "schizophrenia" is really a single homogeneous condition. An alternative view is that "schizophrenia" is a term comparable to "fever" in representing a condition that can arise in different ways. On this view a schizophrenic psychosis implies a constitutional lability of CNS function, which can be thrown out of balance by an effective combination of metabolic, toxic or other intrinsic and environmental factors. If this picture is correct, one would not expect to find a uniform biochemical abnormality present in every case, which could be detected by the statistical comparison of groups of schizophrenics and controls. Clinical investigation might aim either at defining the common neurological mechanisms by which the

TABLE 2

Conditions in which schizophrenia-like psychoses are liable to arise

A. *Tissue damage*
  Tumours of temporal lobe
  Viral encephalitis
  Huntington's chorea
  Trypanosomiasis

B. *Toxic agents*
  Carbon monoxide poisoning
  Bacterial toxins
  Copper in Wilson's disease (hepatolenticular degeneration)
  Amphetamines

C. *Metabolic disorders*
  Myxoedema
  Porphyria
  Nicotinamide deficiency (pellagra)
  Homocystinuria

D. *Functional disorders*
  Temporal lobe epilepsy
  Narcolepsy

symptoms of CNS inbalance are produced, or it could seek to identify further sub-groups in which the psychosis is attributable mainly to a major metabolic, toxic or other cause. Some evidence on the first point is afforded by the data on conditions in which schizophrenia-like psychoses are specially liable to arise (Table 2). It is noteworthy that several of these commonly involve lesions in the gray matter of higher brain-stem structures including the striatal nuclei: this is true of Huntington's chorea, porphyria, Wilson's disease (hepato-lenticular degeneration) and carbon monoxide poisoning. One might include lesions of the temporal lobe, but here it may be relevant that FEINDEL and PENFIELD (3) found that the behavioural automatism characteristic of temporal lobe epilepsy occurs only when the epileptic discharge extends centrally into the higher brain-stem structures. Recent work on the probable points of action of the amphetamines and phenothiazines again draws attention to the relation of schizophrenia-like psychoses to the dopaminergic and adrenergic transmitter mechanisms operating in the upper brain-stem region (15).

In considering the causal factors that operate in schizophrenia we have a few fairly well-authenticated clues. The genetic data on the risk of schizophrenia in one-egg and two-egg twins, and in the adopted children of schizophrenic mothers, give convincing evidence of a genetic causal factor important in the severe, chronic types of psychosis but relatively unimportant in the milder types of illness. The data would be consistent with the existence of sub-groups differing widely in genetic predisposition. We do not know the nature of the genetic factors or the time of life when they are operative, but several studies have given independent evidence of the inheritance in the offspring of schizophrenics of characteristics variously described as "neurotic personality disorder" or "schizoid personality".

The importance of environmental factors is evident from the limited role of genetic influences in many cases, but again we do not know what they are: stress, nutritional factors, infections, and endocrine factors have all been suspected. In this connection an interesting clue is the shape of the age-incidence curve, which shows a marked peak in late adolescence at about the age of 20. This suggests the possible involvement of endocrine factors associated with sexual function. The fact that mescaline and certain other drugs produce hallucinations has suggested the possibility that an abnormal hallucinogenic metabolite of this type might be concerned: but hallucinations appear to be a secondary symptom rather than a primary process in schizophrenia. Greater interest therefore attaches to the action of drugs such as the amphetamines which produce, not only a symptom, but a full schizophrenia-like psychosis.

While the statistical comparison of patients with controls is generally inappropriate for the investigation of a mixed population, it is valid for studying the characteristics of a homogeneous sub-group selected on the basis of any particular criteria. This approach may be illustrated by a recent attempt in the author's laboratory to identify a sub-group in which genetic factors play a dominant role (13). The patients were selected on the basis that each had a severe schizophrenic psychosis of early onset (before the age of 25) requiring hospital treatment for not less than 1 year. Further, each had one or more first-degree relatives with a similar schizophrenic psychosis. A psychosis of this type might result from an inherited predisposition depending on a genetically-determined metabolic deviation. However a comparison of groups of 10—20 such patients with matched controls showed no significant deviation from the normal in haptoglobin type, erythrocyte fragility, plasma taurine level or other factors reported to be abnormal in schizophrenics.

Among the other suggested sub-groups of schizophrenia interest attaches to one characterized by delayed maturation, abnormal body-build and low urinary excretion of androgens (1). The possible existence of a further sub-group of "post-encephalitic schizophrenia" is suggested by the observation that schizophrenia-like psychoses not infrequently follow an attack of encephalitis; and a proportion of schizophrenics have a raised CSF protein level which could be due to a subacute viral infection (8, 12). An observation that may be relevant in this connexion is a recent finding by MacSweeney, Johnson and Timms (10) of a high incidence of stillbirths and miscarriages in the mothers of schizophrenics. This could be due to an increased incidence of genes causing metabolic errors, but it could also be caused by increased susceptibility to a neurotropic virus such as genital herpes which kills some of the foetuses and leaves others permanently impaired. While some still hold to the view that schizophrenia is a single homogeneous condition, an entity *per se*, the evidence appears to point increasingly to the view that schizophrenic psychoses can arise in a number of different ways.

References

1. Brooksbank, B. W. L., MacSweeney, D. A., Johnson, A. L., Cunningham, A. E., Wilson D. A. and Coppen A. J. (1969) Androgen excretion and physique in schizophrenia. Brit. J. Psychiat. **117**, 413.
2. Davison, K. and Bagley, C. R. (1969) Schizophrenia-like psychoses associated with organic disorders. In: Current Problems in Neuropsychiatry. Edited by R. N. Herrington. Headley Bros., Ashford, Kent. p. 113.
3. Feindel, W. and Penfield, W. (1954) Localization of discharge in temporal lobe automatism. A.M.A. Arch. Neurol. Psychiat. **75**, 400.
4. Frohman, C. E., Beckett, P. G. S., Grissell, J. L., Latham, L. K. and Gottlieb, J. S. (1966) Biologic responsiveness to environmental stimuli in schizophrenia. Comprehens. Psychiat. **7**, 494—500.
5. Heath, R. G. and the Department of Psychiatry and Neurology, Tulane University (1954) Studies in Schizophrenia, Cambridge, Mass. Harvard University Press, 610 pp.
6. Heath, R. G. and Krupp I. M. (1967) Schizophrenia as an immunologic disorder. Arch. gen. Psychiat. **16**, 1.
7. Hoffer, A. (1965) A review of serum ceruloplasmin in schizophrenia. Dis. nerv. Syst. **26**, 25.
8. Hunter, R., Jones, M. and Malleson, A. (1969) Cerebrospinal fluid proteins in newly-admitted patients. J. neurol. Sci. **9**, 11.
9. Lewis, N. D. C. (1936) Research in dementia praecox. The National Committee for Mental Hygiene, New York.
10. MacSweeney, D. A., Johnson, A. L. and Timms (1972) Characteristics of the mothers of Schizophrenics. Psychol. Med. in the press.
11. Osmond, H. and Smythies, J. (1952) Schizophrenia: A new approach. J. ment. Sci. **98**, 309.
12. Richter, D. (1970) The biological investigation of schizophrenia. Biol. Psychiatr. **2**, 153.
13. Richter, D. and Ricard, O. (1967) Genetic factors predisposing to schizophrenia. In: Biological Research in Schizophrenia. Academy of Medical Sciences of the U.S.S.R. Moscow. p. 264.
14. Slater, E., Beard, A. E. and Glithero, E. (1963) The schizophrenia-like psychoses of epilepsy. Brit. J. Psychiat. **109**, 95.
15. Snyder, S. H. (1970) Catecholamines in the brain as mediators of amphetamine psychosis. Arch. gen. Psychiat. **27**, 169.
16. Stein, L. (1971) Neurochemistry of reward and punishment: Some implications for the etiology of schizophrenia. J. psychiat. Res. **8**, 345.
17. Wyatt, R. J., Termini, B. A. and Davis, J. (1971) Biochemical and sleep studies of schizophrenia. Schizophrenia Bull. **4**, 10.

D.R., Medical Research Council, Neuropsychiatry Unit, Carshalton, Surrey, England

THE RELATIONSHIP OF THE AMPHETAMINE MODEL PSYCHOSIS TO SCHIZOPHRENIA

E. H. ELLINWOOD, Jr. and A. SUDILOVSKY

Behavioral Neuropharmacology Section, Duke University Medical Center, Durham, North Carolina

INTRODUCTION

In this review we will explore the relationship of amphetamine psychosis to schizophrenia, especially the possible common mechanisms involved. We will be drawing primarily on research out of our laboratory but will also be using information from other sources including extensive contributions from the laboratory of RANDRUP and MUNKVAD and others.

Amphetamine psychosis provides a rare case of pharmacologically induced psychosis that so closely mimics a functional psychosis, paranoid schizophrenia, that diagnostic errors are frequent. Because of this marked correspondence several authors, KETY (27), RANDRUP and MUNKVAD (36), ELLINWOOD (12, 15), and GRIFFITH (23) have commented on amphetamine intoxication as heuristic model of functional psychosis and the applicability of studying the behavioral manifestations. Such studies in chronic intoxicated experimental animals can be relevant to evaluate not only the comparative neurochemical alterations but also to assess the pathologically related behavioral phenomena.

We have previously reported on the analogy to paranoid phenomena of behavioral constellations evolving over a period of time in chronically intoxicated cats. Briefly, amphetamine intoxication primarily induces stereotyped behavior (15, 16, 31, 36, 37). A common denominator of the amphetamine induced stereotyped behaviors across species is that they are comprised of patterns of searching and examining; at least the motor components of these attending processes are present in stereotypies of all species (17). The stereotypies are noted in humans not only in perceptual motor patterns but also in stereotyped thinking which often involves rather intense curiosity and searching behavior, then later suspiciousness. As we have reported previously, this suspiciousness often sets the stage for later paranoia.

Chronic amphetamine induced changes in the latter part of this report were re-evaluated on the basis of behaviors not necessarily consistent with the paranoid model. We wish to draw attention to the bizarre manifestations; loss of motor initiative, frozen postures, dysjunctive posture and dyssynchrony of movements, stereotyped activity, cataleptic phenomena, pupillary changes, known to appear in the catatonic form of the human psychosis as well as in the so-called experimental catatonia. A paranoid-catatonic continuum is proposed as a "clinical" expression of the chronic amphetamine intoxication in lower animals, and the need for earlier observation of the process in humans is stressed. *We are postulating that perseveration and distortions of postural-motor-attitudinal sets are common to both paranoid as well as the catatonic pathways of the "psychotic" process.*

We need to explain our concept of postural-motor-attitudinal sets. For example, amphetamine induces not only a state of persistent frozen posture and motor patterns, i.e., stereotypies, but also persistent attitudes. This can in turn be related to abnormal stimulation of catecholamine systems primarily in the dopamine system. The relationship of posture to attitude and thus to attentive mechanisms can be understood in terms of the behaviors induced. One of the main behaviors that we see stimulated in primates by amphetamines is the pincer grasp (both humans and monkeys). The pincer grasp shows up in stereotyped picking phenomena; both picking the body in grooming patterns or picking at various segments of their environment. In tracing the ontogeny of the pincer grasp in humans we note that at birth the tonic neck reflex turns the head in relation to the outstretched hand and later at approximately nine months of age, one notes this head turning in relationship to the outstreched hand but with the advent of the pincer grasp and probing forefinger. At this stage of development one notes that the child is suddenly attentive to small details in his environment. Increasingly crumbs, specks of dust, and any number of small objects are all the main perceptual hangups of the infant. Just prior to this stage the infant completely disregarded minute objects. Thus we see a "telekinetic" postural mechanism leading to a predominant perceptual mode, in fact, it is more than just attention to details, it is a perseverative attitude of searching out small details in the environment.

With amphetamine intoxication one notes a similar perseveration of attitude which we are speculating is based on these sustained attitudes such as searching behavior and suspiciousness, which set the stage for the eventual paranoia. In macronosomatic animals the primary "stereotyped" mode is that of sniffing (biting and licking are also noted). As one moves up the phylogenetic scale to cats, one not only notices sniffing movements, but head movements associated with looking are also prominent. In primates a new dimension is added; that is, the advent of eye-hand examination patterns. These hand movements are quite specific and consist primarily of forefinger probing, picking, pincer grasp, palm clasping and hand examining. An individual motor-component of these searching-examining patterns can be integrated into several stereotypies and may be directed towards external objects or towards the animal's own body as patterns of grooming.

Observations of, and histories from amphetamine abusers demonstrate a remarkable correspondence to these patterns of examining behavior. In humans the amphetamine induced "grooming behavior" is not unlike that noted in rhesus monkeys and is usually manifest as an incessant examining, rubbing and picking (using forefinger probe and pincer grasp) which results in raw blemishes and scars. At other times the individual may spend up to an hour examining various parts of the body, probing and looking at visually accessible parts (one way screen observations by the author). These same behaviors demonstrate that the time dimension is important in that there is a gradual organization of behavior, thought, and feeling about the acute experiences leading to the formation of delusions. For example, many of the patients with "grooming responses" developed marked delusions of parasitosis and spent many hours examining their skin and digging out imagined encysted parasites. These delusions appeared to develop out of earlier sequences of skin sensations and repetitive "grooming responses" that evolved over time. Thus in our observations of both man and lower animals we have noted sequences of behavior, like the grooming response, that take on an autonomy and centrality of their own, and in man at least this often further evolves into a corresponding delusion. Other repetitious examining, searching and sorting behaviors are directed towards the external environment and are often associated with an intense feeling of curiosity by the individual. These repetitious behaviors have been variously called pundning (38), obsessive-compulsive tendencies (12, 29) and knick-knacking by the inhabitants of the Haight-Asbury scene. Most often the individual engages in repetitious examining, dismantling, rearranging or cleaning tasks which primarily involve small bits or minutia. Thus there is a marked enhancement of perceptual acuity associated with minute objects. Amphetamine addicts frequently state that the scanning, prying and probing behaviors subsequently evolve into what is at first a pleasurable sense of suspiciousness in the old meaning of suspiciousness; that is, looking beneath the surface for the truth or meaning (literally, to look from below). They describe looking for meaningful details and the relationship between details, or they often impart great meaning to trivial details. One patient, for example, stated "I looked everywhere for clues, under the rugs, behind pictures, and I took things apart. I read magazines looking at the periods with a magnifying glass, looking for codes. It would have helped me solve the mystery (of a boyfriend's behavior)." Later there was a manifest change in the direction of the spying behavior in which the amphetamine addicts felt that other people were probing, watching and spying on them. Progressing from this stage the previous suspiciousness flourished to a more paranoid form and still later the patient was often fearful and not infrequently panic-stricken, agitated and over-reactive. At this point it is not unusual for patients to suddenly misinterpret stimuli and often have delusions and hallucinations. They not infrequently present themselves to an emergency room or to a police station in a paranoic panic.

TABLE 1

The triple-layered model with amphetamine psychosis

Functional paranoid psychosis	Human model psychosis Chronic amphetamine intoxication		Animal model psychosis Chronic amphetamine intoxication
Paranoid tendencies ▼	Curiosity ▼	Repetitious examining Searching Sorting behavior	Abnormal investigatory attitude with repetitious activity ▼
	Sustained pleasurable suspiciousness ▼	Looking for meanings Minutia	Restricted repetitious activity ▼
Paranoid psychosis	Ideas of reference ▼ Persecutory delusions and hallucinations	Fearful Panic stricken Agitated Over reactive	Reactive attitude

The symptoms most eminently related to the evolving paranoid psychosis, because of the cognitive-perceptual nature, are difficult to directly correlate with behavioral manifestations in lower animals. However, various remarkable similarities do exist, and in general we have observed that the evolution of behavior in animal models follows a partially analogous path with that noted in human studies. Table 1 presents our triple layered model with amphetamine psychosis serving as a model of functional paranoid psychosis and chronic intoxication studies of animals serving as a behavioral model of amphetamine psychosis. Investigatory stereotypies in animals evolve into more restricted, repetitious activities with the behavior finally deteriorating into a psychologically disruptive state. This final stage is best illustrated with what we have called the reactive attitude, a state in which the animal appears to be hypersensitive to minor stimuli and often appears to be reacting to imaginary stimuli. At this point the animal most frequently is in an agitated muscular tense state and often manifests akathisia-like movements of the extremities.

There are special problems of chronic intoxication studies. Difficulties in controlling variables rise at an exponential rate, especially when variables have both time and drug dose progressing as is the case in chronic amphetamine intoxication in humans. Also, behavior for given individual animals may evolve in several distinct paths, further adding to the problem of interpretation. Because of these problems, behavior itself becomes the anchor to which correlative studies must be related and not the parameters of time or absolute drug dose. This necessitates an accurate quantifiable description of behavior and one that takes into consideration the multi-dimensional nature of behavioral changes which reflect underlying complex metabolic and neurophysiological changes.

METHODS

As we stated previously the main problem arises from the fact that it is impossible to measure a multivariate overlapped and patterned phenomena like motor behavior with a univariate tool. We have thus tried to confront this problem by using in our experiments a detailed phenomenological description combined with a multivariate rating chart (19). In the present report we will comment on the results of our behavioral studies with cats intoxicated over a two week period with increasing doses of methamphetamine. The various phenomenological descriptions are based on amphetamine intoxication in over sixty animals. The behavioral rating charts are based on 22 female cats weighing between 2.5 kg to 4 kg that were chronically administered gradually increasing doses of methamphetamine from 15/mg/kg/day to 35/mg/kg/day injected i.p. in two divided doses at 8:00 a.m. and 4:00 p.m. Sixteen hours between days were allowed for recovery and for the same reason cats were not given methamphetamine on the sixth and seventh days. This schedule is comparable to runs noted in human speed addicts. TV tape recordings were made on days 1, 3, 11, and 12 of the intoxication cycle. Each day, except for day 12, was divided into three minute recording sessions taken prior to injection and at 10, 20, 30 and 90 minutes after the first injection of the day. The pre-injection period of day one represents the pre-drug control.

The 178 items used in the behavioral rating chart reflect motor displays or units of behavior that have been repeatedly observed in previous phenomenologically oriented studies. Each unit of behavior was operationally defined. The various items were distributed into eight selected categories of behavior: (1) physical location (place and orientation), (2) relation with environment (attitude), (3) activity level, (4) motor displays, (5) looking activity, (6) sniffing activity, (7) grooming activity, (8) autonomic responses, and

(9) miscellaneous. A more detailed account of this behavior rating chart has been presented elsewhere (19).

In rating the behavior each three minute observation period was divided into eighteen ten-second observation intervals. Individual items were scored on the basis of their occurrence. For example, when a head, side-to-side stereotypy was present for the entire three minute period there would be a code letter in each of the ten second observational spaces indicating that this behavior had occurred.

BRIEF REVIEW OF RESULTS

Stereotypies, the hallmark of amphetamine intoxication, in these studies were noted to be greatest at 90 minutes on day 1 (Fig. 1). Stereotypies developed much less rapidly on day 1 than on days 3 and 11. However, stereotypies were noted to fall off conspicuously

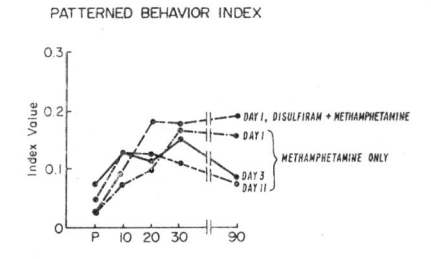

Fig. 1. Stereotypies after methamphetamine intoxication.

at the 90 minute interval on days 3 and 11. We have speculated previously that this accelerated fall-off represents an inability of dopamine synthesis to sustain the amphetamine induced response. We strongly suspect that the dopamine action in the relative absence of norepinephrine is responsible for the more intense stereotypy as well as much of the bizarre dystonic postures to be described later. Rats or cats pretreated with disulfiram prior to amphetamine administration developed more intense stereotypies and also developed dramatically bizarre cataleptic postures.

GUNNE and LEWANDER (24) using biochemical assays demonstrated that primarily norepinephrine is depleted in acutely intoxicated animals whereas extensive norepinephrine and more moderate dopamine depletion is noted in chronic amphetamine intoxication. If according to our thesis norepinephrine has an inhibitory influence on the development of stereotypies then on days 3 and 11 with a relatively greater depletion of norepinephrine one would expect to find a more rapid onset of stereotypies and this is indeed the case. Also if dopamine is partially depleted one would expect the duration of stereotypies would be significantly shorter on days 3 and 11 which was the case. In addition pretreatment with disulfiram, a dopamine β-hydroxylase inhibitor, which blocks norepinephrine synthesis, results in a more accelerated onset of stereotypies on day 1 when methamphetamine is administered. Thus on day 1 with metamphetamine alone there may need to be an initial norepinephrine "blow-off" before the more intense dopamine mediated stereotypies can develop.

Attitudinal scales more consistently than either posture or stereotypy, demonstrate the perseveration of a single mode of relating to the environment (Fig. 2). The investigative abnormal attitudinal scale reflects the persistent "compulsive" searching out of restricted "stimuli", often even when the animal may have broken from a patterned (investigatory) motor stereotypy. Like stereotypy this is most intense on day one, 90 minute period. The interested abnormal scale is defined as a restricted interest in the environment with

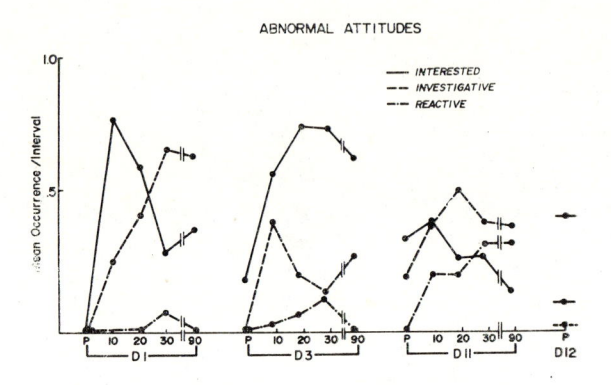

Fig. 2. The attitudinal scales.

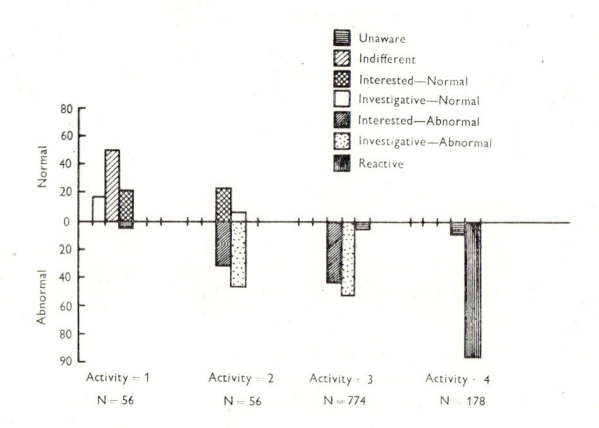

Fig. 3. The activity level.

a nervous, tense or apprehensive quality. As can be noted on day 1, this dramatically drops with the large increase in investigatory behavior yet increases on day 3. The reactive attitude reflects a behavioral state in which the animal suddenly reacts to restricted stimuli without proportion and with a jumpy, agitated, jittery quality while maintaining general body posture. As can be noted the reactive category increased most markedly on day 11, and is correlated best with disorganized behavior such as ataxia and akathisia-like movements. Figure 3 demonstrates that there is an absolute relationship ($P > 0.001$) between the activity level and the attitudinal scale which along with the other behaviors indicated that in the reactive phase there was a gradual hyperexcitable breakdown in organized behavior.

BEHAVIORS DISPARATE WITH PARANOID MODEL

One group of behaviors which does not appear to be analogous to the model of paranoid psychosis that we presented earlier is the various dysjunctive and dyskinetic behaviors that were noted with increasing frequency towards day 11. For example, dyssynchrony of movement was an often noted phenomenon, that is, one body part or body segment moving without proper relation or tempo to other body parts to make a flowing vector of behavior.

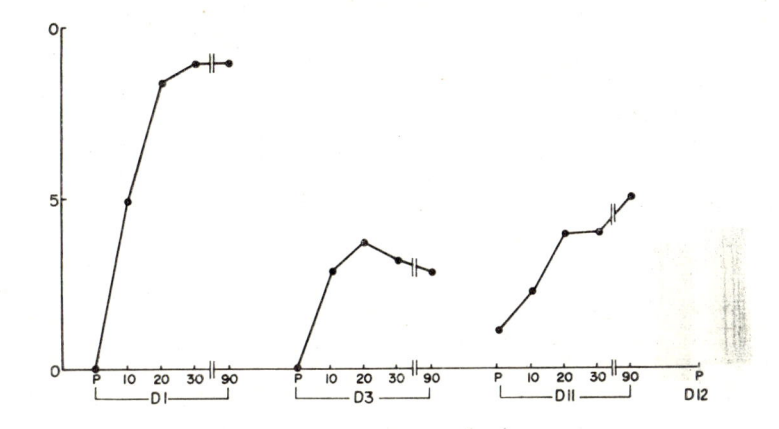

Fig. 4. Stereotypy of head-neck ensemble.

Similarly as a posture, one body segment out of proper relationship to others was often noted and called dysjunctive posture. Ataxia and akathisia were especially frequent during the later stages of intoxication and appeared to be a mixture of hyperactivity, and loss of coordination.

Dyssynchrony as we have defined it in our observations represents a given body segment taking on an autonomous movement which did not seem to have a purpose or relatedness to other body segments. For example, a repetitious repositioning of, or raising movements of the foreleg occurred on many occasions and had little or no relation to the sniffing or looking pattern that was taking place at the head and neck ensemble. The three major body ensembles; head-neck, shoulder-foreleg, and hip-hindleg, were also relatively more independently active at different parts of the drug cycle (Fig. 4). On day one the head-neck ensemble is obviously much more active but recedes over the ensuing days, whereas the shoulder-foreleg ensemble increases dramatically over the latter days of intoxication. The hip-hind leg movements make their appearance primarily during the third day of intoxication but never really become as active in the same way as the foreleg and head region. More often the hind leg was noted to be frozen in a hyperextended postural position. This particular behavioral configuration, active forelegs, and frozen hindlegs, often resulted (in the standing animal) in one of the abnormal movements of the trunk, that is, hunching and a dysjunctive posture called "camel" since the active forelegs would back up against the relatively resistant hindlegs to produce a hunch or camelback phenomenon. In another behavior form, it appeared that the cat had forgotten where a leg was positioned, thus, for example, a leg would remain in an awkward dysjunctive position while the cat goes about other activities (Fig. 5e). Other dysjunctive postures include abnormally twisted, uncomfortable sitting and lying positions. We have made similar observations in monkeys and rats chronically intoxicated. These postures are not unlike those noted in human catatonic patients.

Obstinate progression was noted in three cats on day 10 and 11. When facing a wall these particular cats would continue treading against it rather than turning to one side. One of these cats demonstrated emprosthotonus and a plastic rigidity which cleared when it was raised to a standing position. Other cats demonstrated what could be called obstinate retrogression. First they would alternate a few steps forward and then a few steps backwards, finally ending with the rear-end against a wall pushing backwards with much effort of the forelegs. Four other cats were noted to lean against the wall of the cage,

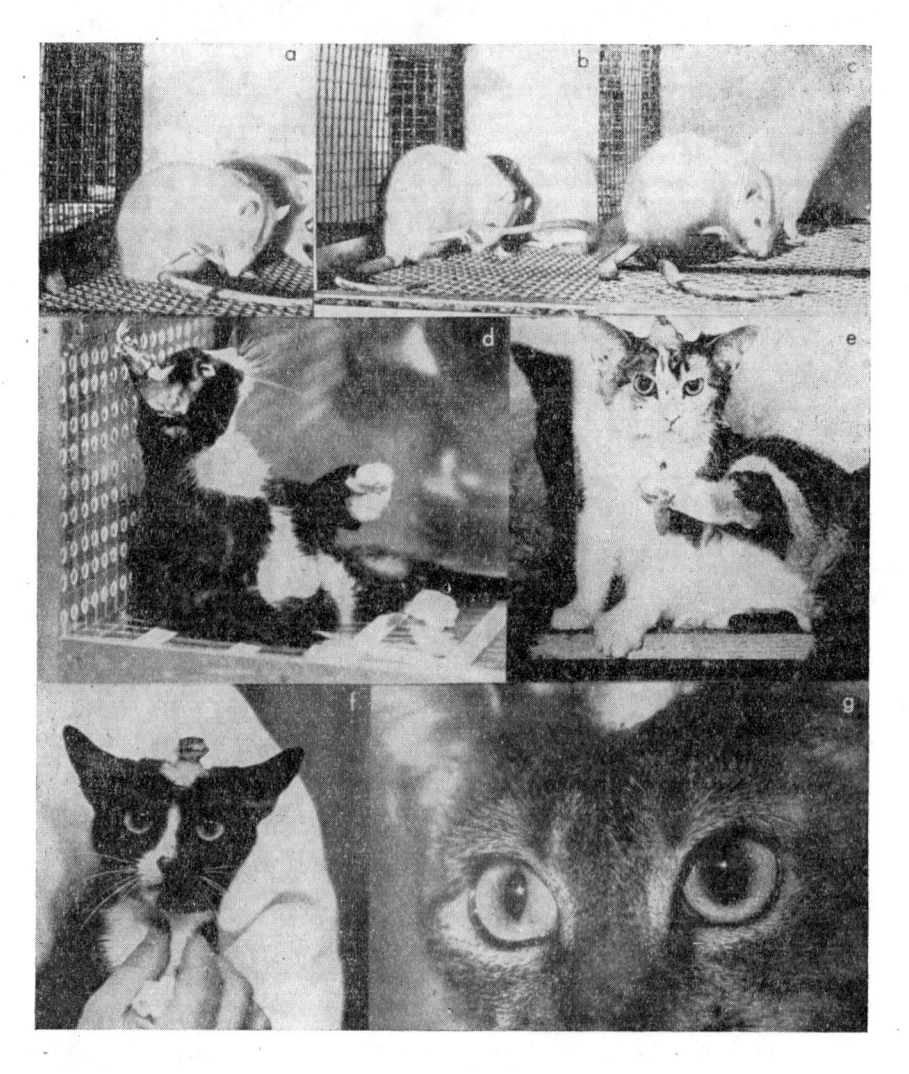

Fig. 5. Chronic methamphetamine and disulfiram intoxication manifestations. a, b, c, d – bizarre postures; e – bizarre posture with chronic methamphetamine alone; f, g – unequal pupils.

gradually allowing their legs to slide out from under them almost as if they were not aware that it was happening to them. The eventual fall did not appear to be the result of weakness in that they quickly righted themselves after the fall. From these observations as well as the general nature of the stereotypies and the chronically sustained attitudes that have been described we have operationally classified these behaviors not on the basis of ataxia but on a basis of loss of initiative in changing attitudes or postural-movements sets. Previous findings in our laboratory are also difficult to reconcile with the model of paranoid schizophrenia alone. These included observations (15) that righting reflexes are lost during the chronic intoxication cycle and that this is associated with a marked loss of catecholamine fluorescence in and around the vestibular nuclei. In addition many of these animals were noted to have some features not unlike a mild waxy flexibility.

The paranoid model: a reconsideration

In an attempt to resolve our model to fit the bizarre motor behaviors noted in the final stages including dysjunctive behaviors and posture, frozen postures, obstinate progression, catalepsy and loss of righting reflexes, we asked ourselves if these features of the model might not be more reminiscent of human catatonic behavior as has been previously mentioned by RANDRUP and MUNKVAD (36). On perusing the literature on catatonic and paranoid schizophrenia one notes many points of commonality especially since both syndromes appear in different phases in the course of an individual's illness (28). As KRAEPELIN (28) mentions "Catatonic states may further appear suddenly in each period of dementia praecox... but lastly the catatonic symptoms may be present in morbid picture in all possible grades and groupings." CONRAD (8) points out that with paranoid and catatonic schizophrenia one can resolve into the other. He however feels that catatonia always goes through the paranoid state first. He cites a case in which there is a long course of body delusions, general sensations of sickness, corporal sensitivities and suspiciousness, which evolved successively through paranoid and catatonic states. As a correlate TATETSU (42) has described amphetamine addicts that manifested catatonic and paranoid syndromes. KRAMER et al. (29) also describe the state of amphetamine "overamping" which is essentially a state of hyperaroused immobility not unlike that noted in catatonia. In examining the "catatonic" manifestations and their parallels with the paranoid manifestations, it appeared that stereotypy might be a common mode in both conditions as BLEULER (4) pointed out. The associated sustained attitudes and thinking modes, could well be common to both catatonic and paranoid schizophrenia and possibly, as well, with other forms of schizophrenia. Figure 6 represents a general progression of phases of catatonic states compared with the level of arousal. In general this evolution would compare analogously with the amphetamine induced states. BLEULER (4) listed a variety of motor disorders noted in catatonic schizophrenia but which also appeared in other schizophrenic forms. Under stereotypies BLEULER included: posture, attitude, thinking and movement. He also mentioned stereotypies of drawing, writing, music and speech (verbigeration). BLEULER also included other signs under motor disorders such as: muscular tension or rigidity, loss of spontaneous movement or initiative, negativistic attitude, automatic obedience, hyperkinesis, and stupor. The catatonic group of schizophrenic first were recognized because of the motor tension states. In addition BLEULER describes the relative autonomy of singular muscular groups including contractions. Tremors may be present and persist. He describes the general incoordination of body segments or dyssynchrony, for example, frequently between the arm and leg movements that do not relate in a synchronous fashion while walking; often even the two feet step irregularly in regard to time and space. Unilateral increase in tendon reflexes has been noted. In addition absence of pupillary reactions to both light and accomodation is frequent. Differences of size are noted between the two pupils, which vary rapidly, often several times in the course of the day, with a result that at times first one, then the other pupil, become wider. BLEULER describes the stereotypies of posture showing marked persistence. At times they would appear painful and impossible

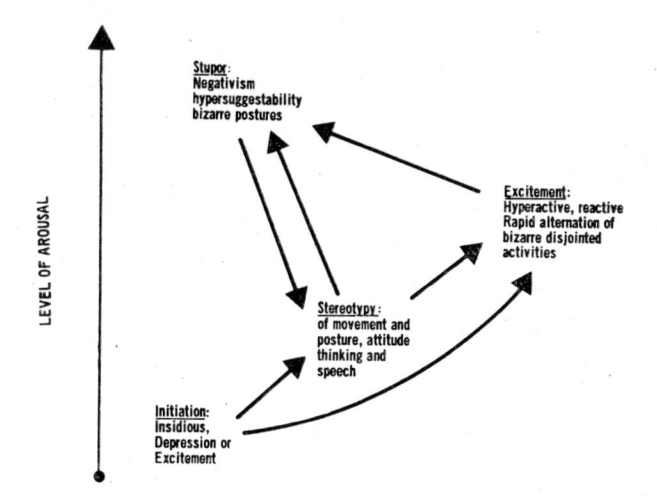

Fig. 6. Evolution of catatonic states compared with level of arousal.

for a normal person. For example, catatonics may stare at the same spot with the eyes in the most extraordinary position for weeks at a time. In a similar manner to our chronic amphetamine cats, stereotypies of position are expressed in two ways in that the patients always select the same corner of the room, the same place in the garden and will actually fight for these places if accidentally or intentionally someone happens to claim the spot. Or the patient always goes to the same place to carry on a particular activity, for example, always striking three times on an identical spot on the wall of the corridor. We have reported similar position postural preferences in amphetamine intoxicated cats previously (16).

The model as a paranoid catatonic continuum

In attempting to ascertain which of the neurotransmitter states might most accurately reflect the "catatonic" phase of the amphetamine intoxication we have hypothesized a stimulated dopamine system in relative absence of norepinephrine action (19). To test this hypothesis we administered disulfiram prior to chronically intoxicating several cats and rats with methamphetamine. Dysjunctive postures and dyssynchronous behaviors were increased even on day 1 in this condition (Figures 5a, b, c, and d). In addition such phenomenon as pupil size discrepancy not infrequently shows up over a period of days with, first one pupil, then the other, being larger. This discrepancy is noted through a full range of diameters and not just when the pupils are dilated. The pupils show a diminished light reaction and at times unilateral failure to react. This is similar to WESTPHAL (43) and BUMKE (5) findings in schizophrenia; they also noted distinct differences in pupil size and reactiveness to light and accomodation.

Chronic amphetamine intoxication preceeded by disulfiram treatment also produces a much more marked reduction in righting reflexes. In many of these same animals we noted a unilateral postural preference. These animals would lie on one side and resist attempts to have them change the laterality of their posture. They showed a marked tendency to circle in one direction. These behavioral manifestations would be in keeping with the more marked depletion of norepinephrine in the vestibular nuclei following the release of norepinephrine by amphetamine and blocking of synthesis by disulfiram.

Analogous phenomena are present in humans. ANGYAL and SHERMAN (2) reported that postural reactions to vestibular stimulation were inhibited in schizophrenia. They noted that rotation, and response to caloric stimulation in schizophrenics was less than one-half of normals. FREEMAN and RODNICK (22) demonstrated significantly less swaying induced by rotation in schizophrenics suggesting reduced activity of the vestibulo-spinal mechanisms. It has been known for years that oculo-motor reactions (nystagmus) to vestibular stimulation is inhibited in schizophrenics. This inhibition is primarily seen in catatonic patients and is noted either to caloric or galvanic stimulation (7, 25, 35). LOWENBACH (32) correlated the decrease of nystagmus following caloric stimulation with the onset and duration of catatonic stupor in periodic catatonia. ANGYAL and BLACKMAN (1) in a study of 58 schizophrenics found that the response hypoactivity was most marked in those patients that showed the greatest apathy, poverty of mental content, and paresthesias, suggesting distortion of perception of the body in relationship to space. FITZGERALD and STENGEL (21) also noted that there was frequently a directional predominance and abnormal differences between the responses of the left and right irrigation. More recently ORNITZ (34) has pointed out that the experimental evidence suggests the vestibular dysfunction is common both to schizophrenic adults as well as autistic children and that autistic children have a heightened awareness and seek out vestibular stimulation as well as paradoxically being fearful and agitated by antigravity play including acceleration and deceleration. This follows the general conclusions of BENDER (3) that in most of the children diagnosed as childhood schizophrenics rotating and whirling motor play was noted in all planes. Additionally there was a tendency to seek a dependable center of gravity, to develop fearful reactions to rather rapid movements such as trains and elevators and intolerance of sensations arising from gravity changes. ORNITZ (34) postulates that pathological vestibular mechanisms would be manifested in an inability to initiate and carry out purposeful actions which are ordinarily automatically regulated. This would lead in adult schizophrenics to the observed psychomotor slowing and catatonic episodes as have been so eloquently described to be related to vestibular and proprioceptive disturbances by McGHIE and CHAPMAN (33) and CHAPMAN (6). We have postulated earlier: (A) that disturbances in visual and vestibulo-postural mechanisms were related to the behavioral manifestation in amphetamine psychosis (13), and (B) that chronic amphetamine induced symptoms in cats are associated with both stimulating release as well as depletion of norepinephrine especially in those brain systems mediating vestibulo-postural and visuo-postural mechanisms (15).

Because of the additional findings of dysjunctive posture, dyssynchronus behavior, loss of righting reflexes, along with other features of catalepsy and frozen posture, there is a need to reconsider the "catatonic syndrome" in any amphetamine model of psychosis. Certainly models of catatonia are not new. DE JONG and BARUK (10) and SCHALTENBRAND (40) have detailed descriptions of behavior in a variety of animals following various experimental conditions. The primary means of producing experimental catatonia was by administration of bulbocapnine, a psychotomimetic amphetamine. The features of experimental catatonia are listed in Table 2. Most authors have emphasized more the dramatic catalepsy, waxy flexibility, and frozen posture, as the major manifestations.

TABLE 2

Features of experimental catatonia

	Chronic intoxication		Acute intoxication			
	Amphetamine	Disulfiram and amphetamine	Bulbocapnine	Mescaline	Apomorphine	6-OH-dopamine and MAO inhibitor
Loss of motor initiative	+	+	++	+	+	+
Frozen posture	+	++	++	+	+	++
Stereotypy	++	++			++	
Stupor		+	+			
Bizarre posture and movements	+	++	+			+
Catalepsy	+	++	++	+		++
Active negativism		+	+	++		
Hyperkinesia	++	+	+			

+   Occurrence of behavior
++ A predominant behavior

However, this appears to reflect an end-point rather than the gammute of behaviors that may be a part of the experimental model. A loss or inability of initiative might well be a common denominator that cuts across many of the syndromes, including the frozen postures and stereotypies. DE JONG emphasizes the active negativism as a symptom perhaps most related to the catatonic schizophrenia and states that mescaline is the drug most remarkable in producing this behavior.

Stereotypy is a major sign of catatonic schizophrenia and we have included it in figure 8 although it is not usually emphasized in experimental catatonia. As one scans the pharmacological agents producing the various signs of experimental catatonia, several of these are known to affect catecholamine mechanisms or at least they have a catechole structure. Several conditions listed either deplete norepinephrine or stimulate dopamine receptors.

CONCLUSIONS

Thus we are faced with a dilemma in which the chronic amphetamine intoxication model induces behavior that may have analogies both with paranoid as well as catatonic phenomenon. If the model is to resolve this association of behaviors, then one needs to understand the relationship between the two types of manifestations, both on a clinical and experimental basis. Certainly, definitive answers to these questions are not available; there are, however, pertinent possibilities based on the nature of the induced behavior itself.

As mentioned previously the most striking findings in our studies are those of dyssynchrony of movement and the postural dysjunction of body segments towards the end of the chronic intoxication. Normally behavior is a symphony of changes and sequences of motivative actions all with their proper lability of attitude and spontaneous initiative for subsequent changes. There are proper relationships and smooth flow of control and autonomy not only in a spacial sense but also in a temporal sense. These relationships become increasingly autonomously independent and/or fixed over the period of intoxication. In others words, they appeared to be islands of separate organization, each establishing its own repetitious autonomy or anarchy without relation to the larger behavioral symphony. Also at the final stage of amphetamine intoxication the dystonic movements tend to be made up of more gross postural mechanisms. Thus it would appear that we also would have a phenomenon of regression to lower levels of behavioral organization.

Even in the initial states of amphetamine intoxication components of behavior became relatively fixed over time and showed a loss of cohesive flow among initiatives with their relative priorities. We found that not only the fixed postures and movement patterns (stereotypies) but also fixed attention-emotive attitudes; that is, animals would continue to maintain set attitudes even after the accompanying stereotypy had broken. These fixed attitudes are quite similar to the same phenomenon in speed freaks who become "hung-up" in a puzzle or examining-sorting compulsions for hours, or in the grossly suspicious or fearful attitudes that are so commonly associated with repetitious scanning eye movements. Thus in both animals and man one finds a marked tendency to maintain attitude-emotional set as well as the accompanying attention-examining modes and background postural set following amphetamine intoxication.

As we mentioned earlier the loss of initiative or distortion of the mechanisms that regulate this smooth flow of behavior from one set to another may be the underlying factor that is associated not only with stereotypies but also with maintenance of perceptual-cognitive attitudinal sets. This process may be triggered with a combination of norepinephrine depletion and dopamine receptor stimulation, even though the eventual end-point behaviors may be due to other derangements of neurotransmitters. Whatever the underlying neurotransmitter mechanisms the most easily *observed* behavioral phenomenon remains the motor stereotypy. We have pointed out previously that the amphetamine induced stereotypies are comprised primarily of the *postural-motor components* of the patterns of attending and examining (18). We proposed that these components represent the ground plan of perceptual-cognitive behaviors, perhaps as an intrinsic scaffolding of behavior that is programmed in the limbic-extrapyramidal catecholamine systems. We in the behavioral sciences need to broaden our concept of postural mechanisms from strictly passive responses providing orientation in space to that of a more vigorous outgoing behavior that is acting on and projecting sensory-motor apparatus on to the environment. Postural mechanisms can be conceived of as reaching out and selecting parts of space and its objects to be acted on. Qualitatively, the nature of these mechanisms might fall somewhere between posture, attitude, and initiation of movement. These mechanisms appear to coordinate the many modes of attention, and might be seen as the leading edge of attention, searching and orientation to the outside world. Conversely these mechanisms may direct attention between various external as well as internal cognitive sets.

In viewing amphetamine induced behavior in this way the induced constraint or restriction of attitude or perception would have the same underlying mechanism as in a postural-motor stereotypy. Similarly, thinking itself could become repetitious secondary to perseveration in one of the same systems subserving perception and cognition. Thus a beginning or insipient paranoid schizophrenic or an individual in the beginning phase of the amphetamine psychosis might start out with an all pervasive attitude of curiosity and/or suspiciousness which would become increasingly constricted. Under the influence of increasing arousal and/or agitation the individual's behavior might then evolve into a paranoid state. Alternately taking off from the same branching point of either stereotypy or restricted attitude the catatonic pathway may have a predilection to move in a motor or postural form because of the more intensive arousal or more marked regression to lower levels of organization. Both pathways, however, are based on distortion and inertia in postural-motor-attitudinal sets. Understanding these postural-attitudinal sets including the underlying nervous system mechanisms that serve as a substrate, as well as the neurotransmitters involved, may not only help in elucidating mechanisms involved in certain forms of schizophrenia but may well have much to say about the underlying principles of behavioral organization.

REFERENCES

1. ANGYAL, and BLACKMAN, N. (1940) Vestibular reactivity in schizophrenia. Arch. Neurol. Psychiat. **44,** 611.
2. ANGYAL, A. and SHERMAN, M. A. (1942) Postural reactions to vestibular stimulation in schizophrenic and normal subjects. Amer. J. Psychiat. **98,** 857.
3. BENDER, L. (1947) Childhood schizophrenia. Clinical study of one hundred schizophrenic children. Amer. J. Orthopsychiat. **17,** 40.
4. BLEULER, E. (1924) Textbook of Psychiatry. New York, McMillian.
5. BUMKE, M. (1910) Münch. med. Wschr. Also quoted by Kraepelin, Dementia Praecox, **55,** p. 77.
6. CHAPMAN, J. (1967) Visual imagery and motor phenomena in acute schizophrenia. Brit. J. Psychiat. **113,** 711.
7. CLAUDE, H., BARUK, H. and AUBRY, M. (1927) Contribution à l'étude de la demence precoce catatonique: Inexcitabilité labyrynthique au cours de la catatonie. Rev. Neurol. **1,** 976.
8. CONRAD, K. (1959) Die dringende Schizophrenie. Versuch einer Gestaltanalyse des Wahns. Georg Thieme Verlag, Stuttgart.
9. CONNELL, P. H. (1958) Amphetamine Psychosis. London, Chapman & Hall.
10. DE JONG, H. and BARUK, H. (1930) La catatonie expérimentale par la bulbocapnine. Masson et Cie, Paris.
11. EASTHAM, R. D. and COX, P. H. E. (1965) Screening test for urinary amphetamines. Brit. med. J. **3,** 924.
12. ELLINWOOD, E. H., JR. (1967) Amphetamine Psychosis: A description of the individuals and process. J. nerv. mental. Dis. **144,** 273.
13. ELLINWOOD, E. H., JR. (1968) Amphetamine Psychosis II: Theoretical implications. J. Neuropsychiat. **4,** 45.
14. ELLINWOOD, E. H., JR. Amphetamine Psychosis: A multi-dimensional process. Seminars in Psychiat., **1,** 208.
15. ELLINWOOD, E. H. JR. and ESCALANTE, O. (1970) Behavioral and histopathological findings during chronic methedrine intoxication. Biol. Psychiat. **2,** 27.
16. ELLINWOOD, E. H., JR. and ESCALANTE, O. (1970) Chronic amphetamine effect on the olfactory forebrain. Biol. Psychiat. **2,** 189.
17. ELLINWOOD, E. H., JR. (1971) Effect of chronic methamphetamine intoxication in Rhesus monkeys. Biol. Psychiat. **3,** 25.
18. ELLINWOOD, E. H., JR. (1971) Comparative methamphetamine intoxication in experimental animals. Pharmakopsychiat. **24,** 351.
19. ELLINWOOD, E. H., JR., SUDILOVSKY, A. and NELSON, L. (1972) Behavioral analysis of chronic amphetamine intoxication. Biol. Psychiat. **4,** 215.
20. ESCALANTE, O. and ELLINWOOD, E. H., JR. (1970) Central nervous system cytopathological changes in cats with chronic methedrine intoxication. Brain Res. **21,** 151.
21. FITZGERALD, G. and STENGEL, E. (1945) Vestibular reactivity to caloric stimulation in schizophrenics. J. ment. Sci. **91,** 93.
22. FREEMAN, H. and RODNICK, E. H. (1942) Effect of rotation on postural steadiness in normal and in schizophrenic subjects. Arch. Neurol. Psychiat. **48,** 47.
23. GRIFFITH, J. D., FANN, W. E. and OATES, J. A. (1970) The amphetamine psychosis: Comparison

of clinical and experimental manifestations. Proceedings of Symposium on Current concepts of amphetamine abuse. In press.
24. GUNNE, L. M. and LEWANDER, T. (1967) Long-term effects of some dependence-producing drugs on the brain monoamines. In: WAHASS, D. (Ed.) Molecular Basis of Some Aspects of Mental Activity. Academic Press, New York, 75.
25. JOO, B., and VON MEDUNA, L. (1935) Labyrinthreizungsuntersuchungen bei Schizophrenie. Psychiat. Neurol. Wschr. **37**, 26.
26. KALANT, O. J. (1966) The amphetamines — toxicity and addiction. Toronto University of Toronto Press.
27. KETY, S. S. (1960) Recent biological theories of schizophrenia. In: Etiology of Schizophrenia, JACKSON, E. D. (Ed.) 137, Basic Books, New York.
28. KRAEPELIN, E. (1971) Dementia praecox and paraphrenia. Translated by BARCLAY, R. M. and ROBERTSON, G. M. Robert Krieger Publishing Company, Huntington, N. Y.
29. KRAMER, J. C., FISCHMAN, V. S. and LITTLEFIELD, D. C. (1967) Amphetamine abuse — pattern and effects of high doses taken intravenously. J. Amer. med. Ass. **201**, 305.
30. LÁT, J. (1965) The spontaneous exploratory reactions as a tool for psychopharmacological studies. In: Proceedings of Second International Pharmacological Meeting, Vol. 1, MIKHELSON, M. and LONGO, V. (Eds.), Pergamon, London and Praha, 47.
31. LÁT, J. and GOLLOVÁ, E. (1964) Drug induced increase of central nervous excitability and the emergence of spontaneous stereotype reactions. Activ. nerv. sup. (Praha) **6**, 200.
32. LOWENBACH, H. (1936) Messend Untersuchungen über die Erregbarkeit des Zentralnervensystems von Geisteskranken, vor allem von periodisch Katatonen, mit Hilfe quantitativer Vestibularisreizung. Arch. Psychiat. **105**, 313.
33. MCGHIE, A. and CHAPMAN, J. (1961) Disorders of attention and perception in early schizophrenia. Brit. J. med. Psychol. **34**, 103.
34. ORNITZ, E. (1970) Vestibular dysfunction in schizophrenia and childhood autism. Comprehens. Psychiat. **11**, 159.
35. PEKELSKY, A. (1921) Transitorischer Nystagmus bei Katatonie. Ist der Nystagmus willkürlich unterdrükbar? Rev. neuropsychopath. **18**, 97.
36. RANDRUP, A. and MUNKVAD, I. (1967) Stereotyped activities produced by amphetamine in several animal species and man. Psychopharmacologia, **11**, 300.
37. RANDRUP, A., MUNKVAD, I. and UDSEN, P. (1963) Adrenergic mechanisms and amphetamine-induced abnormal behavior. Acta pharmacol. **20**, 145.
38. RYLANDER, G. (1966) Preludin narkomaner från klinisk och medicinsk-kriminologisk synpunkt. Svenska Läk.-Tidn. **63**, 4973.
39. SCHALTENBRAND, G. (1924) Über die Bewegungsstörungen bei akuten Bulbocapninvergiftung. Naunyn-Schmiedeberg's Arch. exp. Path. Pharmak. **103**, 1.
40. SCHALTENBRAND, G. (1925) Die wirkung des Bulbocapnins auf unverletzte Katzen. Pflügers Arch. ges. Physiol. **209**, 623.
41. SOURKES, T. L. (1971) Possible new metabolites mediating actions of L-Dopa. Nature, **299**, 413.
42. TATETSU, S. (1963) Methamphetamine psychosis. Folia psychiat. neurol. Jap. 377.
43. WESTPHAL, E. (1909) Dtsch. med. Wschr. Quoted in Dementia Praecox, by KRAEPELIN, E., p. 77 of translation by BARCLAY, R. M. and ROBERTSON, G. M., Robert Krieger Publishing Company, 23.

E.H.E., Behavioral Neuropharmacology Section, Dept. of Psychiatry, Duke University Medical Center, Box 3355, Durham, North Carolina 27710, U.S.A.

PROTEINS IN BLOOD AND CEREBROSPINAL FLUID IN SCHIZOPHRENIC PATIENTS

A preliminary report.*)

ELISABETH BOCK and O. J. RAFAELSEN

Psychochemistry Institute, Rigshospitalet, Copenhagen

Proteins in plasma from schizophrenic patients have been extensively investigated. Applying ultracentrifugal, electrophoretic, immunologic, enzymatic, and non-specific chemical techniques, evidence for abnormalities in serum proteins has been obtained. The literature has been reviewed by FESSEL (4) and WEIL-MALHERBE (12). The results are contradictory and may be summarized as an increase of α- and γ-globulins and a decrease of albumin and β-globulins.

Some authors have attempted to isolate plasma proteins claimed to be specific for schizophrenia (5, 9, 10). These proteins seem to be present in blood in very small quantities, and can for this reason not account for the gross deviations reported.

The present study was undertaken in the light of the many conflicting reports, and because quantitative determination of individual serum proteins has been considerably improved in recent years by means of immunochemical techniques (2, 6, 7).

A pilot study was performed determining 20 serum proteins in 32 normal persons, 16 schizophrenic patients, and 11 manic-depressive patients (1). The patients had been off drugs for at least one month before the study. They were acutely psychotic and did not suffer from any somatic disease. The control group had the same age and sex distribution as the schizophrenic patients, whereas there was an overweight of elder females in the manic-depressive patients. In Table 1 the changes during acute phase reaction of the determined proteins are listed.

This reaction is seen in a multitude of conditions ranging from infections, malignant diseases, and surgical trauma to autoimmune diseases and pregnancy (3, 13).

The changes found in the psychiatric patients were with a few exceptions compatible with an acute phase reaction. The exceptions were ceruloplasmin, which was low in both patient groups, and immunoglobulin M, which was low in the schizophrenic patients only, both compared to the control group and compared to the manic-depressive patients. β_{1C}/β_{1A}-Globulin, the C'3 complement, was also low in the schizophrenic group alone. The manic-depressive patients had on the other hand very increased values of the two glycoproteins: hemopexin and β_2-glycoprotein.

To determine whether these results were specific, we decided to repeat the investiga-

---

*) This investigation was in part supported by grants from Statens laegevidenskabelige Forskningsråd.

Table 1

Variation of plasma proteins during acute phase reaction

Protein	Increase	Decrease	Unchanged	Protein	Increase	Decrease	Unchanged
Prealbumin		+		Ceruloplasmin	+		
Orosomucoid	+			α_2-Macroglobulin			+
Albumin		+		α_2-Glycoprotein			?
α_1-Antitrypsin	+			Hemopexin	+		
Easily precipitable glycoprotein	+			β_{1C}/β_{1A}-Globulin	+		
				Transferrin		+	
α_1-Antichymotrypsin	+			β-lipoprotein		+	
Gc-globulin	+			IgG			+
α_2-HS globulin		+		IgA			+
Haptoglobin	+			IgM			+

tion, and this time we included a determination of the same proteins in the cerebrospinal fluid (BOCK and RAFAELSEN, unpublished data). Changes in serum protein concentrations in this fluid could indicate an altered blood-cerebrospinal fluid-barrier or a local production. Furthermore, the sera were tested for precipitating antibodies against water-soluble human brain proteins by means of crossed immunoelectrophoresis with intermediate gel (11), a newly developed, very sensitive technique. The patients were chosen after the same criteria as in the first study. Cerebrospinal fluid from normal persons was not available, so we had to use a control group consisting of 22 patients suffering from minor psychiatric and neurological disorders. The patients consisted of 17 schizophrenic, 12 demented, and 19 manic-depressive individuals.

When the *serum* values of the schizophrenic patients were compared to normal persons, a pattern of acute phase reaction was found. This was also found in the control group and in the demented and manic-depressive patients.

When the schizophrenic patients were compared to the control group and the demented and the manic-depressive patients, the schizophrenic patients turned out to have significantly lower values of β_{1C}/β_{1A}-globulin, hemopexin, ceruloplasmin, and immunoglobulin M. These findings were in accordance with our first study.

In the *cerebrospinal fluid* the dominating feature was very low amounts of haptoglobin in the schizophrenic patients when compared to the other groups. We therefore had the haptoglobins typed and found the explanation in an increased occurrence of the high molecular forms haptoglobin 2—1 and 2—2 in the schizophrenic patients. However, in larger populations of schizophrenic patients a normal distribution of the haptoglobin types has been found (8).

When the schizophrenic patients were compared to the manic-depressive patients, the latter had high values of haptoglobin, immunoglobulin G and A, and the two glycoproteins hemopexin and Zn α_2-glycoprotein and prealbumin.

When the schizophrenic patients were compared to the demented patients, the latter exhibited high values of haptoglobin and several other proteins. This in connection with a high total protein content of the cerebrospinal fluid in the demented patients could be explained as an increased permeability of the blood-cerebrospinal fluid-barrier in this patient group.

Finally, the sera were tested for precipitating antibodies against water-extractable brain antigens. Such antibodies were not found in any case.

Conclusion

In *serum* from schizophrenic patients, a pattern of acute phase reaction was found. However, β_{1C}/β_{1A}-globulin, ceruloplasmin, hemopexin, and IgM were low in the schizophrenic patients, both in comparison to control groups and in comparison to manic-depressive and demented patients. No antibodies against water-extractable proteins of human brain were found in any patient.

In *cerebrospinal fluid* the schizophrenic patients had low amounts of haptoglobin as most of the patients belonged to haptoglobin type 2—1 and 2—2.

References

1. Bock, E., Weeke, B. and Rafaelsen, O. J. (1971) Serum proteins in acutely psychotic patients. J. Psychiat. Res. **9**, 1.
2. Clarke H. G. M. and Freeman T. (1968) Quantitative immunoelectrophoresis of human serum proteins. Clin. Sci. **35**, 403.
3. Clarke, H. G. M., Freeman, T. and Pryse-Phillips, W. (1971) Serum protein changes after injury. Clin. Sci. **40**, 337.
4. Fessel, W. J. (1962) Blood proteins in functional psychoses. Arch. gen. Psychiat. **6**, 132.
5. Frohman, C. E., Goodman, M., Beckett, P. G. S., Latham, L. K., Senf, R. and Gottlieb, J. S. (1962) The isolation of an active factor from serum of schizophrenic patients. Ann. N. Y. Acad. Sci. **96**, 438.
6. Laurell, C.-B. (1965) Antigen-antibody crossed electrophoresis. Analyt. Biochem. **10**, 358.
7. Laurell, C.-B. (1966) Quantitative estimation of protein by electrophoresis in agarose gel containing antibodies. Analyt. Biochem. **15**, 45.
8. Lovegrove, T. D. and Nicholls, D. M. (1965) Haptoglobin subtypes in a schizophrenic and control population. J. nerv. ment. Dis. **141**, 195.
9. Pennell, R. B. and Saravis, C. A. (1962) A human factor inducing behavioural and electrophysiological changes in animals: I. Isolation and chemical nature of the agent. Ann. N. Y. Acad. Sci. **96**, 462.
10. Sanders, B. E., Smith, E. V. C., Flataker, L. and Winter, C. A. (1962) Fractionation studies of human serum factors affecting motor activity in trained rats. Ann. N. Y. Acad. Sci. **96**, 448.
11. Svendsen, P. J. and Axelsen, N. H. (1972) A modified antigen-antibody crossed electrophoresis characterizing the specificity and titre of human precipitins against *Candida albicans*. J. immunol. Methods, **1**, 169.
12. Weil-Malherbe, H. (1967) The biochemistry of the functional psychoses. Advanc. Enzymol. **29**, 479.
13. Werner, M. (1969) Serum protein changes during the acute phase reaction. Clin. chim. Acta **25**, 299.

E. B., Psychochemistry Institute, Rigshospitalet, 9, Blegdamsvej, DK-2100 Copenhagen, Denmark

TRYPTOPHAN METABOLISM AND SCHIZOPHRENIA

H. H. BERLET

Institute of Pathochemistry and General Neurochemistry of the University, Heidelberg

Tryptophan as the precursor of tryptamine and serotonin in the body and the structural similarity of its indole nucleus to LSD and some other indolealkylamines with psychotropic properties are the main reasons for the heightened interest of investigators in the metabolism of tryptophan in schizophrenia. To elucidate a possible causative role of tryptophan in schizophrenia the following questions have been the subject of numerous studies, past and present. Is there an overt or latent metabolic defect of tryptophan metabolism along known enzymatic pathways in terms of an inborn error of metabolism (72) and secondly, do there exist as yet unknown metabolic steps of tryptophan that may lead to the formation of psychoactive indole derivatives in man and in particular in schizophrenics? From a theoretical viewpoint one may also consider a defect in cellular control mechanisms regulating not only enzyme reactions but also cellular parameters concerned with homeostatic functions like uptake, transport, binding, and storage of tryptophan, its apportioning to the different metabolic channels, and the inactivation and elimination from the cell of biosynthetic material, reflecting a molecular basis of the disease in a more general way. The unifying aspect of these approaches remains of course that of the cause effect relationship of possible abnormalities to the underlying disease process.

There has been a rapid progress of research on several of these aspects, especially with regard to the ramifications of the metabolism of tryptophan and its indole moiety and a brief review of some recent data will be presented and their implications in schizophrenia discussed. A number of review articles and comprehensive summaries are available, broadly covering various biological aspect of mental disease (32, 92, 184, 185), and special topics including general accounts of tryptophan metabolism in normal and pathological conditions (41, 140, 145, 164), indoleamines and schizophrenia (40, 91), and the biochemistry and pharmacology of indolic psychotomimetics (2, 36, 135, 159).

SCHIZOPHRENIA, AN INBORN ERROR OF METABOLISM?

It is now generally agreed upon that there is a genetic basis of both schizophrenia and schizoid disease (111), the latter being considered an attenuated form of the major illness (90), and that schizophrenia is determined by polygenic traits although the transmission of the disease may also suggest a single gene mutant of autosomal dominance, with environmental events or polygenic factors modifying the genotype and possibly accounting for the variability seen among schizophrenics. A biological cause of schizophrenia would therefore appear to be a reasonable assumption, and its cause may eventually be unravelled in the realm of biochemistry by applying appropriate analytical methods. However, of approximately 1500 human diseases known to be genetically determined by defect genes only a small number of some 90 genetic disorders have so far been found to be associated causally with an enzyme deficiency (69). In assuming an enzyme deficiency the following general metabolic alterations may be inferred from other well documented inborn errors of metabolism to become manifest:

1. Increase of substrate of the blocked enzyme reaction in body fluids and tissues.
2. Accumulation of precursor(s) of substrate because of backing up of substrate and its negative feedback effect on preceding reactions.
3. Decrease or disappearance of normal product of blocked enzyme reaction and possibly of other subsequent enzyme reactions due to lack of substrate.
4. Increase of reaction product(s) of one or several alternative *normal* enzyme reactions of substrate.
5. Possible nonenzymatic products through condensation or complex formation of accumulated substrate in storage diseases.

The alterations outlined above usually serve as basis of diagnostic measures which take advantage of increases of substrates or intermediates in body fluids and tissues, a slow rate of disappearance from plasma of substrate given orally or intravenously like in the detection of heterozygotes in phenylketonurics (37), reduced or absent enzyme activity in plasma or its particulate constituents (leukocytes, erythrocytes) (24) or in urine, biopsy specimens and fibroblast cultures as in lipid storage diseases (35) as well as increases in reaction products of alternative pathways as for instance phenylpyruvic acid in phenylketonuria (102).

The traditional approach in schizophrenia has been to study tryptophan metabolites, mainly indoles in body fluids, i.e. primarily in urine, and to search for „abnormal" metabolites; with the advent of more refined and sensitive techniques, however, main emphasis of recent work has shifted to studies of enzyme activities and the search for products of alternative metabolic steps (see below). Some confusion may arise from the usage of the term "abnormal" as it seems to imply a metabolic potentiality in schizophrenics that does not exist in normals. Although there are "abnormal" genes, a term used to designate mutant genes, it was clearly stated some ten years ago (143) that there are in general no "abnormal" metabolites even in inborn errors of metabolism. As discussed by Harris (84) most mutations that alter the genetic code of DNA occur as a single base changes which in turn will alter the amino acid sequence within a small portion only of the whole length of the protein molecule to be synthesized by ribosomes, rather than the entire molecule. Due to the complexity of the transcriptional message imparted by a particular base triplet the ensuing overall alterations of the protein molecule concerned may be diverse affecting both the primary and tertiary structure and thus altering both its physicochemical properties and catalytic activities while its basic character though distorted will be retained.

Accordingly, with the only exception of the enzyme 5-amino-levulinate synthetase (180) exhibiting increased activity in a condition known as acute intermittent porphyria, all enzyme defects hitherto known to be of genetic cause appear to be related to an impaired or faulty synthesis of enzyme proteins rather than to an overproduction of protein or an enhanced enzyme activity due to lack of regulatory factors. In contrast, proteins with novel catalytic activities are the result of evolutionary changes that are of no significance in this context.

In some inborn errors of metabolism due to enzyme failure there may be a rare chance of "abnormal" compounds to arise nonenzymatically from accumulated precursors or intermediates. This hypothetical event has in fact been suggested regarding the cyclization of melatonin or an aldehyde condensation to yield β-carbolines (118) while a toxic compound could be synthesized corresponding to a complex formed from 5-methoxytryptamine and pyridoxal, exhibiting neurological and behavioral effects (172, 175). The latter compound has also been claimed to occur as a urinary constituent in schizophrenics (98).

The marked melanosis found in some schizophrenics was recently again pointed out to have a possible bearing on this point (82).

Aside from enzyme deficiencies, genetic factors may exert their effects on tryptophan indirectly at a molecular level, interacting with the synthesis of transport proteins or carriers, activators of enzyme reactions, or with the structure and function of cell membranes. In this connection the observations of GOTTLIEB et al. (78) are of interest. They isolated a plasma protein (α_2-globulin) from blood of schizophrenics promoting the cellular uptake of tryptophan and other precursor amino acids of important neurotransmitters by erythrocytes *in vitro*. Another alpha-helical protein from schizophrenic plasma called S-protein was later reported to enhance the enzymatic N-methylation of indoleamines incubated *in vitro* with bovine brain homogenates (70).

Tryptophan metabolites of body fluids

In order to demonstrate metabolic aberrations of tryptophan metabolism in disease states and in particular in mental illness, levels of oxidative and deaminated tryptophan metabolites in plasma and urine have been investigated in many cases. Some changes were claimed to occur along the kynurenine pathway in schizophrenics, especially when given an oral load of DL- or L-tryptophan; others have noted changes in levels of indoles in plasma or urine. Rather than discussing the large body of somewhat conflicting data it may be referred to several comprehensive discussions of this subject by students of this field (41, 138, 140, 143, 145, 164). At present the general consensus of opinion prevails that the data does not warrant the assumption of a fundamental disorder of tryptophan metabolism in schizophrenia. Yet, it should be borne in mind that studies of tryptophan metabolism are difficult to conduct because of a number of extraneous factors that are usually beyond rigid experimental control as discussed by FRIEDHOFF (68) and KETY (105), not the least important variable being the adaptive activity of the enzyme tryptophan pyrrolase. All this may obscure a possible though minor metabolic aberration involving tryptophan in schizophrenia.

Besides, reports on the occurrence of new metabolites derived from tryptophan in man continue to appear indicating the action of hitherto entirely unknown metabolic enzyme reactions both in normal and pathological conditions. Furthermore, only 10 to 20% of the dietary tryptophan may be accounted for as urinary excretion products with total indole metabolites comprising as little as 1—2%, leaving a large portion of tryptophan for other metabolic pathways (156, 161).

The likelihood of such disorders to be found is not very great, however, if one remembers that clear-cut changes of tryptophan were indeed found in several conditions other than schizophrenia, like Hartnup's disease (5), Down's syndrome with low levels of 5-hydroxytryptamine (5-HT) in blood (18), or an increased excretion of hydroxykynurenine in a state associated with a deficient kynureninase activity in tissues (108), as well as in migraine and some others (145).

Most notably is the observation of an apparent disturbance of indole metabolism in polar and bipolar depression as summarized by COPPEN and SHAW (48), with low levels of urinary tryptamine and 3-indole-3-acetic acid (3-IAA) (50) as well as low urinary 5-HT and 5-hydroxyindole-3-acetic acid (5-HIAA) (137, 143). Complementary to these findings is the observation that the oxidative metabolism of tryptophan appeared to be potentiated in depressed patients receiving an oral load of L-tryptophan, possibly due to an increased pyrrolase activity in these patients (52).

Indoles of the central nervous system comprise only a small portion of the total indole pool of the human organism. Attempts to deduce changes of levels or turnover of indoles or other tryptophan metabolites in brain from quantitative data of urinary excretion studies are not likely to yield conclusive and unequivocal results unless there would be metabolic changes of a more general or basic nature as discussed above, or changes that are brought about by pharmacological or dietary factors (see below). In contrast, cerebrospinal fluid (CSF) may be more directly affected by metabolic and functional changes of the central nervous system because of its intimate contact with various parts of the brain by ways of simple diffusion. Cerebrospinal fluid has been indeed found to contain measurable amounts of acidic catabolites of catecholamines, especially of dopamine as well as of indoleamines (3, 7, 23, 73, 183), and based on experimental evidence levels of these catabolites in CSF are considered to reflect to some extent levels and turnover of monoamines in brain and spinal cord (55, 56, 57, 83, 120).

Quantitative data on levels of 5-HIAA and 3-IAA in cerebrospinal fluid is now available in various human diseases like parkinsonism (22), dementias (39, 77) and in others.

In schizophrenia quantitative studies of 5-hydroxyindoles of CSF have so far failed to reveal striking changes compared to normal controls (132, 141). In a small number of schizophrenics, however, low levels of 5-HIAA of CSF were also reported and found statistically tenable when the patients were compared to age-matched controls (34) or when a distinction was made between acute and chronic schizophrenic subjects (6). It appears that further data is needed to eventually settle this issue definitely.

In contrast to schizophrenia low levels of 5-HIAA have rather consistently been found in CSF of depressive patients (7, 53, 119 and others) along with reduced 5-HIAA levels in brain of depressive suicidal subjects on autopsy (33, 152). These findings support and are compatible with the serotonin hypothesis of depression, suggesting a malfunction in the metabolism regulating serotonin levels in the brain and possibly peripheral tissues as well (47).

Probenecid, an inhibitory substance of the active transport of organic acids from CSF into the blood was introduced as an experimental tool to study turnover rates rather than concentrations of monoamines in brain (83). While levels of 5-HIAA, for instance, in CSF of untreated subjects merely reflect a steady-state turnover of 5-HT to 5-HIAA the actual rate of synthesis and inactivation of 5-HT in brain may be computed from the accumulation of 5-HIAA in CSF when its outflow is inhibited by probenecid (127). In depressive patients this technique has produced evidence of a low rate of synthesis and turnover of 5-HT in brain (136, 144, 157).

Results of similar studies in schizophrenia are not yet available.

As regards urinary indoles and behavior a somewhat more meaningful pattern emerges from longitudinal studies on the quantitative excretion of indoles in schizophrenic patients. BRUNE and HIMWICH first observed a correlation between the degree of behavioral worsening and the daily amount of urinary tryptamine, indole-3-acetic acid and

5-hydroxyindoleacetic acid in schizophrenics receiving placebo or iproniazide or reserpine (42, 43). Later, similar observations were made in a small number of untreated patients during acute episodes of behavioral exacerbations (17, 20). In these studies striking daily fluctuations of urinary creatinine were also observed to which the urinary excretions of tryptamine and 3-IAA seemed to correlate (19, 139). These fluctuations were considered to result from states of a negative nitrogen balance since periods of behavioral exacerbations were accompanied by dramatic weight losses in these patients. This interpretation was further corroborated by positively correlating urinary indoles with creatinine, amino acids and other parameters (21).

A mobilization of endogenous substrates in schizophrenics was therefore suggested to provide precursors for the formation of psychotoxic indole derivatives like bufotenin and N,N-dimethyltryptamine, which in turn would aggravate psychotic symptoms. It is obvious that this interpretation of the experimental results places the metabolic defect in schizophrenia not with tryptophan itself but another mechanism triggering periods of metabolic imbalances.

ENZYMATIC MODIFICATIONS OF TRYPTAMINE AND SEROTONIN

The first reports on the occurrence of bufotenin in the urine of man (44, 63) have at first raised some controversy in view of the methodology then available and the lack of evidence in support of the presence of respective enzymes in mammals. Meanwhile, methods have been greatly improved, and experimental findings on N-methyltransferases and hydroxylases acting on indole substrates in man and animals are now affording a rational basis for the biosynthesis of indolealkylamines.

The classical indoleamines tryptamine and 5-hydroxytryptamine may be converted to N- or O-methylated compounds following prior hydroxylation along metabolic pathways depicted in Fig. 1, which is also showing some known or hypothetical detoxication mechanisms. Tryptamine and 5-HT are N-methylated to form N-methyltryptamine and N-methylserotonin, respectively, *in vitro* by an enzyme first isolated from rabbit lung tissue

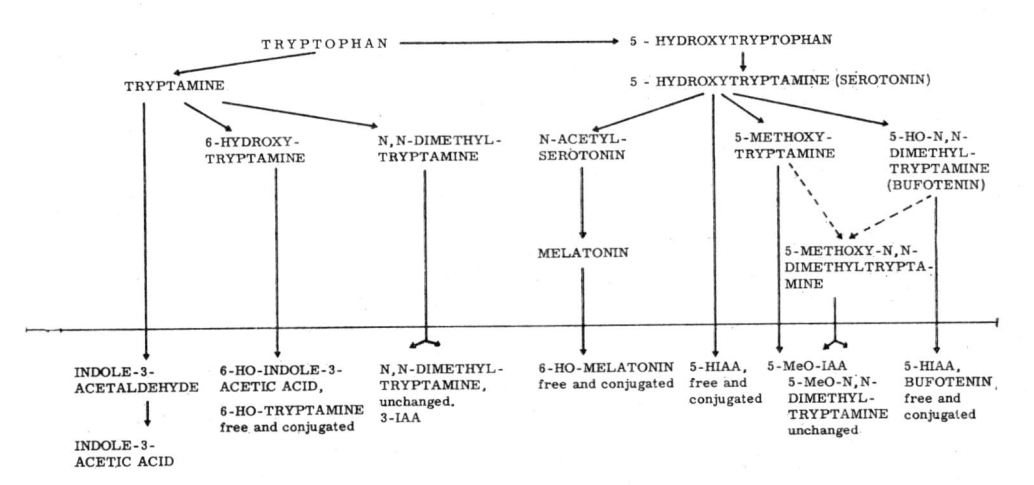

Fig. 1. Biosynthesis and catabolism of indoleamines. For explanation see text. Dotted lines indicate putative pathways. Abbreviations: 5-HIAA—5-hydroxyindole-3-acetic acid; 5-MeO-IAA—5-methoxyindole-3-acetic acid.

(8, 9). The purified enzyme exhibited low substrate specificity, and both catechol- and indoleamines were found to serve as substrates of the enzyme with variable degrees of turnover rates. Aside from 4-hydroxytryptamine and 6-hydroxytryptamine the highest activities were observed with serotonin, tryptamine and N-methylserotonin as substrates. Recently the N-methyltransferases of rabbit lung and chick brain were reinvestigated, and contrary to previous studies the enzyme displayed a high specificity for indoleamines following its purification by gel filtration, methylating N-methyltryptamine, 5-HT and tryptamine in this order of affinity (179), and N-methyltryptamine, N-methylserotonin, tryptamine and 5-HT, respectively (115).

Significantly, similar transferase activities have been found not only in human tissue (182), but also in brain of both animals and man, as well as in serum of schizophrenic patients (88, 126).

Methyltransferase

Morgan and Mandell (121) first described a soluble enzyme activity in chick brain of high specificity toward the indoleamines 5-HT (100%), 5-methoxytryptamine (88%), tryptamine (60%), N-methyltryptamine (47%), while not reacting with norepinephrine or bufotenin. In addition evidence of the presence of this enzyme in man was obtained from studies on biopsy specimens of human brain, to be later confirmed by the demonstration of the enzyme activity in human as well as sheep brain (116). These observations were corroborated independently by another group of investigators studying the formation of N-methyltryptamine and N,N-dimethyltryptamine from radioactive tryptamine injected intracisternally in the rat or incubated with tissue preparations of human brain specimens obtained in the course of neurosurgical procedures (148). The authors reported furthermore the presence of potent endogenous inhibitors, including S-adenosylhomocysteine, of the N-methyltransferase in brain, that might affect the N-methylation of tryptamine in specific brain areas.

Heller (88) and Narahimsachari et al. (126) have evaluated the indoleethylamine N-methyltransferase activity in plasma of schizophrenic patients and normal controls. In one study plasma was incubated with 5-HT, and N-methylserotonin could be isolated as the reaction product. No activity was found in the plasma of 4 normal controls (88). In a more extensive study either 5-HT or 5-methoxytryptamine were incubated again in plasma of acute and chronic schizophrenic patients and of normal controls (126). There was a very high incidence of positive findings as judged from the formation of either bufotenin or 5-methoxy-N,N-dimethyltryptamine in both acute and chronic schizophrenic patients as opposed to negative findings throughout in the controls.

The dialkyl substitution of the amine group of indoles appears to be a necessity for indoleamines to become psychoactive to a significant extent as may be inferred from studies on structural implications of indolic psychotomimetics (60, 74, 149, 159, 167, 171). Potent psychotomimetics of this series include N,N-dimethyltryptamine, N,N-diethyltryptamine and 5-hydroxy-N,N-dimethyltryptamine (bufotenin). Indoleamines will also attain psychotropic properties when hydroxylated on the ring in the 4 or 6 position (168, 170). The significance of the hydroxylation of N,N-dimethyltryptamine has been challenged however (45, 146, 173) and the suggestion that some indolealkylamines may be converted *in vivo* to more potent agents by 6-hydroxylation has yet to be further substantiated. An even greater role appears to play the hydroxylation in the 4 position of the ring, represented by the highly psychotomimetic compounds psilocybin and psilocin, both 4-hydroxyl-dialkyl-indoleamines with hallucinogenic effects in man (95, 104, 186).

From early reports on the urinary excretion of 6-hydroxy-skatole in mental patients and normal subjects (54, 97, 110, 160) hydroxylation of the 6 position of the indole ring would appear to represent a common pathway for the detoxication of indole metabolites in man, especially since it was shown that the excretion of 6-hydroxy-skatoles was not peculiar of schizophrenics. More refined chromatographic separation techniques revealed that urinary skatoles were composed of a mixture of 5-, 6-, 7-hydroxyl isomers, illustrating the wide range of enzymatic potentialities of tissue enzymes in substituting the indole molecule with hydroxyl groups (86). Microsomal 6-hydroxylation of tryptamine and related compounds has been shown by others (101, 100) and was found to take place in human liver as well (99). Furthermore, 6-hydroxylation was found to represent a major metabolic pathway of melatonin, leading to the urinary excretion of 5-methoxy-6-hydroxy--N-acetylserotonin, free and conjugated (109).

When injecting tryptamine-^{14}C intraperitoneally in the rabbit LEMBERGER et al. (114) not only demonstrated the presence of tryptamine in brain as a normal constituent in accordance with other recent studies (117, 148) but also the formation of 6-hydroxytryptamine in brain and other tissues. In urine 6-hydroxyindoleacetic acid was found in addition to free and conjugated 6-hydroxytryptamine.

Notwithstanding conflicting findings on the psychotropic effect of 6-hydroxy-indolealkylamines (see above) the presence of tryptamine in brain and the potentiality of its being converted to 6-hydroxytryptamine in the body enzymatically appears to be significant, especially when considering that the latter is taken up by brain tissue slices and stored in serotonergic neurons (94). This and the effect of reserpine on the release and deamination of 6-hydroxytryptamine seem to suggest that 6-hydroxytryptamine may exert neurotropic effects by replacing neuronal serotonin (114). Another congener of serotonin, 5,6-dihydroxytryptamine was recently shown to cause a long-lasting depletion for up to 30 days of serotonin from rat brain after intraventricular injection, and electron microscopic and fluorescence microscopic findings indicate that serotonergic nerve terminals of neurons are selectively destroyed (15).

Another important molecular modification of indoleamines is the 0-methylation of ring hydroxyl groups. In studying the effects of several 0-methylated dialkylamines in trained rats 5-methoxy-dialkylindoleamines were found to be most effective in disrupting conditioned behavior, followed by 4-methoxy-N,N-dialkylamines and 6-methoxydialkylamines with 7-methoxy-dialkylamines being the least effective (74). Potent effects of 5-methoxy-N,N-dimethyltryptamine had been observed before by other investigators (76, 173), and were summarized by AIRAKSINEN and McISAAC (2), apart from the fact that 5-methoxy-indolealkylamines have come to be known as the active ingredients of hallucinogenic snuffs used by indian natives (96).

As much reason as there is to consider 0-methylated indoleamines potent hallucinogens and psychotomimetics, there is as yet little evidence available to suggest their endogenous formation in animals or man to an appreciable extent. An O-methyltransferase acting upon N-acetylserotonin occurs in the pineal gland of amphibians and mammals (12); however, its activity appears to be strictly confined to this gland as a careful scrutiny for its activity in other brain areas was unsuccessful (11).

Yet a microsomal enzyme was found in rabbit liver, capable of O-methylating dihydroxyindoles among other substrates (10). In view of the much enhanced lipid solubility and rapid uptake by brain of some 5-methoxy-dialkylamines as compared to hydroxyl precursors (46, 74, 150) psychotoxic compounds need not arise from O-methylation in brain, but may be formed peripherally and subsequently enter the brain with relative ease.

Furthermore, most of tryptamine and serotonin of the body is located in tissues and body fluids other than the central nervous system, and are precluded from freely entering it (58, 81, 114), apparently due to their poor lipid solubility. If occurring in high concentrations in the body, e.g. due to a tryptophan load, an appreciable portion of tryptamine and serotonin may be rendered more lipid soluble in the periphery by substitution and thus become centrally active.

INACTIVATION OF INDOLEAMINES

Attention has been drawn to the excretion of free and conjugated bufotenin as an important variable in schizophrenic behavior (177). Conjugation serves to detoxicate and to speed up renal excretion of waste products from the body, and mechanisms which inactivate endogenous as well as exogenous amines in man have indeed important implications in various behavioral states related to biogenic amines. In general, monoamines undergo rapid deamination and subsequent oxidation, catalyzed by a monoamine oxidase and acetaldehyde dehydrogenase, respectively (26). In addition to tissue monoamine oxidase (MAO) there is a MAO activity of plasma as well as of platelets that were found to react with tryptamine and serotonin (27, 129). Substitution of the aminoethyl nitrogen will reduce the reactivity of monoamines with MAO, depending on both the substituent and the degree of substitution. Monoalkyl substitution has little effect, while markedly lower activities of the enzyme were found *in vitro* with tertiary and quaternary indoleamines as substrates like bufotenin and bufotenidine (28, 75, 79). Ring hydroxylation does not alter the reactivity compared to the parent compound.

Somewhat different results with regard to deamination were observed *in vivo*. In man, N,N-dimethyltryptamine was recovered to a large extent from urine as 3-IAA (167, 169), and similar results were obtained in rats (59). Even with N,N-diethyltryptamine about 1/10 of an oral dose was found in urine as 3-IAA (171). The administration of bufotenin resulted in the excretion of a small portion of the total dose as 5-HIAA (59, 150). 5-Methoxy-N-methyltryptamine was almost quantitatively converted to 5-methoxyindole-3-acetic acid in rats (174). The oxidation of dialkylindoleamines *in vivo* may either indicate a slow though measurable turnover by direct deamination, or an N-demethylating process possibly preceding deamination. Inactivation of monoamines by N-demethylating enzymes is considered possible (1). Furthermore, N-demethylation of N-alkyloxindoles was shown to be catalyzed *in vitro* by a microsomal enzyme preparation from liver (16). This type of reaction therefore appears to be a common detoxicating mechanism in the organism; it is not known, however, to what extent indolealkylamines will react with this or related enzyme systems.

In addition to unchanged dialkylamine a large portion of bufotenin will be excreted unchanged as conjugates with glucuronic or sulphuric acid radicals (59, 150).

INDOLEALKYLAMINES AND SCHIZOPHRENIA

The following indolealkylamines with psychotropic effects when tested experimentally have been reported to occur in human plasma or urine or both: Bufotenin or a bufotenin-like substance (44, 64, 65, 66, 67, 87, 89, 124, 125, 176, 177); N,N-dimethyltryptamine (67, 89, 125), and 5-methoxy-N,N-dimethyltryptamine (89, 124, 125). Other investigators were unable to confirm these results (131, 142, 147, 154), and still others found bufotenin and/or N,N-dimethyltryptamine in urine both of normal subjects and mental patients (61, 62, 64, 65, 66, 155).

Depending on the respective outcome of such studies different conclusions may be drawn as to the relevance of psychotomimetics of endogenous origin in either normals or schizophrenics or in both. Also, discussants of these studies have attributed both positive and negative findings to a number of factors unrelated to schizophrenia, like differences in methodology, variability among schizophrenic patients, dietary influences, etc. At present the question of how to reconcile contradictory findings and how to weigh them against each other remains unsettled as yet, although some guidelines in this direction seem to emerge from the enzyme studies outlined above. Thus the formation of various substituted indolealkylamines in the body may be nothing more than an indication of alternative, yet physiological metabolic pathways of little quantitative and functional significance in healthy persons. It follows that these alternative reactions may attain greater significance in certain disease conditions, and the question to be answered is therefore how schizophrenics differ quantitatively rather than qualitatively from normal subjects in their excretion of indolealkylamines. On the same premises the dispute over the significance of negative or positive findings in schizophrenics and normal subjects may eventually be resolved.

In order to prove this point quantitative rather than qualitative studies are desirable. Most of the recent studies do in fact provide quantitative excretion data in schizophrenic patients and normal controls (62, 65, 66, 155). Significantly greater amounts of bufotenin were found in urine of schizophrenics than in control urines in 3 of these studies (65, 66, 155). In addition acute schizophrenics seem to excrete more bufotenin than chronic schizophrenics (65, 66).

It may be yet too soon to draw final conclusions from the relatively small number of reports on quantitative data, and to try to answer the question of how increases in indolealkylamines are brought about and what their causal relationship is to the underlying disorder. MURPHY and WYATT (123) have recently reported reduced activities of a monoamine oxidase from platelets of schizophrenic patients. It would therefore be conceivable that the detoxication of some monoamines is impaired in mental illness. The observation may also be relevant in this context that MAO inhibition seemed to increase urinary bufotenin rather specifically in schizophrenics (87).

Since indolealkylamines are poor substrates of monoamine oxidase other detoxicating mechanisms may be adversely affected as well in schizophrenia, including the formation of conjugates (177).

AMINO ACIDS AND SCHIZOPHRENIA

The implications of the endogenous formation of psychotomimetic indoleamines were tested by means of experimental diets containing large amounts of one or two particular amino acids. Following the early studies by LAUER et al. (113) and SHAW et al. (153) POLLIN and co-workers systematically studied the interaction between certain amino acids, the inhibition of monoamine oxidase and behavior in schizophrenic patients (133). They were the first to demonstrate that the amino acids methionine and tryptophan induce and aggravate psychotic symptoms in chronic patients in a rather specific way. These results were confirmed by most of the subsequent studies of other investigators on the effects of methionine and tryptophan, and as a further result L-cysteine was added to the list of apparently "psychotoxic" amino acids. Experimental details and the results of these and additional studies were recently reviewed by HIMWICH (91) and WYATT et al. (187).

The rationale in designing these studies and in using the above listed amino acids was threefold. Tryptophan was postulated to induce high tissue levels of tryptamine and

5-hydroxytryptamine as it was amply shown to do, especially in conjunction with an MAO inhibitor. The physiological amines would then serve as precursors of possible N- or O-methylated psychotoxic indoleamines. L-methionine was thought to enhance the endogenous transmethylation by raising tissue levels of S-adenosylmethionine and providing "activated" methyl groups (13). Because of the inhibitory effect of agents blocking sulfhydryl groups N-methyltransferases are considered to contain active sulfhydryl groups (9). The administration of the reducing amino acid cysteine could therefore enhance the activity of SH enzymes in tissue.

Whatever the exact mechanism of these amino acids might be in producing psychotic symptoms in schizophrenics the results of these studies are of current significance in three different respects. First, most studies along these lines have shown that the amino acids exert little or no behavioral effect unless an MAO inhibitor is given simultaneously. Secondly, in addition to tryptophan methionine (18, 166) and cysteine (162) were found in man to specifically increase indole levels of body fluids, especially that of urinary tryptamine. With methionine these increases well surpassed those brought about by MAO inhibition alone and the increases of urinary tryptamine appeared to be dose related (18). In animals methionine, but not cysteine or homocysteine also produced specific increases of urinary tryptamine and other indoles even in the absence of an MAO inhibitor (155). Thirdly, parallel studies on urinary indoles, the excretion of indolealkylamines and behavior in schizophrenics receiving cysteine together with an MAO inhibitor have suggested a relationship between behavioral exacerbations and the urinary elimination of methylated indoleamines (124, 162, 178). All these observations are well in line with the working hypotheses at the outset of the experimental studies.

The question now is whether they support the transmethylation hypothesis in schizophrenia in terms of an intrinsic metabolic defect. It is obvious that the results of the studies are open to interpretation in a number of ways, and it is felt that within the scope of this discussion and in view of untoward effects of massive amounts of amino acids on the nitrogen balance and cellular metabolism as well, the observations in schizophrenics may not be taken as strictly indicating an impaired metabolic handling of tryptophan or its metabolites in but one specific way leading to the formation of toxic products as opposed to healthy controls. Also, the need of MAO inhibition in these experiments seems to detract from the view that inactivation of methylated indoleamines might be impaired in schizophrenics. As will be shown in the following paragraphs mere changes in levels of brain biogenic amines are equally unlikely to produce symptoms as severe and as typically seen quite consistently with the regimen of amino acids and an MAO inhibitor. It would therefore appear that schizophrenics are more susceptible to the psychotoxic effects of these diets for reasons that may be metabolically related to tryptophan not as closely as hitherto assumed. A "biological factor" was suggested to contribute to the behavioral reaction of schizophrenics in such studies (93).

Tryptophan and behavior

The discussion of the metabolism of tryptophan would be incomplete without considering some of the pharmacological effects of tryptophan in animals and man in relation to brain biogenic amines and behavioral states (Table 1). In doing so it becomes apparent that L-tryptophan has more than just one action, depending on the baseline situation of the individual under investigation.

5-HT is involved in the regulation of sleep (103) and its selective depletion by p-chlorophenylalanine (107) will cause insomnia and increased "reactivity" (38, 122). These

TABLE 1

Mental states and brain levels of 5-HT and other monoamines

	M'amines involved	Experimental/ Therapeutic	Behavior	Effects M'amines
Sleep	5-HT/NE	p-Chlorophenylalanin	Insomnia	5-HT ↓
		L-Tryptophan	Sleep	5-HT ↑
Depression	5-HT ↓	MAOI+5-HTP/TP	Improvement	5-HT/NE ↑
		ECT	Improvement	5-HT ↑
		Reserpine	Depression	5-HT/NE ↓
Parkinsonism	DA ↓	L-DOPA+Dec. inhib.	Improvement	DA ↑, 5-HT ↓
Park.+L-DOPA- induced psychosis	DA ↑, 5-HT ↓ SAMe ↓	+ L-Tryptophan	Improvement	DA ↑, 5-HT ↑
Schizophrenia	—	L-Tryptoph., L-Meth. DL-Cysteine	No change	5-HT ↑
		+ MAOI	Exacerbation	M'amines ↑
		Low trypt. intake	No change	5-HT ↓
Model psychoses	5-HT ↑	Psychotomim. indoleamines	Disruption	5-HT ↑

Arrows denote increased (↑) or descreased (↓) levels of monoamines.

effects may be reversed by the administration of L-tryptophan. In the light of these observations L-tryptophan has been used successfully as a mild sedative or hypnotic in man (85). Reserpine will deplete both 5-HT and noradrenaline causing sedation and depressive mood changes (151). The administration of tryptophan or 5-HTP together with an MAO inhibitor to depressed patients entails clinical improvement (49, 106). Both lithium and ECT used in the treatment of depression seem to raise the endogenous 5-HT levels (71, 130).

A reduction of dietary tryptophan will quickly lower plasma tryptophan and tissue levels of 5-HT (51) resulting in hyperactivity followed by sedation and motor disturbances in rats (31). In contrast, hyperactivity was also observed in rats receiving L-tryptophan together with an MAO inhibitor (80). Drowsiness and some euphoria were reported from normal subjects taking L-tryptophan without an MAO inhibitor (158), and euphoria and predominantly neurological disturbances from healthy volunteers receiving MAO inhibitor in addition to tryptophan (128).

Diets low in tryptophan and methionine have been given to schizophrenics in an attempt to favorably affect their psychotic behavior, however, without apparent effect, either to the better or to the worse (20, 30).

For the treatment of Parkinson's disease L-DOPA is given in fairly large doses for prolonged periods of time. The side effects of this regimen were observed to include mania-like or psychotic symptoms in some patients (25, 112) that might be related to changes of brain amine levels due to L-DOPA. In animal experiments L-DOPA was found to lower brain 5-HT as well as S-adenosylmethionine (14, 187). It was recently reported that 1 to 2 g of oral L-tryptophan will overcome psychotic symptoms completely in these patients within less than one day of the administration (25).

A number of indolic psychotomimetics will raise 5-HT levels as well, presumably due to their inhibitory effect on MAO (36). Conversely, experimentally lowering 5-HT levels of the brain prior to administration of LSD will enhance the sensitivity to the effect of LSD disrupting behavior (4). On the other hand, it has been speculated that 10% of the normal brain 5-HT will suffice to maintain normal function of the nervous system (29).

These examples will illustrate that L-tryptophan may hardly be considered a pharmacological agent in a strict sense, but it will interfere with the delicate equilibrium of biogenic amines at strategic sites of the nervous system and thus bring about profound effects. It is obvious — and this view was expressed by others before (134) — that our concept of behavioral states and biogenic amines of the brain must take into account not only absolute levels of but one amine but also the delicate balance between several amines, and the dynamics of changing levels of one or several amines.

Conclusion

It was the purpose of this discussion to examine the question of whether there is a aberration of the metabolism of tryptophan in schizophrenia, which may allow one to causally relate one to the other. From the perusal of the pertinent literature it appears that the assumption of an overt metabolic or functional disorder affecting tryptophan directly or indirectly is not warranted by the available evidence. This is not to say that tryptophan is not at all involved in schizophrenia. Its metabolism appears to be severely affected by behavioral disturbances, either of spontaneous origin or brought about by drugs and certain amino acids. The distribution of tryptophan to the various metabolic ramifications is subject to a large number of homeostatic control mechanism relevant to levels and turnover of tryptophan at strategic sides in the central nervous system, which are difficult to assess in man. The metabolic disturbance at this level may be only slight, yet its impact on behaviour may be profound.

Our knowledge of the biological basis of the many delicate nuances of human behavior is very scarce as yet. It is in schizophrenia that the most bizarre and aberrant forms of human behavior may be found. If we only knew more about the normal physiology of human behavior better insight might also be gained into causes of abnormal behavior and there is no doubt that tryptophan is at least one among a number of factors involved.

References

1. AHLBORG, G., HOLMSTEDT, B. and LINDGREN, J. E. (1968) Fate and metabolism of some hallucinogenic indolealkylamines. Advanc. Pharmacol. **6B**, 213.
2. AIRAKSINEN, M. M. and McISAAC, W. M. (1968) Indolealkylamines and Behavior. Annal. Med. exp. Fenn. **46**, 367.
3. ANDEN, N. E., ROOS, B.-E. and WERDENIUS, B. (1963) On the occurrence of homovanillic acid and 3-methoxy-4-hydroxy-mandelic acid in human cerebrospinal fluid. Experientia, **19**, 359.
4. APPEL, J. B., LOVELL, R. A. and FREEDMAN, B. X. (1970) Alterations in the behavioral effects of LSD by pretreatment with p-chlorophenylalanine and α-methyl-p-tyrosine. Psychopharmacologia (Berl.) **18**, 387.
5. ASATOOR, A. M., CRASKE, J., LONDON, D. R. and MILNE, M. D. (1963) Indole production in Hartnup disease. Lancet, **i**, 126.
6. ASHCROFT, G. W., ECCLESTON, D., SHARMAN, B. F., MAC DOUSAL, E. J., STANTON, J. B. and BINNS, J. K. (1966) 5-Hydroxyindole compounds in the cerebrospinal fluid of patients with psychiatric or neurological diseases. Lancet **ii**, 1049.
7. ASHCROFT, G. and SHARMAN, D. F. (1960) 5-Hydroxyindoles in human cerebrospinal fluids. Nature (Lond.) **186**, 1050.

8. AXELROD, J. (1961) Enzymatic formation of psychotomimetic metabolites from normally occurring compounds. Science, 134, 343.
9. AXELROD, J. (1962) The enzymatic N-methylation of serotonin and other amines. J. Pharmacol. exp. Ther. 138, 28.
10. AXELROD, J., INSCOE, J. K. and DALY, J. (1965) Enzymatic formation of O-methylated dihydroxy derivatives from phenolic amines and indoles. J. Pharmacol. exp. Ther. 149, 16.
11. AXELROD, J., MACLEAN, P. D., ALBERS, R. W. and WEISSBACH, H. (1961) Regional distribution of methyl transferase enzymes in the nervous system and glandular tissues. In: Regional Neurochemistry, S. S. KETY and J. ELKES, Eds., New York, p. 307.
12. AXELROD, J. and WEISSBACH, H. (1961) Purification and properties of hydroxyindole-O-methyltransferase. J. biol. Chem. 236, 211.
13. BALDESSARINI, R. J. (1967) Factors influencing S-adenosylmethionine levels in mammalian tissues. In: HIMWICH, H. E., KETY, S. S. and SMYTHIES, J. R., Eds. Amines and Schizophrenia. Oxford, 199.
14. BALDESSARINI, R. J. (1971) Effects of L-dopa on brain amine metabolism. Third Int. Meeting of the Int. Soc. for Neurochemistry, Budapest (Abstr.).
15. BAUMGARTEN, H. G., BJORKLUND, A., LACHENMAYER, L., NOBIN, A. and STEVENI, U. (1971) Long-lasting selective depletion of brain serotonin by 5,6-dihydroxytryptamine. Acta physiol. scand., Suppl. 373, 1.
16. BECKETT, A. H. and MORTON, D. M. (1967) The metabolism of N-alkyloxindoles. Biochem. Pharmacol. 16, 1787.
17. BERLET, H. H., BULL, C., HIMWICH, H. E., KOHL, H., MATSUMOTO, K., PSCHEIDT, G. R., SPAIDE, J., TOURLENTES, T. T. and VALVERDE, J. M. (1964) Endogenous metabolic factor in schizophrenic behavior. Science, 144, 311.
18. BERLET, H. H., MATSUMOTO, K., PSCHEIDT, G. R., SPAIDE, J., BULL, C. and HIMWICH, H. E. (1965) Biochemical correlates of behavior in schizophrenic patients. Arch. gen. Psychiat. 13, 521.
19. BERLET, H. H., PSCHEIDT, G. R., SPAIDE, J. K. and HIMWICH, H. E. (1964) Variations of urinary creatinine and its correlation to tryptamine excretion in schizophrenic patients. Nature (Lond.) 203, 1198.
20. BERLET, H. H., SPAIDE, J., KOHL, H., BULL, C. and HIMWICH, H. E. (1965) Effects of reduction of tryptophan and methionine intake on urinary indole compounds and schizophrenic behavior. J. nerv. ment. Dis. 140, 297.
21. BERLET, H. H., SPAIDE, J. K., MATSUMOTO, K. and HIMWICH, H. E. (1967) Studies on the association of urinary tryptamine with the excretion of amino acids and 17-ketosteroid hormones in schizophrenic patients. Amines and Schizophrenia, H. E. HIMWICH, KETY, S. S. and SMYTHIES, J. R., Eds. Pergamon Press, Oxford. p. 69.
22. BERNHEIMER, H., BIRKMAYER, W. and HORNYKIEWICZ, O. (1966) Homovanillinsäure im Liquor cerebrospinalis: Untersuchungen beim Parkinson-Syndrom und anderen Erkrankungen des ZNS. Wien. klin. Wschr. 78, 417.
23. BERTILSSON, L. and PALMÉR, L. (1972) Indole-3-acetic acid in human cerebrospinal fluid: Identification and quantification by mass fragmentography. Science, 177, 74.
24. BEUTLER, E. (1968) Hereditary disorders of erythrocyte metabolism. Grune and Stratton, New York.
25. BIRKMAYER, W. and MENTASTI, M. (1972) Parkinsonkranke mit L-Dopa behandeln. Dtsch. Ärzteblatt, 69, 686.
26. BLASCHKO, H. (1952) Amine oxidase and amine metabolism. Pharmacol. Rev. 4, 415.
27. BLASCHKO, H., FRIEDMAN, P. J., HAWES, R. and NILSSON, K. (1959) The amine oxidases of mammalian plasma. J. Physiol. (Lond.) 145, 384.
28. BLASCHKO, H. and PHILPOT, F. J. (1953) Enzymic oxidation of tryptamine derivatives. J. Physiol (Lond.) 122, 403.
29. BLOOM, F. E. and GIARMAN, N. J. (1968) Physiologic and pharmacologic considerations of biogenic amines in the nervous system. Ann. Rev. Pharmacol. 8, 229.
30. BOGOSCH, S. (1957) Effect of synthetic diet low in aromatic amino acids on schizophrenic patients. Arch. Neurol. Psychiat. (Chic.) 78, 539.
31. BOULLIN, D. J. (1963) Behaviour of rats depleted of 5-hydroxytryptamine by feeding a diet free of tryptophan. Psychopharmacologia (Berl.) 5, 28.
32. BOULTON, A. A. (1971) Biochemical Research in schizophrenia. Nature (Lond.) 121, 22.
33. BOURNE, H. R., BUNNEY, Jr., W. E., COLBURN, R. W., DAVIS, J. W., DAVIS, J. N., SHAW, M. and COPPEN, A. J. (1968) Noradrenaline, 5-hydroxytryptamine, and 5-hydroxyindole acetic acid in hindbrains of suicidal patients. Lancet ii, 805.
34. BOWERS, JR., M. B., HENINGER, G. R., and GERBODE, F. (1969) Cerebrospinal fluid 5-hydro-

xyindoleacetic acid and homovanillis acid in psychiatric patients. Int. J. Neuropharmacol. **8**, 255.
35. BRADY, R. O. (1970) Prenatal diagnosis of lipid storage diseases. Clin. Chem. **16**, 811.
36. BRAWLEY, P. and DUFFIELD, J. C. (1972) The pharmacology of hallucinogens. Pharmacol. Rev. **24**, 31.
37. BREMER, H. J. and NEUMANN, W. (1966) Tolerance of phenylalanine after intravenous administration in phenylketonurics, heterozygous carriers, and normal adults. Nature (Lond.) **209**, 1148.
38. BRODY, JR., J. F. (1970) Behavioral effects of serotonin depletion and of p-chlorophenylalanine (a serotonin depletor) in rats. Psychopharmacologia (Berl.) **17**, 14.
39. BRODY, J. A., CHASE, T. N. and GORDON, E. K. (1970) Depressed monoamine catabolite levels in cerebrospinal fluid of patients with parkinsonism dementia of Guam. New Engl. J. Med. **282**, 947.
40. BRUNE, G. G. (1965) Biogenic amines in mental illness. Int. Rev. Neurobiol. **8**, 197.
41. BRUNE, G. G. (1967) Tryptophan metabolism in psychoses. Amines and Schizophrenia, HIMWICH, H. E., KETY, S. S. and SMYTHIES J. R., Eds. Pergamon Press, Oxford. p. 87.
42. BRUNE, G. G. and HIMWICH, H. E. (1961) Biphasic action of reserpine and isocarboxazide on behavior and serotonin metabolism. Science, **20**, 190.
43. BRUNE, G. G. and HIMWICH, H. E. (1962) Indole metabolites in schizophrenic patients. Arch. gen. Psychiat. **6**, 324.
44. BUMPUS, F. M. and PAGE, I. H. (1955) Serotonin and its methylated derivatives in human urine. J. biol. Chem. **212**, 111.
45. CERLETTI, A., TAESCHLER, M. and WEIDMAN, H. (1968) Pharmacological studies on the structure-activity relationship of hydroxyindole alkylamines. Advanc. Pharmacol **6B**, 233.
46. COHEN, I. and VOGEL, W. H. (1972) Determination and physiological disposition of dimethyltryptamine in rat brain, liver and plasma. Biochem. Pharmacol. **21**, 1214.
47. COPPEN, A. (1967) The biochemistry of affective disorders. Brit. J. Psychiat. **113**, 1237.
48. COPPEN, A. and SHAW, D. M. (1970) Biochemical aspects of affective disorders. Pharmakopsychiat. Neuropsychopharmakol. **3**, 36.
49. COPPEN, A., SHAW, D. M. and FARRELL, J. P. (1963) Potentiation of the antidepressive effect of a monoamine oxidase inhibitor by tryptophan. Lancet **i**, 79.
50. COPPEN, A., SHAW, D. M., MALLESON, A., ECCLESTON, E. and GUNDY, G. (1965) Tryptamine metabolism in depression. Brit. J. Psychiat. **111**, 993.
51. CULLEY, W. J., SAUNDERS, R. N., MERZT, E. T. and JOLLY, D. H. (1963) Effect of a tryptophan deficient diet on brain serotonin and plasma tryptophan level. Proc. Soc. exp. Biol. Med. **113**, 645.
52. CURZON, G. and BRIDGES, P. K. (1970) Tryptophan metabolism in depression. J. Neurol. Neurosurg. Psychiat. **33**, 698.
53. DENCKER, S. J., MALM, U., ROOS, B.-E. and WERDENIUS, B. (1966) Acid monoamine metabolites of cerebrospinal fluid in mental depression and mania. J. Neurochem. **13**, 1545.
54. DOHAN, F. C., EWING, J., GRAFF, H. and SPRINCE, H. (1964) Schizophrenia: 6-hydroxyskatole and environment. Arch. gen. Psychiat. **10**, 420.
55. DUNNER, D. L. and GOODWIN, F. K. (1972) Effect of L-tryptophan on brain serotonin metabolism in depressed patients. Arch. gen. Psychiat. **26**, 364.
56. ECCLESTON, D., ASHCROFT, G. W. and CRAWFORD, T. B. B. (1970) Effect of tryptophan administration on 5-HIAA in cerebrospinal fluid in man. J. Neurol. Neurosurg. Psychiat. **33**, 269.
57. ECCLESTON, D., ASHCROFT, G. W., MOIR, A. T., PARKER-RHODES A., LUTZ, W. and O'MAHONEY, D. P. (1968) A comparison of 5-hydroxyindoles in various regions of dog brain and cerebrospinal fluid. J. Neurochem. **15**, 947.
58. ERSPAMER, V. (1954) Pharmacology of indolealkylamines. Pharmacol. Rev. **6**, 425.
59. ERSPAMER, V. (1955) Observations on the fate of indolealkylamines in the organism. J. Physiol. (Lond.) **127**, 118.
60. FABING, H. D. and HAWKINS, J. R. (1956) Intravenous bufotenine injection in the human being. Science, **123**, 886.
61. FAURBYE, A. and PIND, K. (1968) Occurrence of bufotenin in the urine of schizophrenic patients and normal persons. Nature (Lond.) **220**, 489.
62. FAURBYE, A. and PIND, K. (1971) The presence of N-methylated and N-acetylated indole amines in the urine of patients with schizophrenia and of normal individuals. Ugeskr. Laeg. **133**, 1356.
63. FISCHER, E., LAGRAVERE, T. A. F., VASQUEZ, A. J. and DISTEFANO, A. O. (1961) A bufotenin-like substance in the urine of schizophrenics. J. nerv. ment. Dis. **133**, 441.

64. FISCHER, E. and SPATZ, H. (1967) Determination of bufotenin in the urine of schizophrenics. Int. J. Neuropsychiat. 3, 226.
65. FISCHER, E. and SPATZ, H. (1970) Studies on urinary elimination of bufotenine-like substances in schizophrenia. Biol. Psychiat. 2, 235.
66. FISCHER, E., SPATZ, H. and FLEDEL, T. (1971) Bufotenin-like substances in form of glucuronide in schizophrenia. Psychosomatics, 12, 278.
67. FRANZEN, F. and GROSS, H. (1965) Tryptamine, N,N-dimethyltryptamine, N,N-dimethyl-5-hydroxytryptamine and 5-methoxytryptamine in human blood and urine. Nature (Lond.) 206, 1052.
68. FRIEDHOFF, A. J. (1967) Biochemical effects of experimental diets. J. psychiat. Res. 5, 265.
69. FRIEDMAN, T. and ROBLIN, R. (1972) Gene therapy for human genetic disease? Science, 175, 949.
70. FROHMAN, C. E. (1971) 26th Nat. Meet. Society of Biological Psychiatry, Washington, D. C. (Abstr.).
71. GARATTINI, S., VALSECCHI, A. and VALZELLI, L. (1957) Variations in encephalic and intestinal serotonin after electrical shock. Experientia, 13, 330.
72. GARROD, A. E. (1909) Inborn errors of metabolism. Oxford University Press, Oxford.
73. GERBODE, F. A. and BOWERS, M. B. (1968) Measurement of acid monoamine metabolites in human and animal cerebrospinal fluid. J. Neurochem. 15, 1053.
74. GESSNER, P. K., GODSE, D. D., KRULL, A. H. and MCMULLAN, J. M. (1968) Structure-activity relationships among 5-methoxy-N:N-dimethyltryptamine, 4-hydroxy-N:N-dimethyltryptamine (psilocin) and other substituted tryptamines. Life Sci. 7, 267.
75. GESSNER, P. K., KHAIRALLAH, P. A., MCISAAC, W. M. and PAGE, I. H. (1960) The relationship between metabolic fate and pharmacological actions of serotonin, bufotenine and psilocybin. J. Pharmacol. exp. Ther. 130, 126.
76. GESSNER, P. K. and PAGE, I. H. (1962) Behavioral effects of 5-methoxy-N:N-dimethyltryptamine, other tryptamines and LSD. Amer. J. Physiol. 203, 167.
77. GOTTFRIES, C. G., GOTTFRIES, I. and ROOS, B.-E. (1970) Homovanillic acid and 5-hydroxyindoleacetic acid in cerebrospinal fluid related to rated mental and motor impairment in senile and presenile dementia. Acta psychiat. scand. 46, 99.
78. GOTTLIEB, J. S., FROHMAN, C. E. and BECKETT, P. G. S. (1969) A theory of neuronal malfunction in schizophrenia. Amer. J. Psychiat. 126, 149.
79. GOVIER, W. M., HOWES, G. B. and GIBBONS, A. J. (1953) The oxidative deamination of serotonin and other 3-(beta-aminoethyl)-indoles by monoamine oxidase and the effect of these compounds on the deamination of tyramine. Science, 118, 596.
80. GRAHAME-SMITH, D. G. (1971) Studies *in vivo* on the relationship between brain tryptophan, brain 5-HT synthesis and hyperactivity in rats treated with a monoamine oxidase inhibitor and L-tryptophan. J. Neurochem. 18, 1053.
81. GREEN, H. and SAWYER, J. L. (1960) Correlation of tryptamine-induced convulsions in rats with brain tryptamine concentration. Proc. Soc. exp. Biol. Med. 104, 153.
82. GREINER, A. C. (1970) Schizophrenia and the pineal gland. Canad. psychiat. Ass. J. 15, 433.
83. GULDBERG, H. C., ASHCROFT, G. W. and CRAWFORD, T. B. B. (1966) Concentrations of 5-hydroxyindoleacetic acid and homovanillic acid in the cerebrospinal fluid of the dog before and during treatment with probenecid. Life Sci. 5, 1571.
84. HARRIS, H. (1970) Genetical theory and the "inborn errors of metabolism". Brit. med. J. 1, 321.
85. HARTMANN, E., CHUNG, R. and CHIEN, C.-P. (1971). Tryptophan and sleep. Psychopharmacologia (Berl.) 19, 114.
86. HEACOCK, R. A. and MAHON, R. A. (1965) The colour reactions of the hydroxyskatoles. J. Chromatog. 17, 338.
87. HELLER, B. (1966) Influence of treatment with a monoamine oxidase inhibitor on the excretion of bufotenin and the clinical symptoms in chronic schizophrenic patients. Int. J. Neuropsychiat. 2, 193.
88. HELLER, B. (1971) N-methylating enzymes in blood of schizophrenics. Psychosomatics, 12, 273.
89. HELLER, B., NARASIMHACHARI, N., SPAIDE, J., HAŠKOVEC, L. and HIMWICH, H. E. (1970) N-dimethylated indoleamines in blood of acute schizophrenics. Experientia, 26, 503.
90. HESTON, L. L. (1970) The genetics of schizophrenic and schizoid disease. Science, 167, 249.
91. HIMWICH, H. E. (1970) Indoleamines and the schizophrenias. Biochemistry, Schizophrenias, and Affective Illnesses. HIMWICH, H. E., Ed. Williams and Wilkins Co., Baltimore, p. 79.
92. HIMWICH, H. E. Ed. (1970), Biochemistry, Schizophrenias, and Affective Illnesses. Williams & Wilkins Co., Baltimore.
93. HIMWICH, H. E., NARASIMHACHARI, N., HELLER, B., SPAIDE, J., HAŠKOVEC, L., FUJIMORI, M. and TABUSHI, K. (1970) Comparative behavioral and urinary studies on schizophrenics and

normal controls. Biochemistry of brain and behavior. BOWMAN, R. E. and DATTA, S. P. Eds., Plenum Press. p. 207.
94. HÖKFELDT, T. (1969) Ultrastructural studies on the uptake and accumulation of monoamines in peripheral and central neurones. Abstracts of the Fourth International Congress on Pharmacology. Schwabe & Co., Basel. p. 70.
95. HOFMAN, A., HEIM, R., BRACK, A. H. and KOBEL, H. (1958) Psilocybin, ein psychotroper Wirkstoff aus dem mexikanischen Rauschpilz Psilocybe mexicana Heim. Experientia, **14**, 107.
96. HOLMSTEDT, B. and LINDGREN, J.-E. (1967) Chemical constituents and pharmacology of South American snuffs. Ethnopharmacologic Search for Psychoactive Drugs. EFRON, D. H., HOLMSTEDT, B. and KLINE, N. S., Eds. Public Health Service Publication N. 1645. Government Printing Office, Washington D. C. p. 339.
97. HORNING, E. C., SWEELEY, C. C., DALGLIESH, C. E. and KELLY, W. (1959) Mammalian hydroxylation in the 6-position of the indole ring. Biochim. biophys. Acta, **32**, 566.
98. HUSZÁK, I. and DURKÓ, I. (1964) Formation of indole-pyridoxal complex in the urine of schizophrenics. Acta biochim. pol. **11**, 389.
99. JACCARINI, A. and JEPSON, J. B. (1968). The 6-hydroxylation of tryptamines by microsomal preparations from human liver tissue obtained at routine autopsy. Experientia, **24**, 29.
100. JEPSON, J. B., UDENFRIEND, S. and ZALTZMAN, P. (1959) The enzymic conversion of tryptamine to 6-hydroxytryptamine. Fed. Proc. **18**, 254.
101. JEPSON, J. B., ZALTZMAN, P. and UDENFRIEND, S. (1962) Microsomal hydroxylation of tryptamine, indoleacetic acid and related compounds, to 6-hydroxy derivatives. Biochim. biophys. Acta, **62**, 91.
102. JERVIS, G. A. (1952) Studies on phenylpyruvic oligophrenia. Phenylpyruvic acid content of blood. Proc. Soc. exp. Biol. Med. **81**, 715.
103. JOUVET, M. (1969) Biogenic amines and the states of sleep. Science **163**, 32.
104. KEELER, M. H. (1965) Similarity of schizophrenia and the psilocybin syndrome as determined by objective methods. Int. J. Neuropsychiat. **1**, 630.
105. KETY, S. S. (1970) Dietary factors in schizophrenia. Chemical Influences on Behaviour. A Ciba Symposium. PORTER, R. and BIRCH, J., Eds. J&A. Churchill, London. p. 76.
106. KLINE, N. S. and SACKS, W. (1963) Relief of depression within one day using and MAO inhibitor and intravenous 5-HTP. Amer. J. Psychiat. **120**, 274.
107. KOE, B. K. and WEISSMAN, A. (1966) p-Chlorophenylalanine: A specific depletor of brain serotonin. J. Pharmacol. exp. Ther. **154**, 499.
108. KOMROWER, G. M., WILSON, V., CLAMP, J. R. and WESTALL, R. G. (1964) Hydroxykynureninuria. Arch. Dis. Childh. **39**, 250.
109. KOPIN, I. J., PARE, C. M. B., AXELROD, J. and WEISSBACH, H. (1960) 6-Hydroxylation, the major metabolic pathway for melatonin. Biochim. biophys. Acta **40**, 377.
110. KRALL, A. R., LEVER, G., VILLAVERDE, R. and BILLETT, B. (1963) Studies on urinary indoles in mental patients. J. Amer. med. Ass. **184**, 280.
111. KREITMAN, N. and SMYTHIES, J. R. (1968) Schizophrenia: Genetic and psychological factors. Biological Psychiatry. SMYTHIES, J. R., Ed. William Heinemann (Medical Books) Ltd., London p. 1.
112. LANDY, P. J. (1970) L-dopa in the treatment of Parkinson's disease. Med. J. Aust. **57**, 632.
113. LAUER, J. W., INSKIP, W. M., BERNSOHN, J. and ZELLER, E. A. (1958) Observations on schizophrenic patients after iproniazid and tryptophan. Arch. Neurol. Psychiat. (Chic.) **80**, 122.
114. LEMBERGER, L., AXELROD, J. and KOPIN, I. J. (1971) The disposition and metabolism of tryptamine and the in vivo formation of 6-hydroxytryptamine in the rabbit. J. Pharmacol. exp. Ther. **177**, 169.
115. MANDEL, L. R., ROSENZWEIG, S. and KUEHL, JR., F. A. (1971) Purification and substrate specificity of indoleamine-N-methyltransferase. Biochem. Pharmacol. **20**, 712.
116. MANDELL, A. J. and MORGAN, M. (1971) Indole(ethyl)amine N-methyltransferase in human brain. Nature (Lond.) **230**, 85.
117. MARTIN, W. R., SLOAN, J. W., CHRISTIAN, S. T. and CLEMENTS, T. H. (1972) Brain levels of tryptamine. Psychopharmacologia (Berl.) **24**, 331.
118. MCISAAC, W. M. (1961) Formation of 1-methyl-6-methoxy-1,2,3,4-tetrahydro-2-carboline under physiological conditions. Biochem. biophys. Acta, **52**, 607.
119. MENDELS, J., FRAZER A., FITZGERALD, R. G., RAMSEY, T. A. and STOKES, J. W. (1972) Biogenic amine metabolites in cerebrospinal fluid of depressed and manic patients. Science, **175**, 1380.
120. MOIR, A. T. P., ASHCROFT, G. W., CRAWFORD, T. B. B., ECCLESTON, A. and GULDBERG, H. C. (1970) Cerebral metabolites in cerebrospinal fluid as a biochemical approach to the brain. Brain, **93**, 357.

121. Morgan, M. and Mandell, A. J. (1969) Indole(ethyl)amine N-methyltransferase in the brain. Science, 165, 492.
122. Mouret, J., Bobillier, P. and Jouvet, M. (1968) Insomnia following parachlorophenylalanine. Europ. Pharmacol. J. 5, 17.
123. Murphy, D. C. and Wyatt, R. J. (1972) Reduced monoamine oxidase activity found in blood platelets from schizophrenic patients. Nature (Lond.) 238, 225.
124. Narasimhachari, N., Heller, B., Spaide, J., Haškovec, L., Fujimori, M., Tabushi, K. and Himwich, H. E. (1971) Urinary studies of schizophrenics and controls. Biol. Psychiat. 3, 9.
125. Narasimhachari, N., Heller, B., Spaide, J., Haškovec, L., Meltzer, H., Strahilevitz, M. and Himwich, H. E. (1971) N,N-dimethylated indoleamines in blood. Biol. Psychiat. 3, 21.
126. Narasimhachari, N., Plaut, J. M. and Himwich, H. E. (1972) Indoleethylamine N-methyltransferase in serum samples of schizophrenics and normal controls. Life Sci. 11, 221.
127. Neff, N. H., Tozer, T. N. and Brodie, B. B. (1967) Application of steady-state kinetics to studies of the transfer of 5-hydroxyindoleacetic acid from brain to plasma. J. Pharmacol. exp. Ther. 158, 214.
128. Oates, J. A. and Sjoerdsma, A. (1960) Neurologic effects of tryptophan in patients receiving monoamine oxidase inhibitor. Neurol. (Minneap.) 10, 1076.
129. Paasonen, M. K. (1961) Inactivation of 5-hydroxytryptamine by mammalian blood platelets. Biochem. Pharmacol. 8, 241.
130. Perez-Cruet, J., Tagliamonte, A., Tagliamonte, P. and Gessa, G. (1970) Stimulation of brain serotonin turnover by lithium. Pharmacologist, 12, 257.
131. Perry, T. L., Hansen, S., MacDougall, L. and Schwarz, C. J. (1966) Urinary amines in chronic schizophrenia. Nature (Lond.) 212, 146.
132. Persson, T. and Roos, B.-E. (1969) Acid metabolites from monoamines in cerebrospinal fluid of chronic schizophrenics. Brit. J. Psychiat. 115, 95.
133. Pollin, W., Cardon, W. P. V. and Kety, S. S. (1961) Effects of amino acid feeding in schizophrenic patients treated with iproniazid. Science, 133, 104.
134. van Praag, H. M. (1969) Monoamines and depression. Pharmakopsychiat. Neuro-Psychopharmakol. 2, 151.
135. van Praag, H. M. (1970) Indoleamines and the central nervous system. Psychiat. Neurol. Neurchir. 73, 9.
136. van Praag, H. M., Korf, J. and Puite, J. (1970) 5-Hydroxyindoleacetic acid levels in the cerebrospinal fluid of depressive patients treated with probenecid. Nature (Lond.) 225, 1259.
137. van Praag, H. M. and Leijnse, B. (1963) Die Bedeutung der Monoaminoxydasehemmung als antidepressives Prinzip. Psychopharmacologia (Berl.) 4, 1.
138. Price, J. M., Brown, R. R. and Peters, H. A. (1959) Tryptophan metabolism in porphyria, schizophrenia, and a variety of neurologic and psychiatric disorders. Neurol. (Minneap.) 9, 456.
139. Pscheidt, G. R., Berlet H. H., Spaide, J. and Himwich, H. E. (1966) Variations of urinary creatinine and its correlation to excretion of indole metabolites in mental patients. Clin. chim. Acta 13, 228.
140. Richter, D. (1967) Tryptophan metabolism in mental illness. Amines and Schizophrenia. Himwich, H. E., Kety, S. S. and Smythies, J. R., Eds. Pergamon Press, Oxford. p. 167.
141. Rimon, R., Roos, B.-E., Rakkolainen, V. and Alanen Y. (1971) The content of 5-hydroxyindoleacetic acid and homovanillic acid in the cerebrospinal fluid of patients with acute schizophrenia. J. psychosom. Res. 15, 375.
142. Rodnight, R. (1956) Separation and characterization of urinary indoles resembling 5-hydroxytryptamine and tryptamine. Biochem. J. 64, 621.
143. Rodnight, R. (1961) Body fluid indoles in mental illness. Int. Rev. Neurobiol. 3, 251.
144. Roos, B.-E. and Sjöström, R. (1969) 5-Hydroxyindoleacetic acid and homovanillic acid levels in the cerebrospinal fluid after probenecid application in patients with manic-depressive psychosis. Pharmacol. Clin. 1, 153.
145. Rose, D. P. (1972) Aspects of tryptophan metabolism in health and disease: a review. J. clin. Path. 25, 17.
146. Rosenberg, D. E., Isbell, H. and Miner, E. J. (1963) Comparison of a placebo, N-dimethyltryptamine and 6-hydroxy-N-dimethyltryptamine in man. Psychopharmacologia (Berl.) 4, 39.
147. Runge, T. M., Lara, F. Y., Thurman, N., Keyes, J. W. and Hoerster, S. H. (1966) Search for a bufotenin-like substance in the urine of schizophrenics. J. nerv. ment. Dis. 142, 470.
148. Saavedra, J. M. and Axelrod, J. (1972) Psychotomimetic N-methylated tryptamines: Formation in brain *in vivo* and *in vitro*. Science, 175, 1365.
149. Sai-Halasz, Brunacker, G. and Szara, S. (1958) Dimethyltryptamin: eine neues Psychoticum. Psychiat. Neurol. 135, 285.
150. Sanders, E. and Bush, M. T. (1967) Distribution, metabolism and excretion of bufotenine

in the rat with preliminary studies of its O-methyl derivatives. J. Pharmacol. exp. Ther. **158**, 340.
151. SCHILDKRAUT, J. J. (1965) The catecholamine hypothesis of affective disorders: A review of supporting evidence. Amer. J. Psychiat. **122**, 509.
152. SHAW, D. M., CAMPS, F. E. and ECCLESTON, E. (1967) 5-Hydroxytryptamine in the hindbrain of depressive suicides. Brit. J. Psychiat. **113**, 1407.
153. SHAW, C. R., LUCAS, J. and RABINOVITCH, R. D. (1959) Metabolic studies in childhood schizophrenics. Arch. gen. Psychiat. **1**, 366.
154. SIEGEL, M. (1965) A sensitive method for detection of N,N-dimethylserotonin (bufotenin) in urine; failure to demonstrate its presence in the urine of schizophrenic and normal subjects. J. psychiat. Res. **3**, 205.
155. SIREIX, D. W. and MARINI, F. A. (1969) Bufotenine in human urine. Biol. Psychiat. **1**, 189.
156. SJOERDSMA, A., OATES, J. A., ZALTZMAN, P. and UDENFRIEND, S. (1959) Identification and assay of urinary tryptamine: Application as an index of monoamine oxidase inhibition in man. J. Pharmacol. exp. Ther. **126**, 217.
157. SJÖSTRÖM, R. and ROOS, B.-E. (1972) 5-Hydroxyindoleacetic acid and homovanillic acid in cerebrospinal fluid in manic-depressive psychosis. Europ. J. Clin. Pharmacol. **4**, 170.
158. SMITH, B. and PROCKOP, D. J. (1962) Central-nervous-system effects of ingestion of L-tryptophan by normal subjects. New Engl. J. Med. **267**, 1338.
159. SMYTHIES J. R., BENINGTON, F. and MORIN, R. D. (1970) The mechanism of action of hallucinogenic drugs on possible serotonin receptor in the brain. Int. Rev. Neurobiol. **12**, 207.
160. SOHLER, A., NOVAL, J. J. and RENZ, R. H. (1963) 6-hydroxyskatole sulfate excretion in schizophrenia. J. nerv. ment. Dis. **137**, 591.
161. SOURKES, T. L. (1962) Biochemistry of Mental Disease. (Hoeber Medical Division) Harper & Row, Publishers. p. 79.
162. SPAIDE, J., TANIMUKAI, H., BUENO, J. R. and HIMWICH, H. E. (1968) Behavioral and biochemical alterations in schizophrenic patients. Arch. gen. Psychiat. **18**, 658.
163. SPAIDE, J., TANIMUKAI, H., GINTHER, R., BUENO, J. and HIMWICH, H. E. (1967) Schizophrenic behavior, and urinary tryptophan metabolites associated with cysteine given with and without a monoamine oxidase inhibitor (Tranylcypromine). Life Sci. **6**, 551.
164. SPRINCE, H. (1961) Indole metabolism in mental illness. Clin. Chem. **7**, 203.
165. SPRINCE, H. (1967) Metabolic interrelationship of tryptophan and methionine in relation to mental illness. Amines and Schizophrenia. HIMWICH, H. E., KETY, S. S. and SMYTHIES, J. R., Eds. Pergamon Press, Oxford. p. 97.
166. SPRINCE, H., PARKER, C., JAMESON, D. and ALEXANDER, F. (1963) Urinary indoles in schizophrenic and psychoneurotic patients after administration of tranylcypromine (Parnate) and methionine or tryptophan. J. nerv. ment. Dis. **137**, 246.
167. SZARA, S. (1956) Dimethyltryptamin: Its metabolism in man; the relation of its psychotic effect to the serotonin metabolism. Experientia, **12**, 441.
168. SZARA, S. (1967) Hallucinogenic amines and schizophrenia. Amines and Schizophrenia, HIMWICH, H. E., KETY, S. S. and SMYTHIES, J. R., Eds. Pergamon Press, Oxford. p. 181.
169. SZARA, S. and AXELROD, J. (1959) Hydroxylation and N-demethylation of N,N-dimethyltryptamine. Experientia, **15**, 216.
170. SZARA, S. and HEARST, E. (1962) The 6-hydroxylation of tryptamine derivatives: a way of producing psychoactive metabolites. Ann. N. Y. Acad. Sci. **96**, 134.
171. SZARA, S., ROCKLAND, L. H., ROSENTHAL, D. and HANDLON, J. H. (1966) Psychological effects and metabolism of N,N-diethyltryptamine in man. Arch. gen. Psychiat. **15**, 320.
172. TABORSKY, R. G. (1967) Long-term behavioral aberration produced in mice by a pharmacological agent. Nature (Lond.) **215**, 752.
173. TABORSKY, R. G., DELVIGS, P. and PAGE, I. H. (1966) 6-Hydroxylation: Effect on the psychotropic potency of tryptamine. Science, **153**, 1018.
174. TABORSKY, R. G. and MCISAAC, W. M. (1964) The relationship between the metabolic fate and pharmacological action of 5-methoxy-N-methyltryptamine. Biochem. Pharmacol. **13**, 531.
175. TABORSKY, R. G. and MCISAAC, W. M. (1964) The synthesis and preliminary pharmacology of some 9H-pyrido (3,4-b)indoles (β-carbolines) and tryptamines related to serotonin and melatonin. J. med. Chem. **7**, 135.
176. TANIMUKAI, H., GINTHER, R., SPAIDE, J., BUENO, J. R. and HIMWICH, H. E. (1967) Occurrence of bufotenin (5-hydroxy-N,N-dimethyltryptamine) in urine of schizophrenic patients. Life Sci. **6**, 1697.
177. TANIMUKAI, H. GINTHER, R., SPAIDE, J. and HIMWICH, H. E. (1967) Psychotomimetic indole compound in the urine of schizophrenic and mentally defective patients. Nature (Lond.) **216**, 490.

178. TANIMUKAI, H., GINTHER, R., SPAIDE, J., BUENO, J. R. and HIMWICH, H. E. (1970). Detection of psychotomimetic N,N-dimethylated indoleamines in the urine of four schizophrenic patients. Brit. J. Psychiat. **117**, 421.
179. THITHAPANDHA, A. (1972) Substrate specificity and heterogeneity of N-methyltransferases. Biochem. Biophys. Res. Commun. **47**, 301.
180. TSCHUDY, D. P., PERLROTH, M. G., MARVER, H. S., COLLINS, A., HUNTER, JR., G. and RECHCIGL, JR. M. (1965) Acute intermittent porphyria: the first "overproduction disease" localized to a specific enzyme. Proc. Acad. Sci. U.S. **53**, 841.
181. TU, J.-B. and ZELLWEGER, H. (1965) Blood-serotonin deficiency in Down's syndrome. Lancet **ii**, 715.
182. WALKER, R. W., AHN, H. S., MANDEL, L. R. and VANDENHEUVEL, W. J. A. (1972). Identification of N,N-dimethyltryptamine as the product of an *in vitro* enzymatic methylation. Anal. Biochem. **47**, 228.
183. WATERBURY, L. D. and PEARCE, L. A. (1972) Separation and identification of neutral and acidic metabolites in cerebrospinal fluid. Clin. Chem. **18**, 258.
184. WEIL-MALHERBE, H. (1967) The biochemistry of functional psychoses. Advanc. Enzymol. **29**, 479.
185. WEIL-MALHERBE, H. and SZARA, S. (1971) The biochemistry of functional and experimental psychoses. C. C. Thomas, Publisher. Springfield, Ill.
186. WOLBACH, A. B., MINER, E. J. and ISBELL, H. (1962) Comparison of psilocin with psilocybin, mescaline and LSD-25. Psychopharmacologia (Berl.) **3**, 219.
187. WURTMAN, R. J., ROSE, C. M., MATTHYSE, S., STEPHENSON, J. and BALDESSARINI, R. (1970) L-Dihydroxyphenylalanine: Effect on S-adenosylmethionine in brain. Science, **169**, 395.
188. WYATT, R. J., TERMINI, B. A. and DAVIS, J. (1971) Biochemical and sleep studies of schizophrenia: a review of the literature 1960—1970. Part I. Biochemical studies. Schizophrenia Bulletin No. 4. National Institute of Mental Health, Rockville, Maryland. p. 10.

H.H.B., Institute of Pathochemistry and General Neurochemistry of the University, Box 1368, 69 Heidelberg, F.R.G.

EFFECTS OF L-DOPA ON SCHIZOPHRENIA

K. INANAGA and M. TANAKA

Department of Psychiatry and Institute of Brain Diseases, Kurume University School of Medicine, Kurume

It has been well demonstrated that an important biochemical disturbance associated with parkinsonism is a marked decrease of the dopamine content in the brain. On the basis of this finding, L-DOPA, an amino-acid precursor of dopamine, has been successfully used to help patients suffering from this disease, presumably by increasing the concentration of dopamine in the brain. However, it has been reported that in the treatment of Parkinson's disease psychotic symptoms appear as the side effects of L-DOPA administration. It is widely known that L-DOPA exacerbates the schizophrenic symptoms with drug-induced parkinsonism. On the other hand, however, it is suggested that L-DOPA has a positive effect on some psychotic conditions.

We have been thus initially interested in whether or not L-DOPA could effectively prevent pharmacological parkinsonism induced in schizophrenic patients given a supporting administration of neuroleptics. During the course of the administration of L-DOPA together with neuroleptics to schizophrenic patients, we have experienced that it occasionally improves or exacerbates the psychic conditions of schizophrenic patients. An interesting finding was that relatively small doses of L-DOPA had a favorable effect on schizophrenia. We have reported this finding in three cases of schizophrenia, which showed a remarkable improvement of psychic conditions by the administration of L-DOPA together with neuroleptics. These cases led us to make an extensive trial of L-DOPA treatment of schizophrenia.

L-DOPA was administered to 84 cases of schizophrenia together with major tranquilizers which had been given previously.

Patients suffering from lack of spontaneity, abulia, apathy, and disturbance of rapport were chosen as subjects in this research. The cases with hallucination, delusion and disturbance of the self were also included. Duration of illness is as follows: Ill for within one year 2 cases, 2—3 years 4 cases, 3—5 years 8 cases, 5—10 years 17 cases, more than 10 years 53 cases. The subjects are in most cases 20—50 years old (Table 1).

Initial daily dose was 100—600 mg, then gradually increased to maximum dose 1200 mg. Maintenance dose was 400—600 mg, and continued administration was at most for 3 months in the longest administered cases. Symptom-changes including amelioration and exacerbation were seen at 400—800 mg daily dose.

Remarkable amelioration was seen in 8 cases (9.5%), moderate in 17 cases (20.2%), and slight in 20 cases (23.8%). Aggravation was seen in 5 cases (6.0%), no change was

Table 1

Duration of illness

Duration	Number of cases
Within one year	2
1—2	0
2—3	4
3—5	8
5—10	17
More than 10	53
Total	84

seen in 34 cases (40.5%). Remarkable and moderate amelioration were noted in 25 cases (29.8%) (Table 2). Most remarkable amelioration was seen at L-DOPA 600 mg administration: Remarkable amelioration 6 cases, moderate 11 cases, and 17 cases (20.2%) in all. Next was seen at 400 mg administration: Remarkably ameliorated cases are 2, moderately 2; total 4 cases. However 4 cases exacerbated at 600 mg. The relation between duration of illness and therapeutic effects is as follows. In the cases ill for more than 10 years, which show personality deterioration, any amelioration is hopeless. Generally speaking it is effective for the cases ill for within 10 years.

The evaluation result on 74 cases is as follows. Disturbance of rapport was the most improved: Remarkably ameliorated cases were 5, moderately 18, and amelioration rate was 31.5%. Disturbance of emotional expression was also ameliorated: remarkable ameliorated cases were 8, moderately 11; the rate was 26.4%.

As exacerbated cases, 10 cases of excitement were noted.

Table 2

Duration of illness and treatment

Duration of illness	Cases	Remarkable amelioration	Moderate	Total (%)
—1	2	0	0	0
1—2	0	0	0	0
2—3	4	0	2	2 (50)
3—5	8	3	2	5 (62.5)
5—10	17	2	7	9 (52.9)
10—	53	3	6	9 (17.0)
Total	84	8	17	25 (29.8)

Next, double blind study was done on 105 schizophrenic patients with successful results. In the L-DOPA group, 200—600 mg L-DOPA was given together with neuroleptics and in the placebo group, placebo was given with neurolptics. The final results are shown in Table 3. There was no statistical significant difference between the two

TABLE 3

Improvement	L-DOPA	Placebo
+++	5	0
++	5	9
+	15	9
±	27	33
—	2	0
Total	54	51

+++, ++, + $P < 0.01$

groups. But five cases of remarkable amelioration were found in the L-DOPA group and none in the placebo group. However, if we select the patients whose duration of illness is within 5 years, 12 patients of L-DOPA group responded favourably as compared to 4 cases of placebo group, statistically significant at the level of 0.01 (Table 4). Responses

TABLE 4

Improvement	L-DOPA	Placebo
+++	2	0
++	2	1
+	8	3
±	2	8
—	0	0
Total	14	12

+++, ++, + $P < 0.01$

to questions improved 3 weeks later (Fig. 1). Facial expression improved as well. Significant difference was found 4 weeks later (Fig. 2). Disturbance of rapport was significantly improved 4 weeks later (Fig. 3). Abulia was significantly improved 3 weeks later.

These results show that a small dose is important in the treatment of psychotic symptoms in schizophrenia. Comparatively safe and effective dosage, though different in individuals, is 400—600 mg daily. Unfavorable effects were noted at dosages of 600 mg and above.

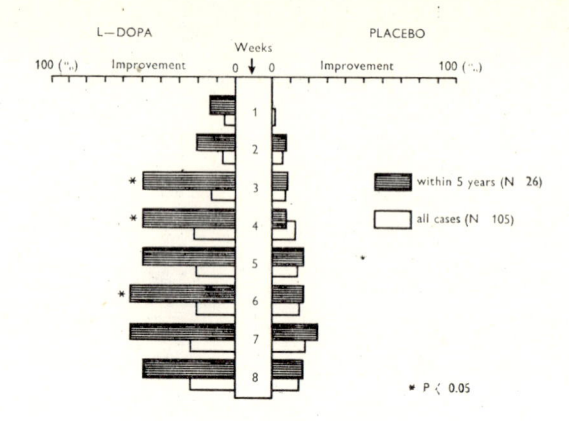

Fig. 1. Responses to questions.

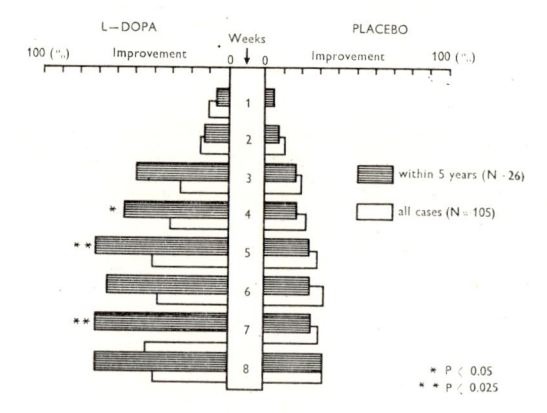

Fig. 2. Facial expression.

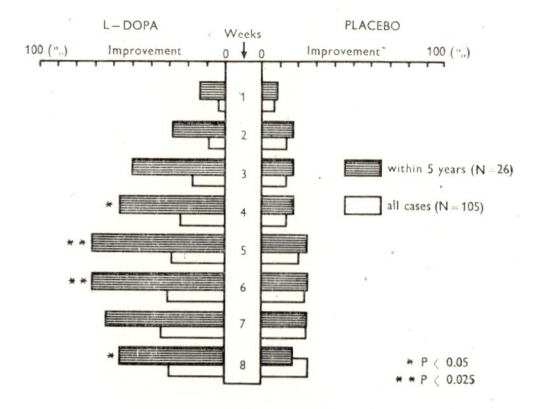

Fig. 3. Disturbance of rapport.

Disorder of rapport and emotional blunting were remarkably ameliorated with L-DOPA administration. Autistic patients showed improvements towards increased rapport and spontaneous activity. Generally they became more active in daily life.

As behavior was much more ameliorated, abnormal experiences decreased. This amelioration indicates that the fundamental symptoms of schizophrenia may be affected by L-DOPA. Our impression is that L-DOPA does not have any favorable effect on paranoid types, but does have an effect on some types of hebephrenics.

Symptoms such as visual hallucination, delusion and excitement seen in catatonia were suppressed with neuroleptics. L-DOPA can be administered to the cases which show lack of spontaneity, autism, abulia, and volitional weakness. Such a small dose of L-DOPA as we used is very characteristic and effective. The problem is the decision on the dosage of L-DOPA. How does L-DOPA work on psychotic conditions after all? The mechanism should be investigated in the future.

K.I., Department of Psychiatry and Institute of Brain Diseases, Kurume University School of Medicine, 67, Asahi-machi, Kurume-shi, Japan

N-METHYLATION OF BIOGENIC AMINES IN THE BRAIN WITH 5-METHYLTETRAHYDROFOLIC ACID AS THE METHYL DONOR: A POSSIBLE IMPLICATION IN SCHIZOPHRENIA

P. LADURON

Department of Neurobiochemistry, Janssen Pharmaceutica Research Laboratories, Beerse

INTRODUCTION

Among several catecholamines, dopamine, noradrenaline and adrenaline have been of special importance in studies dealing with the biochemical and physiological mechanisms of neurotransmission, as well as in those concerning the mechanism of action of many drugs. If it is generally accepted that these three amines are enzymatically synthesized according to the sequence dopamine ⟶ noradrenaline ⟶ adrenaline, each of them, nevertheless, can be considered or used as a neurotransmitter according to its tissular or regional localization, as for instance dopamine in the cerebral dopaminergic areas, noradrenaline in the sympathetic nerves and adrenaline in the adrenal medulla. Up to recently, noradrenaline was thought to be the immediate precorsor of adrenaline, and nearly all the biochemical data seemed to converge to this view (3). Nevertheless, this central dogma of the adrenergic neurotransmission has been questioned and, before considering more specifically the problem in the brain, I shall provide a brief survey of our recent data concerning the N-methylation of dopamine in the adrenal medulla.

In studying the intracellular localization of enzymes involved in the biosynthesis of catecholamines, we concluded that tyrosine hydroxylase is not contained within the catecholamine granules (14) as it was previously interpreted erroneously by NAGATSU, LEVITT and UDENFRIEND (20). A more selective method of tissue fractionation, led us to propose a model for the intracellular pathway of catecholamines. It implies that the first two steps, i.e. hydroxylation of tyrosine and decarboxylation of DOPA occur outside the granules in the cytoplasmic sap and that, after being taken up in the granules, dopamine is converted into noradrenaline by the dopamine-β-hydroxylase, which is certainly within the granules. Finally, it was suggested that, in the adrenal medulla, a certain amount of noradrenaline, when coming out of the granules, is N-methylated into adrenaline which, afterwards, should return to the granules to be stored. It is precisely this point that raised difficulties in forwarding a valid interpretation for the intracellular pathway of catecholamines.

Why such translocation? What is the physiological meaning of such a translocation from an intragranular to an extragranular compartment and vice-versa? How can the granular membrane possess a so highly elaborate screening mechanism, capable of recognizing one specific kind of amine and allowing it to cross in a given direction? There are as many questions but no answers.

Although experimental evidence to support the view of specific translocation mechanism for noradrenaline and adrenaline is still lacking, it remained the only one possible model in 1968, since "N-methyltransferase, as AXELROD (3) claimed, shows an absolute specificity towards phenylethanolamine derivatives, none of the phenylethylamine being N-methylated." Therefore dopamine might not be enzymatically N-methylated *in vitro* and under these experimental conditions. Nevertheless this model seemed unlikely to us and even incompatible with the concept of exocytosis which is opposed to diffusion of neurotransmitters from subcellular structures through the cytoplasmic compartment (27). Moreover, it also seemed incompatible with the latency of dopamine-β-hydroxylase which has been attributed to the lack of permeability of granular membranes toward a given substrate like dopamine or tyramine (4). Therefore, the classical picture described in many textbooks and showing a diffusion phenomenon of catecholamines between an intragranular and a hypothetical extragranular pool remains purely speculative and inconsistent since it is not based on experimental evidence. In this regard, the introduction of the concept of exocytosis into the field of catecholamines has radically changed the way of thinking the problems of adrenergic neurotransmission.

The foregoing considerations, particularly the location in a given intracellular compartment of each enzyme involved in the biosynthesis of catecholamines, have prompted us to find out whether the formation of adrenaline could not be provided through another biosynthetic pathway, apparently more logical than that by which noradrenaline must leave the granules and adrenaline must be taken up again in the same subcellular structures. Our recent experiments have shown that the methyl group of S-adenosylmethionine can be transferred *in vitro* to the amine group of dopamine by means of an enzyme preparation from the bovine adrenal medulla (10, 11). Although this enzymatic formation of epinine has already been reported more in detail, I should like to draw the attention once more to some important aspects of this reaction.

First, in contrast to normetanephrine, dopamine is known to be very sensitive to oxidative processes at neutral or alkaline pH. As the maximum activity of N-methyltransferase occurs at pH 8.0, certain precautions must be taken. By adding metabisulfite and EDTA to the reaction mixture, experimental conditions which prevent the oxidation of catecholamines, we were able to demonstrate the enzymatic conversion of dopamine to epinine in adrenal medulla. Secondly, the Km's determination for different substrates like noradrenaline and dopamine raises difficulties in accepting a prominent physiological role of epinine in the biosynthesis of adrenaline. It must be recalled however that a comparison of two Km's, the first one equal to 10^{-3}M for dopamine and the other one 10^{-5}M for noradrenaline is not possible because a substrate inhibition occurs with high concentration of noradrenaline so that a classical hyperbolic curve showing the velocity as function of substrate concentration cannot be obtained in this case. Therefore these Km's values are not comparable to those for dopamine where a classical saturation curve was obtained. It is worth noting also that a lower Km for a substrate does not always mean a higher affinity towards a given enzyme and that consequently this substrate is indeed the natural substrate *in vivo*. Furthermore, it seems to us that a comparison of two Km's can only have a value if one takes into account the intracellular localization of the enzyme and possible substrates. In this respect, it is beyond doubt that dopamine is present in the cytosol, since the DOPA-decarboxylase is certainly located into this same compartment whereas no evidence supports the view that noradrenaline is also localized in an extragranular pool. The recent interpretations about the release of catecholamines by exocytosis make this latter possibility rather unlikely (27). Therefore in taking into account the laying out of enzyme and possible substrate through the different intracellular compartments, it seems more logical to accept an N-methylation of dopamine in the biosynthesis of adrenaline rather than an N-methylation of noradrenaline.

All this led us to propose a new model in which epinine rather than noradrenaline is the immediate precorsor of adrenaline in adrenal medulla (Fig. 1 B). This model has the great advantage of excluding translocations of noradrenaline and adrenaline from the granular to the extragranular space and vice-versa.

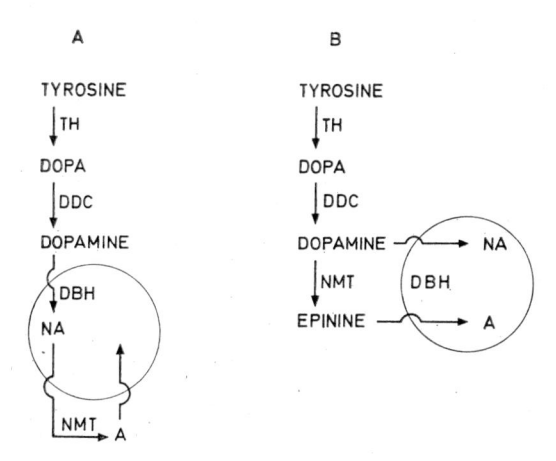

Fig. 1. Intracellular pathway for the biosynthesis of catecholamines in adrenal medulla.
A. Previous model illustrating the "ballet" of catecholamines (noradrenaline coming out granule and adrenaline returning again).
B. Improved and more simplified model involving the N-methylation of dopamine. The first three steps are extragranular while the last one is intragranular.

TH — tyrosine hydroxylase; DDC — DOPA decarboxylase; NM — N-methyltransferase; DBH — dopamine-β-hydroxylase; NA — noradrenaline; A — adrenaline.

Properties of N-methylating enzyme in the brain

Although different types of N-methyltransferase in the brain have already been described (2, 6, 17, 19, 23, 25), the possiblity of N-methylation of dopamine in this organ has never been considered. Two main reasons prompted us to investigate this latter possibility. First, as dopamine is considered as a very important neurotransmitter in the brain, namely in the dopaminergic areas, one might suspect epinine to play a more or less similar role in neurotransmission, if evidence is provided for this *in vitro* formation from a brain enzyme. Secondly, although the origin of schizophrenia remains still unknown, one among numerous hypothesis suggests that the disease should be due to an excessive N-methylation process in the brain. Thirdly, the antipsychotic action of neuroleptics seems related to a dopamine-receptor blocking activity so that dopamine or other compounds, perhaps more specific, but structurally related to dopamine, could either induce schizophrenia or perhaps and more likely, constitute intermediate neurotransmitters for the manifestations of clinical symptoms. In other words, dopamine or its congeners could play a prominent role in this disease if the concept of dopamine-receptor blocking for the neuroleptics is correct.

When beginning this work, we believed that only replacing an enzyme preparation from the adrenal gland by one from rat brains, should have been enough to obtain significant enzyme activities. In fact, our first attempts to convert dopamine into epinine *in vitro* by using S-adenosylmethionine as methyl donor, were unsuccessful. Nevertheless this formation of epinine became possible only when 5-methyltetrahydrofolic acid replaced S-adenosylmethionine in the incubation mixture. This methyl donor, a congener of folic

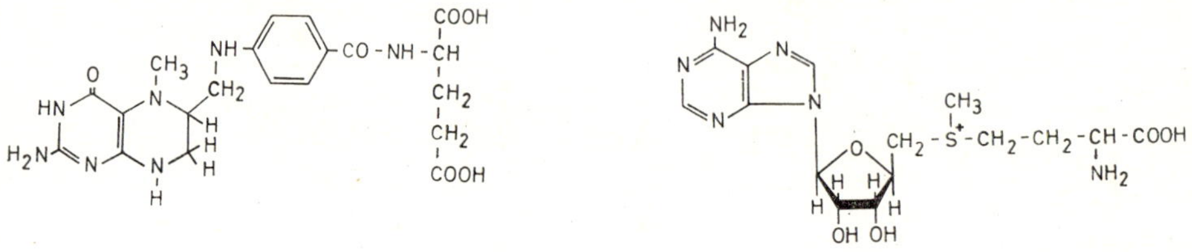

Fig. 2. Chemical structure of S-adenosyl-methionine (left) and 5-methyltetrahydrofolic acid (right).

acid, was completely unusual for biogenic amines, but very common in single-carbon transfer reactions, for instance in the bacterial systems. It is pteridine moiety linked to *p*-aminobenzoic acid which is in turn joined to glutamic acid via a peptide-like linkage (Fig. 2). Our recent work provided the first evidence that 5-methyltetrahydrofolic acid is able to transfer its methyl group to dopamine by means of a N-methylating enzyme (13). The reaction may be written as follows:

N-methyltransferase

dopamine + 5-methyltetrahydrofolic acid ⟶ epinine + tetrahydrofolic acid

If this reaction has been originally studied with dopamine as a substrate, several other amines were also tested (Table 1). Many properties of the reaction have already been investigated. First, the reaction products formed in the incubation mixtures were identified by means of several chromatographic procedures and various enzyme kinetic studies were performed in order to assess the enzymatic formation of epinine (12, 15). Maximum activity was found to occur between pH 8.2 and 8.4 when dopamine or noradrenaline were incubated in a mixture containing also metabisulfite. More recently, however, in absence of this reducing agent, we observed an optimum activity at about pH 6.5 for dopamine as well as for noradrenaline. In contrast, for 3-hydroxy-4-methoxyphenyl-ethylamine, the optimum pH of 6.5 remained unaltered by adding metabisulfite. This suggests that the reducing agent might only interfere with certain substrates or with the enzyme-substrate binding while a structural modification of the enzyme itself cannot be completely excluded (15).

Up to two hours, the rate of dopamine conversion to epinine was found to increase linearly as a function of time or of enzyme concentration. The Km value for 5-methyl-tetrahydrofolate with dopamine as a substrate is equal to 6×10^{-5}M.

Various substrates were tested for their ability to be N-methylated by means of N-methyltransferase from rat brain. As shown in Table 1, the three main amines which act as neurotransmitters in the brain, exhibit high enzyme activities which cannot be compared with the very low conversion rate, previously observed by using S-adenosyl-methionine (17, 25). A comparison of the enzyme activities (Table 1), which were all

TABLE 1

N-methyltransferase activity in rat brain with different substrates

Substrate	Enzyme activity mµmoles . h^{-1} . mg^{-1} protein
Dopamine	0.172
3-Hydroxy-4-methoxyphenethylamine	0.149
N-methyldopamine (epinine)	0.119
Mescaline	0.119
3,4-Dimethoxy N-methylphenethylamine	0.099
N-N'Dimethyldopamine	0
3-Hydroxy-4-methoxy-N,N'-dimethylphenethylamine	0
Amphetamine	0.098
N-methylamphetamine	0.054
N,N'-dimethylamphetamine	0.006
Tryptamine	0.094
N-methyltryptamine	0.052
Serotonin	0.365
Bufotenin	0.071
Noradrenaline	0.642
Adrenaline	0.145
Normetanephrine	0.059

Experimental conditions of enzyme assay: 10 µmoles substrate, buffer pH 6.4, 9 mµmoles 5-MTHF^{C14} as methyl donor. Reaction products were isolated on Al$_2$O$_3$ column for the catecholamines and extracted in toluene-isoamylalcohol for the other amines.

carried out at pH 6.4 and in the presence of 10 µmoles of substrate, enabled us to rule out the occurrence of the methylation process otherwise than by a transfer of the methyl group from 5-methyltetrahydrofolate to the nitrogen of amines. For instance, higher activities were obtained with dopamine than with epinine and with this latter did again higher than with N-dimethyldopamine. Furthermore, for this latter, a tertiary amine, enzyme activity was not even detectable. For bufotenin or dimethylamphetamine, little activity and perhaps not significant can be detected. This should probably be due to the use of an extraction procedure with toluene-isoamylalcohol which is less specific than the absorption of dopamine and its congeners upon aluminium oxide. Nevertheless a higher N-methylation appears in the order following: primary amine > secondary amine > > tertiary amine. It is worth noting also that normetanephrine, a very good substrate in the adrenal medulla is nearly not N-methylated in the brain. As for the substrate specificity, it is too early to decide whether serotonin, tryptamine or dopamine can be considered as more specific substrates. This needs further investigation, especially through kinetic studies.

A striking property of this N-methylating enzyme of the brain is that it requires 5-methyltetrahydrofolate as a methyl donor. It seems also, that this methyl donor is even more specific for N-methylation in the brain than S-adenosylmethionine. This latter must probably be restricted to O-methylation. The analysis of both these enzymes through a sedimentation gradient supports this view (Fig. 3). In this experiment, dopamine was used as a substrate for the determination of COMT as well as for that of

N-methyltransferase. Only the methyl donor was different. The fact that the distribution pattern of both enzymes presents a unique peak, suggests a kind of specificity for the methyl donor.

The foregoing observations are taken as evidence that catecholamines and indoleamines are converted to their corresponding N-methyl- or N-dimethyl derivatives by an N-methyltransferase present in the brain and with an unusual methyl donor for catecholamines. We therefore assume that folic acid and its congeners, namely 5-methyltetrahydrofolic acid could play a role in the metabolism of catecholamines in the brain.

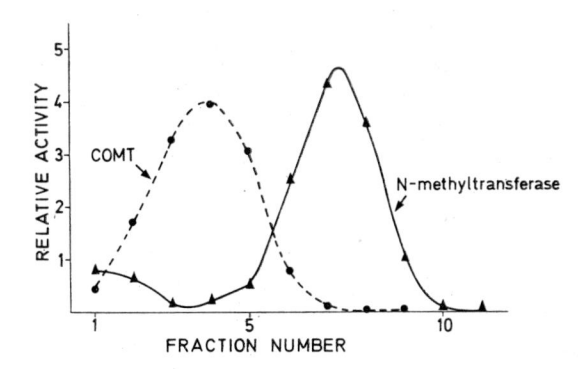

Fig. 3. Sedimentation pattern of N-methyltransferase and catechol-O-methyltransferase (COMT) through a sucrose gradient. An enzyme preparation from rat brain was layered onto 5 ml of a 5 to 20% sucrose gradient and centrifuged for 17 hrs at 50.000 RPM. Fractions were assayed for N-methyltransferase with 5-methyltetrahydrofolic acid as methyl donor, and COMT with S-adenosylmethionine. Sedimentation is from left to right.

N-METHYLATED COMPOUND AND FOLATE CONGENERS IN SCHIZOPHRENIA: A NEW MODEL

The fact that the *in vitro* formation of epinine and other N-methylated amines in the adrenal medulla and brain is well established now, does not imply that such a formation also occurs *in vivo*. However, if for instance, epinine could be isolated from adrenergic tissues, one might put forward a more extended concept of the physiological role of this catecholamine. Up to now, endogenous epinine has been isolated from three different tissues. The first isolation was carried out in the venom and parotid of the South American toad (Bufo Marinus) where an "unspecific" N-methyltransferase for dopamine has also been reported (18). More recently, we isolated endogenous epinine in bovine adrenal medulla after three runs of column chromatography and, final, separation of dopamine and epinine by means of thin layer chromatography (LADURON, unpublished results). Epinine has also been isolated in the rabbit lung (26). These results taken together with our previous *in vitro* experiments (10—12) support the view that epinine is probably endowed with an important role in the adrenergic system and may be considered as the immediate precursor of adrenaline in adrenal medulla.

Nevertheless, the role of epinine or dimethyldopamine, in the central nervous system, if they exist either in normal or pathological conditions, requires further elucidation.

In summing up the different papers dealing with the pharmacological activity of epinine in the peripheral system, one may conclude that dopamine and epinine are generally considered as equipotent and that the difference, if any, is relatively small and only qualitative (8, 22). For instance, it was found that epinine provokes a neurogenic vasodilation in the isolated perfused hind leg of the dog, similar to that induced by dopamine, but in contrast to this latter, a small increase in systemic blood pressure was also detected (30). The same authors have shown also that a neuroleptic like haloperidol could antagonize the epinine-induced vasodilation, indicating that dopamine blocking agents are not only restricted to dopamine and apomorphine but can also interfere with pharmacological activities of N-methylated dopamine. As far as structures are concerned, it must be stressed that epinine resembles apomorphine much more than dopamine does.

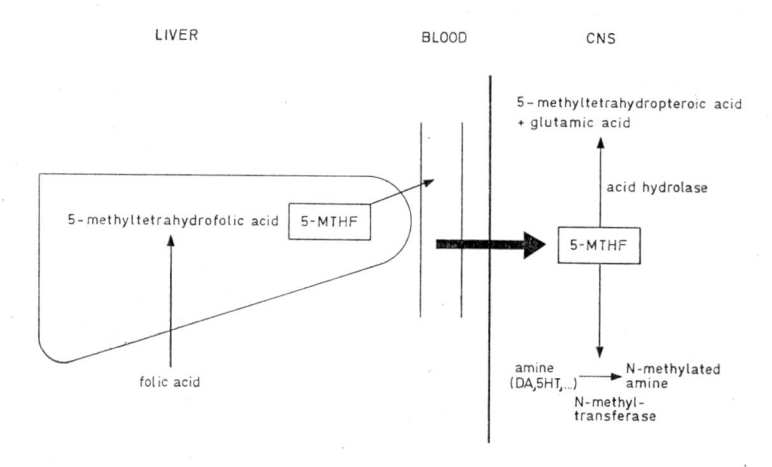

Fig. 4. Metabolic pathways of 5-methyltetrahydrofolic acid and his relationships with the N-methylation process in the brain.

From these data one may assume that epinine and dopamine can be bound to the same kind of receptors. Nevertheless, after the analogy of noradrenaline and adrenaline, both amines could display slight qualitative differences in inducing for example some typical or specific behaviour. With regard to this, it is not unlikely, that epinine and dimethyldopamine can play a prominent role in schizophrenic disorders.

Among all the hypotheses proposed to explain the causes of schizophrenia, one has already received some indirect experimental support. According to this model, schizophrenia should be due to an excessive N-methylation process involving the production of hallucinogen compounds, most of them being N- or N-N'-methylated products (see review 29). Two kinds of investigations support this view; firstly, bufotenin and N,N-dimethyltryptamine were found in the urine of schizophrenic patients (5, 7, 21). The second approach was performed in clinical experiments in which a methyl donor, L-methionine, was fed to schizophrenic patients. This amino acid was found to have no effect when given alone, but when combined with an inhibitor of MAO, some chronic schizophrenic patiens responded with behaviour changes consisting of an increase in psychotic symptoms (24).

Our new working hypothesis to explain the schizophrenic disorders, is based on the fact that the methyl donor responsible for N-methylation in the brain, is not S-adenosylmethionine but 5-methyltetrahydrofolic acid. Fig. 4 illustrates the metabolism of folic acid of which at least 65% is converted to 5-methyltetrahydrofolate in the liver. After having spread through circulation, this folate congener is taken up preferentially in neural tissues (1). This folate retaining capacity in the brain tissue explains why high concentrations of 5-methyltetrahydrofolic acid were found in the spinal fluid (9, 16). Therefore, although up to now the role of the folate coenzymes in neural metabolism has been unknown, our recent findings suggest that this methyl donor plays a role in the metabolism of catecholamines in the brain. It is postulated that in schizophrenic disorders, an excess of folate coenzymes could give rise to an increased or unusual formation of N-methylated amines not only epinine and dimethyldopamine but also N-methyl- and N-dimethyltryptamine and N-methylserotonin and bufotenin. This concept has already received some indirect support. In a preliminary clinical experiment, 10 schizophrenic patients, already treated with neuroleptics, received also 15 mg of folic acid daily for one month; four among them responded with behaviour changes consisting of an increase in psychotic symptoms (28). It should be emphasized that the experimental conditions were against us as the patients concomitantly received neuroleptics which could prevent the effects of folic acid.

What could be the metabolic defect responsible of this excess of folate congeners in schizophrenia? According to the model presented in Fig. 4, one may assume for instance an increased uptake process or modification of permeability in certain areas of the brain. Another possibility should be that the folate coenzymes undergo a metabolic degradation. Very recently, we described a lysosomal enzyme in the brain able to hydrolyze 5-methyltetrahydrofolic acid (13). This enzyme could act as a regulatory factor to maintain a constant level of folate congeners in the neural tissue.

It is tempting to attribute to this enzyme a prominent role in schizophrenic disorders. One is inclined to assume that such a lysosomal enzyme could be defective or decreased in schizophrenia. If this is true, this metabolic or genetic defect should involve an increase in folate congeners, the degradative pathway being so deficient that a subsequent increased production of N-methylated compounds should finally occur. Further investigation dealing with this hypothesis is now in progress.

REFERENCES

1. ALLEN, C. D. and KLIPSTEIN, F. A. (1970) Brain folate concentrations in rats receiving diphenylhydantoin. Neurology, **4**, 403.
2. AXELROD, J. (1962) Purification and properties of phenylethanolamine-N-methyltransferase. J. biol. Chem. **237**, 1657.
3. AXELROD, J. (1966) Methylation reactions in the formation and metabolism of catecholamines and other biogenic amines. Pharmacol. Rev. **18**, 95.
4. BELPAIRE, F. and LADURON, P. (1968) Tissue fractionation and catecholamines. 1. Latency and activation properties of dopamine-β-hydroxylase in adrenal medulla. Biochem. Pharmacol. **17**, 511.
5. BRUNE, G. G., HOHL, H. H. and HIMWICH, H. E. (1963) Urinary excretion of bufotenin-like substance in psychotic patients. J. Neuropsychiat. **5**, 14.
6. CIARANELLO, R. D., BARCHAS, R. E., BYERS, G. S., STEMMLE, D. W. and BARCHAS, J. D. (1969) Enzymatic synthesis of adrenaline in mammalian brain. Nature, **221**, 368.
7. FISCHER, E., FERNANDEZ LAGRAVERE, T. A., VAZQUEZ, A. J. and DI STEFANO, A. O. (1961) A bufotenin-like substance in the urine of schizophrenics. J. nerv. ment. Dis. **133**, 441.
8. GOLDBERG, L. I., SONNEVILLE, P. F. and MCNAY, J. L. (1968) An investigation of the structure requirements for dopamine-like renal vasodilatation: phenylethylamines and apomorphine. J. Pharmacol. exp. Ther. **163**, 188.
9. HERBERT, V. and ZALUSKY, R. (1961) Selective concentration of folic acid activity in cerebrospinal fluid. Proc. Amer. Soc. exp. Biol. **20**, 453.
10. LADURON, P. (1972) N-methylation of dopamine to epinine in adrenal medulla: a new model for the biosynthesis of adrenaline. Arch. int. Pharmacodyn. **195**, 197.
11. LADURON, P. (1972) N-methyldopamine (epinine), a precursor of adrenal medulla. Arch. int. Pharmacodyn. **196**, 304.

12. LADURON, P. (1972) N-methylation of dopamine to epinine in brain tissue using N-methyltetrahydrofolic acid as the methyl donor. Nature, 238, 212.
13. LADURON, P. (1972) A lysosomal enzyme hydrolysing N-methyltetrahydrofolate in the brain. Biochem. biophys. Res. Commun. (in preparation).
14. LADURON, P. and BELPAIRE, F. (1968) Tissue fractionation and catecholamines. 2. Intracellular distribution pattern of tyrosine hydroxylase, dopadecarboxylase, dopamine β-hydroxylase, phenylethanolamine N-methyltransferase and monoamine oxidase in adrenal medulla. Biochem. Pharmacol. 17, 1127.
15. LADURON P. M., GOMMEREN W. R. and LEYSEN J. E. (1973) N-methylation of biogenic amines; characterization and properties of a N-methyltransferase in rat brain using 5-methyltetrahydrofolic acid as the methyl donor. Europ. J. Biochem. (in press).
16. LEVITT, M., NIXON, P. F., PINCUS, J. H. and BERTINO, J. R. (1971) Transport characteristics of folates in cerebrospinal fluid; a study utilizing doubly labeled 5-methyltetrahydrofolate and 5-formyltetrahydrofolate. J. clin. Invest. 50, 1301.
17. MANDELL, A. J. and MORGAN, M. (1971) Indole(ethyl)amine N-methyltransferase in human brain. Nature, 230, 85.
18. MARKI, F., AXELROD, J. and WITKOP, B. (1962) Catecholamines and methyltransferases in the South American toad (Bufo Marinus). Biochim. biophys. Acta 58, 367.
19. MCGEER, P. L. and MCGEER, E. G. (1964) Formation of adrenaline by brain tissue. Biochem. biophys. Res. Commun. 17, 502.
20. NAGATSU, T., LEVITT, M. and UDENFRIEND, S. (1964) The initial step in norepinephrine biosynthesis. J. biol. Chem. 239, 2910.
21. NARASIMHACHARI, N., HELLER, B., SPAIDE, J., HASKOVEC, L., FUJIMORI, M., TABUSHI, K. and HIMWICH, H. F. (1971). Urinary studies of schizophrenics and controls. Biol. Psychiat. 3, 9.
22. PALM, D., LANGENECKERT, W. and HOLTZ, P. (1967) Bedeutung der N- und α-Methylierung für die Affinität von Brenzcatechinaminen zu den adrenergischen Receptoren. Arch. Pharmak. exp. Path. 258, 128.
23. POHORECKY, L. A., ZIGMOND, M. J., KARTEN, H. and WURTMAN, R. J. (1969) Enzymatic conversion of norepinephrine to epinephrine by the brain. J. Pharmacol. exp. Ther. 165, 190.
24. POLLIN, W., CARDON, P. V., JR, and KETY, S. S. (1961) Effects of amino acid feedings in schizophrenic patients treated with iproniazid. Science, 133, 104.
25. SAAVEDRA, J. M. and AXELROD, J. (1972) Psychotomimetic N-methylated tryptamines formation in brain in *in vivo* and *in vitro*. Science, 175, 1365.
26. SCHEEL-KRUGER, J. (1972) Personal communication.
27. SMITH, A. D. and WINKLER, H. (1972) Fundamental mechanisms in the release of catecholamines. In: Catecholamines. Ed.: Blaschko H. and Muscholl, E., Springer Verlag Berlin, p. 538.
28. VAN LOMMEL, R. (1972) Unpublished results.
29. WEIL-MALHERBE, H. and SZARA, S. I. (1971) The biochemistry of functional and experimental psychoses. Charles C. Thomas. Springfield, Ill.
30. WILLEMS, J. L. and BOGAERT, M. G. (1972) Neurogenic vasodilatation: dopamine and related substances. Arch. int. Pharmacodyn. 197, 412.

P.L., Department of Neurobiochemistry, Janssen Pharmaceutica, Research Laboratories, B-2340 Beerse, Belgium

STRATEGY OF TREATMENT OF CHRONIC PATIENTS (PHARMACOLOGICALLY)

Chairmen: O. Vinař and M. Schou

Associate chairman: J. D. Christensen

WHOM DO NEUROLEPTIC DRUGS HELP?

O. VINAŘ

Institute of Psychiatry, Prague

If I may answer the question whom do neuroleptic drugs help, I would like to omit such obvious answers as that they help most the drug manufacturers, doctors, or more specifically nurses and attendants who have to spend most of their working time at the hospital together with the patients — who were some twenty years ago considered as dangerous. I would like to limit my questions to what kind of chronic schizophrenic patients the neuroleptic drugs may be helpful, where they are useless and whether we can recognize what patients can become worse on them.

When I speak about neuroleptic drugs I refer to the group of drugs which have some common traits from the chemical and pharmacological point of view as defined by JANSSEN (10). Although phenothiazincs still represent the central group of neuroleptic drugs, thiaxanthenes and other tricyclic compounds with a seven-member central ring (clothiapin, oxilapin, oktoclothepin, clozapine), butyrophenones and new substances like pimozide, fluspirilene, penfluridol, oxypertine and sulpiride have grown in importance in the past few years. There has been discussion about their mechanism of action and whether their effects are only symptomatic or something more, whether the adjective antipsychotic is correct etc. Two analogies have been expressed in Czechoslovakia: VONDRÁČEK compares their effects with the effects of cardiac glycosides in heart failure which is neither etiological nor only symptomatic and calls these effects regulative, VENCOVSKÝ speaks about psychosostatic effects and compares it with the bacteriostatic effects of sulfonamides. What is common to all members of this class of drugs is their capacity to produce the neuroleptic syndrome which was described in a classical way be DELAY and DENIKER (7). It seems that the psychic phenomena of this syndrome have gradually become more important than the neurological ones: all neuroleptics produce a special state of psychomotor indifference which only exceptionally cannot be observed distinctly in apathetic and withdrawn patients where sometimes the apparent oposite — a desinhibitory action—can be seen. On the other hand, different neuroleptic drugs differ substantially in the production of extrapyramidal and autonomic symptoms and in some of them (e.g. clozapine) these effects are claimed to be practically reduced to zero.

Many of the therapeutic effects of the neuroleptic drugs in psychoses could be explained by the neuroleptic syndrome they induce also in healthy volunteers. A pronounced state of psychomotor indifference is incompatible with psychomotor agitation, aggressivity, affective tension and to a certain extent also with behavioral phenomena connected with hallucinations and delusions. In this way, the therapeutic efficacy of neuroleptics on so-called productive or plus symptoms of schizophrenic psychoses can be understood purely on a phenomenological basis.

It can be assumed that this understanding was the major reason for some of the older notions that phenothiazines with an aliphatic side chain such as e.g. chlorpromazine and levopromazine have a better effect in calming the agitated, excited, over-active psychotic whereas phenothiazines with a piperazine side-chain are more effective in patients with delusions, hallucinations and that they are also able to activate withdrawn, immobile patients. This opinion is still deep-rooted in routine practice although it has not stood up to objective scrutiny of controlled clinical research (68).

A great deal of the controversy between the conviction of doctors engaged in routine practice and the results of controlled trials can be explained by neglecting of one of the classical methodological considerations of KARL JASPERS (11): we can understand some obvious relationships of psychic phenomena but this understanding has nothing to do with the explanation of casual relationships in the physical world. The biological effects of drugs belong to the physical world where casual relationships can be studied and explanations can be found for many of our behavioral observations. On the other hand, the fact that most psychiatrists can understand the incompatibility of psychomotor indifference (which is expressed more after aliphatic phenothiazines than after the piperazine ones) with psychomotor excitement does not imply a casual relationship between these two psychic phenomena. Much of the misunderstanding in clinical psychopharmacology could be removed if the distinction between understanding (Verstehen) and explanation (Erklären) were respected.

We have to deal with drug treatment of chronic patients. What is the definition of chronicity? How long has the illness to last before we call the patient chronic? What about patients with a periodic course? Is a manic depressive who had 5 psychotic episodes lasting 2 month each in the last 10 years a chronic patient? Automated processing of medical prescriptions in one of the Prague districts (14) enabled us to find that many patients who were prescribed anxiolytics for a neurotic condition in January 1970 have got at least one prescription on anxiolytics for the same diagnosis in January 1971 as well. Does this mean that many neurotic patients are chronic and that they are treated by some kind of maintenance medication?

I am not able and do not wish to answer all these questions. I just would like to demonstrate that the problems concernig the definition of chronicity and the necessity of maintenance treatment are not at all specific for schizophrenia or for other psychoses.

In most of the studies, chronicity is defined operationally, e.g., by the length of continuous hospitalization. Two years have been used extensively as a dividing point in this respect and it has been shown that the symptomatology of chronic schizophrenic patients differs from the symptomatology of the acute ones. Without knowing the past history of the patient, an experienced psychiatrist can tell an acute patient from a chronic one only on the basis of the current symptomatology. This can be confirmed by using rating scales: e.g. on the Brief Psychiatric Rating Scale (BPRS) profiles (12), more pathology can be found in the items emotional withdrawal, conceptual disorganization and blunted affect with the increasing duration of illness. These symptoms belong more to the so-called deficiency symptoms than to the productive ones and are close to what BLEULER has called "fundamental" symptoms. It is true that the greatest amount of clinical change during psychiatric treatment — and not only on drug treatment — occurs in the so-called accessory symptoms such as in hallucinations, delusions, excitement. However, in these cases significant improvement occurs also on placebo: and drugs seem merely to induce a quantitative increase in placebo effect. On the other hand, the fundamental symptoms do not react to placebo and if these symptoms are more characteristic for a chronic patient, then significant amelioration of symptomatology in chronic patients can be considered a really pharmacological effect (6).

If we consider the effectiveness of phenothiazines in terms of the difference they effect in comparison with placebo, symptoms characteristic for chronic schizophrenia are reduced even more than the productive or accessory symptoms which predominate in acute patients. Nevertheless, this does not mean that we can be too optimistic in our expectations of a favourable outcome in chronic schizophrenics. A statistically significant reduction of psychopathology does not mean that it is practically significant for the fate of the patient, e.g. that he can be discharged from the hospital and that he will begin to work, earn and lead a socially well adjusted life in his family. The broad usage of rating scales in the evaluation of drug efficacy has led to an overestimation of the symptomatology, we may even see that the symptom becomes a fetish whose disappearance is considered as the unique goal of therapy. If we used the release rate as the criterion of outcome of the treatment in chronic schizophrenia, the percentage would be rather low: 5—15% depending on the criteria of chronicity and the hospital policy.

The study which will be reported further is one of the series of our attempts to predict the outcome of neuroleptic treatment in schizophrenic patients. In the first paper (15) of this series, some clinical and EEG criteria were used as predictors of differential action of five neuroleptic drugs. The equations were based on canonical correlation analysis and could be validated on a second sample of patients — however, the second attempt to cross-validate this result on a third and larger group of patients has failed.

In our further work, we tried to use two different approaches to prediction distinguished also by GOLDBERG (9) in a similar way:

1. First, we grouped the patients according to some reliable criteria and only afterwards we tried to find out whether these groups differ in their response to drugs and placebo. In one study (17) the groups of patients were obtained by a cluster analysis of the data based on the results of a standardized interview (13), in another study similarly obtained groups were based on the results of the examination by means of the Cattel's PF 16 (3, 4).

2. We tried to find a correlation between some pretreatment clinical or experimental criteria and the outcome of the treatment. Together with BAŠTECKÝ (1), we found records of the voice of patients using the method of delayed auditory feedback (DAF) and EMG of mimic muscles to be of predictive value.

The present report deals with the possibility to predict the therapeutic response to chlorpromazine on the basis of the pretreatment symptomatology rated by the BPRS of OVERALL and GORHAM (12). Data related to the social background, past history etc. are the subject of another study not yet finished.

In-patients of the Psychopharmacological Department of the Institute of Psychiatry in Prague yielded data for this study. The city of Prague is the catchment area of the Psychiatric hospital in Prague 8 and our patients are chosen at random from all its admissions using criteria of selection which permit the inclusion only of patients with functional psychoses. Only patients treated with neuroleptic drugs with a duration of illness over five years were included in the present study.

All patients were treated in conditions of the continuous controlled trial applied in the Depatrment during the past 8 years. Its main characteristics are double blind evaluation of the clinical state of patients in one week's intervals and randomized assignment of drugs which is not introduced again and again at new for each trial but goes on continuously according to the research program of the Department. Once a patient has been admitted, he is treated according to this system as long as it is necessary from the therapeutic point of view and the double blind treatment goes on also in discharged patients where the maintenance treatment is studied. When there is a relapse of the psychosis which necessitates rehospitalization, the patient is admitted to the ward of the Department again and the treatment goes on fulfilling an analogous research program as during the preceding hospitalization. Information about the long term course of the illness treated under controlled conditions becomes available.

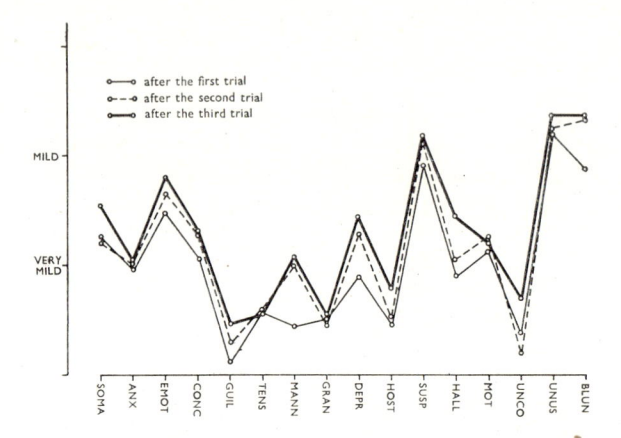

Fig. 1. Post-treatment BPRS profiles. Items of the BPRS (Overall and Gorham): Soma — somatic concern; Anx — anxiety; Emot — emotional withdrawal; Conc — conceptual disorganization; Guil — guilt feelings; Tens — tension; Mann — mannerisms and posturing; Gran — grandiosity; Depr — depressive mood; Host — hostility; Susp-suspiciousness; Hall — hallucinatory behavior; Mot — motor retardation; Unco — uncooperativeness; Unus — unusual thought content; Blun — blunted affect (these abbreviations refer also to Figs. 2, 4, 6, 8 and 9).

107 patients admitted in the years 1967 and 1968 were rated by the BPRS at admission, 52 of them were admitted before 1969 twice and 25 of them three times.*) If we now compare their BPRS profiles after the first six week trial after each admission we can see (Fig. 1), that our therapeutic success decreases with the duration of illness especially in the items somatic concern, emotional withdrawal, uncooperativeness, blunted affect, but also in depression and hallucinatory behavior. If we extrapolate this result, we may assume that these are the symptoms where the outcome of drug treatment will be worse with the duration of illness — or with increasing chronicity. On the other hand, the scores of the items anxiety, tension, grandiosity, motor retardation and unusual thought content remain nearly the same on the end of the three compared trials indicating that in these symptoms the effects of neuroleptic drugs do not decrease with increasing chronicity. Distinction between these two groups of symptoms does not compare with the distinctions which we usually meet in the differentiation of symptoms not sensitive to drugs. Especially surprising is the splitting of the hallucinatory-paranoid syndrome: according to these data, the delusions do not lose their susceptibility to disappear under the influence of neuroleptics with increasing chronicity whereas the hallucinations do lose this susceptibility.

The knowledge about what symptoms in chronic schizophrenic patients disappear or diminish, and what symptoms do not, does not sufficiently answer the question whom neuroleptic drugs help: it cannot be excluded that there is some characteristic trait which

---

*) This analysis was performed during the stay of the author in the Biometric Laboratory George Washington University, Washington, D.C., under the guidance of Dr. R. S. Bonato.

has nothing to do with symptomatology which improves the prognosis e.g. the fact that the patient is worried and the family does not lose interest in him. Social background is decisive already among the causes of chronicity and can play a substantial role in the outcome of treatment. Nevertheless, data about the social background have not yet been used in the study I am reporting about. We were interested in the question whether we can predict the drug response on the basis of the current pretreatment symptomatology.

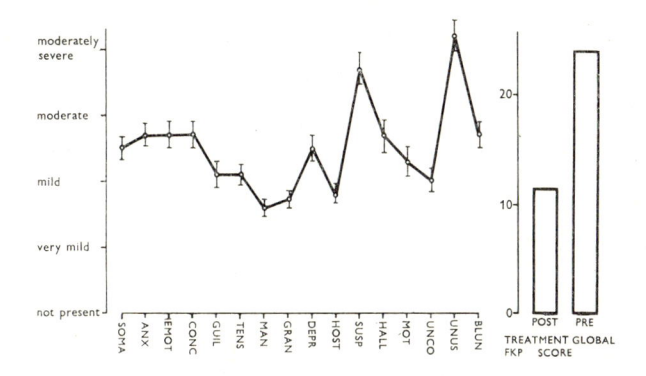

Fig. 2. Mean pretreatment BPRS profiles. Sample of patients (N = 174).

The introduction of multivariate statistical techniques which can test hypotheses involving the combined interrelationships of a number of variables has been recommended in the last 10 years (e.g. 5). The multiple regression approach was closest to help to answer our question whether a single measure in a group of patients can be predicted from a group of other measures. This group of measures (independent variables) were the pretreatment scores of the items of the BPRS of OVERALL and GORHAM (12), the single measure (dependent variable) which had to be predicted was the amount of improvement after six-weeks treatment with chlorpromazine. The weighted global score of the rating scale FKP (Quantification of psychotic symptomatology for the evaluation of drug treatment— Farmakoterapeutická Kvantifikace Psychos) (16) was used for measuring the treatment effects. The FKP is a rating scale with 18 items developed for the evaluation of the treatment at our Institute. In our previous work, we found that the individual items of the FKP do not correlate high with the individual items of the BPRS — nevertheless the canonical correlation between the items of both scales was 0,939. We assume that both rating scales are measuring nearly identical phenomena but from different standpoints.

174 chronic schizophrenic patients treated in conditions of the system of continuous controlled trial with chlorpromazine 400—950 mg/day during six weeks yielded data for this analysis. Their pretreatment BPRS scores can be seen in Fig. 2. The patients were younger than comparable samples of chronic patients of other authors: only 19 patients were older than 40 years, all the other ones were younger.

When predicting the amount of change using the relative decrease of the global FKP score as dependent variable (criterion of response) we obtained a not sufficiently high multiple regression coefficient:

MULTIPLE REGRESSION COEFFICIENT: 0.43

$x_1, x_2 \ldots x_{16}$ pretreatment BPRS scores
y relative decrease of the weighted global score FKP

$$y = 75.02 + 0.61x_1 - 3.22x_2 - 7.66x_3 - 0.92x_4 + 4.98x_5 + 3.41x_6 + 8.72x_7 - 6.29x_8 - 7.77x_9 - 2.87x_{10} + 3.48x_{11} - 0.76x_{12} - 5.46x_{13} - 7.34x_{14} - 1.30x_{15} + 12.45x_{16}$$

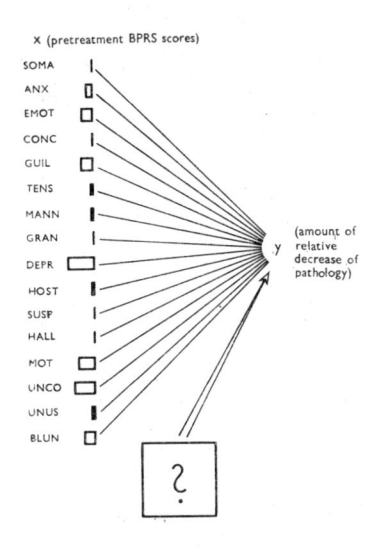

Fig. 3. Multiple regression analysis. Contribution of individual items to the prediction of the outcome. Analysis of the pathological symptoms. y — amount of relative decrease of pathological symptoms.

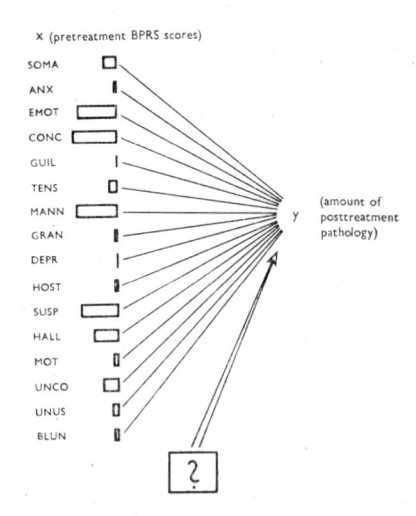

Fig. 4. Multiple regression analysis. Contribution of the individual items to the prediction of the outcome. Results of the pathological analysis. y — amount of post-treatment pathological symptoms.

A path analysis (Fig. 3) shows the contribution of individual items to the prediction: emotional withdrawal, guilt, depression, motor retardation, uncooperativeness and blunted affect contributed most, but approximately 60% of the influence is still dependent on other factors than BPRS pretreatment scores.

A better result can be seen (Fig. 4) when we tried to predict the post-treatment global FKP score. Here, less than 40% of the prediction is due to other factors than to pretreatment psychopathology defined by the BPRS scores.

MULTIPLE REGRESSION COEFFICIENT: 0.618

$x_1, x_2 \ldots x_{16}$ pretreatment BPRS scores
y post-treatment weighted global score FKP

$$y = -3.92 + 0.85x_1 - 1.25x_2 - 2.02x_3 + 1.6x_4 + 0.31x_5 + 1.04x_6 + 2.81x_7 - 0.34x_8 - 0.31x_9 + 0.20x_{10} + 1.25x_{11} + 0.75x_{12} - 0.37x_{13} - 1.49x_{14} + 0.4x_{15} + 2.33x_{16}$$

Theoretically, the comparison of the contributions of the individual BPRS items to the prediction of the drug response is interesting in relation to the two dependent variables which were used. Thus, e.g. depression seems to be very important when predicting the amount of change but does not greatly contribute in predicting the amount of post-treatment psychopathology. The low contribution of the pretreatment score of the item blunted affect to the prediction of the amount of post-treatment psychopathology is surprising.

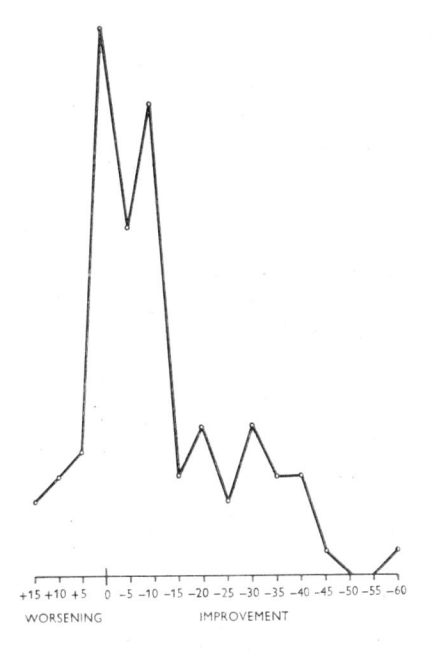

Fig. 5. Frequency distribution of the raw change scores (pre- vs. post-treatment weighted global score).

Fig. 5 demonstrates the reason for abandoning our original idea to use a discriminant function to differentiate chlorpromazine responders from chlorpromazine nonresponders. It would have been only an arbitrary decision by which we could set apart patients with positive and negative drug response.

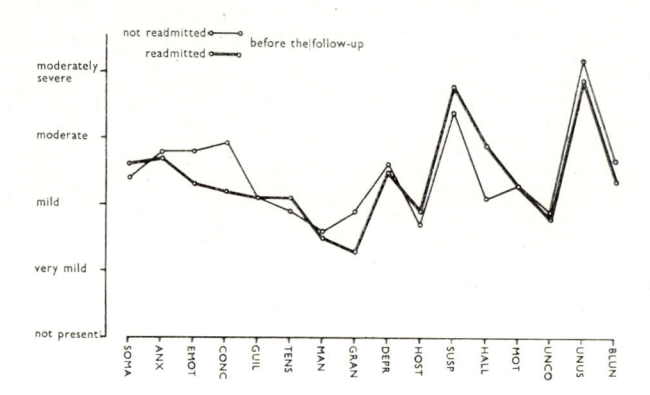

Fig. 6. Average BPRS pretreatment scores.

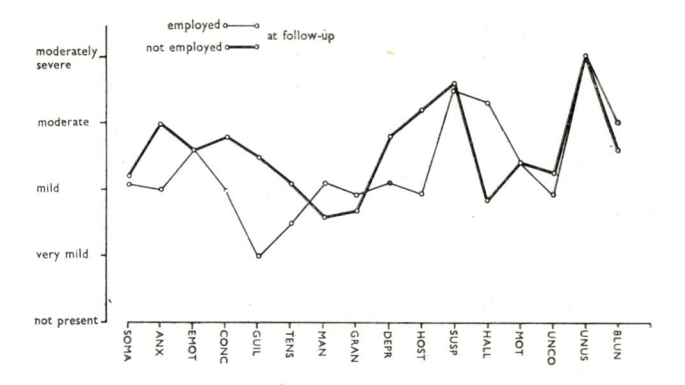

Fig. 7. Average BPRS pretreatment scores.

In 112 patients of the original sample of 174, data were available about the state of the patient one year after the six-weeks chlorpromazine trial. For the purpose of this study, we asked simply whether the patient was at home or in hospital and using the discriminant function analysis we tried to know what combination of BPRS pretreatment scores best discriminates between the patients which were at home at the follow-up (N = 57) and the patients which were still — or again in a psychiatric hospital (N = 55) (Fig. 6). The same question was asked for two similar subgroups of patients: those who one year after the chlorpromazine trial were employed and worked (N = 37) and those who did not (N = = 73) (Fig. 7). Here, both discriminant function coefficients were insignificant statistically.

Although we did not expect this result it is not greatly surprising. The pattern of psychopathology at one of the pretreatment periods does not predict with sufficient probability the state of the patient after one year if this state is defined by his social functioning. Hospital policy in discharging patients, the attitude of the family members and the level of out-patient care can be more important than the current or past psychopathology in deciding whether the patient is at home or in the hospital. The attitudes of the employer, interpersonal atmosphere at work and the efforts of the social worker can again be stronger determinants of the fact whether the patient works or not than his past symptomatology.

Our equations cannot be used yet as a prediction tool for newly admitted chronic patients: it is necessary to validate them on other patient samples.

In conclusion, I would like to stress the importance of controlled clinical research. Only controlled research can e.g. help to avoid treating an illness which disappears spontaneously — or to quote EUGEN BLEULER (2): "Wir geben uns große Mühe, Krankheiten zu behandeln, die von selbst heilen."

REFERENCES

1. BAŠTECKÝ, J., VINAŘ, O. and TOŠOVSKÝ, J. (1972) Delayed auditory feedback: a predictor of the outcome of drug treatment in schizophrenic psychoses. Paper read at the VIII. Congress of the Collegium Internationale Neuro-Psychopharmacologicum, Copenhague, August 11—15.
2. BLEULER, E. (1966) Das autistisch-undisziplinierte Denken in der Medizin und seine Überwindung. Springer, Berlin.
3. BOLELOUCKY, Z., VINAR, O. and ROTH, Z. (1972) Placebo response of schizophrenic patients and Cattell's personality factors. Paper read at the VIII. Congress of the Collegium Internationale Neuro-Psychopharmacologium, Copenhague, August 11—15.
4. BOLELOUCKÝ, Z., VINAŘ, O., TOŠOVSKY, J. and ROTH, Z. (1972) Cluster analysis of the 16 P.F. test data from schizophreniopatients. Relation to the prediction of results of pharmacotherapy. Paper read at the VIII. Congress of the Collegium Internationale Neuro-Psychopharmacologicum, Copenhague, August 11—15.
5. COLE, J. O. (1065) The impact of psychopharmacology on research in psychiatry. In: KLINE, N. S., LEHMANN, H. E. (Eds.): Psychopharmacology (p. 925). Little, Brown and Comp., Boston.
6. COLE, J. O. and DAVIS, J. M. (1968) Clinical efficacy of the phenothiazines as antipsychotic drugs. In: EFRON, D. H., COLE, J. O., LEVINE, J., WITTENBORN, J. R. (Eds.): Psychopharmacology. A review of progress 1957—1967 (p. 1057). Publ. Health Service Publication No. 1836, Washington, D. C.
7. DELAY, J. and DENIKER, P. (1957) Caractéristiques psycho-physiologiques des médicaments neuroleptiques. In: GARATTINI, S., GHETTI, V. (Eds.): Psychotropic drugs (p. 485). Elsevier, Amsterdam.
8. GOLDBERG, S. C. (1968) Prediction of response to antipsychotic drugs. In: EFRON, D. H., COLE, J. O., LEVINE, J., WITTENBORN, J. R. (Eds.): Psychopharmacology. A review of progress 1957—1967 (p. 1101). Publ. Health Service Publication No 1836, Washington, D. C.
9. GOLDBERG, S. C. (1969) Paranoid and withdrawal symptomatology: simple but useful predictors in schizophrenia. In: MAY, P. R. A., WITTENBORN, J. R. (Eds.): Psychotropic drug response (p. 29). CC. Thomas, Springfield.
10. JANSSEN, P. A. J. (1970) Chemical and pharmacological classification of neuroleptics. In: Bobon, D. P., Janssen, P. A. J., Bobon, J. (Eds.): The Neuroleptics (p. 33). S. Karger, Basel.
11. JASPERS, K. (1953) Allgemeine Psychopathologie. Sechste Auflage. Springer, Berlin.
12. OVERALL, J. E. and GORHAM, D. R. (1962) The Brief Psychiatric Rating Scale. Psychol. Rep. **10**, 799.
13. SPITZER, R. L., BURDOCK, E. I. and HARDESTY, A. S. (1964) Mental Status Schedule. Biometric Research, N. Y. State Dept. of Mental Hygiene and Dept. of Psychiat., Columbia Univ., New York.
14. ŠTIKA, L., HOVOROVÁ, M. and KRATOCHVÍL, J. (1971) Automated processing of medical prescriptions. Activ. nerv. Super. (Prague) **13**, 228.
15. VINAŘ, O., MATOUŠEK, M., ROUBÍČEK, J. and VOLAVKA, J. (1969) Importance of some clinical and EEG criteria for drug selection. In: CERLETTI, A., BOVÉ, F. J. (Eds.): The present status of psychotropic drugs (p. 409). Excerpta Medica, Amsterdam.

16. VINAŘ, O., VÁŇA, J. and GROF, S. (1966): Rating scale FKP. Activ. nerv. Super. (Prague) 8, 405.
17. VINAŘOVÁ, E., VINAŘ, O. and TOŠOVSKY, J. (1972): Diagnosis made by cluster analysis and its relation to the outcome of drug treatment. Paper read at the VIII. Congress of the Collegium Internationale Neuro-Psychopharmacologium, Copenhague, August 11—15.

O.V., Institute of Psychiatry, Prague 8, Bohnice 95, Czechoslovakia

LANGJÄHRIGE BEHANDLUNG MIT NEUROLEPTIKA BEI CHRONISCH SCHIZOPHREN KRANKEN MÄNNERN

F. ECKMANN

Landeskrankenhaus Schleswig-Stadtfeld und Abteilung für epidemiologische und statistische Psychiatrie, Dokumentationszentrale der Landeskrankenhäuser Schleswig-Holsteins

Bei der Wiedereingliederung chronisch schizophren Kranker in die menschliche und berufliche Gemeinschaft sind „persönliche, soziale, mitmenschlich-familiäre sowie berufliche Situationen" (3) zu beachten. Darüberhinaus spielt hierbei die Behandlung mit Neuroleptika eine nicht unwesentliche Rolle.

Zur Klärung eines möglichen Zusammenhanges zwischen diesen Faktoren stellten wir uns im Juni 1965 folgende Fragen:

I. Lassen sich hinsichtlich der Merkmale „soziale Stellung der Eltern", „soziale Stellung des Patienten", „Familienstand", „Schulbildung", „Unterbringungsart", „Schizophrenieformen", „Kontakt mit den Familienangehörigen" Unterschiede zwischen den entlassenen und nicht entlassenen bzw. wiederaufgenommenen chronisch schizophren kranken Männern feststellen?

II. Lassen sich hinsichtlich der Art und Potenz der verabreichten Neuroleptika Unterschiede zwischen den entlassenen und nicht entlassenen bzw. wiederaufgenommenen chronisch schizophren kranken Männern feststellen?

Entsprechend formulierten wir die Null- und Alternativhypothesen. Unsere Untersuchungen führten wir in der Zeit vom Juni 1965 bis Juni 1972 an 502 schizophren kranken Männern einer Abteilung des Landeskrankenhauses Schleswig durch. Die Untersuchung war prospektiv geplant. Alle Daten wurden auf einen Lochbeleg aufgenommen.

Als statistische Testmethoden wählten wir den Vierfelder-Test mit nach c transformierten Werten und die Berechnung nach IRWIN — SNEDECOR für eine 2 × a — Tafel. Bei dieser Methode wird mit dem χ^2 - Test untersucht, wieweit die relativen Häufigkeiten in den einzelnen Klassen von der durchschnittlichen relativen Häufigkeit, berechnet über alle Klassen, abweichen. Das Signifikanzniveau wurde auf $\alpha = 0{,}05$ festgelegt.

Bereits bei der Planung der Untersuchung war uns bewußt, daß ein klinisch-psychiatrisches Krankengut *a priori* selektiert ist. Durch die Tatsache, daß nur Patienten mit einer bestimmten Diagnose in die Untersuchung einbezogen werden konnten, war die endliche Grundgesamtheit um ein weiteres selektiert. Damit konnte ein systematischer Fehler in die Beziehungen zwischen Stichprobe und Grundgesamtheit eingehen, der in seiner Größenordnung nur schwer abschätzbar war. Die Klärung der Wechselbeziehungen zwischen entlassenen und nicht entlassenen bzw. wiederaufgenommenen chronisch schizophren kranken Männern und den eingangs aufgeführten Faktoren schien uns aber doch so wichtig, daß den Problemen trotzdem nachgegangen werden sollte.

Zunächst war festzustellen, ob die beiden Kollektive „entlassene" und „nicht entlassene" bzw. „wiederaufgenommene" hinsichtlich der Merkmale „Altersklassenaufteilung" und „Verweildauer" vergleichbar waren. Die entsprechenden Berechnungen ergaben, daß das mittlere Alter in beiden Gruppen bei 47,8 Jahren lag; die Verweildauer lag in der Gruppe der Entlassenen bei 4,5 Jahren, in dem anderen Kollektiv bei 4,4 Jahren. Damit war die Vergleichbarkeit der beiden Untersuchungsgruppen — soweit prüfbar — gegeben.

Nun zu den Ergebnissen:

TABELLE 1

Soziale Stellung der Eltern der entlassenen und nichtentlassenen bzw. wiederaufgenommenen chronisch schizophren kranken Männer (Untersuchung Juni 1965—Juni 1972)

Soziale Stellung der Eltern	Entlassen ja a	Entlassen nein b	$\sum n$	a . p
Selbständig	36	112	148	8,748
Mithelf. Fam.-Angehörige	5	25	30	0,830
Beamte	7	22	29	1,687
Angestellte	14	27	41	4,774
Lohnempfänger	22	46	68	7,106
Arbeitslos	18	58	76	4,248
Rentner, Pensionär	22	88	110	4,400
Summe	124	378	502	31,793

$\chi^2 = 6,263$;
$\chi^2_{(6; 0,05)} = 12,592$.   Die Null-Hypothese läßt sich nicht verwerfen.

Tabelle 1 läßt erkennen, daß die Nullhypothese nicht zu verwerfen ist, d.h. es besteht hinsichtlich des Merkmales „soziale Stellung der Eltern" kein Unterschied in den Gruppen „entlassene" und „nicht entlassene" bzw. „wiederaufgenommene".

Tabelle 2 macht deutlich, daß kein Zusammenhang zwischen der „sozialen Stellung der Patienten" und den beiden Kollektiven nachzuweisen ist ($\chi^2 = 5,752$; $\chi^2_{(6; 0,05)} = 12,592$).

Wie Tabelle 3 zeigt, läßt sich auch kein Zusammenhang zwischen dem „Familienstand" und den beiden Kollektiven sichern ($\chi^2 = 6,079$; $\chi^2_{(3; 0,05)} = 7,815$).

Ebenso ließen sich keine Zusammenhänge zwischen den Merkmalen „Schulbildung" (Tabelle 4), „Unterbringungsart" (Tabelle 5) und den beiden Kollektiven „entlassene" und „nicht entlassene" bzw. „wiederaufgenommene" sichern.

Wie aus Tabelle 6 hervorgeht, war die Alternativhypothese anzunehmen. Der berechnete χ^2 — Wert betrug 8,516; der kritische Abszissenpunkt beträgt bei einer Signifikanzschranke von 5 % und einem Freiheitsgrad 3,841, d.h. „nicht entlassene" bzw. „wiederaufgenommene" haben einen schlechteren Kontakt zu ihren Familienangehörigen als „entlassene" chronisch schizophren kranke Männer. Dieses Ergebnis weist auf die Bedeutung des mitmenschlich familiären Faktors für eine erfolgreiche Rehabilitation hin.

Die in Tabelle 7 aufgeführte Unterteilung in vorwiegend „produktive" und „unproduktive" Schizophrenieformen stimmen mit der von HAASE definierten Plus- und Minussymptomatik überein. Ein Zusammenhang ließ sich auch hier nicht sichern ($\chi^2 = 1{,}010$; $\chi^2_{(1;\ 0{,}05)} = 3{,}841$).

TABELLE 2

Soziale Stellung der entlassenen und nichtentlassenen bzw. wiederaufgenommenen chronisch schizophren kranken Männer vor der Erstmanifestation ihrer Erkrankung (Untersuchung Juni 1965—Juni 1972)

Soziale Stellung	Entlassen ja a	Entlassen nein b	$\sum_n$	a · p
Selbständig	9	20	29	2,790
Mithelf. Fam.-Angehörige	9	28	37	2,187
Beamte	6	18	24	1,500
Angestellte	23	59	82	6,440
Lohnempfänger	52	160	212	12,740
Arbeitslos	14	72	86	2,268
Rentner, Pensionär	11	21	32	3,773
Summe	124	378	502	31,698

$\chi^2 = 5{,}752$;
$\chi^2_{(6;\ 0{,}05)} = 12{,}592.$ Die Null-Hypothese läßt sich nicht verwerfen.

TABELLE 3

Familienstand der entlassenen und nichtentlassenen bzw. wiederaufgenommenen chronisch schizophren kranken Männer (Untersuchung Juni 1965—Juni 1972)

Familienstand	Entlassen ja a	Entlassen nein b	$\sum_n$	a · p
Ledig	71	255	326	15,407
Verheiratet	24	44	68	8,448
Verwitwet	11	21	32	3,773
Geschieden	18	58	76	4,248
Summe	124	378	502	31,876

$\chi^2 = 6{,}709$;
$\chi^2_{(3;\ 0{,}05)} = 7{,}815.$ Die Null-Hypothese läßt sich nicht verwerfen.

Tabelle 4

Schulbildung der entlassenen und nichtentlassenen bzw. wiederaufgenommenen chronisch schizophren kranken Männer (Untersuchung Juni 1965—Juni 1972)

Schulbildung	Entlassen ja a	Entlassen nein b	$\sum_n$	a . p
Sonderschule	22	60	82	5,896
Volksschule	61	204	265	14,030
Mittelschule	20	48	68	5,880
Höhere Schule	12	30	42	3,420
Hochschule	9	36	45	1,800
Summe	124	378	502	31,026

$\chi^2 = 2,139$
$\chi^2_{(4;\,0,05)} = 9,488.$ Die Null-Hypothese läßt sich nicht verwerfen.

Tabelle 5

Unterbringungsart der entlassenen und nichtentlassenen bzw. wiederaufgenommenen chronisch schizophren kranken Männer (Untersuchung Juni 1965—Juni 1972)

Unterbringungsart	Entlassen ja a	Entlassen nein b	$\sum_n$	a . p
Freiwillig	22	76	98	4,928
Vormundschaft	46	144	190	11,132
Pflegschaft	10	36	46	2,170
Unterbringungsgesetz	46	122	168	12,558
Summe	124	378	502	30,788

$x^2 = 0,879$
$x^2_{(3;\,0,05)} = 7,815.$ Die Null-Hypothese läßt sich nicht verwerfen.

Mit Tabelle 8 kommen wir zur 2. Fragestellung, nämlich inwieweit Art und Potenz der Neuroleptika für die Gruppe der „entlassenen" und „nicht entlassenen" bzw. „wiederaufgenommenen" von Bedeutung ist.

Es zeigt sich, daß hier (Tabelle 8) ein Unterschied statistisch gesichert werden kann ($\chi^2 = 19,387$; $\chi^2_{(1;\,0,05)} = 0,841$). Nicht mit Neuroleptika behandelte chronisch schizophrenen kranke Männer werden häufiger nicht entlassen bzw. wiederaufgenommen.

Tabelle 9 bestätigt in gewisser Weise dieses Ergebnis und läßt darüber hinaus erkennen, daß die Verabreichung von Kurzzeit- oder Langzeit-Neuroleptika im Hinblick auf die Entlassung keine gesicherte Rolle spielen.

Tabelle 6
Kontakt mit Familiengehörigen der entlassenen und nichtentlassenen bzw. wiederaufgenommenen chronisch schizophren kranken Männer (Untersuchung Juni 1965—Juni 1972)

Kontakt mit Familienangehörigen	Entlassen ja a	Entlassen nein b	$\sum_n$	a . p
Ja	112	296	408	30,688
Nein	12	82	94	1,524
Summe	124	378	502	32,212

$\chi^2 = 8{,}516$;
$\chi^2_{(1;\,0{,}05)} = 3{,}841$.   Die Alternativ-Hypothese ist anzunehmen.

Tabelle 7
Schizophrenieformen der entlassenen und nichtentlassenen bzw. wiederaufgenommenen schizophren kranken Männer (Untersuchung Juni 1965—Juni 1972)

Schizophrenieformen	Entlassen ja a	Entlassen nein b	$\sum_n$	a . p
Produktiv	40	145	185	8,640
Unproduktiv	84	233	317	22,176
Summe	124	378	502	30,816

$\chi^2 = 1{,}010$;
$\chi^2_{(1;\,0{,}05)} = 3{,}841$.   Die Null-Hypothese läßt sich nicht verwerfen.

Tabelle 8
Behandlung mit Neuroleptika der entlassenen und nichtentlassenen bzw. wiederaufgenommenen chronisch schizophren kranken Männer (Untersuchung Juni 1965—Juni 1971)

Behandlung mit Neuroleptika	Entlassen ja a	Entlassen nein b	$\sum_n$	a . p
Ja	82	163	245	27,388
Nein	42	215	257	6,846
Summe	124	378	502	34,234

$\chi^2 = 19{,}387$;
$\chi^2_{(1;\,0{,}05)} = 3{,}841$.   Die Alternativ-Hypothese ist anzunehmen.

TABELLE 9

Art der verabreichten Neuroleptika bei entlassenen und nichtentlassenen bzw. wiederaufgenommenen chronisch schizophren kranken Männer (Untersuchung Juni 1965—Juni 1972).

Art der Neuroleptika	Entlassen ja a	Entlassen nein b	$\sum n$	a · p
Keine	42	215	257	6,846
Kurzzeit — N.	37	72	109	12,543
Langzeit — N.	45	91	136	14,850
Summe	124	378	502	34,239

$\chi^2 = 19{,}413$
$\chi^2_{(2;\,0,05)} = 5{,}991$.   Die Alternativ-Hypothese ist anzunehmen.

TABELLE 10

Potenz der verabreichten Neuroleptika bei entlassenen und nichtentlassenen bzw. wiederaufgenommenen chronisch schizophren kranken Männer (Untersuchung Juni 1965—Juni 1972)

Potenz der Neuroleptika	Entlassen ja a	Entlassen nein b	$\sum n$	a · p
Schwach	10	21	31	3,220
Mittelstark	13	34	47	3,588
Stark	11	11	22	5,500
Sehr stark	48	97	145	15,888
Summe	82	163	245	28,196

$\chi^2 = 3{,}639$;
$\chi^2_{(4;\,0,05)} = 9{,}488$.   Die Null-Hypothese läßt sich nicht verwerfen.

Schließlich ist aus Tabelle 10 zu ersehen, daß sich kein Zusammenhang zwischen den Potenzklassen und den beiden Kollektiven ergibt ($\chi^2 = 3{,}639$; $\chi^2_{(6;\,0,05)} = 12{,}592$).

In Tabelle 10 können naturgemäß nur Patienten eingehen, die Neuroleptika erhalten haben. Andererseits wäre diese Prüfung überflüssig gewesen, wenn in den Tabellen 8 und 9 die Null-Hypothese nicht hätte verworfen werden können. Bei derartigen „Folgetests" muß besonders konservativ getestet, d.h. also der kritische Punkt möglichst hoch angesetzt werden. Daher wird der kritische Punkt für *die* Zahl der Freiheitsgrade aufgesucht, die für die ursprüngliche Tabelle gegolten hätten. Diese hatte 5 Zeilen und 2 Spalten, daher nach $(s-1) \cdot (z-1) = 4$ Freiheitsgrade.

Zusammenfassend läßt sich für das hier ausgewertete Patientengut von 502 langjährig hospitalisierten schizophren kranken Männern einer Abteilung folgendes feststellen:

1. Ein Zusammenhang zwischen „entlassenen" und „nichtentlassenen" bzw. „wiederaufgenommenen" und Merkmalen wie „Soziale Stellung der Eltern", „Soziale Stellung der Patienten", „Familienstand", „Schulbildung" „Unterbringungsart", „produktive und unproduktive Schizophrenieformen" ließ sich statistisch nicht sichern.

2. Zwischen der Gruppe der „Nichtentlassenen" und dem Merkmal „Kein Kontakt mit Familienangehörigen" ließ sich ein Zusammenhang sichern.

3. Nicht mit Neuroleptika behandelte schizophren kranke Männer werden gesichert häufiger „nichtentlassen" bzw. „wiederaufgenommen". Dagegen ließ sich für die Art (Kurz- oder Langzeit-Neuroleptika) und Potenz der verabreichten Neuroleptika in den beiden Kollektiven kein Zusammenhang sichern.

4. Die Untersuchungen machen erneut die Diskrepanz zwischen praktischen Gegebenheiten in der Klinik und theoretisch wissenschaftlichen Forderungen deutlich. Es erhebt sich hier die Frage, inwieweit der Arzt berechtigt ist, einem chronisch schizophren Kranken eine Behandlung mit Neuroleptika vorzuenthalten, nur um den theoretischen Forderungen einer streng zufälligen Zuteilung zu genügen.

5. Die vorgebrachten Ergebnisse beziehen sich auf die endliche Grundgesamtheit der mir zugängigen Patienten und lassen sich auf diese hin verallgemeinern. Es bleibt offen, ob man hieraus eine Verallgemeinerung für sämtliche vergleichbaren chronisch schizophren kranken Männer ziehen kann. Somit ergibt sich erneut ein typisches Beispiel dafür, wie schwierig es ist, verallgemeinernde und wirklich für alle Situationen zutreffende Aussagen zu gewinnen aus Untersuchungen über Ergebnisse, die im täglichen klinischen Ablauf besondere diagnostische und therapeutische Überlegungen voraussetzen. Diese Art der Betrachtungen gilt natürlich auch für die Ergebnisse anderer Autoren.

LITERATURVERZEICHNIS

1. F. ECKMANN (1967) Rehabilitationsversuche bei langjährig hospitalisierten Schizophrenen. Mod. Krankenpflege, **6**.
2. F. ECKMANN (1969) Neuroleptische Potenz und Rehabilitationsversuche bei langjährig hospitalisierten Schizophrenen. In: Sozialpsychiatrische Aspekte bei der Langzeittherapie Schizophrener. Schleswiger Symposium Mai 1969, Janssen, Düsseldorf.
3. D. SPAZIER (1966) Gedanken zur nachgehenden Fürsorge und Rehabilitation bei psychisch Kranken. Nervenarzt, **9**, 381.

F.E., Landeskrankenhaus, 2380 Schleswig-Stadtfeld, B.R.D.

RELATIVE SAFETY AND EFFICACY OF HIGH AND LOW DOSE ADMINISTRATION OF FLUPHENAZINE-HCl TO PSYCHOTIC PATIENTS

R. P. DE BUCK

Psychopharmacological Research Unit, Institute of Psychiatry, University of Brussels

OBJECTIVE

The study was designed to test the following hypotheses:

1. Patients who do not respond adequately to the usual (low) fluphenazine dosage regimen improve on a high dose fluphenazine regimen.
2. The incidence of side-effects, particularly extrapyramidal symptoms, is comparable on low-dose and high-dose fluphenazine therapy.
3. The onset of remission of "psychopathology" is earlier with high dose fluphenazine than with low dose and greater remission is associated with the high-dose regimen.

METHODOLOGY

Patient selection:

To be selected for this study patients had to be:

Males and/or females from age 20 to 55 in good physical condition, in a satisfactory state of nutrition with no debilitating disease.

Any psychoses were acceptable with the exception of "chronic organic psychosis" with superimposed non-psychotic symptomatology, and endogenous depression with retardation and apathy, and "acute organic psychosis".

Chronic patients who had been sick for more than one year and responded inadequately to other forms of treatment (patients who showed only some minor improvement in their behavior but still presented gross psycho-pathology were eligible).

Acute patients who had been sick for less than six months and presented acute symptoms of psychoses (patients who relapsed after satisfactory improvement in their condition might be included in this group).

DESIGN OF THE STUDY

The design called for in this study is summarized below:

Two equal groups of patients were selected at random from the same in-patient population.

One group (the high dose group) started at a dose level of 100 mg per day which was increased by 50 mg every two days. When the daily dosage reached 200 mg, 400 mg, 600 mg and eventually 800 mg each (never higher), patients were maintained on the dosage for a period of 10 days. On the 10th day, if improvement was inadequate, the dosage was increased to the next plateau. If the improvement was satisfactory, however, the patient was kept on the same dosage for 20 more days and then reduced to an adequate maintenance dosage.

This reduction in dosage was progressive, i.e., reduced by 25 mg every 4 days. Since fluphenazine is reported to be rapidly acting and is slowly eliminated, the drug was given twice a day.

The second group received for the first month 5 to 20 mg per day according to the doctor's choice and 20 mg per day for the second month. After the second month, if no satisfactory improvement was observed, the patients were placed on the same high-dosage regimen as was administered to the first group (such patients are said to be members of the cross-over group). If there was satisfactory improvement, no further observations were made (such patients were said to belong to the low-dose-only-group).

The study had the following breakdown of treatment groups:

Group	Number of patients
Low dose only	8
Hig dose only	23
Cross-over	11

Five additional patients could not be classified into any of the dosage regimens listed above because the dosage regimen did not fit into any of the three categories.

OBSERVATIONS MADE

1. *Rating scales*

Each rating scale was completed before treatment began and then every two weeks for the first month of treatment, and once a month thereafter, the last rating coinciding with the end of the trial.

    A. *Global Rating Scales*

Improvement was rated on a seven point scale. The degree of illness was also rated on a seven point scale.

    B. *Brief Psychiatric Rating Scale* (BPRS)
    C. *Nurses Observation Scale for In-patient Evaluation* (NOSIE)
    D. *Side-Effects Rating Scale*

Each side-effect was rated as mild, moderate or severe. Only symptoms recognizable by psychiatrists or nursing staff were recorded. In addition to the rating scale, patients' complaints were recorded only when volunteered by the patients.

2. *Laboratory examinations*

Laboratory examinations were carried out before treatment, on day 15 and thereafter every month. These studies included:

A. Hemogram — including hemoglobin, RBC, WBC and differential.
B. Liver function tests — including SGPT and bilirubin.
C. Urine analysis and blood urea.

3. *Physiological measurements*

A. Weight — recorded every other week.
B. Blood pressure and pulse — sitting and supine, once a day for one week, once a week for one month, and thereafter every two weeks.

Data preparation

All data were coded into computer formats, key-punched and key-verified for computer processing. The data cards were then listed and edited to assure maximum accuracy. Both computer programming and manual systems were used in the edit phase.

All questions of medical interpretation in the coding were resolved under the supervision of George M. Simpson, M.D.

Statistical analysis

The statistical analyses were planned so as to test the hypotheses outlined under "OBJECTIVE".
1. A two-way analysis of variance (patients × time) was performed on each BPRS item and factor, on the NOSIE factors and on the "degree of illness". Patients included in this analysis were selected on the basis of having failed to respond to low dose treatment.

This analysis was carried out to test the null hypothesis that there are no differences in the responses measured at the end of the low dose period and of the high dose period.

2. For the low-dose group and the high-dose group, two-way analyses of variance (time × patients) were performed for each BPRS item and factor, for each NOSIE factor and for the "degree of illness".

These analyses tested the null hypothesis of no differences in psychopathology over time, i.e., the drug was ineffective.

One-way analyses of covariance were performed in order to compare the low-dose-only-group and high-dose-only-group in terms of the end of treatment measurement for each BPRS item and factor, each NOSIE factor and the "degree of illness". The null hypothesis of no difference in the effect of the dose level on psychopathology was tested.

3. The incidence and severity of side-effects were summarized separately for the low-dose-only-patients, the high-dose-only-patients and the low and high dose periods of the cross-over patients.

4. Abnormalities in laboratory data are summarized for each dosage group and their clinical significance is commented on.

5. Analyses of covariance were performed to test the null hypothesis that the low-dose, high-dose and cross-over treatments do not differ in their effect on physiological measurements.

Results

Forty-two patients, 36 of whom were schizophrenics, were evaluated, eight on low dose only, twenty-three on high dose only, and eleven as cross-over patients. Five additional patients could not be assigned to any of these groups and were therefore not included in the analysis. The distributions of age and sex of the patients in each group were summarized in Table 1.

TABLE 1

Fluphenazine high dose investigation
Age vs. sex

Age	Male L.D.	Male H.D.	Male C.	Female L.D.	Female H.D.	Female C.	Total
1—10							0
11—20	1			1			2
21—30	1	10		2	4	1	18
31—40	1	3	1		2	1	8
41—50		2	2	1	2	2	9
51—60			2	1			3
61—70							0
71—80							0
Over 80							0
Total	3	15	5	5	8	4	40

L.D. — Low Dose; H.D. — High Dose; C. — Cross-over.

EFFICACY

1. While eleven patients crossed over from low to high dose, only five of these were low-dose-failures (no greater than "minimally improved" in global rating) with sufficiently complete data for analysis. The analysis of variance contrasting with the baseline, end of low-dose and end of high-dose rating scale results was not evaluated because of the small sample. Only 2 of the 11 cross-over patients had improved in global rating at the end of the low-dose period and 4 of 11 were improved at the end of high-dose.

2. Table 2 summarizes the results of the analysis of covariance comparing the final low-dose ratings (low-dose-only-patients and low-dose period of cross-over patients) with the final ratings of the high-dose-only patients. It can be seen from the table that the groups did not differ significantly on any BPRS items or factors, on any NOSIE factors or on the global rating of improvement or degree of illness. It can be noted that the high-dose group was significantly improved over the baseline on eleven BPRS items, 4 BPRS factors, 5 NOSIE factors and on the degree of illness, while the low-dose patients were significantly improved only on 6 BPRS items, 3 BPRS factors, 1 NOSIE factor and on the degree of illness. An analysis of data was made to attempt to differentiate the onset of response between high- and low-dose fluphenazine therapy. There is no significant indication of a more rapid onset of activity in the high-dose group.

TABLE 2

Fluphenazine high dose investigation.
Analyses of covariance — Summary

BPRS items	Low dose group Baseline	Low dose group Final	No.	High dose group Baseline	High dose group Final	No.
Somatic concern	1.9	2.4	17	2.1	2.0	23
Anxiety	2.9	2.1	18	3.3	2.7	23
Emotional withdrawal	5.8	4.0*	18	5.0	3.3*	23
Conceptual disorganization	5.6	3.4*	18	4.7	2.8*	23
Guilt feelings	1.6	1.1	18	1.7	1.2	23
Tension	3.1	2.7	18	3.8	2.4*	23
Mannerisms and posturing	4.4	4.0	18	4.7	3.2*	23
Grandiosity	2.1	1.5	18	2.8	1.2*	22
Depressive mood	1.8	1.3	18	3.1	1.8*	23
Hostility	2.5	1.6	18	2.8	2.1	23
Suspiciousness	4.7	2.8*	18	3.5	1.9*	22
Hallucinatory behavior	3.5	2.6	17	3.3	1.6*	23
Motor retardation	4.3	3.1*	18	4.0	3.1	23
Uncooperativeness	2.9	2.1	17	3.2	2.2	23
Unusual thought content	5.1	1.9*	18	5.0	3.0*	23
Blunted affect	5.1	3.6*	17	5.7	3.6*	23
Excitement	2.3	1.9	18	3.0	1.4*	23
Disorientation	1.6	1.3	18	2.1	1.7	23
BPRS factors						
Thinking disturbance	13.9	7.7*	17	13.0	7.4*	23
Withdrawal retardation	15.2	10.6*	17	14.7	10.0*	23
Paranoid interpersonal	9.8	6.6*	17	9.4	5.8*	22
Depressive disturbance	9.3	7.2	18	11.9	8.1*	23
NOSIE factors						
Social competence	29.8	30.9	16	23.9	31.7*	22
Social interest	15.6	16.9	16	11.0	20.4*	23
Personal neatness	27.2	23.1	18	18.5	22.9	22
Irritability	11.9	10.8	18	17.5	9.3*	22
Manifest psychosis	8.7	9.8	18	11.1	4.9*	21
Retardation	12.6	7.5*	16	10,5	7.5	22
Total patient assets	142.8	160.3	12	110.2	147.4*	18
Degree of illness						
Global	5.8	4.4*	18	5.8	3.8*	23
Change evaluation		2.8	17		2.3	23

* Significantly different from corresponding baseline at 0.05 level of confidence

3. No sex or diagnosis-related differences are apparent.

In summary, it can be seen from the efficacy data that while no statistically significant advantage of high dose over low dose as a starting regimen is apparent, trends in BPRS, NOSIE and global ratings all point to a superiority of the high-dose treatment. The effect of high-dose treatment on low-dose failures could not be evaluated due to the small sample size.

TABLE 3

Number of significant changes from the baseline

	Number of patients analyzed BPRS NOSIE		Total number of significant changes	Number of significant changes			Number with no significant time contrast
				7—21 days	up to 45 days	up to 90 days	
Low dose	7	3*	5	0	3	4	1
High dose	9	5	15	0	1	13	2

* Not evaluated due to small sample size.

RESULTS

Side-effects

No relationships between age and incidence of side-effects are apparent for any of the treatment groups. No sex-related differences are noted.

Side-effects have been evaluated by dosage group and by the two periods of dosage for the cross-over patients. The incidence rates of side-effects are summarized in Table 4.

TABLE 4

Group (N)	Incidence of all side-effects	Incidence of extra-pyramidal side-effects
Low dose only (8)	2.6	1.5
High dose only (23)	3.7	1.9
Cross-over low period (11)	0.5	0.2
Cross-over high period (11)	1.3	0.5
Low dose* (19)	1.3	0.7

* Including low dose only + cross-over low period.

It can be seen that the high-dose-only-patients reported more side-effects than the low-dose-patients and the cross-over patients reported more side-effects during the high-dose-period than during the low-dose-period.

The extrapyramidal symptoms were of special interest in this study. Dystonic symptoms (including difficulty in swallowing, in standing, spasms of neck or tongue) and akathisia were reported with greater frequency by the high-dose-only-patients than by the low-dose patients (including the cross-over patients' low-dose period).

Since the vast majority of patients in these studies were of the same diagnosis (schizophrenia), no relationship between diagnosis and side-effects was noted.

A higher proportion of side-effects reached the rating "severe" of high-dose-only-treatment (28.9%) than on low-dose (including low-dose period of cross-over patients) treatment (3.8%). The proportion of "moderates" was about the same for low dose (50.0%) and high dose (51.8%) treatment.

For the cross-over patients, of the five side-effects reported on low dose, four were reported by the same patient(s) on high dose. Ten of the fourteen high-dose-reports were made only during the high-dose period.

In summary, analysis of the side-effect data indicates that high-dose Fluphenazine therapy is associated with a higher incidence and greater severity of side-effects than a low dose regimen of the same compound.

Laboratory and physiological findings

TABLE 5

Summary of laboratory abnormalities

Group	WBC	Neutro-phils	Eosinophils 6 or less	Eosinophils over 6	SGPT 40 or less	SGPT over 40	Bilirubin 1 or less	Bilirubin over 1	N
Low dose only	1		4					1	8
High dose only	2		6	1	4	7	1		23
Cross-over-low-dose-period			1		1		1		11
Cross-over-high-dose-period						2			11
Unknown	1				1			1	5

From Table 5 it is noticeable, in particular, that eleven patients exhibited abnormally high SGPT on high-dose-only-treatment compared to only one slight elevation by patients starting therapy on low dose. No other differences between groups were noted.

As to the bi-weekly observation of weight, blood pressure and pulse, while occasional significant changes from the baseline may be noted on these variables, at no time did the groups differ significantly from each other, and in no case was the change of such size as to be of clinical concern.

DISCUSSION

While the sample size of the low-dose failure group was small, and no significant differences between groups were found on the efficacy measures, one should note that most of the results imply trends which indicate a preference for high-dose therapy. High-dose patients as a group improved on more individual parameters than did the low-dose patients.

In summary, it was noted that:

1. While patients improve on both dose regimens, patients are slightly more likely to improve on high-dose fluphenazine therapy.
2. The incidence and severity of side-effects, and particularly extrapyramidal signs, is higher on high dose than on low dose.
3. No significant differences between groups were found in weight, blood pressure on pulse.
4. Except for increased SGPT in several high-dose patients, no differences between groups were noted on liver function or haematology.

SUMMARY

This evaluation was made in 42 psychiatric in-patients, 36 of whom were schizophrenics. Each patient was entered into one of two groups: the low-dose group (5—20 mg fluphenazine per day) and the high dose-group (100—800 mg fluphenazine per day). Patients in each group were treated for up to two months under specific dose titration schedules. Behavioral improvements were measured by Brief Psychiatric, NOSIE-30 and Global Rating Scales. Side-effects were rated. Laboratory examinations and physiological measurements were carried out. All data were coded for computer processing.

Results:

1. Fluphenazine-HCl was an effective treatment in both groups.
2. Trends indicated a preference for high-dose therapy.
3. The incidence and severity of side effects and particularly extrapyramidal signs was higher on the high-dose regimen than on the low-dose regimen.
4. No significant differences between groups were found in weight, blood pressure or pulse.
5. Except for increased SGPT in several high-dose patients, no differences between groups were noted on liver function or haematology.

ACKNOWLEDGEMENT

The author wants to thank SQUIBB Laboratories whose help has been very valuable particularly for the analysis of data which has been performed by Medicine Studies, Inc.

R.P.D.B., Psychopharmacological Research Unit, Institute of Psychiatry of the University, 1020 Brussels, Place Van Gehuchten, 4, Belgium

DIE KOMBINATION VON RATING SCALES UND HANDSCHRIFTTEST ZUR OBJEKTIVIERUNG UND QUANTIFIZIERUNG NEUROLEPTISCHER EFFEKTE. EINE DOPPELBLINDSTUDIE MIT FLUSPIRILENE UND PENFLURIDOL

K. J. LINDEN, M. KNAACK und W. EDEL

Psychiatrische Klinik der Universität, Rheinisches Landeskrankenhaus, Düsseldorf

Bei der Prüfung neuroleptischer Substanzen wirft die Befunderhebung nach wie vor erhebliche Probleme auf. Ein Ziel ist es, im psychopathologischen Bereich abnorme seelische Zustände so objektiv wie möglich zu erfassen und gleichzeitig zu quantifizieren. Erst unter dieser Voraussetzung können intra- und interindividuelle Vergleiche angestellt und statistisch gesichert werden.

Daneben gibt es Bestrebungen, im somatischen Bereich neuroleptische Effekte zu erfassen und als Kriterien zu verwenden, um möglicherweise weitaus zuverlässigere Meßwerte im Zentimeter-Gramm-Sekunden-System zu gewinnen.

In der Psychopathologie gehören inzwischen mehrdimensionale Schätz- oder Bewertungsskalen wie die Wittenborn Psychiatric Rating Scales zum festen Bestand. Solche Skalen basieren meist auf einer größeren Zahl in sich gestufter Symptome, die analog zum klinischen Syndrom faktorenanalytisch zu Clustern oder Symptomenkomplexen zusammengefaßt werden und ein anschauliches Bild des psychopathologischen Querschnitts vermitteln. Die Wittenborn-Skalen (WPRS) haben sich besonders im Bereich der endogenen Psychosen sowohl im anglo-amerikanischen wie im französischen und auch deutschen Sprachraum bewährt.

Weniger erfolgreich sind bisher die Bemühungen verlaufen, im somatischen Bereich Meßgrößen zu finden, die mit den psychischen Effekten der Psychopharmaka korrelieren.

HAASE hat zur Klassifizierung der Neuroleptika die Wirkung auf das extrapyramidale System herangezogen. Er kam nach umfangreichen Untersuchungen zu dem Ergebnis, daß erst mit dem Einsetzen feinmotorischer extrapyramidaler Veränderungen, wie sie sich zuerst und am besten im Schriftbild erkennen lassen, antipsychotische Effekte im engeren Sinne zu erwarten seien. Unterhalb dieser "Schwelle" könne nur mit Tranquilizer-Effekten der Neuroleptika gerechnet werden.

HAASE ging methodisch so vor, daß er an standardisierten Schriftproben in Vers- und Strophenform typische extrapyramidale Schriftveränderungen wie Verkürzung und Verkleinerung etc. durch optischen Vergleich der Schriftbilder abschätzte und in 3 Schweregrade einteilte. Nach seinen Angaben stimmten die Schätzwerte von 3 unabhängigen Auswertern hoch signifikant überein. Die unter diesen Kriterien gewonnenen Schriftveränderungen wurden in Beziehung zu psychopathologischen Befunden anhand einer Symptomenliste gesetzt.

Ausgehend von den Befunden von HAASE hatten die Autoren das Ziel zu prüfen, ob sich statistisch Korrelationen zwischen den psychopathologischen Zustandsbildern und den in der Schrift faßbaren extrapyramidalen feinmotorischen Veränderungen unter neuroleptischer Medikation sichern lassen.

Eine solche Prüfung setzt eine Quantifizierung beider Dimensionen — der psychopathologischen und der somatischen — voraus. Im psychischen Bereich erschien die WPRS nach zahlreichen Vorstudien am besten geeignet.

Zur Vermessung des standardisierten Schriftbildes mußten neue Meßgrößen entwickelt werden.

Als Untersuchungsmodell erschien zu diesem Zweck eine Doppelblindstudie mit 2 Langzeit-Neuroleptika, Fluspirilene und Penfluridol an einer Gruppe von dauerhospitalisierten männlichen Patienten mit chronisch verlaufender Schizophrenie am besten geeignet. Dieses Krankengut bot den Vorteil, daß die Symptomatik der einzelnen Patienten und ihre diagnostische Zuordnung bereits gut bekannt war und daß spontane Änderungen der psychopathologischen Symptomatik kaum zu erwarten waren.

METHODIK

Es handelte sich um 25 männliche Patienten im Alter zwischen 21 und 55 Jahren, die bereits 2 bis 15 Jahre hospitalisiert waren. Von 2 unabhängigen Untersuchern wurde die Diagnose einer chronisch verlaufenden Schizophrenie gestellt. Alle Patienten befanden sich in derselben Krankenabteilung.

Untersuchungsanordnung: In einer ersten etwa 7 Tage dauernden Phase wurde langsam ausschleichend das Medikament, das vorher gegeben worden war (alle Patienten erhielten vorher Neuroleptika), abgesetzt. Es folgte eine Placebo-Phase, in der das Placebo in Form der später zu verabreichenden Wirkstoffe gegeben wurde. Placebo wurde solange verabreicht, bis die von früher bekannte psychotische Symptomatik wieder voll zum Vorschein gekommen war.

Darauf folgte die erste Wirkstoff-Phase, in der der Wirkstoff in langsam ansteigender Dosierung bis zum Erreichen der „Schwelle" (s. unten) gegeben wurde. In der vierten Phase wurde die Dosis weiter gesteigert, bis die psychotische Symptomatik optimal zum Abklingen gebracht worden war.

Anschliessend wurde in 20 Fällen noch ein cross-over mit Austausch der beiden Prüfmedikamente durchgeführt. Über diese Phase wird an anderer Stelle berichtet.

Medikation: Die Medikamente wurden vorher randomisiert. Die Verabreichung erfolgte einmal wöchentlich. Da Fluspirilene parenteral und Penfluridol oral gegeben wird, erhielt jeder Patient jeweils eine Injektion und eine Tablette, wobei nur eine der beiden Applikationsformen Wirkstoff enthielt. Dieselbe Applikationsart wurde bereits in der Placebo-Phase angewendet. Die Wirkstofftabletten enthielten 20 mg Penfluridol, die Injektionslösung 2 mg Fluspirilene pro ml. Die Dosierung erfolgte in „Einheiten", wobei 1 ml Lösung jeweils 1 Tablette entsprach.

Untersuchungsdauer: Die Untersuchung erstreckte sich bei den einzelnen Patienten über einen mittleren Zeitraum von 225 Tagen, im kürzesten Fall 168 Tage, im längsten 273 Tage.

Registrierung der Befunde: Zwei- bis dreimal wöchentlich wurde bei jedem Patienten eine Handschriftenprobe nach dem Schema von HAASE (vierzeilige Volksliedstrophe, dreimal untereinander geschrieben) abgenommen. Zu Beginn bzw. bei Abschluß jeder Phase wurde gemeinsam durch 2 Untersucher die Bewertung des psychischen Befundes mit Hilfe der WPRS durchgeführt.

Auswertung der Befunde: Bei der Vermessung der Schriftbilder wurden folgende Größen erfaßt:

1. Länge einer bestimmten Zeile.
2. Diagonale einer vierzeiligen Strophe.
3. Summe beider Diagonalen einer vierzeiligen Strophe.
4. Fläche einer vierzeiligen Strophe.

Die WPRS wurde nach dem von WITTENBORN angegebenen Verfahren in Standard-Clusterwerte umgerechnet. Die statistische Auswertung der Meßgrößen des Handschrifttests sowie der Faktoren der Wittenborn-Skala erfolgte mit Hilfe des Wilcoxon Matched-Pairs Signed-Ranks Tests.

ERGEBNISSE

Psychopathologischer Verlauf

Während der Absetz- und Placebo-Phase reagierten die Patienten, die alle vorher neuroleptisch behandelt worden waren, unterschiedlich. Bis auf einen Kranken, bei dem keine Exacerbation auftrat, fielen alle Patienten wieder in die psychotischen Zustandsbilder zurück, die schon vorher in der Krankengeschichte beschrieben worden waren und die die ganze Breite der für die Schizophrenie typischen psychopathologischen Symptomatik umfaßte. In der WPRS zeigten sich diese Veränderungen in einer hoch signifikanten Erhöhung der Clusterwerte, die chronisch psychotische Zustandsbilder erfassen: Antriebsstörung mit Negativismus, Apathie und Zurückgezogenheit, produktive psychotische Symptomatik im verbalen und motorischen Bereich, Aggressivität, besonders in Form von Tätlichkeiten sowie der „Hebephrenie"-Cluster, bei dem sich die Untergruppe „albern läppisch" besonders hervorhob. Es fiel auf, daß der Faktor „Paranoia" sich nicht signifikant veränderte. Es entspricht dem klinischen Eindruck, daß bei einzelnen Patienten eine stabile, d.h. auch neuroleptisch nicht beeinflußbare Wahnthematik vorhanden war, die auch nach Absetzen der Neuroleptika konstant blieb.

Die Zeiten vom Absetzen der Medikation bis zum Wiederauftreten der psychotischen Symptomatik variierten erheblich. In 4 Fällen exacerbierte das Krankheitsbild bereits in den ersten 10 Tagen. Innerhalb von 3 Wochen waren insgesamt 9 und nach 50 Tagen 18 Patienten, d. h. 75 % psychotisch geworden, ein letzter erst nach 89 Tagen.

Unter der Medikation von Penfluridol und Fluspirilene bildete sich die psychopathologische Symptomatik in allen 24 Fällen — ein Fall fiel aus, da er, wie bereits erwähnt, nach Absetzen der Vormedikation symptomfrei blieb — wieder deutlich zurück.

In der statistischen Analyse (Tabelle 1) zeigte sich, daß Fluspirilene in allen oben genannten Faktoren der Vormedikation signifikant überlegen war, mit Ausnahme der Wirkung auf die Aggressivität, die der Vormedikation entsprach. Darüber hinaus kam es noch zu weiteren positiven Effekten im Bereich der Faktoren „Paranoia" und "zwanghafte Verhaltensweisen".

Penfluridol hob sich signifikant gegenüber der Vormedikation besonders durch Effekte auf die Faktoren „Antriebsstörung/Negativismus/Rückzug" und „hebephrener" Symptomenkomplex, insbesondere Nachlässigkeit ab. Ein Vergleich zwischen Fluspirilene und Penfluridol ergab, daß Fluspirilene produktiv-psychotische Symptome und die Zwangssymptomatik signifikant stärker beeinflusste. Penfluridol dagegen zeigte eine signifikant bessere Wirkung auf den Antriebsbereich. Die effiziente Wochendosis geht aus Tabelle 2 hervor.

Tabelle 1

Statistischer Vergleich der verschiedenen Untersuchungsphasen nach dem Wilcoxon Matched-Pairs Signed-Ranks Tests anhand der Wittenborn-Skalen

P (two-tailed)	1 — 2	1 — F	1 — P	F — P
I	.31	.012	.025	.58
II	.17	.78	.61	.28
III	.42	.22	.83	.35
IV	+.00024	—.0042	—.00045	—.055
a	.00092	.083	.0039	.047
b	.0096	.0029	.0064	.71
c	—.0058	.0058	.00067	.31
d	.021	.37	.011	.047
V	.00033	.0043	.32	+.020
e	.0094	.0040	.16	.055
f	.00042	.064	.76	.029
VI	.0026	.31	.51	—
g	.13	.74	.86	.25
h	.0019	.22	.40	.97
VII	.26	.024	.31	.40
VIII	.00060	.00032	.0096	.33
i	.030	.00052	.0016	.21
j	.00071	.078	.46	.54
k	.67	.48	.58	.78
IX	.0063	.025	.42	.074
X	.0051	.21	.14	.78
XI	.50	.50	.24	.80
XII	.85	.055	.22	.66

Zeichenerklärung: I—XII — Cluster der Wittenborn-Skalen, 1 — Prämedik., 2 — Placebo-Phase, F — Fluspirilene, P — Penfluridol.

Tabelle 2

	min.	max.	Durchschnitt
Penfluridol	40 mg	90 mg	72,5 mg
Fluspirilene	2 mg	14 mg	7,1 mg

Es muß zur Bewertung dieser Dosen betont werden, daß es sich bei allen Patienten um schwerste, chronisch verlaufende Krankheitsbilder handelte.

Der Handschrifttest

Die quantitative Auswertung des Handschrifttestes erforderte noch besondere methodische Vorarbeiten. Nach HAASE wird als neuroleptische Schwelle das Auftreten erkennbarer feinmotorischer Bewegungshemmung in der Handschrift bei einer individuell unterschiedlichen neuroleptischen Dosis definiert. Um eine Maßeinheit zu gewinnen, wurde vor der Untersuchung festgelegt, daß die Schwelle dann erreicht wird, wenn sich die Länge einer bestimmten Verszeile der Schriftproben um 10—20 % verkürzt hat. Dabei mußte vorausgesetzt werden, daß es nach Absetzen der Vormedikation zu einer Vergrößerung des Schriftbildes kommen würde. Das traf in den meisten Fällen auch zu. Häufig ließ sich initial nach dem Absetzen eine Verkleinerung und dann erst eine Erweiterung des Schriftbildes beobachten. In einem Fall kam es zu einer progredienten Schriftverkleinerung während der ganzen Placebo-Phase, der klinisch eine zunehmende psychomotorische Sperrung entsprach.

Als problematisch erwies sich die Tatsache, daß unter zunehmender Aktivierung der Psychose in manchen Fällen die Schriftbilder tageweise außerordentlich stark variierten. Aus diesem Grunde wurde vor Beginn der Behandlung ein Durchschnittswert aus 5 Schriftproben als Basiswert errechnet.

Bei 4 Patienten ließ sich trotz progredienter Dosissteigerung und antipsychotischer Wirkung der Medikamente eine Schriftveränderung im Sinne der neuroleptischen Schwelle nach den angegebenen Kriterien und auch bei einfacher optischer Kontrolle nicht nachweisen.

Bei den übrigen Patienten wurden folgende Schwellendosierungen (pro Woche) ermittelt:

Tabelle 3

	min.	max.	Durchschnitt
Penfluridol	10 mg	80 mg	45,5 mg
Fluspirilene	1 mg	6 mg	2,8 mg

Die statistische Auswertung erfolgte unter der Hypothese, daß sich für die einzelnen Parameter (Zeilenlänge, Fläche, einfache und gekreuzte Diagonalen) Unterschiede zwischen den einzelnen Untersuchungsphasen nachweisen lassen könnten, insbesondere aber zwischen der Placebo-Phase einerseits und den Wirkstoff-Phasen andererseits. Solche signifikanten Beziehungen ergaben sich nur für die planimetrisch ermittelten Flächenmeßwerte der Schriftproben.

Zusammenfassung

Untersuchungen über den Effekt von Langzeitneuroleptika stellen methodisch hohe Anforderungen, da die Krankheitsverläufe über größere Zeiträume möglichst zuverlässig und konstant erfaßt werden müssen. Deshalb wurde in der vorliegenden Studie bei der Doppelblindprüfung von Fluspirilene und Penfluridol ein Krankengut mit weitgehend konstanter Symptomatik in konstantem Milieu gewählt. Als standardisiertes Testverfahren zur Erfassung des psychopathologischen Befundes dienten die klinisch bewährten Wittenborn-Skalen.

Außerdem erschien die Untersuchungsanordnung geeignet, für den Handschrifttest nach Haase Meßmethoden zu entwickeln und ihn damit einer statistischen Bearbeitung zugänglich zu machen.

Die Wittenborn-Skalen lieferten auch über längere Beobachtungsperioden hinweg qualitativ und quantitativ exakte und zuverlässige psychopathologische Daten, aus denen sich das Wirkungsspektrum der geprüften Neuroleptika klar erkennen ließ.

Als Meßgröße zur Auswertung des Handschrifttestes hat sich unter verschiedenen Möglichkeiten nur die Fläche des Schriftbildes als brauchbar erwiesen. Damit steht jetzt eine Methode zur Verfügung, mit deren Hilfe die Beziehungen zwischen psychopathologischen und extrapyramidalen Effekten der Neuroleptika statistisch weiter aufgeklärt werden können.

K.J.L., Im Asemwald 56/11/602, 7 Stuttgart-70, B.R.D.

CLINICAL AND NEUROPHYSIOLOGICAL INVESTIGATIONS OF COMBINED THIORIDAZINE — d-AMPHETAMINE MAINTENANCE THERAPY AND WITHDRAWAL IN CHILDHOOD BEHAVIOR DISORDERS[*]

J. SIMEON, B. SALETU, G. VIAMONTES, M. SALETU and T. ITIL

Department of Psychiatry, St. Louis Division, Missouri Institute of Psychiatry, School of Medicine, University of Missouri-Columbia, St. Louis, Mo.

INTRODUCTION

The use of stimulant drugs such as dextroamphetamine and methylphenidate in children with behavior disorders is based on the drugs' beneficial effects on behavior, performance and learning (2, 6, 11, 21, 36). These and other psychotropic drugs are too often given to both improved and unimproved children for periods that may be either shorter or longer than needed for maximum beneficial effects.

Childhood behavior disorders have been treated with amphetamines for 35 years, but many medical and social issues concerning their use remain unanswered or controversial. An estimated three per cent of elementary school children suffer from moderate or severe hyperkinetic disorders, and the increasing and often indiscriminate use of stimulant medication in such children has aroused public concern.

Thus there seems to be a necessity for more information concerning drugs most effective in the therapy of childhood behavior disorders, the need for maintenance treatment with such drugs, the psychopathological changes during withdrawal and finally an objective indicator of therapy responsiveness in patients. As we have demonstrated in recent years, the latter could very well be found in the quantitatively analyzed EEG and evoked potentials, since alterations in behavior have been found to be directly correlated to neurophysiological changes during psychotropic drug treatment (16—20, 24—26).

The goals of this study were to evaluate the behavioral and neurophysiological effects of a combined d-amphetamine — thioridazine therapy and drug withdrawal in childhood behavior disorders.

METHOD

In the survey of 101 children attending an outpatient psychiatric department, 12 boys 6—13 years (mean, 9 years) of age, suffering from chronic severe behavior disorders, were treated with a combination of thioridazine and d-amphetamine for periods of 8 to 76 weeks (mean, 44). The simultaneous administration of these two drugs was based on the favorable results one of the authors had obtained in clinical practice treating

---

[*] Supported in part by the Psychiatric Research Foundation of Missouri.

children with these disorders, diagnosed as hyperkinetic behavior disorders, but with frequent secondary diagnoses of overanxious or unsocialized aggressive reactions. Maximum daily dosages of thioridazine ranged from 30 to 80 mg (mean, 47 mg), and of d-amphetamine from 10 to 25 mg (mean, 18 mg). To obtain further evidence of thioridazine — d-amphetamine efficacy in hyperkinetic childhood behavior disorders, seven more boys, 8—11 years (mean, 9 years) old, were given this drug combination for a period of 8—16 (mean, 10) weeks. Daily dosages of thioridazine ranged from 20 to 100 mg (mean, 59 mg) and of d-amphetamine from 10 to 20 mg (mean, 13 mg).

To evaluate the need for maintenance treatment with the drug combination, determine the occurrence of any drug withdrawal effects and correlate the behavioral changes to quantitatively analyzed EEG and visual evoked responses (VEP), thioridazine was discontinued first while d-amphetamine was maintained. Four weeks later d-amphetamine was stopped and placebo given instead.

The study called for behavioral and neurophysiological evaluations for at least three weeks after d-amphetamine withdrawal. This was not possible, however, as deteriorating behavior in 16 patients necessitated retreatment with combined drug therapy, which started one week after d-amphetamine withdrawal.

Clinical evaluations were made weekly by the treating psychiatrist using the Clinical Global Impression Rating scale (Early Clinical Drug Evaluation Units — ECDEU) and the Treatment Emergent Rating scale (ECDEU) as well as by the parents using the parent's questionnaire (3, 7).

Neurophysiological investigations were carried out in the second and fourth weeks of d-amphetamine treatment only (thioridazine withdrawal), on the first, third and sixth days of placebo administration (d-amphetamine withdrawal) and during the eighth week of retreatment with combined thioridazine—d-amphetamine. A 10-minute resting EEG was recorded utilizing the 10×20 system. The right occipital-right ear lead was analyzed off-line based on period analysis (4) using a digital computer (PDP-12) (30). This program permits analysis of the primary wave and its first derivative in 10-second epochs at the sampling rate of 320 points per second. Twenty-two EEG measurements were obtained from each EEG epoch (eight different frequency bands, average frequency and frequency deviation of both the primary wave and the first derivative as well as the average amplitude and amplitude variability (DROHOCKI)).

Visual evoked potentials (VEP) were elicited by light flashes produced by a Grass TS-2 photic stimulator at dial intensity 4, which is equivalent to 375,000 candle power at a distance of 10 inches (25 centimeter) with an assumed square pulse of 10 microseconds. The lamp face was centered 6 inches in front of the glabella. The rate of the stimulus presentation was randomized (6 stimuli over 20 seconds). Electrodes were placed over the right and left occipital region with the reference electrodes at the ipsilateral earlobes. VEPs were amplified with two Tektronix type 122 pre-amplifiers in series with two transistorized post-amplifiers and were fed into a CAT 400B for summation. The analysis time was 500 msec. A squared-wave calibration of 9.5 microvolts in series with the recording electrodes was fed into the input of the pre-amplifiers ahead of the evoked responses. Each averaged VEP of 50 stimuli was finally plotted on a Mosely X—Y plotter (five times per session).

Statistical analysis included 1 sample t-test, 2 sample t-test, Wilcoxon test, Spearman Rank correlation, and Pearson Product Moment correlation on an IBM 370.

Results

A. Behavioral investigations

On admission the global degree of illness for the total group of 19 children was evaluated as severe in six patients, marked in ten, and moderate in three (Table 1). Treatment with combined thioridazine and d-amphetamine resulted in marked clinical global improvement in nine, and moderate or slight in five each. The global severity of illness became borderline in three patients, mild in 13, and moderate in two. No adverse effects were noticed during drug administration, and the children apparently tolerated the combination quite well.

TABLE 1

Effects of combined thioridazine — d-amphetamine therapy, withdrawal and retreatment on clinical global severity of illness in childhood behavior disorders
(N=19)

Patient	Admission	Thioridazine and d-amphetamine	d-Amphetamine only (thioridazine withdrawal) Week 2	Week 4	Placebo (d-amphetamine withdrawal) Day 3	Day 6	Thioridazine and d-amphetamine (retreatment) Week 4	Week 8
JTr.	6	3	3	4	4	4	2	2
WB	6	3	3	3	3	4	2	5
CW	6	3	3	4	3	4	4	4
RM	6	3	4	5	5	5	3	5
BSi.	6	3	4	5	5	5	5	4
PP	5	2	3	4	4	5	2	3
RW	5	2	4	3	3	4	4	4
AS	5	2	3	4	4	5	4	4
TB	5	3	4	5	5	6	3	3
KM	5	3	4	5	5	6	3	2
MM	5	3	3	4	4	4	2	2
BSk.	5	3	3	3	4	3	4	5
JTe.	5	3	2	5	4	5	4	5
MD	4	3	2	4	5	5	2b	2b
RS	4	3	4	3	3	3	3	3
JE	5	4	4	5	4	5	5b	5b
SG	4	3	3	3	3	3	3b	2b
WK	5	4	4	4	4	5	2	3
CK	6	5a	4	5	5	6	2	5
Mean	5.1*	2.9*	3.4	4.1	4.1	4.6	3.1	3.6

a) Received d-amphetamine only
b) Received placebo only.
* Patient CK excluded.

Severity of illness:
1. Normal
2. Borderline ill.
3. Mildly ill.
4. Moderately ill.
5. Markedly ill.
6. Severely ill.
7. Most severely ill.

Following thioridazine withdrawal while d-amphetamine administration was maintained, eight of 18 patients*) were worse within two weeks and 13 within four. By the sixth day of d-amphetamine withdrawal, six of these 13 children showed further behavioral deterioration, and three others (including one that received no thioridazine but only d-amphetamine) also relapsed (Table 2). The severity of illness was rated as mild in three

TABLE 2

Relapses (—) during withdrawal of thioridazine and d-amphetamine
(N = 18)

PERIOD / PATIENT	d-AMPHETAMINE (THIORIDAZINE WITHDRAWAL) WEEK 2	WEEK 4	PLACEBO (d-AMPHETAMINE WITHDRAWAL) DAY 6	WEEK 3
CW		—		
JTe.		—		
JE		—		
MM		—		
JTr.		—		
RM	—	—		
BSi.	—	—		
PP	—	—	—	
AS	—	—	—	
TB	—	—	—	
KM	—	—	—	
RW	—	—	—	
RS	—	+	—	
MD	—	—	—	+
WB			—	
WK			—	
BSk.				
SG				

Some patients relapsed during thioridazine withdrawal, others during thioridazine and d-amphetamine withdrawal, while a third group relapsed during d-amphetamine withdrawal only.

children, moderate in five, marked in eight and severe in three. Within three weeks of d-amphetamine withdrawal, two more patients gradually relapsed, while one improved. Only two (MD and SG), rated as borderline mentally ill, continued to do well and still had received no drug therapy 11 weeks after drug withdrawal. After eight weeks of retreating 16 patients with combined thioridazine and d-amphetamine, global improvement was marked in two, moderate in four, slight in three and none in five, while two were worse. The dosages were the same as for the first trial, with individual readjustments when indicated. The lesser degrees of improvement during retreatment as compared to the first trial may have been due to the smaller group mean for the severity of illness than the one during admission. Compared to the first trial, drug combination retreatment resulted in further improvement in four children, no change in two and worsening in nine.

The mean change and distribution of global scores for each of the periods are shown on Table 3. The mean change of global scores for each successive period from admission

---

*) The nineteenth child discontinued the study, and was replaced by another who received d-amphetamine only without thioridazine.

to thioridazine-d-amphetamine therapy, the fourth week of d-amphetamine treatment alone, the sixth day of d-amphetamine withdrawal and fourth week of combined drug retreatment was significant at the $P < .01$ level (Wilcoxon test). The change from the sixth day of d-amphetamine withdrawal to the eighth week of retreatment was significant at the $P < .05$ level (Wilcoxon test).

TABLE 3

Mean change and distribution of clinical global scores in children with behavior disorders during thioridazine — d-amphetamine therapy, withdrawal and retreatment
(N = 19)

PERIOD / SEVERITY OF ILLNESS	ADMISSION	THIORIDAZINE & d-AMPHETAMINE	d-AMPHETAMINE ONLY WEEK 2	WEEK 4	PLACEBO DAY 3	DAY 6	THIORIDAZINE & d-AMPHETAMINE WEEK 4	WEEK 8
1. NORMAL								
2. BORDERLINE		3	2				7	5
3. MILD		13 (2.9)	8	5 (3.4)	5	3	5 (3.1)	4 (3.5)
4. MODERATE	3	2	9	7 (4.1)	8 (4.1)	5 (4.6)	5	4
5. MARKED	10 (5.1)	1a		7	6	8	2	6
6. SEVERE	6					3		
7. MOST SEVERE								

a Received d-Amphetamine only   * $P < .01$ Wilcoxon test

Evaluations done by the parents during the long-term combined thioridazine — d-amphetamine treatment demonstrated that seven symptoms on an 81-item rating scale (3) improved significantly ($P < .05$, Wilcoxon test) as compared to admission: doing poorly in school work; cannot pay attention for a long time; inability to relax and seems tense; always on the go, cannot sit or lie still; nervous, jittery, jumpy; gets angry easily, has a bad temper; temper tantrums. Both global and symptomatic improvement were related to the duration of the therapy: the longer the course of drug therapy, the greater the global improvement ($p < .05$, Spearman Rank correlation) and the larger the percentage of improved symptoms ($P < .05$, Pearson Product Moment correlation).

Based on a 93-item parent's questionnaire (7), 42 symptoms were grouped in eight clusters: 1. conduct, 2. anxiety, 3. impulsivity-hyperkinesis, 4. learning problem, 5. psychosomatic problem, 6. perfectionism, 7. antisocial behavior and 8. muscular tension. Analyses (t-test and Wilcoxon test) demonstrated significant changes after both thioridazine and d-amphetamine withdrawal (Table 4). After thioridazine withdrawal, anxiety, tension, impulsivity, hyperactivity, learning and psychosomatic complaints became worse, while antisocial behavior improved. After d-amphetamine withdrawal, impulsivity-hyperactivity, tension and learning showed further worsening, antisocial

TABLE 4

Mean changes in symptomatology of 18 behaviorally disturbed children during thioridazine and d-amphetamine treatment, withdrawal and retreatment
(based on parent's questionnaire)

Period	Combined treatment before discontinuation of thioridazine				d-Amphetamine only				Placebo		Retreatment	
Symptom cluster	3rd	2nd	1st	Disc.	1st	2nd	3rd	4th	1st	3rd	6th	4th	8th
	Week				Week				Day		Week	
	A	B	C	D	E	F	G	H	I	J	K	L	M
Conduct	0.8	0.8	0.8	1.1	1.1	1.1	0.9	0.9	0.9	0.8	0.9	0.9	1.2
Anxiety	0.3	0.2	0.3	0.2	0.6	0.3	0.3	0.5	0.3	0.3	0.3	0.3	0.3
Impulsive Hyperactive	0.8	0.7[a]	1.1	0.6	0.7	0.7	0.7	0.7	0.8	0.8	0.9	0.9[fc]	1.2[fc]
Learning problem	0.6	0.5	0.5[b]	0.4	0.5	0.6	0.5	0.6	0.6	0.7	0.7[e]	0.5[f]	1.1[jihgd]
Psychosomatic	0.2	0.2	0.1	0.1	0.2	0.2	0.2	0.2	0.2	0.2	0.2	0.2	0.2
Perfectionism	0.2	0.2	0.2	0.2	0.2	0.4	0.3	0.1	0.2	0.2	0.2	0.2	0.4
Antisocial	0.2	0.2	0.2	0.2	0.1	0.1	0.1	0.1	0.1	0.1	0.1	0.1	0.0
Muscular tension	0.3	0.2	0.2	0.1	0.2	0.2	0.2	0.3	0.3	0.3	0.3	0.3	0.3

a ... $P < .05$, t-test (as compared with A)
b ... $P < .05$, Wilcoxon (as compared with A)
c ... $P < .05$, t-test (as compared with D)
d ... $P < .01$, t-test (as compared with D)
e ... $P < .05$, Wilcoxon (as compared with D)
f ... $P < .01$, Wilcoxon (as compared with D)
g ... $P < .01$, t-test (as compared with H)
h ... $P < .01$, t-test (as compared with L)
i ... $P < .05$, Wilcoxon (as compared with H)
j ... $P < .05$, Wilcoxon (as compared with L)

Score code: 0 ... not at all
1 ... just a little
2 ... pretty much
3 ... very much

behavior remained unchanged, while conduct and anxiety improved. Following eight weeks of retreatment with thioridazine — d-amphetamine, impulsivity-hyperactivity, conduct, learning and perfectionism were worse; tension, anxiety and psychosomatic problems remained unchanged, while antisocial behavior improved. A more detailed report of symptomatic changes evaluated by parents and teachers, and psychometric tests will be made elsewhere (31, 32).

B. *Neurophysiological investigations*

1. *Visual evoked potential findings*

Within the first 500 msec. following the photic flash, 10 peaks were identified (Fig. 1). According to the descriptive nomenclature of CIGÁNEK (5), peaks 1, 2 and 3 can be considered as primary response. However, peaks 1 and 2 were not always recognizable and often merged with wave 3, as noted previously by CREUTZFELDT and KUHNT (8) and

SALETU et al. (23), and were thus omitted from statistical analysis. Peak 4 marks the beginning of the secondary response, whereas peaks 8, 9 and 10 can be looked upon as the beginning of the after-discharge.

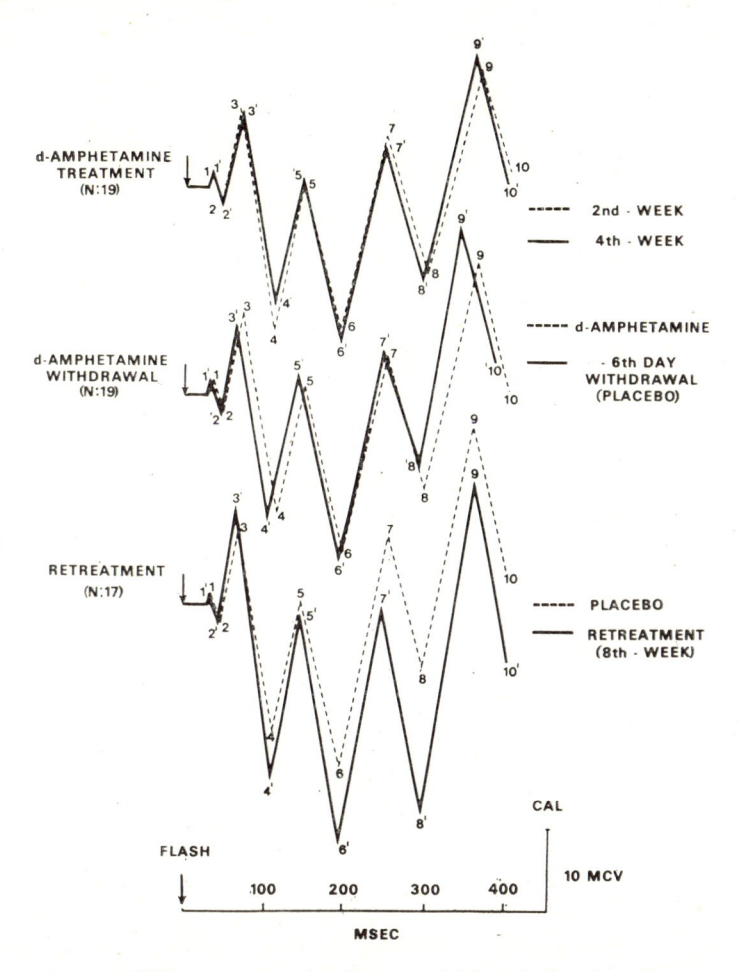

Fig. 1. Schematic mean VEPs of behaviorally disturbed children during d-amphetamine treatment, withdrawal and combined thioridazine and d-amphetamine retreatment.

Statistical analysis demonstrated a slight latency increase and a significant ($P < .05$, t-test) decrease in the late peaks during the fourth as compared with the second week of d-amphetamine treatment (Fig. 2). The amplitude was augmented in peaks 9—10 ($P < .01$). After discontinuation of d-amphetamine, the latency of all peaks decreased, reaching the level of statistical significance ($P < .01$—$.05$) in one variable on the first and sixth days of withdrawal and in four variables on the third day of withdrawal. Thus the latency changes were maximal on the third day. Alterations in amplitudes were unsystematic and not significant. During the eighth week of retreatment with combined thioridazine and d-amphetamine, the latency changes were small as compared with the placebo period, but the amplitude increased significantly in peaks 3—4, 7—8 and 8—9 ($P < .05$).

When the total patient population was divided into therapy responsive and resistant groups on the basis of therapeutic outcome during retreatment as compared with the

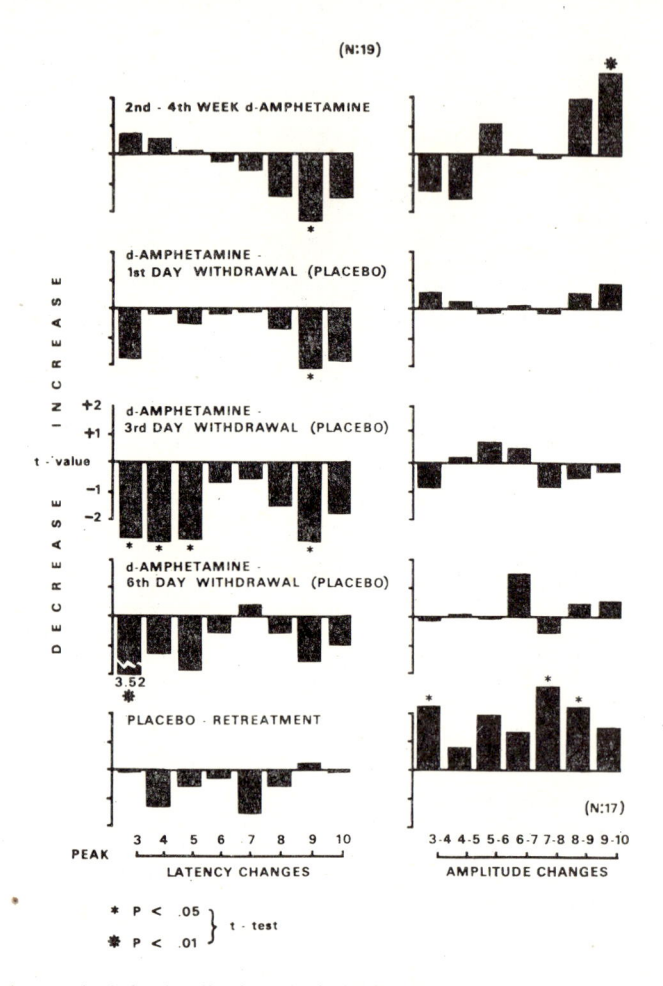

Fig. 2. VEP changes in behaviorally disturbed children during d-amphetamine treatment, withdrawal and combined thioridazine and d-amphetamine retreatment. Combined treatment produced a significant amplitude increase, while withdrawal a significant latency decrease in the evoked potential.

withdrawal phase (therapy responsive patients showed at least one point improvement in global score), a latency decrease (significant at the $P < .05$ level in peak 8) was observed in the responsive group, whereas resistant patients revealed no significant latency changes (Fig. 4). The latter group, on the other hand, showed a greater amplitude augmentation, reaching the level of statistical significance in peaks 3—4. However, there were no statistically significant differences between the changes in the responsive and resistant groups ($P < .05$, two sample t-test).

2. EEG findings

EEG digital computer period analysis demonstrated a significant ($P < .05$, t-test) increase of fast activity during the fourth week as compared with the second week of d-amphetamine treatment (Fig. 3). A slight increase in average frequency and amplitude was observed as well.

After discontinuation of d-amphetamine, theta and alpha activity increased, whereas beta activity, average frequency and frequency deviation decreased. The amplitude showed a tendency to increase further on. These alterations reached their maximum on the third day of withdrawal. During the retreatment with combined thioridazine and

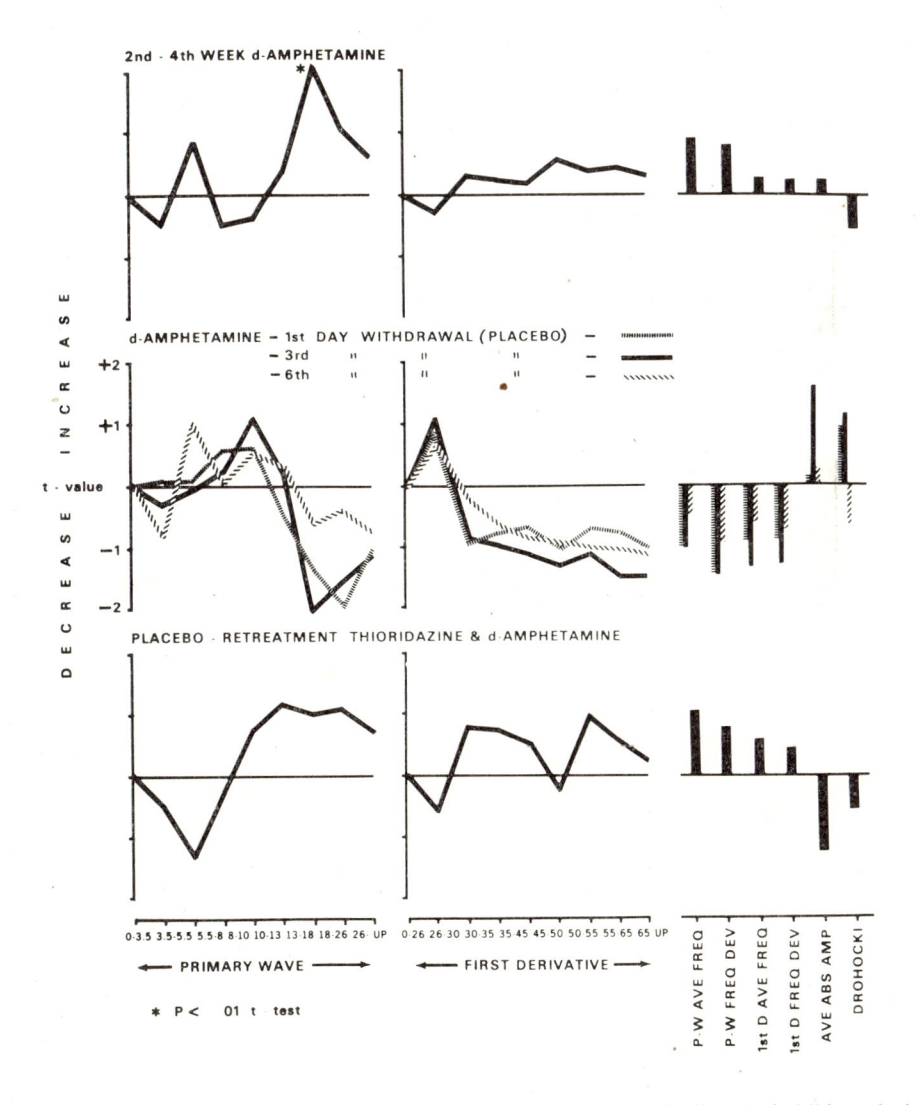

Fig. 3. Changes in EEG period analysis measurements in behaviorally disturbed children during d-amphetamine treatment, withdrawal and combined thioridazine and d-amphetamine retreatment.

d-amphetamine, average frequency, frequency deviation and fast activity again increased, whereas slow activity, amplitude and amplitude variability were attenuated. However, the findings of neither the withdrawal nor the retreatment period reached the level of statistical significance.

Statistical analysis of the EEG data regarding therapy responsiveness during retreatment as compared with the placebo period demonstrated significant differences between the therapy responsive and resistant children (Fig. 4). The former exhibited a marked increase of average frequency, frequency deviation and fast activity as well as a decrease of slow activity, amplitude and amplitude variability, which reached the level of statistical significance in 12 variables ($P < .01$—$.05$, t-test). In contrast, resistant patients revealed

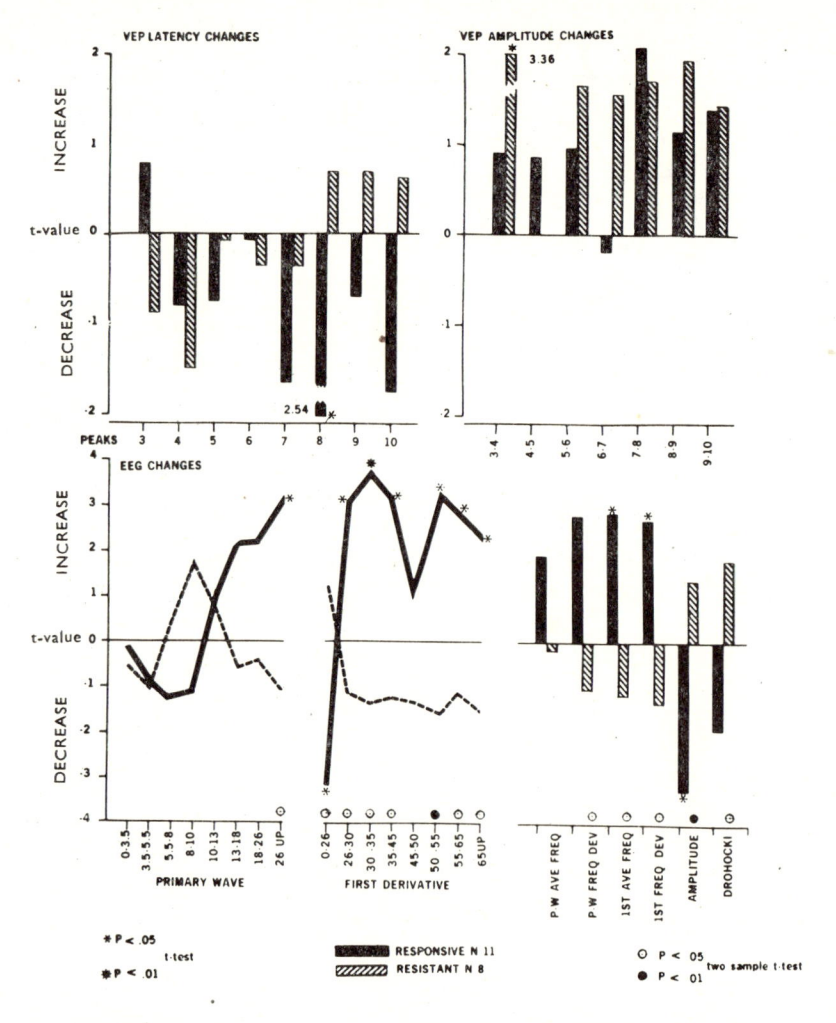

Fig. 4. VEP and EEG changes in therapy responsive and resistant children during retreatment with combined thioridazine and d-amphetamine treatment. Computerized EEG changes were statistically significant in the responsive patients, but not in the resistant ones.

a decrease of average frequency, frequency deviation and fast activity as well as an increase of amplitudes, amplitude variability and slow activity. The differences between these contrasting changes were significant in 13 variables (P < .01—.05, 2 sample t-test).

Discussion

The results of this study suggest that while some children with hyperkinetic behavior disorders benefit most from either minor stimulants or neuroleptic drug therapy, others respond even better to a combination of both. Although in animal studies low doses of chlorpromazine have potentiated the effects of amphetamines on avoidance learning (9), psychomotor stimulation (1, 29, 35) stereotyped behavior (13), and caused an elevation of amphetamine levels in rat brains (1) it is doubtful that the beneficial clinical effects in this study were due to a potentiation of d-amphetamine by thioridazine. Clinical investigators have indicated a greater improvement of irritability, aggressivity and destructiveness in "hyperactive children" and "behavior disorders" treated with phenothiazines than with stimulants (11, 33). It is conceivable that these children suffer from multiple disorders that may respond to the synergistic effect of a "stimulant"-neuroleptic combination.

The high rate of clinical relapses, even after prolonged therapy, was an unexpected finding; it indicates that many children with behavior disorders who respond with improvement to stimulant medication may require long-term drug maintenance, possibly even beyond the usually recommended cut-off age of 12. Other studies in delinquent boys, 11—17 years old, who had improved with d-amphetamine, have also demonstrated clinical relapses when the drug was discontinued (10).

Our neurophysiological findings demonstrated significant alterations in the quantitatively analyzed EEG and VEP during thioridazine and d-amphetamine withdrawal as well as during retreatment. The steady deterioration in clinical symptomatology during both withdrawal phases was accompanied by a continuous decrease in VEP latencies. Although these findings confirmed our previous results concerning a direct correlation between clinical improvement and deterioration on the one hand and EP changes on the other (24—26), they were nevertheless surprising. After discontinuation of d-amphetamine, one would expect changes in the opposite direction from those observed in the second to fourth weeks of d-amphetamine treatment. However, one must bear in mind that all recordings were done after withdrawal from thioridazine. Since major tranquilizers produce latency increases (27), the thioridazine withdrawal might result in a long-lasting attenuation in latencies potentiated by d-amphetamine. Stimulatory drugs have been found to decrease EP latencies in normal adults (28).

Digital computer period analysis of the EEG demonstrated an increase of fast activity from the second to the fourth weeks of d-amphetamine treatment. During d-amphetamine withdrawal, an increase of slow and decrease of fast activity occurred, followed by changes in the opposite direction after the start of retreatment with combined thioridazine and d-amphetamine.

One of the most important findings is the fact that neurophysiological changes preceded the psychopathological alterations. While both EEG and VEP changes reached their maximum on the third day of d-amphetamine withdrawal, clinical changes were greatest on the sixth day. That the quantitative EEG is of considerable value in predicting therapeutic outcome has been stated previously (18). The findings of the present study may be another important step in determining whether or not a patient needs drug therapy maintenance.

A further intriguing result was the contrasting EEG alterations of therapy responsive and resistant patients during the retreatment phase. Neurophysiological differences between such groups of patients have been described repeatedly in schizophrenia utilizing evaluation of the awake EEG (12, 14—16, 34), thiopental-activated EEG (16, 22), and natural all-night sleep (22). The present findings may even elucidate the pharmacodynamics of combined drug treatment with neuroleptic and stimulatory compounds. As we know, slow EEG activity is induced by major tranquilizers, while fast activity is produced by stimulatory drugs. One could hypothesize that therapy responsive children are more susceptible to the therapeutic efficacy of d-amphetamine than therapy resistant ones, who exhibit more major tranquilizer-induced alterations in their brain activity.

Although our clinical findings may have clarified some questions concerning the treatment of behaviorally disturbed children, further neurophysiological investigations of the effects of psychotropic drugs and their withdrawal are necessary in order to allow a better definition of diagnostic sub-types, to determine the length and optimal drug dosage of drug administration and to predict the therapeutic outcome.

Summary

The necessity for maintenance of drug treatment was studied in a group of 19 children suffering from severe and chronic hyperkinetic behavior disorders with frequent secondary diagnosis of over-anxious and unsocialized aggressive reaction. Clinical and behavioral investigations were carried out at admission, during long-term treatment with combined thioridazine and d-amphetamine, after discontinuation of thioridazine and during the subsequent d-amphetamine withdrawal as well as during retreatment with combined thioridazine and d-amphetamine. Based on the global clinical impression as rated by the psychiatrist, it was found that during long-term combined drug treatment the overall symptomatology improved markedly in 9 patients, moderately and slightly in 5 each. In regard to side effects, the drug combination was well tolerated. Within 4 weeks of thioridazine withdrawal (while d-amphetamine was maintained) 13 patients became worse. When d-amphetamine was also discontinued, 6 of the 13 patients deteriorated even further and another 3 also relapsed. In 16 children drug retreatment was necessary, resulting in significant improvement.

A more detailed evaluation of the children's symptomatology by the parents based on the parent's questionnaire generally yielded similar results. Both global and symptomatic improvement was related to the duration of therapy: the longer the course of drug therapy the greater the global improvement and the larger the percentage of improved symptoms.

Neurophysiological investigations were carried out during both withdrawal phases and the retreatment period. A continuous latency decrease was found in the VEP during both withdrawal phases while amplitude changes were not significant. After retreatment, on the other hand, latency changes were small but amplitudes showed a significant augmentation. Digital computer period analysis of the EEG demonstrated an increase of fast activity during thioridazine withdrawal. After discontinuation of d-amphetamine, an increase of slow and decrease of fast activity occurred, followed by changes in the opposite direction during retreatment with combined drugs. Interestingly, both VEP and EEG changes were found to be ahead of psychopathological alterations. When the total patient population was divided into therapy responsive and resistant groups based on the therapeutic outcome during retreatment, significant differences in their drug-induced EEG changes came to the fore: while the therapy responsive group exhibited a marked increase of average frequency, frequency deviation and fast activity as well as a decrease of slow activity, amplitude and amplitude variability, resistant patients showed changes in completely opposite directions.

Acknowledgements

The authors would like to express their thanks to Charles Coffin, M.S., Computer Programmer and Statistician, William Hsu, M.S., Systems Analyst and Statistician, Patricia McDonnell, RN, Coordinating Nurse, Mary Clark, M.S. Editorial Assistant, George Wassilchenko and Timothy Stroop, Medical Illustration and Photography, the EEG staff for their valuable assistance, Barbara McKinney, Secretary.

References

1. Borella, L., Herr, F. and Wojdan, A. (1969) Prolongation of certain effects of amphetamine by chlorpromazine. Can. J. Physiol. Pharmacol. 47, 7.
2. Bradley, C. (1950) Benzedrine and dexedrine in the treatment of children's disorders. Pediatrics, 5, 24.
3. Brugger, T. Problem check-list for psychiatric disorders in children. Washington University Child Guidance Clinic, St. Louis, Missouri.
4. Burch, N. R., Nettleton, W. H., Sweeney, J. et al. (1964) Period analysis of the electroencephalogram on a general purpose digital computer. Ann. N. Y. Acad. Sci. 115, 827.
5. Cigánek, L. (1961) The EEG response (evoked potential) to light stimulus in man. Electroenceph. clin. Neurophysiol. 13, 165.
6. Conners, C. K. (1971) Stimulant drugs and cortical evoked responses in learing. In: Smith, W. L. (ed.): Drugs, Development and Cerebral Function. Charles C. Thomas, Springfield, Illinois, p. 179.
7. Conners, C. K. (1970) Symptom patterns in hyperkinetic, neurotic, and normal children. Child Develop. 41, 667.
8. Creutzfeldt, O. D. and Kuhnt, V. (1967) The visual evoked potential: physiological, developmental and clinical aspects. In: Cobb, W. and Morocutti, C. (eds.): The Evoked Potentials. Amsterdam, Elsevier, p. 4.
9. Del Rio, J. (1970) Facilitating effects of some chlorpromazine-d-amphetamine mixtures on avoidance learning. Psychopharmacologia, 21, 39.
10. Eisenberg, L., Lachman, R., Molling, P., et al. (1963) A psychopharmacologic experiment in a training school for delinquent boys: methods, problems, findings. Amer. J. Orthopsych. 33, 431.
11. Fish, B. (1971) The "one child, one drug" myth of stimulants in hyperkinesis. Arch. gen. Psychiat. 25, 193.
12. Flügel, F., Itil, T. M. and Stoerger, R. (1964) Klinische und elektro-encephalographische Untersuchungen bei therapieresistenten schizophrenen Psychosen. In: Bradley, P. B., Flügel, Hoch, P. H. (eds.): Neuro-Psychopharmacology. Amsterdam, Elsevier, p. 474.
13. Halliwell, G., Quinton, R. M. and Williams, F. E. (1964) A comparison of imipramine, chlorpromazine and related drugs in various tests involving autonomic functions and antagonism of reserpine. Brit. J. Pharmacol. 23, 330.
14. Igert, C. and Lairy, G. C. (1962) Intérêt pronostique de l'EEG au cours de l'evolution des schizophrènes. Electroenceph. clin. Neurophysiol. 14, 183.
15. Itil, T. M. (1961) Die Veränderungen der Pentothal-Reaktion im Electroencephalogramm bei Psychosen unter der Behandlung mit psychotropen Drogen. Proceedings of the III World Congress of Psychiatry, Univ. of Toronto Press, 947.
16. Itil, T. M. (1964) Elektroencephalographische Studien bei endogenen Psychosen und deren Behandlung mit psychotropen Medikamenten unter besonderer Berücksichtigung des Pentothal-Elektroencephalogramms. Istambul, Ahmet Sait Matbaasi.
17. Itil, T. M., Hsu, W., Saletu, B. et al. (1971) Effects of fluphenazine hydrochloride on digital computer sleep prints of schizophrenic patients. Dis. nerv. Syst. 32, 751.
18. Itil, T. M. and Saletu, B. (in press) Quantitative Wach-EEG, Schlaf-EEG und EP-Untersuchungen im schizophrenen Krankengut. Presented at the V World Congress of Psychiatry, Mexico City, Mexico, November 28 — December 4, 1971.

19. ITIL, T. M., SALETU, B., HSU, W. et al. (1971) Clinical and quantitative EEG changes at different dosage levels of fluphenazine treatment. Acta. psychiat. scand. **47**, 440.
20. ITIL, T. M., STOCK, M. J., DUFFY, A. D. et al. (1972) Therapeutic trials and EEG investigations with SCH-12, 679 in behaviorally disturbed adolescents. Curr. ther. Res. **14**, 136.
21. Report of the conference on the use of stimulant drugs in the treatment of behaviorally disturbed young school children sponsored by the Office of Child Development and the Office of the Assistant Secretary for Health and Scientific Affairs, Department of Health, Education and Welfare. Washington, D. C., January 11—12, 1971.
22. SALETU, B. and ITIL, T. M. (1972) Thiopental activation and spontaneous sleep and dream patterns of resistant schizophrenics. Canad. Psychiat. Ass. J. **17**, SS-209.
23. SALETU, B., ITIL, T. M. and SALETU, M. (1971) Evoked responses after hemispherectomy. Confin. Neurol. **33**, 221.
24. SALETU, B., SALETU, M. and ITIL, T. M. (in press) The relationships between psychopathology and evoked responses before, during, and after psychotropic drug treatment. Presented as the A. E. Bennett Clinical Science Award Research paper at the 27th Annual Convention of the Society of Biological Psychiatry, 1972, Biol. Psychiat.
25. SALETU, B., SALETU, M., ITIL, T. M. et al. (1971) Changes in somatosensory evoked potentials during fluphenazine treatment. Pharmakopsychiat. **4**, 158.
26. SALETU, B., SALETU, M., ITIL, T. M. et al. (1971) Somatosensory-evoked potential changes during haloperidol treatment of chronic schizophrenics. Biol. Psychiat. **3**, 299.
27. SALETU, B., SALETU, M. and ITIL, T. M. (1972) Effect of minor and major tranquilizers on somatosensory evoked potentials. Psychopharmacologia, **24**, 347.
28. SALETU, B., SALETU, M., ITIL, T. M. et al. (1972) Effect of stimulatory drugs on the somatosensory evoked potential in man. Pharmakopsychiat. **5**, 129.
29. SETHY, V., NAIK, P. and SHETH, U. (1970) Effect of d-amphetamine sulphate in combination with CNS depressants on spontaneous motor activity of mice. Psychopharmacologia, **13**, 19.
30. SHAPIRO, D., HSU, W. and ITIL, T. M. (1971) Period analysis of the EEG on the PDP-12. In: Wulfsohn N. L. and Sances, A. (eds.): The Nervous System and Electric Currents. Vol. 2, Plenum Press, New York, p. 59.
31. SIMEON, J., SALETU, B., KRETSCHMANN, J. et al. (in press) Does dextroamphetamine produce drug dependence in children? Presented at the Turkish Neuro-Psychiatric Association meeting, September 25—30, 1972, Marmaris, Turkey.
32. SIMEON, J., SALETU, B., VIAMONTES, G. et al. (in press) The mother's role in child psychiatry research. Presented at the Group Without a Name meeting, Seattle, Washington, September 8—10, 1972.
33. SOLOMONS, G. (1965) The hyperactive child. J. Iowa med. Soc. **55**, 464.
34. STERN, J. A. and SMALL, J. G. (1964) Cross correlation and frequency analysis of the EEG in psychiatric research. Presented at the 120th Annual meeting of the American Psychiatric Association, Los Angeles.
35. SULSER, F. and DINGELL, J. V. (1968) The potentiation and blockage of the central action of amphetamine by chlorpromazine. Biochem. Pharmacol. **17**, 634.
36. WERRY, J. S. (1970) Some clinical and laboratory studies of psychotropic drugs in children: An overview. In: SMITH, W. L. (ed.): Drugs and Cerebral Function, Charles C. Thomas, Springfield, Illinois.

J.S., Department of Psychiatry, St. Louis Division, Missouri Institute of Psychiatry, School of Medicine, University of Missouri-Columbia, 5400 Arsenal Street, St. Louis, Mo. 63139, U.S.A.

NIACIN IN THE TREATMENT OF SCHIZOPHRENIAS: ALONE AND IN COMBINATION

T. A. BAN and H. E. LEHMANN

Department of Psychiatry, McGill University

RATIONALE FOR NIACIN TREATMENT IN THE SCHIZOPHRENIAS

The original rationale of nicotinic acid treatment was based on the notion that abnormal mental states are the result of a "faulty" adaptation to "overwhelming" environmental stimulation. Among the first who entertained this notion were OSMOND and SMYTHIES (19), who formulated the hypothesis that schizophrenia is the outcome of stress-induced anxiety and a failure of metabolising adrenaline which results in highly toxic, mescaline-like compounds. HARLEY-MASON (8) suggested that 3,4-dimethoxyphenylethylamine (DMPEA) may be the toxic agent responsible for the psychopathological changes, and put forward the hypothesis that the production of DMPEA is the result of "transmethylation", in which the "physiological" N-methylation of norepinephrine to epinephrine is replaced by the "pathological" O-methylation of the phenol ring of dopamine.

An alternative hypothesis proposed that adrenochrome, a psychotoxic oxidation product of epinephrine, was the (toxic) "M" substance (13). Its production was thought to be the result of increased phenolase (oxidase) activity of schizophrenic serum (10) (Fig. 1). In the absence of specific drugs which interfere with adrenochrome formation, HOFFER (9) suggested the administration of nicotinic acid (which converts into nicotinamide) to prevent excessive epinephrine production under stress, thus restricting the supply of the substance from which the alleged psychotoxic aminochrome is formed. The inhibition of epinephrine formation is thought to occur through the following mechanisms: nicotinamide competes with norepinephrine for available methyl groups which are mainly supplied in the diet by methionine, a sulfur-containing amino acid, to form N-methylnicotinamide, one of its main metabolic end products. Considering that only 1200 mg of methionine (daily intake 2000 mg) is neutralized by 1000 mg of nicotinic acid administration, therapeutic effects of nicotinic acid based on this specific mechanism could only be achieved if rather high — 2000 mg or more — daily doses are given (Fig. 2).

While for some time the only rational basis of nicotinic acid treatment was based on the assumption that nicotinic acid prevents excessive epinephrine and subsequent adrenochrome formation, more recently the possibility was raised that the therapeutic action of nicotinic acid might be explained by the fact that it increases nicotinamide adenine nucleotide (NAD) synthesis. NAD, as a reducing agent, inhibits aminochrome formation, i.e. interferes with the mechanism by which the psychotoxic adrenochrome (and sub-

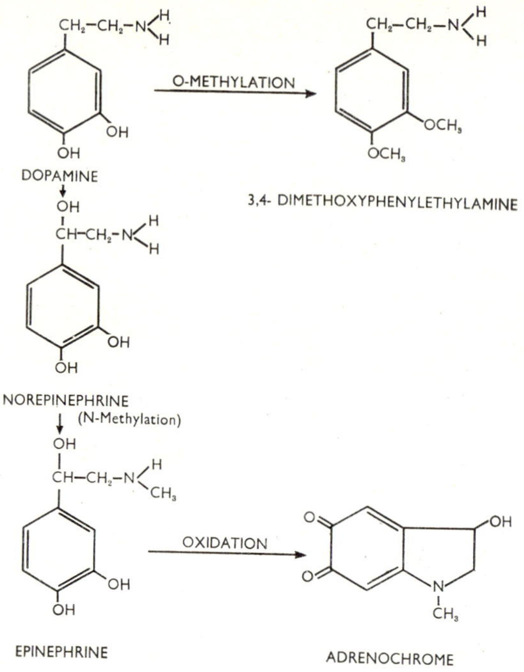

Fig. 1. The formation of 3,4-dimethoxyphenylethylamine (DMPEA) from dopamine and the formation of adrenochrome from epinephrine.

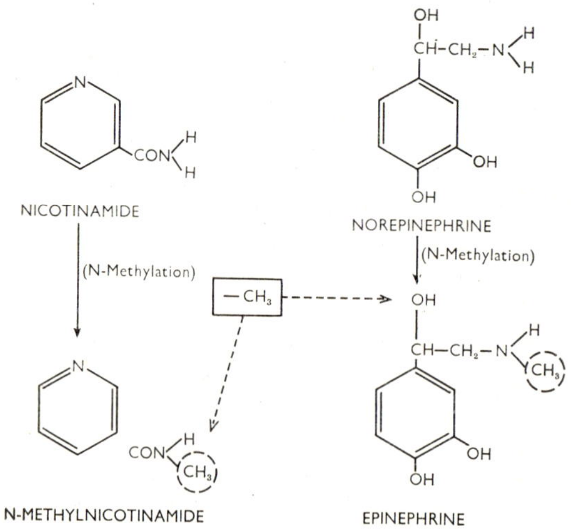

Fig. 2. The formation of N-methylnicotinamide from nicotinamide and the formation of epinephrine from norepinephrine.

sequently adrenolutin) substance is formed. Subsequently, it was speculated that schizophrenia might be a NAD deficiency disease, a form of cerebral pellagra, and the possibility was raised that a patient may have normal quantities of nicotinic acid in the diet but have "cerebral pellagra", because of a failure of NAD synthesis from tryptophan via the quinolinic acid pathway (11).

Findings in Clinical Trials with Niacin

Independent of the theoretical considerations, following the first successful therapeutic trial with nicotinic acid in schizophrenic patients, several other clinical investigations were conducted. As a result, HOFFER (9, 12) suggested that high dosages of nicotinic acid — from 3000 to 30 000 mg per day — have a gradual beneficial effect in acute or subacute schizophrenic patients; and, when combined, with other pharmacological, physical and psychological treatments, nicotinic acid was reported to produce a better therapeutic outcome than that which can be achieved by any of these treatments alone. Nevertheless, at variance with the reported beneficial therapeutic findings (15, 21) with nicotinic acid, ASHBY, COLLINS and BASSETT (2) found no therapeutic effects with nicotinamide in chronic schizophrenic patients; MIRSKY (17) obtained completely negative results in a placebo-controlled study with nicotinic acid; and McGRATH et al. (16) has failed to show any significant difference in therapeutic results between patients on the active (nicotinamide) and inactive (placebo) tablets two years after the commencement of drug administration. The same appplies to O'REILLY (18) and VALLELY, LOVEGROVE an HOBBS (23) who failed to obtain therapeutic changes with nicotinic acid in schizophrenic patients.

In view of this controversy regarding the effectiveness of nicotinic acid treatment, and because schizophrenia is one of the major public health problems — roughly one quarter of all the available hospital beds are taken up by schizophrenic patients — affecting at least one person in three hundred (i.e. approximately 70 000 of Canada's 21 million population), the Board of Directors of the Canadian Mental Health Association (CMHA), approximately five years ago, decided to set up a series of systematic studies to obtain relevant information on nicotinic acid treatment (4—6).

Results of the CMHA Collaborative Studies with Niacin

Since the initiation of the CMHA Collaborative Studies five years have passed, and five of the originally designed 12 clinical trials have been completed (Table 1). Findings in these studies strongly suggest that the administration of nicotinic acid in the dosage of 3000 mg per day has no therapeutic effect, or may even have a negative therapeutic effect, in unselected groups of schizophrenic patients. This statement is based on the following findings:

1. The overall therapeutic efficacy of nicotinic acid as *the sole medication in newly admitted schizophrenic patients* is not superior to the overall therapeutic efficacy of an inactive placebo. In fact, the majority of newly admitted schizophrenic patients — in a placebo controlled two-years study with 30 patients — could not be sufficiently controlled with high dosages — 3000 to 8000 mg per day — of nicotinic acid administration. Although there was a statistically significant improvement with all three treatment regimes — nicotinic acid, nicotinamide, and placebo — in the total scores of the Brief Psychiatric Rating Scale, no significant difference between the groups was found. Further

TABLE 1
The twelve clinical trials which entail the CMHA Collaborative Study and their present status

	General hypothesis	Design	Site	Present status
I	Nicotinic acid has a beneficial action over and above the effects achievable by standard treatments	1. Placebo-controlled 2. Standard-controlled. 3. Placebo-controlled; combined with phenothiazines in acute patients. 4. Placebo-controlled; combined with phenothiazines in chronic patients. 5. Placebo-controlled; five year follow-up.	J.D., H.L., D.H. Undecided D.H. D.H. H.L.	C S C C C
II	Therapeutic efficacy of nicotinic acid is increased by the administration of ascorbic acid, pyridoxine, or d'penicillamine.	6. Placebo-controlled; combined with ascorbic acid. 7. Placebo-controlled; combined with pyridoxine. 8. Placebo-controlled; combined with d'penicillamine.	H.H. D.H. D.H.	C C S
III	The presence of the "mauve factor", "pink spot", or a bufotenin-like substance in the urine indicates a more favorable therapeutic outcome with nicotinic acid.	9. Comparison groups; "mauve spot" present or absent. 10. Comparison groups; "pink spot" present or absent. 11. Comparison groups; bufotenin-like substances present or absent.	L.H. L.H. L.H.	P S S
IV	The exacerbation of psychopathology induced by the associated administration of a methyl-donor and an MAOI in schizophrenia can be prevented or counteracted by nicotinic acid administration.	12. Placebo-controlled.	D.H.	C

J.D. — Hôpital St. Jean de Dieu, Montreal
H.L. — Hôpital des Laurentides, L'Annonciation
H.H. — Hamilton Psychiatric Hospital, Hamilton
L.H. — Lakeshore Psychiatric Hospital, Toronto
D.H. — Douglas Hospital, Montreal

C — Completed
S — To be started
P — In progress

analysis of data revealed that during the two-year investigational period — regardless of whether the patients were kept on the project or not — the average number of days spent in hospital was lowest in the placebo (211 days) and highest in the nicotinamide treated group (353 days). However, the number of days spent in hospital was only slightly higher — 214 days — in the nicotinic acid than in the placebo treated patients (1).

2. The overall therapeutic efficacy of nicotinic acid as *an adjuvant medication in newly admitted schizophrenic patients* is inferior to the overall therapeutic efficacy of an inactive

placebo. In fact, the addition of nicotinic acid, in the dosage of 3000 mg per day, to regular phenothiazine treatment — in a placebo controlled six months study with 30 patients — prolonged the duration of hospital stay and increased the amount of neuroleptic medication required in treatment. Patients in the placebo group received — and presumably required — a significantly lower (analysis of variance $p < 0.05$) total and lower average daily amount of phenothiazine drugs (418 chlorpromazine equivalent units) than those on either of the active substances (i.e. nicotinic acid: 730, and nicotinamide: 705). The same applied to the number of days of hospitalization, although this did not reach the accepted level of statistical significance (placebo: 67, nicotinic acid: 90 and nicotinamide: 88 days) (20).

3. The overall therapeutic efficacy of nicotinic acid — in the dosage of 3000 mg per day — as an adjuvant medication *in chronically hospitalized schizophrenic patients* is inferior to the overall therapeutic efficacy of an inactive placebo. In fact, in a one-year placebo-controlled study with 30 patients, the active treatment groups fared worse than the placebo group by all measures of assessment. It was noted that while on the Clinical Global Impression Scale (CGI) all three groups improved, on the Nurses' Observation Scale for Inpatient Evaluation (NOSIE) two groups improved and one deteriorated, and on the Brief Psychiatric Rating Scale (BPRS) only one group improved and two groups became clinically worse. The least improvement (CGI) and the greatest amount of deterioration (on both BPRS and NOSIE) was seen in the nicotinic acid group. Moreover, it was shown that patients in the placebo group required less increase in their concomitant phenothiazine medication than patients in the two active treatment groups.

4. The overall therapeutic efficacy of *combined administration of nicotinic acid and pyridoxine* as an adjuvant medication in chronically hospitalized schizophrenic patients is inferior to the overall therapeutic efficacy of the component drugs. Although there occurred a statistically significant improvement in groups receiving either nicotinic acid (3000 mg per day) or pyridoxine (75 mg per day) as an adjuvant medication to phenothiazines in the 40 week study, the improvement with the combined treatment fell short of statistical significance.

5. Nicotinic acid in the dosage of 3000 mg per day — *can neither prevent nor counteract the psychopathology induced by the combined administration of a monoamine oxidase inhibitor (tranylcypromine) and methionine*. In fact, during the two weeks of methionine (20 000 mg per day) administration, there was a considerably greater increase in psychopathological symptoms — expressed in mean total scores of the Brief Psychiatric Rating Scale (BPRS) — in the nicotinic acid — than in the placebo-treated group. Furthermore, it was noted that after discontinuation of both, tranylcypromine and methionine administration, there was further deterioration in the nicotinic acid and some improvement in the placebo-treated group.

DISCUSSION OF FINDINGS

In view of the negative therapeutic findings in the CMHA Collaborative Studies, and in view of the absence of verified clinical indicators of therapeutic responsiveness to nicotinic acid in other clinical trials, the recognition of a suspected biochemical heterogeneity within the schizophrenias becomes of crucial importance. As an example, this was demonstrated by SNEZHNEVSKY and VARTANIAN (22) who were able to show that the serum of schizophrenic patients with two different types of development — continuous or periodic — evoked opposite actions on the mitotic activity of cell cultures and consequently covered up meaningful differences between schizophrenic patients and normal subjects. Applying the same concept to the nicotinic acid problem, the crucial question of the identification of biochemically homogeneous subgroups within the schizophrenic population still remains.

In this context, Harley-Mason's (8) idea that transmethylation is the process which may be responsible for the formation of psychotoxic substances regained importance in Kety's (14) formulation of the transmethylation hypothesis of schizophrenia. This hypothesis is based on the assumption that, at least in certain schizophrenics, methylations occur at an abnormally high rate, leading to the formation of hallucinogenic reaction products. Accordingly, one may speculate that at least in those schizophrenics in whom methylations occur at an abnormally high rate, transmethylation could be interfered with and schizophrenic symptoms alleviated by such simple means as nicotinic acid administration which might act as a methyl-trap. Nevertheless, the finding that administration of megadosages of nicotinic acid did not reduce the stress-induced increase in the synthesis of methylated compounds, i.e. epinephrine and creatinine in humans (7), indicates that even if transmethylation processes are disordered in certain schizophrenics, this does not imply that the metabolic disorder in these patients can be successfully interfered with by nicotinic acid treatment.

Summary

The current status of nicotinic acid treatment in schizophrenia has been reviewed. It was pointed out that in all the therapeutic trials in the CMHA Collaborative Studies, completed up to date, nicotinic acid alone or in combination with other substances, had no effect — or had a negative therapeutic effect — in both, newly admitted and chronic schizophrenic patients. Furthermore, it was also pointed out that even if a biochemically homogeneous small group could be identified, e.g. on the basis of NAD deficiency or excessive methylation processes, the chances that such a group will show a beneficial therapeutic response to nicotinic acid is very slim. Nevertheless, without the results of further studies of this kind the therapeutic potential of nicotinic acid in the schizophrenias cannot be considered fully evaluated.

References

1. Ananth, J. V., Vacaflor, L., Kekhwa, G., Sterlin, C. and Ban, T. A. (1972), Nicotinic acid in the treatment of newly admitted schizophrenic patients: A placebo-controlled study. Int. J. clin. Pharmacol. 5, 466.
2. Ashby, W. R., Collins, G. H. and Bassett, M. (1960), The effect of nicotinamide and placebo on the chronic schizophrenic. J. ment. Sci. 106, 1555.
3. Ban, T. A. (1969), Niacin in the treatment of schizophrenias. Psychopharmacol. Bull. 5, 5.
4. Ban, T. A. (1971) Nicotinic Acid in the Treatment of Schizophrenias. Complimentary Report A. Canadian Mental Health Association, Toronto.
5. Ban, T. A. (1971) Nicotinic acid in psychiatry. Canad. psychiat. Ass. J. 16, 413.
6. Ban, T. A. and Lehmann, H. E. (1970) Nicotinic Acid in the Treatment of Schizophrenias. Canadian Mental Health Collaborative Study. Canadian Mental Health Association, Toronto.
7. Ellerbrook, R. C. and Purdy, M. D. (1970) Capacity of stressed humans under megadosages of nicotinic acid to synthesize methylated compounds. Dis. nerv. Syst. 31, 196.
8. Harley-Mason, J. (1952) In: Osmond, H. and Smythies, J.: Schizophrenia: A new approach. J. ment. Sci. 98, 309.
9. Hoffer, A. (1962) Niacin Therapy in Psychiatry. Charles C. Thomas, Springfield.
10. Hoffer, A. (1964) The adrenochrome therapy of schizophrenia: A review. Dis. nerv. Syst. 25, 173.
11. Hoffer, A. (1966) Enzymology of hallucinogens. In: Martin, G. J. and Kisch, B. (Eds.): Enzymes in Mental Health. Lippincott, Philadelphia.
12. Hoffer, A. (1971) Megavitamin B-3 therapy for schizophrenia. Canad. psychiat. Ass. J. 16, 499.

13. HOFFER, A., OSMOND, H. and SMYTHIES, J. (1954) Schizophrenia: a new approach. J. ment. Sci. **100**, 29.
14. KETY, S. S. (1967) Current biochemical approaches to schizophrenia. New Engl. J. Med. **276**, 325.
15. MASLOWSKI, J. (1967) Zastosowanie kwasu nikotynowego w leczeniu schizofrenii przewleklej. Psychiat. Pol. **1**, 307.
16. MCGRATH, S. D., O'BRIEN, P. F., POWER, P. J. and SHEA, J. R. Nicotinamide treatment of schizophrenia — report of a multi-hospital controlled trial. (In press).
17. MIRSKY, A. I. (1967) Personal Letter of Dr. J. D. Griffin.
18. O'REILLY, P. O. (1955) Nicotinic acid therapy and the chronic schizophrenic. Dis. nerv. Syst. **16**, 67.
19. OSMOND, H. and SMYTHIES, J. R. (1952) Schizophrenia: A new approach. J. ment. Sci. **98**, 309.
20. RAMSEY, R. A., BAN, T. A., LEHMANN, H. E., SAXENA, B. M. and BENENTT, J. (1970) Nicotinic acid as adjuvant therapy in newly admitted schizophrenic patients. Canad. med. Ass. J. **102**, 939.
21. SAARMA, J. M. and VASAR, H. (1970) Nicotinic acid as an adjuvant in the treatment of chronic schizophrenic patients with special reference to changes in higher nervous activity. Curr. ther. Res. **12**, 729.
22. SNEZHNEVSKY, A. V. and VARTANIAN, M. (1971) The forms of schizophrenia and their biological correlates. In: HIMWICH, H. E. (Ed.): Biochemistry, Schizophrenias and Affective Illness. The Williams and Wilkins Co., Baltimore.
23. VALLELY, J. F., LOVEGROVE, T. D. and HOBBS, G. E. (1971) Nicotinic acid and nicotinamide in the treatment of chronic schizophrenia. Canad. psychiat. Ass. J. **16**, 433.

T.A.B., Division of Psychopharmacology, McGill University, Montreal, Canada

DOMINANT X-LINKED TRANSMISSION IN MANIC-DEPRESSIVE ILLNESS: LINKAGE STUDIES WITH THE XGa BLOOD GROUP[*]

R. R. FIEVE, J. MENDLEWICZ and J. L. FLEISS

New York State Psychiatric Institute and Columbia University, New York, N. Y.

Although twin studies (2, 10, 17) and studies of morbid risk (2, 11, 14), show that heredity is a major factor in the pathogenesis of manic-depressive illness, the precise mode of transmission is still controversial. Two major lines of evidence have accumulated over the past few years, one supporting the polygenic theory and the other supporting X chromosome transmission. The studies of SLATER et al. (12) and PERRIS (7) have given weight in favor of the polygenic hypothesis. In contrast, the studies of WINOKUR et al. (16), and REICH et al. (8), have pointed to an X-linked transmission.

Two recent studies from our laboratory have added further support in favor of X-chromosome transmission. In the first of these two studies we reported on the distribution of ancestral secondary cases in bipolar patients having a positive family history of mania, and concluded in favor of major gene, rather than polygenic, transmission (4). The second line of evidence from our laboratory in support of X-linkage was based on an analysis of seven families in which manic-depressive illness and either protan or deutan color blindness (recessive X-linked traits) occurred in several generations. Close and statistically significant linkage was found in these seven families between the locus for manic-depressive illness and the loci for both of the X-linked genetic markers studied (5).

SUBJECTS AND METHODS

In this study, six informative families were identified in which manic-depressive illness and the genotypes of the XGa blood group (a dominant X-linked trait) assorted in successive generations. The index cases (probands) were all taken from a sample of over 80 carefully diagnosed manic-depressive patients consecutively admitted during an 18 month period to the Lithium Treatment and Research Clinic at the New York State Psychiatric Institute.

All patients as well as their spouses and available first (sibs, parents and offspring), second (aunts, uncles, grandparents, etc.), and third degree (more distant) relatives on

---

[*] This study was supported by the Lithium Clinic Grant # 6003C from the Division of Local Services. Department of Mental Hygiene, Albany, New York.

both the maternal and paternal sides were examined single-blind for XGa blood type and for psychopathology.

In this study we assume that within given families sharing the genotype for manic-depressive illness, a predisposed individual, depending on his internal and external environment, can develop either depression alone (unipolar illness), or manic-depression (bipolar illness). Although a number of studies have indicated that unipolar and bipolar illness may be genetically different, most of them have found a higher than expected prevalence of unipolar illness in the relatives of bipolar probands (14, 15). Furthermore, in ZERBIN-RUDIN's (17) review of twin studies, a high proportion of pairs of monozygotic twins (25%), both of whom had an effective illness, were such that one member suffered from bipolar and the other from unipolar illness.

Thus, in spite of studies (6, 15) which have demonstrated that unipolar and bipolar illnesses are genetically distinct, we believe that at least in some instances, one's environment (internal or external) may affect the outward expressivity of the bipolar genotype. This is to say that the unipolar relatives of some bipolar probands might, in fact, have the bipolar genotype. We assume in this report, therefore, that *within a family unit* identified by a bipolar proband, bipolar illness and unipolar illness are genetically related and express the same genotype.

The diagnosis of bipolar illness in probands was made separately by two investigators using criteria similar to those of LEONHARD et al. (3), PERRIS et al. (6), and WINOKUR et al. (15). A clinical semi-structured interview (13) was used for the evaluation of current psychopathology and past history in probands and relatives. Bipolar depression was diagnosed in probands and relatives who had a history of clear-cut manic behavior and of depressive episodes severe enough to require treatment or hospitalization, or to cause a disruption in everyday activities for at least 3 weeks. Periodicity of illness with symptom-free intervals were among the criteria used for the diagnosis of bipolar illness. This diagnosis was made, when deemed clinically appropriate, irrespective of the subject's age.

For the purposes of this study, unipolar depression was diagnosed in individuals who had never experienced mania or hypomania but had experienced one or more depressive episodes severe enough to require treatment or hospitalization. In order to exclude possible schizophrenics, a firm diagnosis of unipolar illness was made only if the subject was at least 40 years of age. For both bipolar and unipolar illness, there had to be no personality disintegration before or following psychotic episodes, and no other pre-existing psychiatric or medical disease which might be associated with an affective symptomatology.

The family study method (i.e., personal interview with the relatives) was used because this method has proven to have better reliability than the family history method (i.e., family history data collected from the proband) (9). Pertinent medical and social records were used when available.

Blood samples were collected from all available subjects as follows: Five cc's of blood were collected on E.D.T.A. and refrigerated before being sent to the New York Blood Center for blood group analysis.*)

STATISTICAL METHODS

Each of the female's ova has only one X chromosome. During the process of meiosis, some genetic material from one X chromosome may be exchanged for material from the other (i.e., crossing over may occur). The offspring exhibiting crossing over are called

---

*) The XGa analysis was carried out by Dr. G. Allen of the New York Blood Center.

"recombinants", while those exhibiting no crossing over are called "nonrecombinants".

The relative frequency of "recombinants" versus "nonrecombinants" is a function of the distance between the two loci for the exchangeable genetic materials. The more distant the two loci, the more likely, on the basis of the laws of probability, is recombination to occur. Linkage between pairs of traits is in fact usually assessed by estimating the relative frequency of recombinants to nonrecombinants (technically, the "recombination fraction", denoted θ). The minimum value of θ is 0.0, which indicates that the loci for the two traits coincide. The maximum value is 0.50, which indicates either that the loci for the two traits are on opposite ends of the same chromosome or that they are on two different chromosomes. The closer the value of θ is to 0.0, the stronger the evidence is for linkage. EDWARDS (1) presents tables which facilitate the estimation of θ. If θ is significantly less than 0.50 the inference may be drawn that the loci for the two traits are linked.

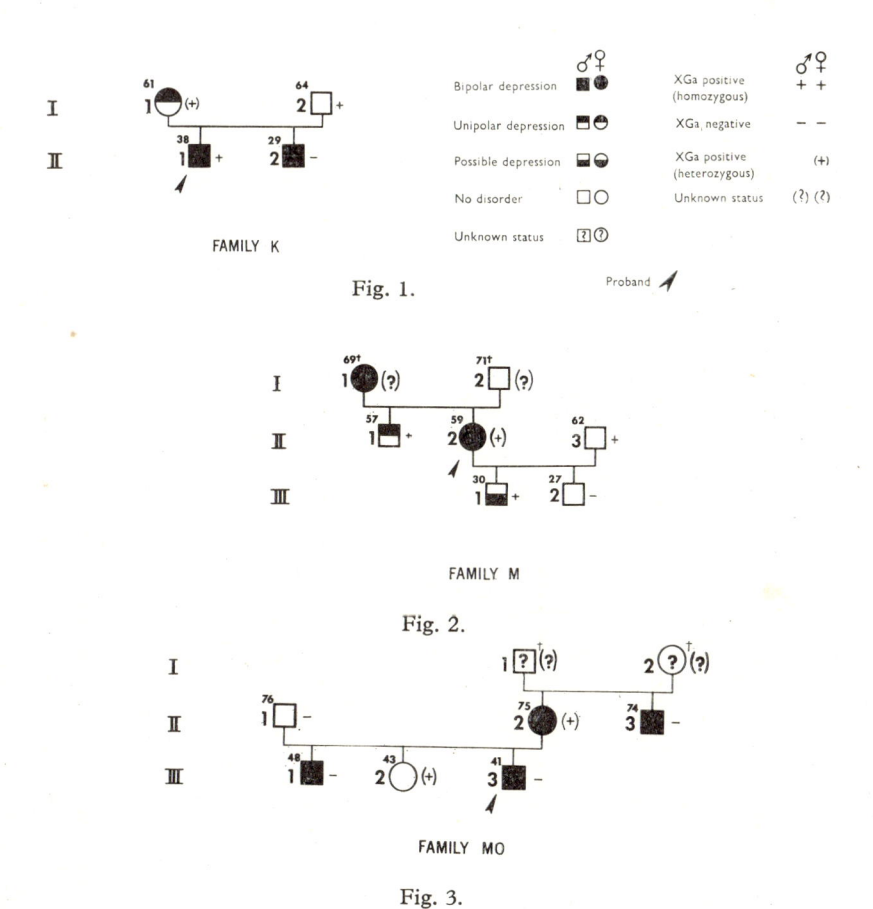

Fig. 1.

Fig. 2.

Fig. 3.

LINKAGE RESULTS

Family K — The proband, II(1), has been hospitalized for manic-depressive illness and is XGa positive. His brother also has manic-depressive illness but is XGa negative. Their mother has suffered from depression and is heterozygous for XGa. Since there was no maternal uncle available and since the maternal grandfather is dead, the linkage phase in the mother (coupling or repulsion) cannot be determined. One of II(1) and II(2) is, therefore, a nonrecombinant, and the other is a recombinant (Fig. 1).

Family M — The proband has two sons, III(1) and III(2). One of them, III(1), is XGa positive and has been hospitalized for depression. He is too young to be considered a definite depressive, however. The other son, III(2), is XGa negative and has no history of affective disorder. The characteristics of the proband's brother, II(1), suggest that she has the traits in "coupling": the alleles for the illness and XGa positive are on one chromosome, and those for no illness and XGa negative are on the other. Therefore, III(1) is counted as a recombinant and III(2) as a nonrecombinant. Had III(1) been considered a definite case of affective illness, both he and his brother would have been counted as nonrecombinants. Counting III(1) as a recombinant, therefore, has the effect of underestimating linkage (Fig. 2).

Family MO — The proband, III(3), has bipolar illness and is XGa negative. He has one brother, III(1), who is XGa negative and also has the illness, and one sister, III(2), who has no evidence of the illness and is XGa positive. This represents an instance where a daughter is informative for X-linkage. Because III(2)'s father, II(1), is XGa negative, therefore III(2) necessarily inherited her XGa positive gene from her mother. The mother, II(2), has bipolar illness and is heterozygous for XGa. Her brother, II(3), is XGa negative and has the illness, suggesting that the mother has the traits in repulsion. All three off-springs are therefore counted as nonrecombinants (Fig. 3).

Family L — The proband, IV(12), is a female who is an identical twin and who is bipolar and heterozygous for the XGa blood group. Her two sons are too young to be counted for purposes of statistical analysis. Her maternal aunt, III(11), is bipolar and is heterozygous for the XGa blood group. She has three sons. IV(7) is depressed and XGa positive; IV(8) has never had an affective episode and is XGa negative; and IV(9) is bipolar and XGa positive. Her brother, III(9), is well and XGa positive, suggesting that the traits may be in repulsion. To be on the safe side (underestimating the degree of linkage), we count IV(7), IV(8), and IV(9) as three recombinants (Fig. 4).

Family S — The proband, III(2), has bipolar illness and is XGa positive. He has a brother, III(1), who has never had an affective episode and is XGa negative. Their mother, II(2), has had serious depressions and is heterozygous for XGa. Both sons, III(1) and III(2), can be counted as nonrecombinants (Fig. 5).

Family SA — The proband, II(3), is bipolar and XGa posi-

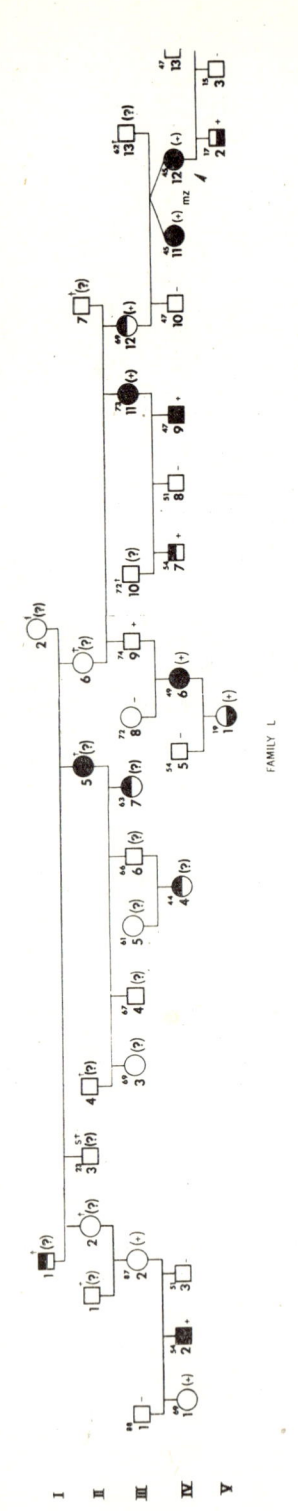

Fig. 4.

tive. His older brother, II(1), and his fraternal twin, II(2), have never had an affective illness and are XGa negative. The mother, I(2), is bipolar and heterozygous for XGa. Individuals II(1)—II(3) are counted as three nonrecombinants (Fig. 6).

The detailed mathematical analysis of the information from these six families, as well as the information from two informative families studied by WINOKUR et al. (16) is available from the authors. Table 1 summarizes the results. These results give a likelihood

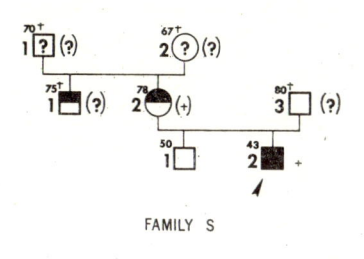

FAMILY S

Fig. 5.

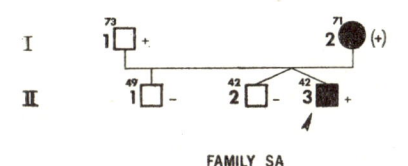

FAMILY SA

Fig. 6.

TABLE 1

XGa blood type and depression: Log odds scores for seven families

Study	Number of		Recombination fraction (Θ)								
	NRC*	RC*	.05	.10	.15	.20	.25	.30	.35	.40	.45
Current	10	5	—1.45	—.48	—.07	.16	.24	.25	.17	.11	.04
(WINOKUR and TANNA) (5)	7	1	.32	.47	.48	.43	.36	.26	.16	.08	.02
Sum	17	6	—1.13	—.01	.41	.59	.60	.51	.33	.19	.06

* NRC = Nonrecombinant $\Theta = .23$, s.e. (Θ) = .10
** RC = Recombinant

estimate of the recombination fraction θ close to .25 ($\theta = .23$), with an estimated standard error of .10. Because the 95% confidence interval for θ is $\theta < .39$, statistically significant linkage is indicated between the loci for the XGa blood type and manic-depressive illness. Even closer linkage would have been inferred had we considered III(1) in Family M as definitely suffering from depression. Ten individuals used in the analysis (six from our series and four from WINOKUR'S) are symptom-free but have not yet passed the age of risk for an affective illness. Reanalysis of all possible $2^{10} = 1024$ patterns of future disease occurrence in these cases confirmed the finding of statistically significant linkage between the loci for manic-depressive illness and the XGa blood group.

Examining all six pedigrees one can see that the transmission of manic-depressive illness fits the model of dominant inheritance: the illness occurs in successive generations and all heterozygous individuals (in this case all women who carry both the dominant or recessive allele for the illness) exhibit the illness. The single exception is individual III(2) in Family L. She has both an ill and a well son, but has not exhibited the illness herself.

DISCUSSION AND CONCLUSIONS

Eight families informative for linkage between the loci for manic-depressive illness and the XGa blood type have been reported in the literature, two by WINOKUR et al. (16), and six in this report. Statistically significant linkage was found. This analysis lends further evidence to the previous linkage studies of WINOKUR et al. (16) and REICH et al. (8), and the recent linkage report from our laboratory by MENDLEWICZ et al. (5), all supporting dominant X-linked transmission in manic-depressive illness.

Several criteria must be met in the identification of a trait as being inherited by an X-linked mode of transmission. First of all, affected males transmit the trait to all of their daughters and none of their sons. Secondly, affected females who are heterozygous transmit the condition to one-half of their children of either sex; and thirdly, affected females who are homozygous transmit the trait to all of their children. Despite the fact that a few manic-depressive fathers appear to have sons with manic-depressive illness, claims of father-son transmission of the illness are still rare (approx. 10% in our population). Family study data from several centers agree to this finding, and studies of illegitimacy or assortative mating are critical where father-son transmission has been presumed. Further use of family history data in mapping out the transmission of the illness is difficult since, unlike with known genetic markers, it is impossible to determine homozygosity or heterozygosity in many instances where the patient has not passed through the age of risk or the family is noninformative. Therefore, the use of genetic markers to establish linkage has become an increasingly important method for establishing mode of genetic transmission.

In recent years particular focus has been given to use of the XGa blood group locus since its crossover frequencies seem to render it an excellent candidate for marker status. In addition, the XGa positive allele occurs in a high proportion of the general population (66%), in contrast to other X-linked markers (color blindness, G6PD, etc.) so that patients with a given condition to be investigated have a high likelihood of also possessing the XGa positive marker. Therefore, other investigators could detect informative families assorting for this marker and the illness in order to test the hypothesis of X-linkage in manic-depressive illness.

Despite our findings of X-linked dominant transmission in manic-depressive illness, it is still possible that in some subgroups a single variant allele at one locus, or an involvement of different alleles at different loci are needed to explain the genetic characterization of this illness. In addition, there may be polygenic inheritance in other subgroups. None of these models can be ruled out and one cannot generalize from the data presented that all cases of manic-depressive illness are X-linked. We, therefore, conclude from the results of six of our informative families, and two from WINOKUR et al. (16), that a dominant X-linked gene is most likely to be involved in the transmission of manic-depressive illness within the families studied.

References

1. Edwards, J. H. (1971) Ann. hum. Genet. Lond. **341**, 229.
2. Kallman, F. J. (1954) In: Depression, Hoch, P. & Zubin, J., Ed., New York, Grune & Stratton, 1.
3. Leonhard, K., Korff, I. and Shulz, H. (1962) Psychiat. Neurol. **143**, 416.
4. Mendlewicz, J., Fieve, R. R., Rainer, J. D. and Cataldo, M. (1972) Brit. J. Psychiat. In press.
5. Mendlewicz, J., Fleiss, J. L. and Fieve, R. R. (1972) J. Amer. med. Ass. **222**, 1624.
6. Perris, C. (1966) Acta. psychiat. scand. Suppl. 194.
7. Perris, C. (1971) Brit. J. Psychiat. **118**, 207.
8. Reich, T., Clayton, P. J. and Winokur, C. (1969) Amer. J. Psychiat. **125**, 1358.
9. Rimmer, J. and Chambers, D. S. (1969) Amer. J. Orthopsychiat. **39**, 760.
10. Rosanoff, A. J., Handy, L. M. and Plesset, I. R. (1935) Amer. J. Psychiat. **91**, 725.
11. Slater, E. (1936) Proc. roy. soc. Med. **29**, 981.
12. Slater, E., Maxwell, J. and Price, J. S. (1971) Brit. J. Psychiat. **118**, 543.
13. Spitzer, R. L., Endicott, J. and Fleiss, J. L. (1967) Compr. Psychiat. **8**, 321.
14. Stenstedt, A. (1952) Acta psychiat. neurol. Scand. Suppl. 79.
15. Winokur, G. and Clayton, P. J. (1967) In: Rec. Adv. Biol. Psychiat. Wortis, J., Ed., 935.
16. Winokur, G. and Tanna, V. L. (1969) Dis. nerv. Syst. **30**, 89.
17. Zerbin-Rudin, E. (1967) In: Becker, P. E. Ed. Human genetic, section 2, Stuttgart, Georg Thieme Verlag, 5.

R.R.F., New York State Psychiatric Institute, 722 West 168th Street, New York, N. Y., U. S. A.

GENETIC ASPECTS OF LITHIUM PROPHYLAXIS IN BIPOLAR MANIC-DEPRESSIVE ILLNESS

J. MENDLEWICZ, R. R. FIEVE and F. STALLONE

New York State Psychiatric Institute and Department of Psychiatry, Columbia University, N. Y.

It has been hypothesized that when lithium is administered chronically to manic-depressive patients, it prevents a recurrence of future episodes of mania and depression, or significantly lessens their severity or duration. This premise has been the subject of international controversy in the last several years. Since its introduction into psychiatry about twenty years ago, lithium therapy has been clearly established as a highly effective and specific treatment for acute manic attacks in many clinical trials in the United States and elsewhere. However, long-term chronic administration of lithium during symptom-free intervals for purposes of preventing subsequent attacks of the illness has been enthusiastically supported by some investigators and seriously questioned by others, and failures on lithium long-term therapy still occur.

The resolution of this controversy rests with carefully designed double-blind controlled studies, several of which have been reported recently. BAASTRUP et al. (1) have recently conducted a double-blind study of lithium prophylaxis. In this study, matched pairs of patients were assigned at random to either lithium or placebo groups and followed closely. After five months, the study was discontinued when 21 placebo patients and no lithium patients developed affective episodes. Evidence for lithium prophylaxis was found in the prevention of manic and depressive episodes in bipolar manic-depressives, and in the prevention of depressive episodes in unipolar endogenous depressives. However, as carefully performed as this study was, it included what might be considered a selective sample since all patients randomized into the study had previously been on lithium, thus constituting a lithium responsive population.

Further evidence of lithium prophylaxis is provided in a British collaborative study reported by COPPEN et al. (3). Sixty-five patients, both bipolar manic-depressives and unipolar recurrent depressives, were randomly assigned to either lithium or placebo treatments, and were followed closely for up to 112 weeks. The results were clearly in support of lithium prophylaxis, in terms of several criteria, including the number of episodes, ratings of severity of episodes, and amounts of antidepressant and antimanic medication when these were needed. Lithium was found to be equally effective in the prevention of manic as well as depressive episodes in bipolar patients and in the prevention of depressive episodes in unipolar patients. This study represented a substantial improvement over previous studies, but also failed to carefully specify whether any of the cases in the 4 samples coming from 4 hospital centers had been treated with lithium prior to entry into the study.

In view of the above findings, the question of lithium prophylaxis needs to be more fully investigated, with particular attention being paid to what effects having a previous lithium regimen might have in biasing a sample to be studied. The present study also focuses on the genetic aspects of manic-depressive illness as related to response in a double-blind study of lithium prophylaxis in manic-depressive bipolar patients attending the Lithium Treatment and Research Clinic for Affective Disorders at the New York State Psychiatric Institute.

METHOD

Selection of patients

Cases for inclusion in the study needed to be diagnosed as bipolar manic-depressives independently by two psychiatrists. Patients were selected only if they had a history of at least three episodes of affective disorder with normal interval functioning between episodes. At least one of these episodes needed to be manic, in which the patient became overactive, overtalkative, had reduced need for sleep, became grandiose in his planning, and became sexually hyperactive. Depressive episodes were variously characterized by depressed and tearful mood, lack of appetite and loss of weight, sleep disturbance, loss of energy, low self-esteem, anxiety, and agitation. Each episode needed to be of at least two weeks' duration and of sufficient severity to impair the patient's usual functioning. Schizo-affective patients were excluded from the study.

In order to maintain comparability with the selection criteria adopted by BAASTRUP and SCHOU (2), patients were included in the study only if at least two episodes occurred within the two years prior to entrance into the trial.

At the time of inclusion into the study, all patients were symptom-free and not being treated with anti-depressant or tranquilizing medications. Two-thirds of the patients (N = 33), however, had been receiving lithium openly as a prophylactic drug at the time they entered the study and this group had been, by and large, successfully treated and followed on lithium for 1—6 years with no adequate record of the percentage of dropouts or failures that had occurred over this time period.

The research plan was implemented in October, 1969. From October, 1969 to January, 1970, 36 patients were started on the study. Sixteen more were subsequently added over the next several months. Among these, 33 patients had been treated with lithium carbonate for 1—6 years prior to their incorporation in this study. Nineteen patients had never received lithium before. Although the study is still in progress, for purposes of this report, the data up to February, 1972, were analyzed. Therefore, lithium prophylaxis for periods up to 28 months is assessed in this report.

Twenty-five patients were randomly assigned to lithium carbonate and twenty-seven patients received a placebo. After the initial administration of the drug, serum levels were monitored once every four weeks and dosage was regulated so as to maintain a serum lithium level between 0.80 meq/l and 1.30 meq/l. If a patient was judged sufficiently ill by at least two independent blind evaluators to require additional medication (other than lithium) or hospitalization, he was considered a failure. Details on the method and clinical results of this double-blind study of lithium prophylaxis are to be presented elsewhere.

RESULTS

The mean ages and sex distributions of the study patients are given in Table 1. No appreciable differences in age or in sex distribution were noted between the lithium and placebo groups.

TABLE 1

Age and sex distribution of study patients in percentage (N = 52)

	Lithium		Placebo	
	Ages male	female	Ages male	female
Mean	54.75	49.46	48.15	50.79
S.D.	11.10	10.45	15.40	9.78
N	12	13	13	14

If lithium exerts a prophylactic effect on manic-depressive illness, those patients assigned to the lithium group would be expected to remain in remission longer than those assigned to the placebo condition. Table 2 shows the number of months in remission from the time of entry into the study to the time of the first episode. Fourteen of the twenty-five lithium patients remained in remission for over two years (up to February, 1972, or 25—28 months). Only 2 of the placebo patients remained in remission for the full time. The mean number of months in remission is nearly three times as great in the lithium group (17.88) as in the placebo group (6.33). The difference between these means is statistically significant below the .001 level.

TABLE 2

Number of months in remission from time of entrance into study to time of first episode

Number of months	Lithium	Placebo
25—28	14	2
19—24	1	1
13—18	0	0
7—12	4	3
1—6	6	21
TOTALS:	25	27
Mean*	17.88	6.33
S.D.	10.47	7.21

* t-ratio for difference between means is: 4.66, df = 50, $p < .001$

At the end of the time interval with which this report is concerned (February, 1971), 31 of the original 52 patients had dropped out of the study. The reasons for dropping out in the lithium and placebo groups are given in Table 3. Twenty-two of the thirty-one drop-outs were in the placebo group. Eighteen of these were directly attributable to the disruptive effects of an acute episode, usually manic. Only three lithium patients dropped out because of an acute episode of illness. It is clear that the placebo patients' proneness to acute episodes made it impossible for them to remain in the study on placebo for the 24 months as was originally intended.

TABLE 3

Reasons for drop-outs

Reasons		Lithium	Placebo
1.	Patient pressed for open treatment after having an acute episode	2	14
2.	Patient terminated study participation during acute manic episode and was hospitalized elsewhere	1	4
3.	Patient withdrew from study in order to undergo different treatment plan	4	2
4.	Patient terminated for reasons unrelated to manic-depressive illness (e.g., physical illness, moved out of area).	2	2
	TOTAL:	9	22

Because of the more rapid drop-out rate in the placebo group, the two groups were not studied for equal durations. The lithium patients were in the study for a mean of 1.840 years, while the placebo patients were in the study for a mean of 0.685 years. Comparisons of the mean number of episodes in the two groups, therefore, had to control for this difference in study time. This was done by computing the mean number of episodes per patient-year. Table 4 gives these data for manic episodes. Without controlling for study time, the mean number of episodes in the lithium and placebo groups are 0.200 and 0.593 respectively. However, controlling for study time, the mean number of episodes per patient-year in the lithium and placebo groups are 0.109 and 0.865 respectively.

TABLE 4

Comparison of frequency of manic episodes in lithium and placebo groups

	Lithium	Placebo
Mean number of episodes	0.200	0.593
Mean number of years in study	1.840	0.685
Mean number of manic episodes per patient-year	1.109	0.865
Number of cases	25	27

The evaluation of the significance of the difference between the mean numbers of episodes per patient-year is by means of the critical ratio of the difference to its standard error (4). The ratio for the comparison of the mean number of manic episodes per patient-year in the lithium and placebo groups was 8.968, which is statistically significant at less than the .005 level.

Similar comparisons between lithium and placebo groups for the number of depressive episodes are shown in Table 5. Comparisons of the mean number of depressive episodes without controlling for study time revealed a very small difference, means of 0.440 and 0.481 episodes in the lithium and placebo groups respectively. However, when controlling for study time, the mean number of depressive episodes per patient-year in the lithium and placebo groups are 0.239 and 0.703 respectively. This difference yielded a critical ratio of 6.48, which is statistically significant at less than the .025 level.

TABLE 5

Comparison of frequency of depressive episodes in lithium and placebo groups

	Lithium	Placebo
Mean number of episodes	0.440	0.481
Mean number of years in study	1.840	0.685
Mean number of depressive episodes per patient-year	0.239	0.703
Number of cases	25	27

However, the hospitalization rates of the lithium and placebo depressed patients are of interest. The decision whether or not to hospitalize a patient was made by a physician, blind to the patient's treatment. Of the thirteen placebo patients who got depressed, seven (53.8%) were hospitalized. In contrast, only two of the seven lithium depressions (28.6%) were hospitalized. While these findings are not statistically significant and need to be interpreted with caution, they suggest that placebo depressed patients are more prone to acute episodes that require hospitalization, while those on lithium, although significantly depressed, could be treated as outpatients.

An analysis of manic failures on placebo or lithium was subsequently made controlling for whether the patient was admitted to the trial having previously been treated with

TABLE 6

Manic failures

Old cases				New cases			
	Lithium	Placebo	Total		Lithium	Placebo	Total
Failure	2	8	10	Failure	3	7	10
No failure	16	7	23	No failure	4	5	9
Total:	18	15	33	Total:	7	12	19

$\chi^2 = 5.05$ (p < .025) $\chi^2 = 0.03$ (ns)

lithium ("old" cases), or whether the patient had been freshly detected and admitted to the trial with no history of previous lithium administration. Table 6 shows that lithium is clearly superior to placebo in preventing future manic failure among the previously lithium treated patient group. However, there is no apparent prophylactic advantage of lithium over placebo in preventing mania among the freshly admitted bipolar patients.

Similarly an analysis of depressive failures is made among the "old" and "new" patient population.

From Table 7, it can be seen that lithium is clearly superior to placebo in preventing future depressive attacks in the "old" previously lithium treated group. However, among fresh cases not previously given lithium, this drug had no advantage over placebo in preventing future depressive attacks over the 28 month period.

TABLE 7

Depression failures

	New cases				Old cases		
	Lithium	Placebo	Total		Lithium	Placebo	Total
Failure	2	7	9	Failure	5	6	11
No failure	16	8	24	No failure	2	6	8
Total	18	15	33	Total	7	12	19

$\chi^2 = 3.58$ (p < .06) $\chi^2 = 0.18$ (ns)

The isolation of a group of patients with affective disorders who do not respond to lithium, perhaps for biological reasons, raises the further possibility that manic-depressive patients who are lithium non-responders might be genetically different from those who are lithium responders.

In order to investigate this hypothesis, we have undertaken a family study of all patients admitted into our on-going double-blind study of lithium prophylaxis in bipolar illness. All the available first degree relatives and spouses of the patients accepted in the study have been personally examined by one of the authors in order to determine the presence of psychopathology in their families. This investigator was blind in that he did not know which probands were assigned to lithium and which to placebo, and in that he was unaware of the patients' treatment response. The methodology of our family history study has been discussed in detail in a recent work (7).

Of the twenty-five manic-depressive patients followed on lithium carbonate, seventeen (70%) were responders, and eight (30%) were long-term failures. Three of the eight failures experienced manic episodes only, three experienced depressive episodes only, and two experienced both kinds of episodes. The lithium plasma levels for the responders as well as the failures were regularly maintained between 0.80 and 1.30 meq/liter. Of the twenty-seven patients followed on placebo, five (18%) were responders, and twenty-two (82%) were long-term failures. Twelve of the twenty-two failures experienced manic episodes only, five experienced depressive episodes only, and five experienced both kinds of episodes. All placebo patients, responders as well as failures, were given fictitious lithium plasma levels between 0.8 and 1.3 meq/liter to help maintain blindness of the treating physician.

Four samples of patients are thus available for further analysis: responders and failures under lithium and responders and failures under placebo. The mean numbers of living first degree relatives were similar in all four samples, ranging from 4.7 to 5.4 per family. The mean numbers of relatives examined were also similar, ranging from 3.7 to 4.4 per family.

Table 8 compares the responders and non-responder to lithium with respect to the presence or absence of bipolar illness in the proband's first degree relatives: eleven out of the seventeen responders to lithium had a positive family history of bipolar illness while only one out of the eight non-responders had a positive family history [p = .019 (Fisher Exact Probability Test)].

TABLE 8

Prophylactic response and family history in first degree relatives
1. Lithium sample

	Responder	Non-responder	Total
Bipolar illness present	11	1	12
Bipolar illness absent	6	7	13
Total	17	8	25

p = .019 (Fisher Exact Probability Test)

Because this association between family history and response to treatment may reflect a decreased frequency of affective episodes in patients with a positive family history, irrespective of treatment, the association was examined separately for the placebo sample. Table 9 shows an absence of any association between family history and response to placebo [p = .351 (Fisher Exact Probability Test)].

TABLE 9

Prophylactic response and family history in first degree relatives
2. Placebo sample

	Responder	Non-responder	Total
Bipolar illness present	2	11	13
Bipolar illness absent	3	11	14
Total	5	22	27

p = .351 (Fischer Exact Probability Test)

Information about second degree relatives was obtained on the basis of the recollections of the interviewed subjects. When this information is taken into account, the association for the lithium sample becomes even stronger (Table 10). Fourteen out of the seventeen responders to lithium had at least one first or second degree relative with a bipolar illness, while again only one out of the eight non-responders to lithium had a positive family history

Table 10

Prophylactic response and family history in first and second degree relatives
1. Lithium sample

	Responder	Non-responder	Total
Bipolar illness present	14	1	15
Bipolar illness absent	3	7	10
Total	17	8	25

p = .001 (Fisher Exact Probability Test)

[p = .001 (Fisher Exact Probability Test)]. Table 11 shows that, in contrast, there is no corresponding association in the placebo sample even when second degree relatives are taken into account [p = .245 (Fisher Exact Probability Test)]. Lithium responders are thus far more likely to have a genetic history of bipolar illness than lithium non-responders.

Table 11

Prophylactic response and family history in first and second degree relatives
2. Placebo sample

	Responder	Non-responder	Total
Bipolar illness present	2	14	16
Bipolar illnes absent	3	8	11
Total	5	22	27

p = .245 (Fisher Exact Probability Test)

Discussion

The overall research findings in this study clearly establish lithium prophylaxis of mania, and also lend support to lithium prophylaxis of bipolar depression. These findings are consistent with those reported by previous investigators (1, 3, 6), and also confirm a previous single-blind prophylaxis study done in this Clinic (5). However, prophylaxis is not a universal finding among all manic-depressives and its demonstration appears to depend on the nature of the sample studied with at least two new important variables being present or absent — a family history of mania, and prior history of adhering to a maintenance lithium regimen in an outpatient clinic.

The findings with respect to lithium prophylaxis of depression are somewhat ambiguous even when not controlling for "old" versus "new" cases. Since a large proportion of placebo patients experienced acute manic episodes, their continuation in the study in order to assess lithium prophylaxis of depression was not possible. Therefore, comparisons of depressive failure rates between lithium and placebo groups did not include a large proportion of placebo patients who had dropped out because of severe manic episodes. A further clarification of the question of lithium prophylaxis of depression ideally requires comparisons between lithium and placebo groups who are followed and studied for approximately equal durations. Further studies are currently under way with patients who are not prone to acute manic episodes and who are, therefore, more likely to complete lengthy trials without dropping out. Such a group, in itself, may constititute another subtype of the illness where depression rather than mania tends to dominate the course of the illness and thus affect the outcome in a prophylactic trial.

The finding that lithium response is related to the presence of mania in the family is consistent with a recent report by MENDLEWICZ et al. (7) showing that manic-depressive patients with a strong genetic background run a more severe course of illness, and exhibit more mania than patients with no family history. We have also found clinically that the greater the total amount of mania, the greater is the overall response to lithium therapy.

From the data it would appear that previously treated lithium patients who have managed to adhere to a lithium regimen in an outpatient clinic are likely to be lithium responders in a double-blind prophylactic trial. Likewise, bipolar patients with a family history of mania are prone to have a clinical course where manic episodes tend to dominate over episodes of depression, and these patients are more likely to show lithium prophylaxis. Although the numbers are small and need to be confirmed by other investigators in controlled longitudial studies where serum lithium levels are monitored on a regular basis, the present genetic findings underscore the need to correlate a patient's response to lithium with his genetic background in order to predict the long-term prognosis of patients on lithium maintenance therapy.

ACKNOWLEDGEMENTS

Thanks are due to Dr. Joseph Fleiss for his advice on the statistical analysis, and for his critical reading of the manuscript.

The assistance of Miss Geraldine Dalesandro and Mr. John O'Brien in tabulating the data is also gratefully acknowledged.

REFERENCES

1. BAASTRUP, P. C., PAULSEN, J. C., SCHOU, M. et al. (1970) Prophylactic Lithium: Double-Blind Discontinuation in Manic-Depressive and Recurrent Depressive Disorders. Lancet, 325.
2. BAASTRUP, P. C. and SCHOU, M. (1967) Lithium as a Prophylactic Agent: Its Effects against Recurrent Depression and Manic-Depressive Psychosis. Arch. gen. Psychiat. **16**, 162.
3. COPPEN, A., NOGUERA, R. BAILY, J. et al (1971) Prophylactic Lithium in Affective Disorders: Controlled Trial. Lancet, 275.
4. DEMING, W. W. (1966) Some Theory of Sampling. New York, Dover, page 177.
5. FIEVE, R. R., PLATMAN, S. R. and PLUTCHIK, R. R. (1968) The Use of Lithium in Affective Disorders: II. Prophylaxis of Depression in Chronic Recurrent Affective Disorders. Amer. J. Psychiat. **125**, 492.
6. MELIA, P. I. (1970) Prophylactic Lithium: A Double-Blind Trial in Recurrent Affective Disorders. Brit. J. Psychiat. **116**, 621.
7. MENDLEWICZ, J., FIEVE, R. R., RAINER, J. D. et al. (1972) Manic-Depressive Illness: A Comparative Study of Patients with and without a Family History. Brit. J. Psychiat. **120**, 523.

J.M., New York State Psychiatric Institute, 722 West 168th Street, New York, N. Y., U.S.A.

LITHIUM EFFECTS ON CARBOHYDRATE
AND ELECTROLYTE METABOLISM

E. T. MELLERUP, P. PLENGE and O. J. RAFAELSEN

Psychochemistry Institute, Rigshospitalet, Copenhagen

Lithium may influence electrolyte metabolism by a simplesubstit ution process, as lithium is similar to sodium and potassium with respect to charge, to magnesium with respect to ionic radius (r), and to calcium with respect to ionic potential $\left(\dfrac{e}{r}\right)$ (Table 1)

TABLE 1

Ion	r	$\dfrac{e}{r}$	Ion	r	$\dfrac{e}{r}$
Li⁺	**0.60**	**1,67**	Be²⁺	0.35	5.71
Na⁺	0.97	1.06	Mg²⁺	**0.66**	3.03
K⁺	1.33	0.75	Ca²⁺	0.99	**2.02**

If lithium replaces one of the four other cations, e.g., at a site on an enzyme where the cation is important for the enzymatic activity, this activity may be changed. Such a concept is supported by the fact that many enzymes influenced by lithium are activated or inhibited by one or more of the other cations. Some of these enzymes are listed in Table 2 (21).

Among the enzymes influenced by lithium are several belonging to carbohydrate metabolism, thus hexokinase is activated (1), whereas pyruvate kinase (1, 11), glycogen transferase kinase (22), and adenyl cyclase (4, 8, 14,) are inhibited. Furthermore, lithium may influence glucose transport across the cell membrane (13) (Fig. 1).

Each of these different effects of lithium may lead to an increased synthesis of glycogen, which in fact also are found in brain, muscle, and adipose tissue after lithium administration (2, 18). In liver, on the other hand, lithium may in acute experiments decrease the glycogen content due to an increase in plasma glucagon (15). As a consequence of the latter lithium effect, blood glucose increases shortly after the lithium administration, but probably due to the increased glycogen synthesis in the other tissues, blood glucose decreases

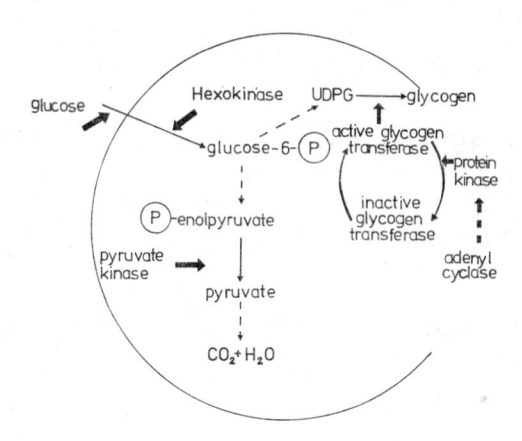

Fig. 1. Lithium influence on intermediary glucose metabolism.

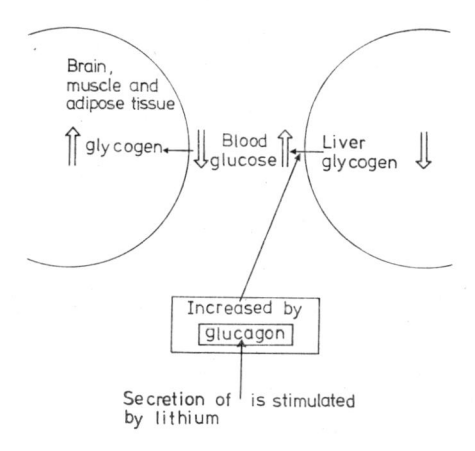

Fig. 2. Effect of lithium on glycogen metabolism and blood glucose.

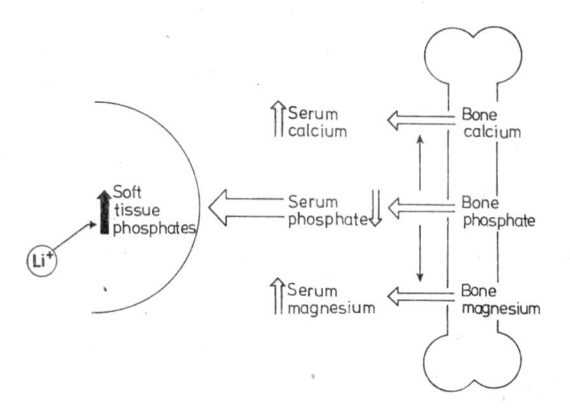

Fig. 3. Effect of lithium on phosphate, calcium and magnesium.

Table 2

Some enzymes, which all have been shown to be influenced by lithium, as well as by the other four cations

	Li+	Na+	K+	Mg²⁺	Ca²⁺
Acetyl thiokinase	i	i	a	a	
Adenosine triphosphatase	a	a		a	
Adenyl cyclase (brain)	i				
Adenyl cyclase (fatt cells)	i			a	i
Adenyl cyclase (kidney)	i			a	i
Aldehyd dehydrogenase	i		a	a	a
Glycogen transferase kinase	i		i		
Hexokinase	a			a	
Lactase	i	a	a		
Phosphotransacetylase	i	i	a		
Pyruvate kinase	i	a	a.	a	i
Tryptophanase	i	i	a	(i)	

a = Signifies activating effect.
i = Inhibitory effect.

some hours later (18). These effects of lithium may explain the weight gain seen in many lithium treated patients (12, 17) and the effect of lithium in the treatment of diabetic patients (23) (Fig. 2).

The increased glucose metabolism after lithium is followed by an increased uptake of phosphate into muscle, brain and liver leading to a lowering of serum phosphate and a decreased uptake of phosphate into the bones (19). Probably due to the stoichiometric relationship between phosphate and calcium in bone tissue, phosphate changes are accompanied by parallel changes in calcium, giving rise to increased serum calcium levels (16). As half of the total body magnesium is deposited in the bones, magnesium may also follow the changes in bone phosphate leading to an increase in serum magnesium (MELLERUP, PLENGE and RAFAELSEN, to be published) (Fig. 3).

As both calcium and magnesium are important for nerve excitability as well as for synaptic transmission (5, 9, 10, 20) it is possible that the influence of lithium on these two divalent cations may bear a relationship to the effect of lithium in manic-depressive psychosis.

References

1. BALAN, G., CERNÁTESCU, D., TRANDAFIRESCU, M. and ABABEI, L. (1970) The influence of lithium ions on the activity of hexokinase and pyruvatekinase. 7th CINP Congress, Prague.
2. BHATTACHARYA, G. (1959) Influence of ions on the uptake of glucose and on the effect of insulin on it by rat diaphragm. Nature, **183**, 324.
3. BHATTACHARYA, G. (1964) Influence of lithium on glucose metabolism in rats and rabbits. Biochim. biophys. Acta, **93**, 644.
4. BIRNBAUMER, L., POHL, S. L. and RODBELL, M. (1969) Adenyl cyclase in fat cells. J. biol. Chem. **244**, 3468.
5. BRINK, F. (1954) The role of calcium ions in neural processes. Pharmacol. Rev. **6**, 243.

6. CLAUSEN, T. (1968) The relationship between the transport of glucose and cations across cell membranes in isolated tissues. Biochim. biophys. Acta, **150**, 66.
7. CLAUSEN, T. (1972) Cations, glucose metabolism, and insulin action. A review.
8. FORN, J. and VALDECASAS, F. G. (1971) Effects of lithium on brain adenyl cyclase activity. Biochem. Pharmacol. **20**, 2773.
9. FRANKENHAEUSER, B. and HODGKIN, A. L. (1957) The action of calcium on the electrical properties of squid axons. J. Physiol. (Lond.) **138**(2), 218.
10. HUTTER, O. F. and KOSTIAL, K. (1954) Effect of magnesium and calcium ions on the release of acetylcholine. J. Physiol. (Lond.) **124**, 234.
11. KACHMAR, J. F. and BOYER, P. D. (1953) Kinetic analysis of enzyme reactions. The potassium activation and calcium inhibition of pyruvic phosphoferase. J. biol. Chem. **200**, 669.
12. KERRY, R. L., LIEBLING, L. I. and OWEN, G. (1970) Weight changes in lithium responders. Acta psychiat. scand. **46**, 238.
13. KOHN, P. G. and CLAUSEN, T. (1972) The relationship between the transport of glucose and cations across cell membranes in isolated tissues. Biochim. biophys. Acta, **255**, 798.
14. MARCUS, R. and AURBACH, G. D. (1971) Adenyl cyclase from renal cortex. Biochim. biophys. Acta, **242**, 410.
15. MELLERUP, E. T., THOMSEN, H. G., PLENGE, P. and RAFAELSEN, O. J. (1970) Lithium effect on plasma glucagon, liver phosphorylase-a and liver glycogen in rats. J. psychiat. Res. **8**, 37.
16. MELLERUP, E. T., PLENGE, P., ZIEGLER, R. and RAFAELSEN, O. J. (1970) Lithium effects on calcium metabolism in rats. Int. Pharmacopsychiat. **5**, 258.
17. MELLERUP, E. T., THOMSEN, H. G., BJØRUM, N. and RAFAELSEN, O. J. (1972) Lithium, weight gain, and serum insulin in manic-depressive patients. Acta psychiat. scand. **48**, 332.
18. PLENGE, P., MELLERUP, E. T. and RAFAELSEN, O. J. (1970) Lithium action on glycogen synthesis in rat brain, liver, and diaphragm. J. psychiat. Res. **8**, 29.
19. PLENGE, P., MELLERUP, E. T. and RAFAELSEN, O. J. (1971) Lithium action on rat phosphate metabolism. Int. Pharmacopsychiat. **6**, 52.
20. RUBIN, R. P. (1970) The role of calcium in the release of neurotransmitter substances and hormones. Pharmacol. Rev. **22**, 389.
21. SCHOU, M. (1957) Biology and pharmacology of the lithium ion. Pharmacol. Rev. **9**, 17.
22. WALAAS, E., WALAAS, O. and HORN, R. S. (1970) The regulatory effect of monovalent cations on protein kinase (glycogen transferase kinase). The mechanism of insulin action. Symposium, Oslo.
23. WEISS, H. (1924) Über eine neue Behandlungsmethode des Diabetes Mellitus und verwandter Stoffwechselstörungen. Wien. klin. Wschr. **37**, 1142.

E.T.M., Psychochemistry Institute, Rigshospitalet, 9, Blegdamsvej, DK-2100 Copenhagen, Denmark

LITHIUM STABILIZATION AND WEIGHT GAIN

P. GROF, E. LOUGHREY, B. SAXENA, L. DAIGLE, and J. QUESNELL

Hamilton Psychiatric Hospital, McMaster University, Hamilton, Ontario

Lithium salts like other psychoactive drugs may in long-term administration lead to weight gain. The body weight increase is usually mild, on the average less pronounced than, for instance, chlorpromazine induced obesity. Yet, in some patients the weight gain on lithium may be excessive and troublesome indeed and exceed 20% of the initial body weight.

Lithium-induced obesity raises several questions which we examined in this study: What, if any, is the relationship between the weight gain and the treatment response? What are the characteristics of the patients who gain excessively on lithium? Can this gain be reversed by a diet?

MATERIAL

The changes of body weight during lithium stabilization have been studied systematically month by month in a sample of 74 patients. The sample consisted of 42 manic-depressives, 28 schizo-affectives and 4 patients with recurring depression. There were more women in the group (42) than men (32). All of them have been placed on lithium

TABLE 1

Response to lithium. Distribution of diagnosis

	R	I	N	Entire group
Manic-depressives	19	22	1	42
Recurrent depressives	3	0	1	4
Schizo-affectives	8	6	14	28
	30	28	16	74

R — complete response, I — intermediate response, N — no response.

because of a long history of frequently relapsing affective disease. The illness lasted prior to the initiation of treatment for 19 years on the average (range 2—45 years) and the mean age at the initiation of lithium stabilization was 46 years, with the range between 18 and 79 years.

TABLE 2

Response to lithium. Age at the initiation of the treatment

	R	I	N	Entire group
Mean ± SD	42.8 ± 13.6	50.2 ± 11.0	40.0 ± 11.4	46.2 ± 12.6
Range	18—69	20—79	19—59	18—79

R — complete response, I — intermediate response, N — no response.

Results

Weight gain and response

In order to investigate the relationship between the benefit from treatment and weight gain, the patients were classified into three groups using arbitrary definitions based on the change of relapse rate. These definitions were as follows. A complete responder has not experienced any relapse on lithium for at least 12 months despite having a high risk for further episodes. A non-responder was defined as a person whose relapse rate has not decreased despite adequate lithium treatment. Intermediate group showed improved relapse rate only. A patient was considered having high risk for relapse if he had more than 4 previous episodes, with at least 2 of them occurring during the 2 years preceding lithium. By methods previously elaborated we felt we had secure grounds on which to define all three groups. Using these definitions, there were 30 complete responders, 28 intermediates and 16 non-responders in our sample.

While the complete responders kept gaining weight during the first year of treatment and the increase of body weight averaged more than 10 pounds, the non-responders during the same time did not put on any weight on the average. The intermediates as a group showed moderate increase of body weight and their values are placed in the middle between complete responders and non-responders. Expressed in percentage of the pretreatment body weight, complete responders gained $6^1/_2\%$ of their weight which is less than the gain usually observed with most phenothiazines or thioxanthines (1).

Using a chi-square, we found a significant association between the weight gain and favourable response to lithium treatment ($p < .01$). Also, there was a significant difference between the weight changes of complete responders and non-responders. The difference was less pronounced when we expressed the changes in terms of the percentage of the pretreatment body weight for each patient. This is because the complete responders with higher body weight prior to the treatment were inclined to gain weight faster. Although there was a great degree of variability in the body weight changes among our patients, it was possible to demonstrate a consistent relationship between clinical response and body weight changes.

It should be emphasized, however, that we were able to prove this relationship statistically only because our criteria for the inclusion of an affective disorder were broad enough to supply us with a relatively large number of non-responders and fairly low count of patients with excessive weight gain. Whereas in Hamilton, only 20% of patients gained weight excessively (over 5 kilograms during the first year), in our previous studies (4, 6) with more stringent criteria more than 30% showed considerable weight gain. If one administers lithium to manic-depressive patients only, 50% may gain weight excessively (7).

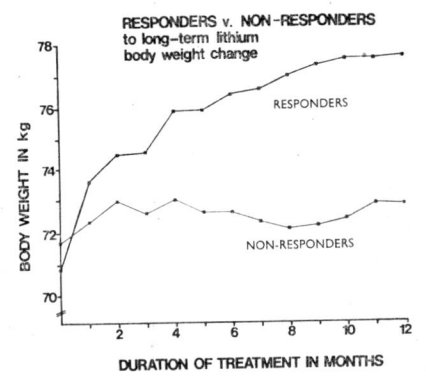

Fig. 1. Changes of body weight during the first year of lithium treatment. Complete responders (n = 30) and non-responders (n = 16) plotted separately.

Naturally, we were wondering whether the non-responders fail to gain weight on lithium because they keep losing the same during relapses. However, the analysis of the weight changes observed in non-responders does not support this hypothesis. The average change of weight in non-responders was only slight during relapses as compared to their weight during free intervals, and could not match the gain observed in complete responders. From our data it seems more likely that in non-responding patients neither relapses nor the mechanisms regulating the body weight were influenced by lithium.

As the non-responders showed no psychiatric benefit along with the lack of weight gain, one has to consider the possibility that they were not treated adequately. However, average serum levels of non-responders were found even slightly higher than those of responders and thus the assumption of inadequate treatment does not hold.

Another piece of evidence concerning the relationship between weight gain and response to lithium came from a configuration analysis conducted on our patients and reported in detail elsewhere (5). Only two clear-cut configurations emerged from the material on our patients: firstly a group of those suffering from a typical affective disorder who gain considerably and respond well. Secondly, those with schizo-affective type who fail in both putting on weight and responding. Thus, although it remains unresolved in the literature on phenothiazines whether there is a relationship between weight gain and clinical response, it appears from our data that such relationship does exist with lithium salts.

It is also worth noticing that the peak of the weight gain coincides with the maximum clinical improvement achieved. Whereas the average weight gain gradually increases and reaches its plateau between the 10th and 12th month of lithium administration, the relapse rate for the groups of patients shows a sharp decline during the first year of treatment (2, 3). During the second year relapse rate for the groups of patients remains at a constant minimum and also the body weight shows a relative stabilization with a slight tendency to lose some of the previously accumulated pounds.

Patients at risk for excessive gain

When placed on long-term lithium many patients do gain some weight. However, only some of them put on pounds excessively and therefore require special attention. We feel that it is clinically important to anticipate who is predisposed to excessive gain on lithium. Who are the people we should be concerned about when placing them on long-term lithium?

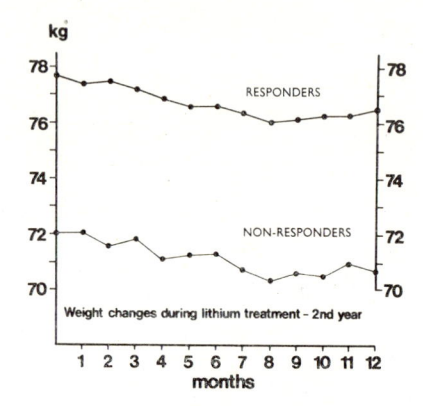

Fig. 2. Changes of body weight during the second year of lithium treatment.

We analyzed our material from this point of view and found significant association between lithium-induced weight gain and the following factors: obesity of the patient prior to starting lithium, one or both parents being overweight. As mentioned before a complete clinical response was also significantly linked up with the weight gain. Patients with parents from continental Europe showed tendency to gain more weight. Unipolar depressions showed a higher average increase of weight than manic-depressives; however, the number in our sample is scarce. Other factors such as the extent of previous weight fluctuations, the country of the patient's origin, etc. appeared unrelated. Apparently, patients with these characteristics are predisposed to obesity in general. However, our observations on the patients who discontinued lithium and showed an immediate and profound loss indicate that we have been dealing with a drug-induced weight gain.

Thus, it would emerge from our data that a typical patient at risk for lithium-induced obesity is a lady who arrives chubby for the lithium screening, her parents came from continental Europe and one or both of them were on the heavy side.

Effects of balanced, low-calorie diet

The question now arises whether the weight gain on lithium can be reversed by dietary measures. Space does not allow our observations to be reported in detail; we are describing them elsewhere.

So far, we have tried a systematic dietetic approach with 21 patients who were overweight during long-term lithium treatment. In each patient, prior to his being placed on a diet, food intake was assessed quantitatively. The average caloric intake was around 1800 calories a day. For each patient, an experienced dietician then tailored a balanced, low-calorie diet. Average caloric value of these diets was around 1200 calories a day. In evaluating the results seen so far our sample can be broken down into three subgroups.

A good third of the patients did cooperate satisfactorily and stuck closely to the proposed restrictions in their food. Paradoxically, scales failed to demonstrate any significant success in terms of reduction of the body weight.

Another third of our patients, after being placed on the diet, lost only their motivation to diet but no pounds. These patients made frequent complaints about their body weight on lithium; however, when they were advised as to the dietary regime they found it difficult to follow the advice, for a variety of reasons.

The remaining third of the patients showed weight loss while following the devised diet. However, we had also data available on six lithium responders with weight gain who for one or another reasons discontinued lithium and were followed up in terms of body weight The weight loss in the dieting patients by far did not match the weight reduction of the patients who went off lithium.

Thus, we have not had much success with a balanced low-calorie diet. One-third of the patients did not cooperate enough, one-third did not lose despite compliance, and only one-third showed some success. However, the only profound weight loss was observed in the patients who went off lithium.

It is worth mentioning that recently we have had a striking success in several patients with a low carbohydrate diet, without any particular caloric restrictions.

Summary

A sample of 74 patients with recurring affective disorder was treated with lithium and followed up for two years; the body weight was regularly checked. A positive association between the weight gain and favourable response to treatment was found. Patients particularly prone to gain weight are those who are obese prior to lithium and have a family history of obesity. A balanced, low-calorie diet was unsuccessful as it led to only marginal weight reduction in one-third of those who gained weight.

References

1. AMDISEN, A. (1964) Drug-produced obesity. Dan. med. Bul. **11**, 182.
2. ANGST, J., WEIS, P. GROF, P., BAASTRUP, P. C. and SCHOU, M. (1970) Lithium prophylaxis in recurrent affective disorders. Brit. J. Psychiat. **116**, 599.
3. COPPEN, A., NOGUERA, G. and BAILEY, J. (1971) Prophylactic lithium in affective disorders — A controlled study. Lancet i, August 7, 275.
4. DOSTAL, T., ANGST, J., DITTRICH, A. and GROF, P. (1971) Profylaktické účinky lithiovych solí u periodickych afektivních psychóz. Cs. Psychiat. **67**, 151.
5. GROF, P., MACCRIMMON, D., STREINER, D., FRITZE, K., ROBERTSON, R. and DOSTAL, T. (1972) Responders and non-responders to long-term lithium. To be published.
6. GROF, P., VINAŘ, O., GRÓFOVÁ, E. and ZVOLSKÝ, P. (1969) Prophylaktische Wirkung von Lithium bei oft rezidivierenden affektiven Erkrankungen. Arzneim. Forsch. **19**, 454.
7. MELLERUP, E. T. (1972) Personal communication.

P. G., Department of Psychiatry, McMaster University,
Hamilton Psychiatric Hospital, Hamilton, Ontario,
Canada

"TECHNICAL FAILURES" IN LITHIUM PROPHYLAXIS

W. WERNER

University Neuropsychiatric Clinic, Homburg-Saar

Our experience with lithium prophylaxis has shown that lithium, in some cases, could not have its intended effect because it had been discontinued after some time. Because of this, some psychiatrists feel that the enormous effort of controlling blood levels is a useless endeavor, since even the most simple conditions ensuring regular lithium intake have not been guaranteed. If one considers that lithium is a drug taken, as it were, by so-called healthy patients and that, furthermore, it shows no abstinence symptoms, such criticism is justified.

Since we have had such disappointing results in our own lithium prophylaxis, we tried to discover the most important factors of such "technical failures". We call such failures "technical" because they were not conditioned by an absence of lithium effect or of an appropriate patient sample. Moreover, these "technical failures" were conditioned by organizational factors and could therefore be influenced.

TABLE 1

Lithium prophylaxis

	CLT	ILT	LS
Male (%)	53.5	38.5	44.4
Female (%)	46.5	61.5	55.6
Age at time of starting (average in years)	44.37	47.38	46.39
Length of illness at time of starting (average in years)	10.91	12.00	12.67
Number of times already ill at time of starting (average)	8.94	9.62	6.97
Illness frequency (pro year)	0.81	0.8	0.54

CLT — Continuous Lithium Takers (71 pat.)   ILT — Intermittent Lithium Takers (13 pat.)
LS — Lithium Stoppers (36 pat.)

In the course of the past five years, we started 149 patients on lithium. The greater majority of these patients were typical manic-depressives and patients who had had repeated depressive phases after the age of 45. In our group of patients, so-called schizo-affective psychoses were a rarity. Almost half of these 149 patients we knew personally. All these patients were asked to fill out a rather complete questionnaire, which could be answered by checking off either "yes" or "no". 120 patients completed the questionnaire. Our results stem from this group of 120 patients. We found that 71 patients, that is 59.2%, took lithium continuously. We shall call this group the "continuous-lithium-takers". 36 patients, that is 30%, completely stopped taking lithium. 13 patients, that is 10.8%, took lithium only intermittently. We called these last two groups the "lithium-stoppers" and the "intermittent-lithium-takers".

In order to discover possible factors determining such differences in lithium intake, we first examined the more obvious possibilities (Table 1). Statistically important deviations are indicated in the tables by a cross and statistically significant deviations are denoted by asterisks. As the results show, no important differences were found either with respect to age or sex. The individual experience of illness played no major role, i.e. the length of the illness and the number of previous phases was almost the same in the various groups. However, in the case of the lithium-stoppers, the phase frequency was seen to be somewhat less.

TABLE 2

Lithium prophylaxis

	CLT	ILT	LS
Hereditary loading with psychosis or suicide (%)	43.1	38.5	58.3
Hereditary loading with suicide (%)	15.3	23.1	27.8 +
Typical psychopathology (%)	73.6	92.3	69.4
Ability to understand lithium instructions (%)	75.0	76.9	66.7

χ^2: [+ $p < 0.1$] * $p < 0.05$ ** $p < 0.01$ *** $p < 0.001$

CLT — Continuous Lithium Takers (71 pat.) ILT — Intermittent Lithium Takers (13 pat.)
LS — Lithium Stoppers (36 pat.)

Initially, we thought that the incidence of a similar illness or a suicide in a patient's close relative might have been the prime motivation to continue lithium prophylaxis (Table 2). In patients with hereditary loading for suicide, there was, an opposite tendency, but no significant difference was found. On the other hand, suicidal attempts on the part of the patient played no motivating role. Initially, it was also thought that "technical failures" might be due to a nosologically inappropriate patient sample. On re-checking all the case histories, we found no significant differences. In general, most of our patients were aware of the importance of continuing lithium prophylaxis. At any rate, in patients aware of this fact, there was no question of mental retardation or dementia.

When we consider the time factor i.e. the time at which the patient was placed on lithium, we find, for the first time, statistically significant differences (Table 3). In general, it was found that the most important factor was the intensity with which the physician attempted to prod the patient to continue taking lithium or to start taking lithium once again. This was the case either when the doctor had a small talk with the patient at the

TABLE 3

Lithium prophylaxis

	CLT	ILT	LS
Conversation with physician at time of starting (%)	54.4	50.0	39.3
Conversation regarding the effect of lithium (%)	41.2	58.3	28.6**
Information about possible lag in lithium effect (%)	48.5	41.7	28.6 +
Information about side-effects (%)	60.3	50.0	32.1*
Information about blood lithium level (%)	54.4	41.7	32.1 +
Written instruction about lithium (%)	42.6	16.7	25.0**

$\chi^2: [+ p < 0.1] * p < 0.05 ** p < 0.01 *** p > 0.001$

CLT — Continuous Lithium Takers (71 pat.) ILT — Intermittent Lithium Takers (13 pat.)
LS — Lithium Stoppers (36 pat.)

time of starting lithium or if the doctor gave more detailed information about the effect of lithium. With respect to these means of providing information, the physicians concerned themselves least with the lithium-stoppers. The same was also the case when the physician provided other forms of information, such as telling the patient that lithium might have its first prophylactic effect after half-a-year to one year, or when the doctor told the patient that lithium might have some side-effects of a temporary nature. Furthermore, only 32.1% of the lithium-stoppers were made aware by the physician that a certain blood lithium level was necessary for lithium to have its effect. Lastly, only one fourth of the lithium-stopper-group was given written instructions by their physicians. This shows that written instructions and conversation giving details about the effects of lithium seem to be of prime importance.

TABLE 4

Lithium prophylaxis

	CLT	ILT	LS
Starting of lithium during depressive phase (%)	61.1	69.2	72.2
Starting of lithium during manic phase (%)	26.4	23.1	11.1*
Starting of lithium during interval between phases (%)	11.1	0.0	8.3

$\chi^2: [+ p < 0.1] * p < 0.05 ** p < 0.01 *** p < 0.001$

CLT — Continuous Lithium Takers (71 pat.) ILT — Intermittent Lithium Takers (13 pat.)
LS — Lithium Stoppers (36 pat.)

We then considered the point of time at which lithium was started (Table 4). The results indicate that patients started on lithium in the manic-phase show the least amount of lithium-stoppers. However, the number of manic-phase patients in our sample was not sufficient for us to make a definite statement on this point.

TABLE 5

Lithium prophylaxis

	CLT	ILT	LS
Patient-trust (%)	57.4	58.3	39.3
Autosuggestion (%)	42.6	41.7	25.0 +
Lithium considered dangerous (%)	35.3	0.0	17.9 +
Lithium considered not dangerous (%)	57.4	58.3	28.6**

χ^2: [+ p < 0.1] * p < 0.05 ** p < 0.01 *** p < 0.001

CLT — Continuous Lithium Takers (71 pat.)   ILT — Intermittent Lithium Takers (13 pat.)
LS — Lithium Stoppers (36 pat.)

We then attempted to analyse the inner commitment of the patient to lithium prophylaxis (Table 5). Our results demonstrated, though, to a statistically insignificant degree that trust in the doctor and autosuggestion play an important role. 42.6% of the continuous lithium takers were certain from the very start that they now had effective medication against a relapse of the illness. It is interesting to note that the fact that lithium might be a dangerous drug played an unimportant role with respect to its discontinuation. The continuous-lithium-takers believed twice as often that lithium was a dangerous drug as did the lithium-stoppers. A bit confusing was the significant result that continuous-lithium-takers were also more often of the opinion that lithium was not a dangerous drug. Our results might be interpreted as follows: that the continuous-lithium-takers had a definite point of view with regard to lithium, but that the lithium-stoppers, on the other hand, did not show such a clearcut attitude.

TABLE 6

Lithium prophylaxis

	CLT	ILT	LS
Regular blood lithium controls (%)	35.3	58.3	35.7*
Regular blood lithium controls plus conversation with physician (%)	61.9	53.8	13.9***

χ^2: [+ p < 0.1] * p < 0.05 ** p < 0.01 *** p < 0.001

CLT — Continuous Lithium Takers (71 pat.)   ILT — Intermittent Lithium Takers (13 pat.)
LS — Lithium Stoppers (36 pat.)

We now considered another aspect of lithium prophylaxis: the time between the starting and stopping of lithium (Table 6). Once again, it was seen that the intensity of the physician's concern was of prime importance. It appears that although regular blood lithium controls were very important for the continuation of lithium intake, it was much more important for such continuation that at the time of the blood-taking the physician had a conversation with the patient. Our results show that only 13.9% of the lithium-stoppers engaged in such conversations which represented opportunities for the physician to discuss side-effects with the patient or warn him that lithium might take some time to work. In addition, if necessary, the physician could immediately treat any affective changes present at that time.

TABLE 7

Lithium prophylaxis

	CLT	ILT	LS
Length of follow-up (average in months)	21.31	36.25	27.21
Length of follow-up until stoppage or intermittent use of lithium (average in months)		12.90	7.37

CLT — Continuous Lithium Takers (71 pat.)   ILT — Intermittent Lithium Takers (13 pat.)
LS — Lithium Stoppers (36 pat.)

Our study then considered why some people discontinued lithium and why others took it only intermittently. It must also be noted that the preponderance of continuous-lithium-takers in our sample was not conditioned by a shorter or too short follow-up. The length of follow-up was almost the same for continuous-lithium-takers and lithium-stoppers (Table 7). Indeed, the period of follow-up in the case of continuous-lithium-takers was three times as long as the time until lithium was stopped and twice as long as the time until lithium started to be used intermittently.

TABLE 8

Lithium prophylaxis

	ILT	LS
Indicated (%)	15.4	16.7
Because of initial side-effects (%)	30.8	44.4
Because of inadequate information concerning necessity of lithium continuation (%)	15.4	25.0
Because of recurrence of illness (%)	23.1	16.6
Not indicated and no reason given by physician (%)	15.4	22.2
Lithium stoppage or intermittent lithium use not indicated by physician (%)	30.8	44.4

ILT — Intermittent Lithium Takers (13 pat.)   LS — Lithium Stoppers (36 pat.)

In analysing the conditions under which lithium was stopped or used intermittently, it was found that only in 16.7% or 15.4% of patients respectively a serious enough indication was present to make such a change: for example, an intoxication, an ECG-change or a pregnancy (Table 8). In almost as many cases lithium was stopped without a medical reason being given by the physician. The patients were given various reasons why they no longer required the drug. Some were told that they were too healthy to continue the use of lithium. In many cases, the physician or the patient discontinued lithium because of initial side-effects, often due to the fact that they were unaware of such side-effects and their temporary nature. Many patients were never told that this was a form of long-term prophylaxis with the necessity of continued lithium intake. Furthermore, just as many patients were of the opinion that lithium had failed because they had been again taken ill, usually during the first year after lithium had been started, and they therefore felt that further intake of lithium was useless.

SUMMARY

The main determinant of so-called "technical failures" in lithium prophylaxis seems to be lack of providing proper information or false decision-making on the part of the physician. For example, we saw that an uncalled for intermittent use of lithium (30.8%) or discontinuation of lithium (44.4%) were directly attributed to the physician. If we further consider the failure to provide information on the part of the physician at the time when lithium intake was first started, the results show that lithium stoppage was necessary in only 6 out of 36 cases of lithium-stoppers and an intermittent use of lithium was necessary in only 4 out of 13 cases of intermittent-lithium-takers. In other words, 83.3% of the lithium-stoppers were denied effective protection against falling ill by factors which could have been prevented. It can be therefore stated that the "technical failures" of lithium prophylaxis were not due to a wrong choice of patient material or specific disadvantages of lithium. An important factor seems to be inadequate concern on the part of the physician at the time of starting lithium. Even more important is the fact that physicians giving follow-up care lack proper information themselves. The practical consequences are self-evident. They are of as great importance as the development of still better tolerated lithium preparations.

W.W., University Neuropsychiatric Clinic,
665 Homburg — Saar, F.R.G.

NEED FOR ADDITIONAL MEDICATION IN OUT-PATIENTS DURING THREE YEARS OF PROPHYLACTIC LITHIUM TREATMENT

S. KANOWSKI and B. MUELLER-OERLINGHAUSEN

Psychiatric Clinic of the Free University, West Berlin

Most studies on the therapeutic or prophylactic efficacy of lithium treatment are based on controlled conditions in such a way that the patients receive only lithium during a limited experimental period (2, 3, 4). Additional drug treatment was not given in those trials except in case of acute relapses. All patients who were in constant need of other psychotropic drugs are considered as non-responders of lithium therapy or drop-outs. Furthermore, in investigations focussing on the prophylactic effect of lithium patients have been selected mainly according to the clinical criteria of recurrent affective disorders (4, 7, 8).

However, these experimental conditions under which reliable drug studies are performed do not meet the everyday problems of non resident psychiatrists treating out-patients. In daily routine work one is rarely concerned with plain and unobjectionable psychiatric diagnoses and has to accept the frequent therapeutic interventions of the patients themselves (5).

We started our lithium investigations in 1967 as an uncontrolled study. Originally only patients with recurrent affective disorders and at least 3 relapses during the last three "prelithium" years were admitted to the study. Our main goal was not to prove the prophylactic action of lithium but to study special problems as e.g. side effects and changes of the EEG (6).

Yet in the long run we learned that it was extremely difficult to follow the rules we had set up formerly, i.e. to prescribe only lithium and no other medication. Initially, there were only a few exceptions to this general rule, but in the mean time they turned up to a considerable percentage of our sample. Therefore, it might be of some interest to analyse the frequency and reasons of combined therapy and how they are related to sex, diagnoses and number of relapses or side effects.

For this retrospective study we selected all patients who have been on lithium treatment for at least three years. They had never been treated with lithium before and most of them started the therapy as in-patients of our department. 16 male and 24 female patients fit these criteria of selection. The age distribution of males and females did not differ in any way, the average age being 49 years.

The most common reasons for combined drug treatment were:

1. Patients had been on neuroleptic or antidepressive treatment before lithium therapy started, — yet the dosage of the former drug therapy could be reduced step by step because the patients were too much afraid of another relapse.

2. Some patients experienced more or less severe relapses and antidepressive or neuroleptic treatment was requested by the patients themselves or their relatives. Social needs and ethic considerations did not allow the withholding of additional medication.

3. In some patients lithium therapy did not suppress all symptoms or complaints and the patients were not willing to do without additional drugs as e.g. hypnotics, minor tranquilizers or antidepressives.

4. Some patients remained under care of general practicioners or non-resident psychiatrists so that the therapeutic strategy was not fully under our control.

TABLE 1

Diagnostic distribution of 40 patients (24 ♀, 16 ♂) treated with lithium only or lithium combined with other drugs over 3 years

Treatment	Recurrent affective psychosis ICD 296.1—3 Unipolar	Recurrent affective psychosis ICD 296.1—3 Bipolar	Schizoaffective psychosis ICD 295.7	Other
Lithium N = 13	6 (1 ♀, 5 ♂)	5 (4 ♀, 1 ♂)	—	2 (1 ♀, 1 ♂)
Lithium + psychopharmaca N = 27	7 (6 ♀, 1 ♂)	12 (7 ♀, 5 ♂)	7 (4 ♀, 3 ♂)	1 (♀)

TABLE 2

Frequency of the different types of combined treatment at the beginning and during the 3rd year of lithium treatment. Additional treatment was given either temporarily (intermit.) or continuously (contin.)

Treatment	Initial	Third year intermit.	Third year contin.	△ pat
Lithium + neuroleptics	10 (6 ♀, 4 ♂)	1 (♀)	7 (4 ♀, 3 ♂)	—2
Lithium + antidepressants	7 (5 ♀, 2 ♂)	4 (2 ♀, 2 ♂)	3 (2 ♀, 1 ♂)	0
Lithium + neuroleptics + antidepressants	5 (♀)	—	3 (♀)	—2
Lithium + sedatives + antidepressants	2 (♀)	—	—	—2
Lithium + sedatives	1 (♀)	2 (1 ♀, 1 ♂)	2 (1 ♀, 1 ♂)	+3
Lithium + miscellaneous	2 (♀)	1 (♀)	—	—1
Σ	27 (21 ♀, 6 ♂)	8 (5 ♀, 3 ♂)	15 (10 ♀, 5 ♂)	—4

△ pat — difference between number of patients at the beginning and during the 3rd year of treatment.

The relation between the diagnostic classifications and the types of treatment can be seen from Table 1. In agreement with the results of other authors (1) we observed that patients with schizoaffective disorders did not well on lithium only and needed additional treatment with psychotropic drugs (mostly neuroleptics).

TABLE 3

Cumulated relapses during 3 years of lithium treatment

Treatment	♀	♂
Lithium $N_1 = 8$ (2 ♀, 6 ♂)	2 (—) $n = 1$	4 (—) $n = 2$
Lithium + psychopharmaca $N_2 = 32$ (22 ♀, 10 ♂)	50 (6) $n = 19$	19 (4) $n = 8$

( ) — number of admissions to a hospital.
N_1 — number of patients treated with lithium exclusively.
N_2 — number of patients receiving any additional treatment during the 3 years period.
n — number of relapsed patients.

TABLE 4

Mean ($\bar{x}$) and median ($\tilde{x}$) values of lithium serum concentration (meq/liter). The figures given are based upon all serum samples of each treatment subgroup taken during the first or 3rd year respectively

Treatment		♀ 1st year	♀ 3rd year	♂ 1st year	♂ 3rd year
Lithium	$\bar{x}$	0.685	0.721	0.729	0.645
	$s_{\bar{x}}$	±0.028	±0.019	±0.027	±0.029
	$\tilde{x}$	**0.67**	**0.75**	**0.76**	**0.66**
	N	3 (33)	9 (81)	9 (91)	8 (44)
Lithium + miscellaneous	$\bar{x}$	0.807	0.746		
	$s_{\bar{x}}$	±0.057	±0.079	—	—
	$\tilde{x}$	**0.80**	**0.71**		
	N	2 (24)	1 (9)		
Lithium + psychopharmaca	$\bar{x}$	0.771	0.699	0.751	0.647
	$s_{\bar{x}}$	±0.016	±0.018	±0.025	±0.028
	$\tilde{x}$	**0.78**	**0.70**	**0.75**	**0.60**
	N	19 (244)	14 (114)	7 (35)	8 (44)

$s_{\bar{x}}$ — s.e.m.
N — number of patients.
N ( ) — number of serum samples.

Table 2 shows the frequency of different types of combined treatment at the beginning of lithium therapy and during the 3rd year. More than 50% of the patients recieved additional psychotropic drugs the ratio being nearly the same during the first and the third year of lithium treatment for both sexes resp. Nevertheless the dosage of the additional drugs given could be reduced in most cases during the 3 years period.

Those patients who needed combined treatment had the highest incidence of relapses (Table 3). However, in a remarkably low amount had these relapsed patients to be treated as in-patients in the hospital. 13 of 75 relapses and 4 of 10 hospital admissions refer to patients with schizoaffective disorders. The patients treated with lithium only showed a smaller total number of relapses and in no case did they need clinical treatment as in-patients (the difference is statistically significant).

The mean and median values of the cumulated lithium serum concentrations for both types of treatment during the first and third year are listed in Table 4. (We preferred the median values for any calculations as a normal distribution of the single values can not be taken for granted). There is a small decrease of the mean and median serum levels during the third as compared to the first year in 3 groups. This difference is significant whereas the increase of serum levels in females treated with lithium only during the third year is not. Whether these changes are of any biological relevance can not be decided at present.

TABLE 5

Number of some registered side effects or complaints calculated as percentage of patients check-ups (see text)

Treatment	Items	♀ 1st year	♀ 3rd year	♂ 1st year	♂ 3rd year
Lithium	Tiredness	51.5	8.3	1.1	2.7
	Thirst	72.7	29.1	7.7	10.8
	Sweating	0	3.1	3.3	—
	Tremor	33.3	6.2	18.7	—
	Insomnia	6.1	1.0	2.2	5.4
	N (patients)	3	9	9	8
	N (Σ check-ups)	33	96	91	37
Lithium + psychopharmaca	Tiredness	30.8	29.8	1.4	—
	Thirst	57.6	36.2	9.6	16.2
	Sweating	6.6	14.5	1.4	8.1
	Tremor	37.9	36.2	20.5	21.6
	Insomnia	39.5	39.5	23.3	29.7
	N (patients)	19	14	7	8
	N (Σ check-ups)	243	124	73	37

If we look at the distribution of the most frequent physical complaints which our patients expressed under lithium therapy (Table 5) the most prominent feature is that female patients have a much higher incidence of physical and other complaints than males. The incidence of each item has been summed up for the three years period of each group of patients.*) Obviously the rate of side effects decreases markedly in those female patients who received only lithium treatment whereas the males show generally smaller changes. It would be of great therapeutic consequence to know whether the higher incidence of complaints during the third year within the group of patients with combined treatment is due to the additional medication itself or to the fact of unresponsive disease. However, on the basis of the present data no decision can be made about this problem.

The results of this investigation indicate that lithium alone is not sufficient as long-term treatment in a high percentage of recurrent affective disorders. However, even in those patients requiring additional psychopharmacotherapy the therapeutic outcome seems to be favorable insofar that hospital admissions have been shown not to be necessary in many cases. Schizoaffective disorders without exception always needed combined treatment and showed the poorest therapeutic results.

REFERENCES

1. ANGST, J., BAASTRUP, P., GROF, P., SCHOU, M. and WEIS, P. (1969) Die Prophylaxe manisch-depressivschizophrener Mischpsychosen. In: Neuroleptische Dauer- und Depottherapie in der Psychiatrie. Ed. K. Heinrich, Konstanz.
2. ANGST, J., WEIS, P., GROF, P., BAASTRUP, P. C. and SCHOU, M. (1970) Lithium-prophylaxis in recurrent affective disorders. Brit. J. Psychiat. 116, 604.
3. BAASTRUP, P. C. and SCHOU, M. (1967) Lithium as a prophylactic agent. Arch. gen. Psychiat. 16, 162.
4. BAASTRUP, P. C., POULSEN, J. C., SCHOU, M., THOMSEN, K. and AMIDSEN, A. (1970) Prophylactic lithium: double blind discontinuation in manic-depressive and recurrent-depressive disorders. Lancet II, 326.
5. FREYHAN, F. A., O'CONNELL, R. A. and MAYO, J. A. (1970) Treatment of mood disorders with lithium carbonate. Int. Pharmacopsychiat. 5, 137.
6. HELMCHEN, H. and KANOWSKI, S. (1971) EEG-Veränderungen unter Lithium-Therapie. Nervenarzt, 42, 144.
7. MELIA, P. I. (1970) Prophylactic lithium: a double-blind trial in recurrent affective disorders. Brit. J. Psychiat. 116, 621.
8. MENDELS, J., SEKUNDA, S. K. and LAUDERBACH, W. (1972) A controlled study of the antidepressant effects of lithium carbonate. Arch. gen. Psychiat. 26, 154.

B.M. — Oe., Psychiatric Clinic of the Free University, West Berlin

---

*) The frequency is expressed as percentage of single check-ups. This procedure has been found necessary because the total number of check-ups is so different between males and females. For this remarkable difference social factors may be mainly responsible.

LONG-TERM EFFECTS OF PSYCHOTROPIC DRUGS

Chairmen: HANNAH STEINBERG and J. P. VON WARTBURG

Associate chairman: E. BECHGAARD

ACKNOWLEDGEMENTS

Help from the following is gratefully acknowledged: the Boston Mental Health Fund, F. Hoffmann-La Roche & Co. and Mrs. E. Lawrence.

LONG TERM AFTER-EFFECTS OF PSYCHOACTIVE DRUGS ON ANIMAL BEHAVIOUR*)

HANNAH STEINBERG and M. TOMKIEWICZ

Department of Pharmacology, University College London

This paper deals with some puzzling after-effects which can follow the administration of psychoactive drugs. "After-effect" is a rag-bag term which, nevertheless, seems to refer to interesting, important and robust phenomena, and our purpose is to draw attention to the need for making it clearer. In its simplest sense it refers to changes which can be detected when there is no reason to suppose that a drug or its active metabolites are still present in the organism, though it must presumably involve anatomical and/or biochemical changes. This paper deals with some after-effects of psychoactive drugs on animal behaviour only.

It has often been observed that the effects of merely a single or of a relatively short-term administration of psychoactive drugs in animals can persist for a surprisingly long time. For example, many studies have shown that various treatments administered to animals when young can profoundly affect their adult behaviour (11). Furthermore, some drug treatment given in infancy not only affect the behaviour of adults (8, 10, 21, 33), but their effects can even be detected in the second and third generations (5, 9). Findings of this kind, although startling, are perhaps not too surprising: not inplausible it is that any important changes in the life circumstances of an *immature* organism are likely to alter the course of its subsequent development. What is much more surprising is that some treatments given to *adults* appear to have extremely long lasting after-effects and to be seemingly ineradicable. For example, in adult rats "tolerance" to a single dose of morphine can persist for several months, and for even as long as a year (5, 6, 12).

In the course of our own work we can distinguish three kinds of circumstances in which drug effects on different forms of behaviour of rats and mice persist for long periods after the original treatment. The particular circumstances are: (1) after-effects of single drug administration on behaviour in novel environments, (2) after-effects of repeated administrations on social behaviour, and (3) the after-effects of long term self-administration of drugs. Examples of each are given below.

---

*) The work was supported by research grants from the National Institute of Mental Health, U. S. Public Health Service, the Medical Research Council and the Foundations Fund for Research in Psychiatry.

After-effects of a single drug experience in a novel environment in rats and mice

In one of our earlier experiments we studied the after-effects of single injections of an amphetamine-barbiturate mixture on the spontaneous activity of rats tested one at a time in a novel environment (23). The drug-mixture was used because it was found that it reliably stimulated activity much more than any dose of the constituent drugs given separately (19), and it therefore provided a suitable baseline for studying behaviour and drug after-effects.

The subjects were four groups of 120 day old female hooded rats which had significantly been reared in standard laboratory conditions and had not been handled or disturbed since weaning. All four groups were tested twice for three minutes in a Y-shaped runway. The main measure of spontaneous activity was the number of times the animals entered the arms of the maze with all four feet. At the first trial, two groups were injected with saline and the other two with an amylobarbitone-amphetamine mixture (15.0 and 0.75 mg/kg respectively). Three days later, one of the saline groups was re-tested with saline and the other with the drug mixture. Similarly, one of the mixture-treated groups was re-tested with saline and the other with the mixture. This was a balanced cross-over design in which the animals were re-tested either with the same treatment as at the first trial or were given the opposite treatment.

The results (Fig. 1) showed that the saline-saline group was markedly less active at the second trial as compared with the first trial. This decline in activity is what one would normally expect when animals are exposed to the same environment for the second time. In the saline-mixture group the expected decrease in activity was counteracted by the drug mixture which was administered at the second trial. However, the stimulant effect of the mixture itself was markedly reduced by the rats' previous experience with saline.

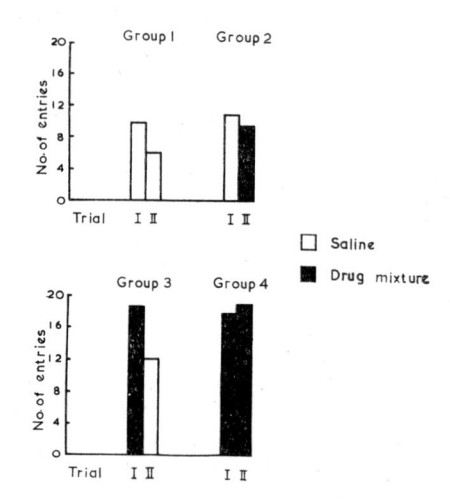

Fig. 1. Effects of a single experience on subsequent behaviour. Rats were given two trials, 3 days apart, in a Y-shaped runway while under the influence of either a drug mixture (amylobarbitone sodium 15.0 mg/kg + amphetamine sulphate 0.75 mg/kg) or of saline. The behaviour measured was the number of entries into the arms of the Y during 3 minutes. Activity at trial 2 (II) depended on the particular treatment administered at trial 1 (I): activity was relatively increased if the first trial had occurred under the influence of the drug mixture and relatively decreased after a first trial under saline. (By courtesy of the British Journal of Pharmacology.)

Thus a single previous saline experience counteracted the large increase in activity normally found with the mixture (19). In the mixture-saline group, activity with saline was somewhat greater than with saline at the first trial. Thus, a previous experience with the mixture counteracted the decline normally found at a second exposure to the same test environment.

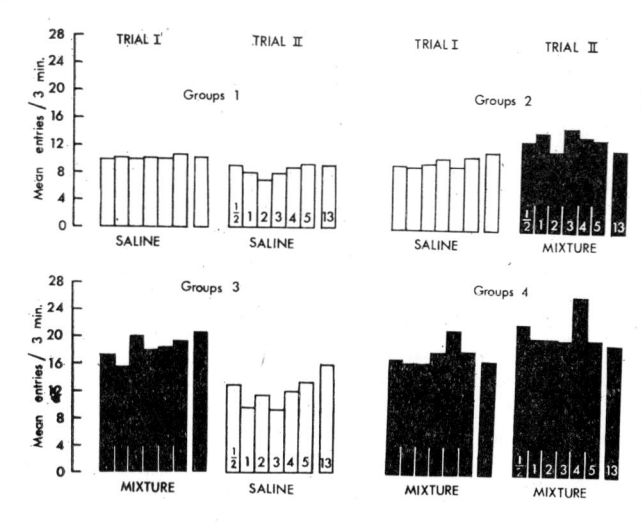

Fig. 2. Effects of a single experience on subsequent behaviour after varying intervals of time. Groups of rats were given two trials in a Y-shaped runway either under the influence of an amphetamine-barbiturate mixture or saline. The behaviour measured was the number of entries into the arms of the runway during 3 minutes. The intervals between the two trials ranged from 1/2 to 13 weeks. Behaviour at the second trial was significantly affected by the treatment the animals received at the first trial (cf. Fig. 1), and these effects persisted for up to 13 weeks. (By courtesy of Nature.)

Later (24, 26) we used a similar experimental design and the same drug mixture, but varied the lengths of the time intervals between the two trials, so that they ranged from 3 days to 13 weeks. Again, different groups of rats were used for each treatment condition and time interval. The aim of this experiment was to find out whether the substantial carry-over effects found after 3 days do in fact persist for longer periods.

At the first trial animals which received the drug mixture were, again, much more active than animals tested with saline (Fig. 2). The results are strictly comparable with the results shown in Fig. 1. At the second trial, as in the previous experiment, the amount of activity seemed to consistently depend on the particular treatment (either the drug-mixture or saline) given in trial 1.

Activity at trial 2 was relatively depressed after a first trial with saline and boosted after a first trial with mixture. Notably, in the mixture-saline groups, saline activity at the second trial was even higher than saline activity at trial 1. Under the most favourable conditions, (the mixture-mixture groups) trial 2 activity was more than two and a half times as great as under the least favourable (saline-saline groups). All the differences were significant at $P < 0.001$. This pattern of carry-over effects remained substantially unchanged even with a 3 months interval between the two trials.

Both experiments show that even a single experience, with or without drugs, lasting only three minutes, significantly alters the behaviour of adult animals for up to three months. For example, in the saline-mixture and mixture-saline groups, activity at trial 2 was roughly the same, even though in one group the second trial occurred under the mixture and in the other group under saline. In the mixture-saline group, one might say, therefore, that at trial 2 the drug was 'conspicuous by its absence'. In the saline-mixture group, the drug more than counteracted the depressant effect of a previous trial; and, in line with this, the ataxia observed at trial 2 with mixture-after-saline, seemed to have been greater than in animals which were given the mixture on both occasions.

The results also show that for some purposes the second dose may be more important than the first. The second mixture dose produced a greater effect than the first and the animals behaved as if the first trial with the drug acted as a 'primer'. Thus in testing for the stimulant effects of the drug-mixture the second dose might have been more appropriate as the second trial yielded clearer results than the first.

To analyse long term effects of single drug experiences further, we used several doses of a different drug mixture, a different species of rodent — the mouse — and a different test environment — a hole board instead of a Y-maze (7). The drug mixture consisted of dexamphetamine combined with chlordiazepoxide. Previous experiments with rats had shown mixtures of these two drugs to stimulate Y-maze activity of rats even more than amphetamine-barbiturate mixtures (22, 27).

Groups of eight naive female adult mice, Porton strain, and housed four per cage, were injected i.p. with one of three doses of a dexamphetamine-chlordiazepoxide mixture in a ratio of 1 : 10 by weight, with the separate constituents, or with saline. This particular ratio of the two drugs was chosen because previous Y-maze experiments with rats (22, 27) and hole board experiments with mice (4, 7, 31) had shown that dose ratios of drugs, which were optimal in rats were also effective in mice. All the four mice in a cage received the same treatments. Twenty minutes after injection the mice were placed one at a time on square horizontal wooden boards with sixteen holes evenly spaced in four rows (3). Behaviour was scored during 3 minutes as follows:

(1) Total number of head dips; a 'dip' was counted whenever the mouse put its head into a hole far enough for both its eyes to disappear below the surface of the board — to explore holes is very natural behaviour for mice: and (2) amount of walking about on the board, determined by drawing on specially prepared paper grids, the path which the mice followed on the board; the number of times the animals' path crossed the grid lines was taken as a quantitative index of the amount of walking. Other forms of behaviour such as grooming, defaecation and urination were also recorded.

After the original 3 minute test on the hole board (trial 1) the mice were replaced in their home cages and were left undisturbed for 1 week; they were then given their second test (trial 2) on the same boards but without any drugs or even injections. Otherwise the procedure was similar to that followed at trial 1.

The results (Fig. 3a) show that at the first trial the separate drugs, with any of the three doses used, hardly affected the number of times that the mice dipped their heads into the holes, as compared with saline controls. With the two smaller doses of the mixture, on the other hand, head-dipping greatly increased. With the highest mixture dose the amount of head dipping was no different from that of the saline controls, and the mice were very ataxic.

When the mice were re-tested without drugs one week later (Fig. 3b) the shapes of the original dose-response curves seemed to re-emerge (Kruskal-Wallis one way analysis of variance for the groups of mice previously tested with the mixtures, $H = 17.68$, d.f. 3, $P < 0.001$) though the absolute scores for all groups were approximately 50% lower than at trial 1. Similar results were obtained with the other measure of behaviour, the amount of walking on the board (Fig. 4), although this measure proved to be more variable than the head-dipping. The greater variability in this measure may be due to the fact that it probably is more difficult to score it unequivocally.

These experiments with mice support the results obtained with rats. In addition, they show that if the circumstances in which drugs are first experienced are appropriate, the after-effects on behaviour which persist for a surprisingly long time can be dose-dependent.

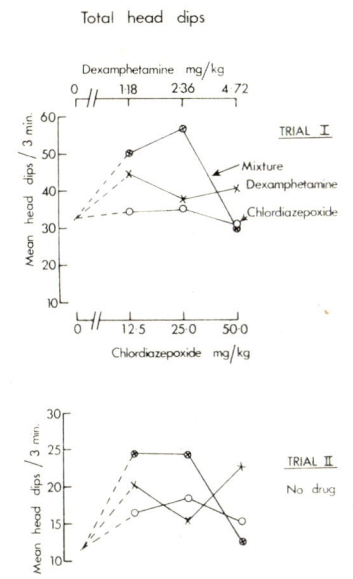

Fig. 3. Dose-related after-effects of a single experience in mice. The behaviour measured was the number of head-dips on a hole-board by different groups of mice which were given three doses of dexamphetamine (X), chlordiazepoxide (O) or a combination of the two drugs (⊕) injected in a constant ratio between the doses of the two drugs, approximately 1 : 10 by weight. The mice were injected at the first trial only. At the second trial, one week after, all animals were re-tested without drugs or injections. "Dose-response" curves, similar in shape but at a uniformly lower absolute level emerged at the second trial without drugs. (By courtesy of Nature.)

A curious feature which emerges from our experiments is that these drugs by themselves do not seem to produce long term effects; it seems that a combination of both the drug effect and an actual experience of the test environment is necessary. Rats which had been injected with an amylobarbitone-amphetamine mixture and then replaced in their home cages without being tested, did not show any detectable drug after-effects when they were subsequently tested (20, 24).

Furthermore, PORSOLT et al. found that daily injections of an amphetamine-barbiturate mixture or of its separate constituents for up to 24 days but without any exposure to the test environment had no appreciable effect on behavioural response to the drugs when the rats were finally tested in a Y-maze (18).

These studies taken together indicate that even single doses of psychoactive drugs can radically alter the behaviour of adult animals for very long periods of time. Drug administration by itself, however, does not appear to be sufficient. Whether long lasting effects occur or not depends on a rather complex interaction between the drugs and the particular environmental setting in which their effects are first experienced.

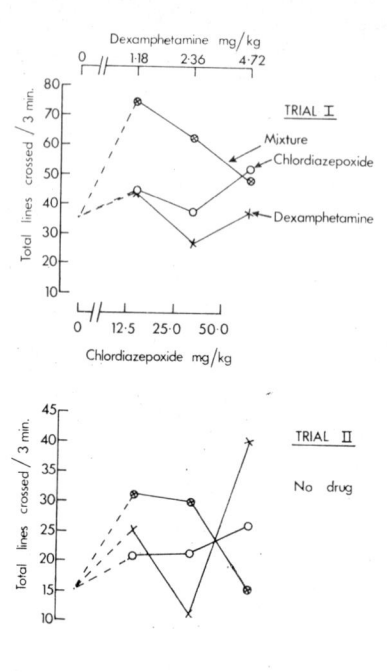

Fig. 4. Dose related after-effects of a single experience in mice treated as described in Fig. 3. The behaviour was the amount of walking over hole-boards during 3 minutes. Again the relative increases in behaviour observed in trial I with the drug mixture re-appeared without any drug treatment one week later. though again activity was about half that of the first trial. (By courtesy of Nature.)

AFTER-EFFECTS OF A SHORT PERIOD OF ADMINISTRATION OF AMYLOBARBITONE ON SOCIAL BEHAVIOUR IN GROUPS OF RATS

Earlier workers have shown that adult dominance behaviour can be affected by repeated administrations of drugs to young animals (10, 33).

We have adapted a technique which enables us to measure simultaneously competitive behaviour in groups of rats in their home-cage environment (1, 30). It also enables the study of the effects of drugs on complex interactions within groups.

One of the first drugs investigated was amylobarbitone since it has been shown that it can, to some extent, reinstate behaviour which had been suppressed by fear (17), and can increase aggression in rats (25) and in mice (13), possibly by decreasing fear. We have carried out experiments to establish whether amylobarbitone can alter dominance hierarchies formed by rats given the opportunity to compete for water.

At weaning, male hooded rats were assigned at random to groups of four with the proviso that there were no litter mates in any group. They were left undisturbed with food and water *ad libitum* for 3 months. The rats were then deprived of water for 21 hr. each day and their behaviour was observed for the first 3 minutes of the daily 3 hr. drinking period, during which they could obtain water from a spout which protruded into the middle of their home cage, and which was specially built in such a way that only one rat could drink at any particular time. This made them compete vigorously and continuously; the rat which spent the longest time drinking during the observation period was considered to be most dominant and the rat which spent the least time at the water spout was considered to be the least dominant. The observation period was limited to three minutes, because after this time the most dominant rat having, presumably, satisfied his immediate thirst ceases to compete and indulges in other forms of behaviour, such as eating or grooming.

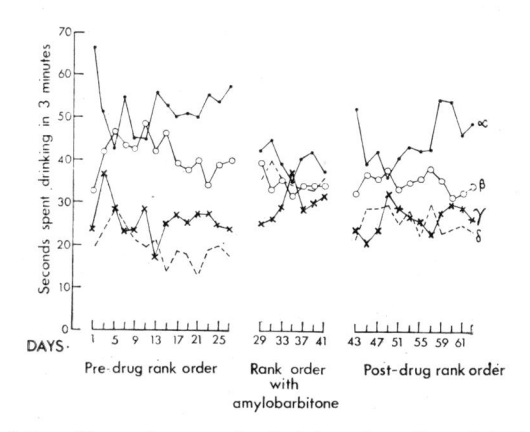

Fig. 5. Persistence of the effects of repeated administration of amylobarbitone (7.5 mg/kg) on subsequent social behaviour of rats. Rats which were forced to compete for water in groups of 4 developed stable dominance hierarchies after approximately 14 days. Amylobarbitone administered on days 29—41 tended to disrupt these hierarchies. When the drug was withdrawn, the disruptive effects persisted until day 59, after which time the original, pre-drug, hierarchies re-emerged. Each line represents a mean of six different rats.

Approximately 2 weeks from the beginning of restricted drinking the rats in each group established a distinct hierarchy and this tended to remain remarkably stable for long periods of time (1, 30). However, i.p. injections of a moderate dose of amylobarbitone (7.5 mg/kg) 20 minutes before the rats were given access to water, completely abolished the previously stable hierarchies (Fig. 5), so that *all* the rats now spent approximately the same amount of time drinking from the water spout.

The injections continued for 14 days but no discernible dominance orders emerged. When amylobarbitone was withdrawn and the rats continued to be injected with saline, the disturbing effect of the drug on the dominance hierarchies persisted for about sixteen days. After this period of time the original, pre-drug, dominance hierarchies re-emerged in a stable form. Thus, repeated administrations of relatively small doses of the drug had a considerable carry-over effect on a complex form of social behaviour (30).

AFTER-EFFECTS OF LONG TERM SELF-ADMINISTRATION OF DRUGS IN RATS

We have developed a method whereby we can teach rats to self-administer opiates and other drugs by drinking solutions of them without previous "passive" premedication by injections (14, 15, 28). Rats are first made thirsty by being given access to water only between 10 a.m. and 5 p.m. each day for a fortnight or so. Both plain drinking water and drug solutions are made available during this drinking period on every third day ("choice trials"), but morphine solutions only on the two intervening days ("forced trials"). With time, rats gradually increase their intake of the initially rejected bitter morphine solutions and eventually they "choose" to take 60—70% of their total fluid intake in the form of

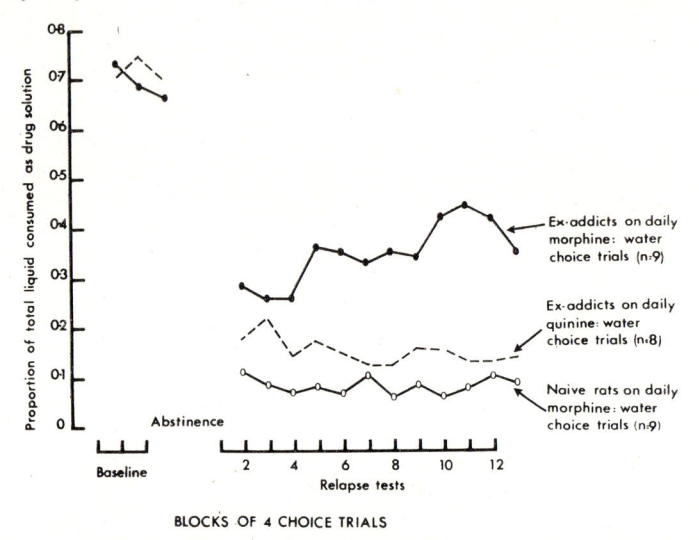

Fig. 6. After-effects of prolonged oral self-administration of morphine. Rats which had been made dependent on morphine by being repeatedly given a choice between water and morphine solutions (0.5 mg/ml) every third day, and morphine solutions only during the intervening two days, were then deprived of morphine solutions for 110 days. Even after this period previously dependent rats spontaneously consumed more morphine solution than controls when given a choice between morphine and water. (By courtesy of the Journal of Comparative and Physiological Psychology.)

morphine solution. When the "forced trials" are omitted at this stage and morphine solutions and plain water are both simultaneously available daily, ("daily choice trials"), this preference for morphine persists.

Human and animal addicts to opioids show a remarkable tendency to resume drug taking even after very long periods of abstinence. This is known only too well to those concerned with the drug-dependence problem.

In our laboratory we have attempted to mimic this phenomenon in rats and to try to modify this tenacious tendency to relapse (16, 16a).

Rats which had been made stably dependent on morphine by the method described, were forced to abstain from morphine by being given only plain drinking water for 110 days. They were then divided into two groups and given daily "choices" either between water and morphine solutions, or between water and quinine solutions. The morphine and quinine solutions were as far as possible matched for bitterness. These two groups were compared with naive rats which were given daily "choices" between water and morphine solutions. Ex-addict rats drank significantly more morphine over 48 daily "relapse tests" than controls (Fig. 6); more surprisingly, the ex-morphine addicted rats drank significantly more quinine solution than the naive controls of morphine though less than the amounts of morphine drunk by ex-addict rats given a choice between water and morphine solutions.

Thus, even after 110 days of abstinence, the animals resumed their previous morphine drinking habit and even started to drink a fluid which resembled morphine solutions in no other respect except in its bitterness.

In another experiment where quinine solutions or methadone injections were given during a period of abstinence, the tendencies to relapse into morphine self-administration were not substantially altered (16). Thus a tendency to resume self-administration of morphine in the form of voluntary drinking by rats which had been made dependent on it is remarkably resistant to extinction and persists for long periods of time. WIKLER and PESCOR (32), for example, found that tendencies to "relapse" can persist for more than a year after morphine withdrawal.

On the other hand, STOLERMAN, KUMAR and STEINBERG (29) found that long term (46 days) self-administration of amylobarbitone, chlordiazepoxide, cocaine, dexamphetamine or ethanol did not substantially alter the rate at which rats subsequently became dependent on morphine. The only exception were rats which had previously been given dexamphetamine. These rats had drunk progressively less and less dexamphetamine solution in successive trials, and this "aversion" seemed to transfer to morphine solutions when these again became available. This group tended for a short time to reject morphine solutions more than any of the other rats (29). In these circumstances therefore previous drug experiences generally failed to alter subsequent drug-taking behaviour.

DISCUSSION

Whether single or repeated drug experiences produce after-effects or not probably crucially depends on the drugs themselves, on the precise circumstances in which the drug experience takes place, on the particular behaviour studied and on the manner in which repeated or chronic drug administration is terminated.

For example, BARRETT et al. (2) have shown that repeated administration of dexamphetamine or of scopolamine can improve a form of avoidance behaviour in rats. If drug administration was abruptly terminated, the beneficial effects of the drugs were lost. If, however, the drugs were withdrawn gradually, by injecting progressively smaller and smaller doses, the behavioural improvements carried over beyond the period of drug administration.

Results of this kind possibly suggest that long term carry-over effects of drugs are more likely to occur in situations where the animal actively participates in the drug experience. We have shown that the subsequent behaviour of animals passively injected with dexamphetamine and amylobarbitone, alone or in combination, is only affected, if the original drug administration is combined with the experience of a novel environment (18, 20, 26). Similarly, "passive" injections of morphine failed to influence the rate at which the rats became dependent on morphine by self-administration. This may reflect the now generally held view that iatrogenic drug dependence in man is relatively rare. On the other end of scale, we have found that when the animals' participation in the morphine administration is greatest, i.e. when they administer the drugs voluntarily by drinking, the carry-over effects were very robust and could not be erased by prolonged forced abstinence or by other treatments. It may well be that "dependence" phenomena are in a class by themselves in that they may involve more definite and permanent irreversible physiological or biochemical changes. This suggestion is reinforced by our findings that self-administration of non-opiate drugs or repeated injections of morphine (14) failed to influence the way in which rats become subsequently dependent on morphine.

As far as we are aware there are no biochemical explanations wich would account for the diverse range of after-effects described in this paper. The fact that "passive" drug administrations failed, in several instances, to produce detectable after-effects on subsequent behaviour indicates that biochemical effects of the drug *per se* may not be the main determinants of the behavioural changes.

These studies may also have significant implications for clinical trials and for the therapeutic use of drugs in man. Nowadays it is rarely, if ever, possible to obtain a "drug naive" human subject, and therefore the study of long-term drug after-effects is of both theoretical and practical importance.

REFERENCES

1. BAENNINGER, L. P. (1970) Social dominance orders in the rat: 'Spontaneous', food, and water competition. J. comp. Physiol. Psychol. **71**, 202.
2. BARRET, R. J., LEITH, N. J. and RAY, O. S. (1972) Permanent facilitation of avoidance behaviour by d-amphetamine and scopolamine. Psychopharmacologia, **25**, 321.
3. BOISSIER, J. R. and SIMON, P. (1962) La réaction d'exploration chez la souris. Thérapie, **17**, 1225.
4. BRADLEY, D. W. M., JOYCE, D., MURPHY, E. H., NASH, B. M., PORSOLT, R. D., SUMMERFIELD, A. and TWYMAN, W. A. (1968) Amphetamine-barbiturate mixture: Effects on the behaviour of mice. Nature, **220**, 187.
5. COCHIN, J. (1970) Possible mechanisms in development of tolerance. Fed. Proc. **29**, 19.
6. COCHIN, J. and KORNETSKY, C. (1964) Development and loss of tolerance to morphine in the rat after single and multiple injections. J. Pharmacol. exp. Ther. **145**, 1.
7. DORR, M., JOYCE, D., PORSOLT, R. D., STEINBERG, H., SUMMERFIELD, A. and TOMKIEWICZ, M. (1971) Persistence of dose related behaviour in mice. Nature, **231**, 121.
8. DOTY, B. A. and DOTY, L. A. (1963) Chlorpromazine-produced response decrements resulting from chronic administration in infancy. Canad. J. Psychol. **17**, 45.
9. GAURON, F. and ROWLEY, V. M. (1971) Cross-generational effects resulting from an early drug experience. Eur. J. Pharmacol. **15**, 171.
10. HEIMSTRA, N. W. and SALLEE, S. (1965) Effects of early drug treatment on adult dominance behaviour in rats. Psychopharmacologia, **8**, 235.
11. KORNETSKY, C. (1970) Psychoactive drugs in the immature organism. Psychopharmacologia, **17**, 105.
12. KORNETSKY, C. and BAIN, G. (1968) Morphine: Single-dose tolerance. Science, **162**, 1011.
13. KRŠIAK, M. and STEINBERG, H. (1969) Psychopharmacological aspects of aggression: A review of the literature and some new experiments. J. psychosom. Res. **13**, 243.
14. KUMAR, R., STEINBERG, H. and STOLERMAN, I. P. (1968) Inducing a preference for morphine in rats without premedication. Nature, **218**, 564.
15. KUMAR, R., STEINBERG, H. and STOLERMAN, I. P. (1969) How rats can become dependent on morphine in the course of relieving another need. In: STEINBERG, H. (Ed.) Scientific Basis of Drug Dependence. Churchill: London, 209.
16. KUMAR, R. and STOLERMAN, I. P. (1972) Resumption of morphine self-administration by ex-addict rats: An attempt to modify tendencies to relapse. J. comp. physiol. Psychol. **78**, 457.
16a. KUMAR, R., STOLERMAN, I. P. and STEINBERG, H. (1972) Resumption of morphine self-administration by ex-addict rats. In: KOSTERLITZ, H. W., COLLIER, H. O. J. and VILLAREAL, J. E. (Eds.). Agonist and antagonist actions of narcotic analgesic drugs. Macmillan: London, 255.
17. MILLER, N. E. (1964) The analysis of motivational effects illustrated by experiments on amylobarbitone sodium. In: STEINBERG, H., de REUCK, A. V. S. and KNIGHT, J. (Eds.) Animal Behaviour and Drug Action. Churchill: London, 1.
18. PORSOLT, R. D., JOYCE, D. and SUMMERFIELD, A. (1969) Lack of tolerance to an amphetamine-barbiturate mixture and its components. Nature, **223**, 1277.
19. RUSHTON, R. and STEINBERG, H. (1963) Mutual potentiation of amphetamine and amylobarbitone measured by activity in rats. Brit. J. Pharmacol. **20**, 145.
20. RUSHTON, R. and STEINBERG, H. (1964) Modification of behavioural effects of drugs by past experience. In: STEINBERG, H., de REUCK, A. V. S. and KNIGHT, J. (Eds.) Animal Behaviour and Drug Action. Churchill: London, 207.
21. RUSHTON, R. and STEINBERG, H. (1965) Early experience and adult reactions to drugs. In: BENTE, D. and BRADLEY, P. D. (Eds.) Neuropsychopharmacology. Elsevier: Amsterdam, **4**, 345.

22. RUSHTON, R. and STEINBERG, H. (1966) Combined effects of chlordiazepoxide and dexamphetamine on activity of rats in an unfamiliar environment. Nature, **211**, 1312.
23. RUSHTON, R., STEINBERG, H. and TINSON, C. (1963) Effects of a single experience on subsequent reactions to drugs. Brit. J. Pharmacol. **20**, 99.
24. RUSHTON, R., STEINBERG, H. and TOMKIEWICZ, M. (1968) Equivalence and persistence of the effects of psychoactive drugs and past experience. Nature, **220**, 885.
25. SILVERMAN, A. P. (1966) Barbiturates, lysergic acid diethylamide and the social behaviour of laboratory rats. Psychopharmacologia, **10**, 155.
26. STEINBERG, H. and TOMKIEWICZ, M. (1968) Drugs and memory. In: EFRON, D. H., COLE, J. O., LEVINE, J. and WITTENBORN, J. R. (Eds.) Psychopharmacology: A Review of Progress. PHS Publication No. 1836. U. S. Government Printing Office: Washington D. C., 879.
27. STEINBERG, H. and TOMKIEWICZ, M. (1970) Animal behaviour models in psychopharmacology and their extrapolation to man. In: PORTER, R. and BIRCH, J. (Eds.) Chemical Influences on Behaviour. Ciba Foundation Study Group No. 35. Churchill: London. 199.
28. STOLERMAN, I. P. and KUMAR, R. (1970) Preferences for morphine in rats: Validation of an experimental model of dependence. Psychopharmacologia, **17**, 137.
29. STOLERMAN, I. P., KUMAR, R. and STEINBERG, H. (1971) Development of morphine dependence in rats: Lack of effect of previous ingestion of other drugs. Psychopharmacologia, **20**, 321.
30. TOMKIEWICZ, M. (1972) Amylobarbitone abolishes social dominance hierarchies in laboratory rats. Brit. J. Pharmacol. **44**, 351P.
31. U'PRICHARD, D. C. and STEINBERG, H. (1972) Selective effects of lithium on two forms of spontaneous activity. Brit. J. Pharmacol. **44**, 349 P.
32. WILKER, A. and PESCOR, F. T. (1970) Persistence of 'relapse tendencies' of rats previously made physically dependent on morphine. Psychopharmacologia, **16**, 375.
33. WOLF, H. H. and ROWLAND, C. R. (1969) Effects of chronic postnatal drug administration on adult dominance behaviour in two genera of mice. Develop. Psychobiol. **2**, 195.

H.S., Department of Pharmacology, University College, Gower Street, London, England

A POSSIBLE ROLE OF BIOGENIC ALDEHYDES IN LONG-TERM EFFECTS OF DRUGS

J. P. VON WARTBURG[*], M. M. RIS and T. G. WHITE

Institute of Medical chemistry, University of Berne, and Wander Research Institute (Sandoz Research Unit), Berne

When a biologically or behaviourally detectable change in the brain outlasts the presence of the drug in the organism one can speak of long-term effects. A wide range of time-scales varying from weeks to months and even up to a year exists. A time scale of hours only is observed, for example, for the nystagmus which outlasts acute alcohol intoxication (10).

The duration of the persistent effect, or the "biological memory" solely depends on the turnover rates of the components of the affected system. In terms of molecular biology, it depends on the half-life time of the macromolecular structures involved. It is important therefore to recognise that the repeated administration of drugs obviously can lead to progressive changes in a system only if the time between two single doses is shorter than that required for the abolition of the first effect by turnover of the systems involved. A change of state by repeated drug administration then becomes a dynamic deviationary process, where each single dose induces a change in a system already containing the various long-term effects of previous single doses. Thus, dependence, the interaction of drug experience with previously stored information, is interconnected with "memory".

Experiments using cycloheximide as a protein synthesis inhibitor, have led to three memory storage processes being postulated: a "short-term" memory storage process which is independent of protein synthesis, with a fixed life time of 3 6 hours, followed by two subsequent "long-term" processes which depend on protein synthesis (21). It has also been shown that the experimental induction of dependence on drugs such as morphine is inhibited by cycloheximide and thus is protein synthesis dependent as well (13). Enzyme proteins, receptor proteins and/or structural membrane lipoproteins used for storage or synaptic membranes all could be involved in the various processes. The general hypotheses put forward to explain the induction of drug dependence with development of withdrawal syndromes and tolerance invoke protein synthesis and include the adaptation of a biological system to repeated drug ingestion by feed-back regulation. The hypothesis of GOLDSTEIN and GOLDSTEIN, (11), for instance, is based on repression and de-repression of enzyme synthesis. An analogous hypothesis based on an induction of the synthesis of receptors has been advanced by COLLIER (5).

---

[*] Supported by Swiss National Science Foundation Grant-No. 3.320.70 and US Public Health Service Grant-No. MH-16202.

These current hypotheses exemplify one principal mechanism for long-term effects of drugs. The drug induces a change in the functional state of the neuron, which in turn provokes an adaptation in the metabolism of neurotransmitters or modulators and/or their interaction with receptors, which involves feed-back regulation of protein synthesis. The duration of the effect, as measured by the outlasting tolerance and withdrawal symptoms, depends on the time required for re-adaptation to normal conditions without drug, that is, on the half-life time of the enzyme or receptor proteins. Another example is given by the storage of information following exposure to a drug which depletes the stores of neurotransmitters. Information related to the exposure lasts until the stores have been refilled. On the other hand, extremely long-term effects are observed with drugs which induce an irreversible, permanent change in the system, such as 6-hydroxydopamine which leads to a degeneration of the adrenergic neurons. Within this context, the question of what mechanisms are involved in long-term effects of intermediate duration is posed.

A possible alternative to the induction of protein synthesis is the storage of information by protein modification. From immunological studies it is well known that information from a single drug exposure can be stored for long periods and it seems that the duration of the effect correlates with the protein modifying capacity of the antigenic drug. The rate of decay of the effect depends on the normal half-life time of the modified protein, provided that there is no alteration in the rate of synthesis by feed-back and that newly synthesized protein has the original, and not the modified structure. Following from the estimate of half-life times for synaptic membrane proteins of one to three weeks (14), a duration of several weeks could be expected for drug induced effects involving a modification of membrane structure. Current knowledge indicates that endogenous neurotransmitters and psychoactive drugs exert their action by modifying protein structure in the sense of induced conformational changes during the short period of the formation of a reversible ligand-protein complex. It is therefore unlikely that permanent modifications of the protein structure can be achieved in this way. Biogenic aldehydes produced in the catabolism of biogenic amines, however, represent a group of compounds likely to exert such effects.

The following scheme represents the catabolism of biogenic amines:

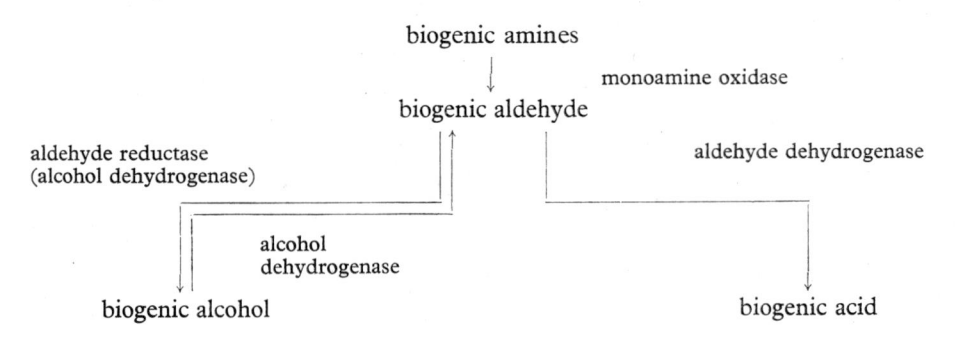

```
                    biogenic amines
                          |
                          |         monoamine oxidase
                    biogenic aldehyde
aldehyde reductase                          aldehyde dehydrogenase
(alcohol dehydrogenase)
            |      alcohol
            |    dehydrogenase
            |
      biogenic alcohol                        biogenic acid
```

Biogenic aldehydes are formed by oxidative deamination of biogenic amines (phenylethylamine, tyramine, octopamine, dopamine, noradrenaline, serotonin) by the action of monoamine oxidase. It seems accepted that these highly reactive products are instantaneously metabolized further, without producing biological effects. However, the enzymes involved and the aldehyde products can be isolated and their properties studied. In liver, the further oxidation of the aldehydes to the corresponding acids seems to predominate and the reduction to the alcohols is probably mainly catalysed by alcohol dehydrogenase (25).

In contrast the reductive pathway predominates in the brain, although the particular pathway also seems to depend on the structure of the aldehyde (23). Three enzyme systems are available to the brain; first, the aldehyde reductase for the reduction of the aldehydes to the alcohol; second, traces of alcohol dehydrogenase carrying out the reverse reaction from the alcohol to the aldehyde; and finally, the aldehyde dehydrogenase which oxidizes the aldehydes to the corresponding acid.

The biogenic aldehydes are chemically very labile and reactive. It has been shown that aldehydes of indoleamines are partly incorporated into acid-insoluble material obtained from brains of experimental animals (1). This type of incorporation is probably due to interaction of the aldehyde with proteolipids of membranous material. The intracellular distribution showed that after intraventricular administration synaptosome ghosts become heavily labelled, while relatively less radioactivity is incorporated into storage vesicles (2).

It is of interest that benzaldehyde, formed by the oxidative deamination of benzylamine by monoamine oxidase can be fixed to bovine serum albumin, resulting in an extensive benzylation of lysyl residues of this protein. Observations in our own laboratory reveal that various biogenic aldehydes produced *in vitro* by monoamine oxidase are bound to proteins, as shown by ultrafiltration, acid precipitation or centrifugation. Fractionation of subsequently extracted aldehydes by thin layer chromatography reveals a mixture of products, of which some are reactive as substrates with aldehyde reductase and liver alcohol dehydrogenase.

It is probable that the binding of biogenic aldehydes to proteins initially involves the formation of Schiff bases. Such a mechanism has been previously postulated for the binding of intact serotonin to proteins (3). In the case of biogenic aldehydes, however, the biogenic aldehyde would represent the carbonyl group donor and amino groups of the protein, the amino group donor. The binding of biogenic aldehydes to membrane proteins can only be of biological interest if conformational changes are induced in the structure of these proteins, thus modifying the properties of membranes, such as permeability to ions, fusion with storage vesicle membranes, or re-uptake of neurotransmitters. Corresponding experiments with biogenic aldehydes and membranous brain proteins are still awaited. In model experiments with human serum albumin, however, it has been shown by measurements of the optical rotary dispersion and by peptide mapping that the binding of aromatic aldehydes induces extensive changes in the protein structure (4).

From these findings one would predict that biogenic aldehydes exert biological activity. Some early work indicated that biogenic aldehydes may be physiologically inactive (6), yet it was later suggested that 5-HO-indolacetaldehyde and/or 5-HO-tryptophol may be involved in some of the sleep mechanisms (8, 20, 24). One would therefore expect that compounds interfering with the metabolism of biogenic aldehydes exert actions on the brain. Characterization of the aldehyde reductases from human brain therefore seems to be of interest.

As shown in Table 1, human brain shows various enzymatic activities using aldehydes as substrates. NADPH-dependent aldehyde reductase activity predominates over the NADH-dependent. The opposite is found for the aldehyde dehydrogenase. In both cases aromatic substrates are favoured. Finally, traces of alcohol dehydrogenase are also detectable. Since this work relates to whole brain homogenates, these observations do not exclude the possibility that higher activities are present in certain regions of the brain. The nucleus caudatus of various animal species was shown to contain more alcohol dehydrogenase than aldehyde dehydrogenase and monoamine oxidase (6). Furthermore it has been proposed that an ethanol-induced adaptation of alcohol dehydrogenase may occur in rat brain (15).

TABLE 1

Pyridine nucleotide dependent enzymes from human brain using aldehydes as substrate. Activities in International Units (μmol/min) per 300 g brain wet weight as measured in homogenate

Enzyme[1]	Coenzyme[2]	Substrate	Activity
Aldehyde reductase	NADPH	Butyraldehyde	5.0
Aldehyde reductase	NADPH	p-NO$_2$-Benzaldehyde	47.7
Aldehyde reductase	NADH	Butyraldehyde	3.9
Aldehyde reductase	NADH	p-NO$_2$-Benzaldehyde	6.2
Aldehyde dehydrogenase	NADP	Butyraldehyde	1.3
Aldehyde dehydrogenase	NADP	p-NO$_2$-Benzaldehyde	13.6
Aldehyde dehydrogenase	NAD	Butyraldehyde	29.4
Aldehyde dehydrogenase	NAD	p-NO$_2$-Benzaldehyde	58.3
Alcohol dehydrogenase	NADP	Butanol	not detectable
Alcohol dehydrogenase	NAD	Butanol	4.3

[1] Assay conditions: Aldehyde reductase, 1×10^{-1}M Na-phosphate pH 7.0, coenzyme 1.6×10^{-4}M, substrate 5×10^{-4}M. Aldehyde dehydrogenase, 1×10^{-1}M Na-pyrophosphate pH 9.5, NAD 5×10^{-3}M, NADP 1×10^{-3}M, substrate 5×10^{-4}M. Alcohol dehydrogenase, Na-pyrophosphate 1×10^{-1}M pH 9.5, NAD 5×10^{-3}M, substrate 1×10^{-3}M.

[2] Coenzymes: NAD, NADH oxidized or reduced nicotinamide adenine dinucleotide; NADP, NADPH, oxidized or reduced nicotinamide adenine dinucleotidephosphate.

TABLE 2

Substrate specificity of the multiple forms of aldehyde reductase from human brain. Activities in percent of activity with p-NO$_2$-benzaldehyde. Mean values of six preparations. For assay conditions see Table 1

Substrate	Concentration (mM)	Enzyme fraction 4.1	4.2	4.3	4.4
Propionaldehyde	0.5	∅	64	8	9
Chloral hydrate	0.5	3	69	∅	22
Glyceraldehyde	0.5	∅	97	14	11
Benzaldehyde	0.5	9	78	6	11
4-NO$_2$-Benzaldehyde	0.5	100	100	100	100
3-NO$_2$-Benzaldehyde	0.5	46	72	10	163
2-HO-Benzaldehyde	0.5	∅	131	60	11
3-Methoxy-4-HO-Benzaldehyde	0.05	∅	8	∅	3
Phenylacetaldehyde	0.05	∅	42	3	17
Benzylmethylketone	0.5	4	∅	∅	25
Indole acetaldehyde	0.5	5	44	4	∅

∅ — no detectable activity.

By chromatography of human brain homogenates on DEAE-cellulose, CM-cellulose and Sephadex G-100, four distinct NADPH dependent fractions of aldehyde reductase (4.1, 4.2, 4.3 and 4.4) can be isolated (17, 18). The two main fractions (4.1 and 4.3) together represent 80—90% of the total activity, which varies from 40 to 70 IU between preparations. Aldehyde dehydrogenase is also fractionated into two distinct forms by the same procedure. Because the aldehyde reductases have molecular weights of about 40,000 and the aldehyde dehydrogenase is much larger, these enzymes are entirely separated by the gel chromatography step. All four multiple molecular forms of aldehyde reductase need NADPH. The NADH-dependent activity found in the homogenate is mainly due to the minor fraction 4.2.

The substrate specificity with regard to aliphatic and aromatic aldehydes differs for the four multiple forms of aldehyde reductase (Table 2). The main fraction 4.1 has a relatively high substrate specificity, p-NO$_2$-benzaldehyde being the best substrate of the model compounds studied. Of the physiological substrates the aldehydes derived from dopamine and noradrenaline seem to be preferred. The minor enzyme fraction 4.2 has a low specificity which includes aliphatic aldehydes. It could be called the all-round enzyme as it can also use NADH as coenzyme. Biogenic aldehydes with a hydroxyl group in the side-chain are good substrates. The substrate specificity of the other main multiple form 4.3 is similar to that of fraction 4.1 with the exception of 2-HO-benzaldehyde. Of the multiple forms, it is the only one showing relatively high activity with 5-HO-indoleacetaldehyde. 3-NO$_2$-benzaldehyde is the best substrate for enzyme 4.4 which also reduces benzyl-methylketone, a metabolite of amphetamine.

TABLE 3

Inhibitors of the multiple forms of aldehyde reductase from human brain. Percent inhibition with p-NO$_2$-benzaldehyde as substrate. For assay conditions see Table 1

Inhibitor	Concentration (mM)	Enzyme fraction 4.1	4.2	4.3	4.4
Na-Barbital	1.0	8	23	91	19
Glutethimide	0.5	7	3	57	7
Diphenylhydantoin	0.5	30	60	28	35
Chlorpromazine	1.0	47	55	61	69
Butyraldoxime	0.5	12	50	36	11
p-Chloromercuribenzoate	0.1	100	0	10	0
3,4-Dihydroxyphenylacetic acid	0.5	8	55	53	38

The effect of inhibitors is shown in Table 3. It was previously reported that phenobarbital inhibits aldehyde reductase from bovine brain (7, 22). It is of interest to note that only the main fraction 4.3 is strongly inhibited by barbital. Analogous inhibitions are obtained with phenobarbital, allobarbital, pentobarbital, carbromal, bromisoval and abasin. Barbituric acid is not an inhibitor of these enzymes, while glutethimide follows the pattern of barbital. Diphenylhydantoin mainly inhibits enzyme 4.2 but hydantoin is inert in this respect. Chlorpromazine produced non-specific inhibitions of all multiple forms. Imipramine does not affect the human enzymes although it is an inhibitor of rat brain aldehyde reductase (23). A typical inhibitor of alcohol dehydrogenase, pyrazole, is inactive.

Butyraldoxime apparently inhibits some aldehyde reductases as well as alcohol dehydrogenase. The inhibitors of aldehyde dehydrogenase and dopamine hydroxylase, disulfiram and diethyldithiocarbamate, have little effect on aldehyde reductase. The inhibition by 3,4-dihydroxyphenylacetic acid is one example of typical inhibitions observed with biogenic acids, the products of oxidation of biogenic aldehydes by aldehyde dehydrogenase. A regulatory function through this inhibition at the metabolic bifurcation of biogenic aldehyde to alcohol or acid cannot be excluded.

It is of interest to note that both barbiturates and acetaldehyde or ethanol have similar actions on the brain *in vivo*. From this one could expect that some biogenic aldehydes decrease excitability of synapses. Conversely, a lack of these aldehydes should lead to increased excitability. Indeed, it is an old observation that carbonyl trapping agents such as hydrazines, semicarbazide or thiosemicarbazide induce convulsive seizures, although other interpretations have been offered for this phenomenon (19). Furthermore, convulsions induced as withdrawal symptoms after alcohol treatment have been interpreted as a latent hyperexitability of the brain following depression by ethanol (9, 12). A disturbance in the removal of biogenic aldehydes including an adaptive increase of the enzymes fully explains this observations.

Thus, it has been indicated that the aldehyde metabolites of biogenic amines can be physiologically active, and that they have the potential to produce functional changes through a modification of protein structure. Our biochemical studies have shown that the enzyme processes governing the metabolism of these aldehydes are highly differentiated, both with respect to substrate specificity and to sensitivity towards inhibitors known to affect brain function acutely and chronically. Nonetheless, the hypothesis that biogenic aldehydes participate in short-term and, especially, long-term changes of brain function is still highly speculative and requires further experimental verification.

References

1. ALIVISATOS, S. G. A. and UNGAR, F. (1968) Incorporation of radioactivity from labeled serotonin and tryptamine into acid insoluble material from subcellular fractions of brain. Biochemistry, **7**, 285.
2. ALIVISATOS, S. G. A. (1970) Aldehyde derivatives. Neurosciences Res. Proj. Bull. **8**, 34.
3. ALIVISATOS, S. G. A., UNGAR, F., SETH, P. K., LEVITT, L. P., GEROULIS, A. J. and MEYER, T. S. (1971) Receptors: Localization and specificity of binding of serotonin in the central nervous system. Science, **171**, 809.
4. BAGDASAR'JAN, S. N. and TROITSKII, G. V. (1971) Study of albumin-aldehyde complexes by the optical rotary dispersion and peptide map methods. Biochemistry, Russian original, **36**, 615.
5. COLLIER, H. O. J. (1969) Humoral transmitters, supersensitivity, receptors and dependence. In: "Scientific basis of drug dependence", Ed. STEINBERG, H., p. 49, Churchill, London.
6. DUNCAN, R. J. S. and SOURKES, T. L. (1972) Enzymology of aldehyde metabolism in caudate nucleus. Trans. Amer. Soc. Neurochem. **3**, 73.
7. ERWIN, V. G., TABAKOFF, B. and BRONAUGH, R. L. (1971) Inhibition of a reduced nicotinamide adenine dinucleotide phosphate-linked aldehyde reductase from bovine brain by barbiturates. Mol. Pharm. **7**, 169.
8. FELDSTEIN, A. and KURCHASKI, J. M. (1971) Pyrazole and ethanol potentiation of tryptophol-induced sleep in mice. Life Sci. **10**, 961.
9. FREUND, G. and WALKER, D. W. (1971) Sound-induced seizures during ethanol withdrawal in mice. Psychopharmacologia **22**, 45.
10. GOLDBERG, L. (1961) Alcohol, tranquilizers and hangover. Quart. J. Stud. Alc. Suppl. **1**, 37.
11. GOLSTEIN, A. and GOLDSTEIN, D. B. (1968) Enzyme expansion theory of drug tolerances and physical dependence. In: The Addictive States, Vol. 46, p. 265, Ed. WIKLER, A. J. Williams and Wilkins, Baltimore.

12. GOLDSTEIN, D. B. (1972) Relationship of alcohol dose to intensity of withdrawal signs in mice. J. Pharmacol. exp. Ther. **180**, 203.
13. LOH, H. H., SHEN, F. H. and WAY, E. L. (1969) Inhibition of morphine tolerance and physical dependence development and brain serotonin synthesis by cycloheximide. Biochem. Pharmacol. **18**, 2711.
14. MAHLER, H. R. (1969) Protein turnover and synthesis: relation to synaptic function. In: Advances in biochemical psychopharmacology, Ed.: COSTA, E. and GREENGARD, P., Raven Press, New York, Vol. I, p. 49.
15. RASKIN, N. H. and SOKOLOFF, L. (1972) Ethanol-induced adaptation of alcohol dehydrogenase activity in rat brain. Nature, **236**, 138.
16. RENSON, J., WEISSBACH, H. and UDENFRIEND, S. (1964) Studies on the biological activities of the aldehydes derived from norepinephrine, serotonin, tryptamine and histamine. J. Pharmacol. exp. Ther. **143**, 326.
17. RIS, M. M., SCHENKER, T. M. and VON WARTBURG, J. P. (1972) Heterogeneity of pyridine nucleotide dependent aldehyde reductase in human and rat brain. Experientia, **28**, 738.
18. RIS, M. M. and VON WARTBURG, J. P. (1972) Pyridine nucleotide dependent aldehyde reductases and dehydrogenases from brain. FEBS Meeting, Abstr. 236.
19. ROBERTS, E., WEIN, J. and SIMONSEN, D. G. (1964) Aminobutyric acid, vitamin B_6, and neuronal function — a speculative synthesis. Vitamin. and Horm., **22**, 503.
20. SABELLI, H. C., GIARDINA, W. J., ALIVISATOS, S. G. A., SETH, P. K. and UNGAR, F. (1969) Indoleacetaldehydes: Serotonin-like effects on the central nervous system. Nature, **223**, 73.
21. SQUIRE, L. R. and BARONDES, S. H. (1972) Variable decay of memory and its recovery in cycloheximide-treated mice. Proc. nat. Acad. Sci. **69**, 1416.
22. TABAKOFF, B. and ERWIN, V. G. (1970) Purification and characterization of a reduced nicotinamide adenine dinucleotidephosphate-linked aldehyde reductase from brain. J. biol. Chem. **245**, 3263.
23. TABAKOFF, B., ANDERSON, R., UNGAR, F. and ALIVISATOS, S. G. A. (1972) Disposition of biogenic aldehydes: oxidation or reduction depends on chemical structure. Trans. Amer. Soc. Neurochem. **3**, 126.
24. TABORSKY, R. G. (1971) 5-Hydroxytryptophol: Evidence for its having physiological properties. Experientia, **27**, 929.
25. von WARTBURG, J. P. (1971) The metabolism of alcohol in normals and alcoholics: enzymes. In "The Biology of Alcoholism", Vol. I. p. 63, Ed. KISSIN, B. and BEGLEITER, H., Plenum Press, New York.

J.P.v.W., Institute of Medical Chemistry, University of Berne, Switzerland

THE ROLE OF PERSONALITY FACTORS IN THE DEVELOPMENT OF DEPRESSIVE CONDITIONS IN THE COURSE OF PSYCHOPHARMACOTHERAPY

O. TESAŘOVÁ

Department of Psychiatry, Institute of Postgraduate Medical and Pharmaceutical Studies, Bratislava

When applying different psychopharmacological drugs therapeutically we face the phenomenon that in addition to the therapeutically desired effect, in the course of therapy there develop new psychopathologic symptoms, for example unrest, stupor, disturbances of consciousness, depressive symptoms and deliriant syndromes, which do not fall into line with the basic disease. From this point of view the action of the psychopharmacologic drugs has not yet been cleared. According to several authors (1, 3—7, 9, 10), as well as the action of drug itself, an important part in the development of accompanying psychopathological symptoms is played by factors such as constitution, disposition, age, and organic factors.

This paper focuses on the problems of accompanying depressive symptoms of psychopharmacotherapy. PETRILOWITSCH (12) explains the origin of depressive states in the course of long-term neuroleptic therapy in schizophrenics as the consequence of protracted therapy. The basic reactivity of personality, which shows itself in some patients by depression, is damped by the reduction of productive psychotic symptoms. A similar opinion is presented by JANZARIK (8). GRAHAM and PETERS, (2) LEMIEUX, (19) and others assume that reserpine does not play the main part in the development of depression in the course of reserpine treatment but that there are additional factors at work. In their opinion it is a predisposition to depression which is important.

These hypotheses are proved by our own experience with experimental depressions, which were published (13, 14, 15, 16, 18, 19) and presented at the CINP Congress in 1970 in Prague (17). We took the experimental production of apomorphine and phenoharmane depressions and dysphory in neurotics without depression, as well as the characteritic image of depression in neurotics without depression, and its spontaneous recession in the majority of test persons after the experiment, for proof of direct dependence of the developed depression upon the action of the drug. We found at the same time that in the manifestation of the depressant effect of the drug the drug alone is not responsible. The depressogenic effect of both drugs showed only in individuals with a latent disposition to react depressively, which was proved by the statistically highly significant interdependence between the presence of a latent depressivity in psychodiagnostic tests (Beck-test, M-test, Zulliger-Z-test-22), carried out before the application of apomorphine and phenoharmane, and following manifestation of apomorphine and phenoharmane depression or dysphory in the clinical experiments. (Fig. 1 and 2).

Group	Positivity of psychodiagnostic test before application of apomorphine			Evocation of depression after application of apomorphine
	Z-test	M-test	Beck-test	
Neurotics II showing manifestation of depression after application of apomorphine	●●●●●● ●●●●●● ●●●●●● ●●●●	●●●●●●● ●●●●●●● ○○○○	○○○○○○ ○○○○○○ ○○○○○○ ○○○○	●●●●●●● ●●●●●●● ●●○○○○○
Neurotics II devoid of manifestation of depression after application of apomorphine	●	● ○	○	
Mentaly healthy II showing depression after application of apomorphine	●●●●● ●●●●● ●●●	●●●●●●○	○○○○○ ○○	●●●●●● ●●●●● ●●○○○○
Mentaly healthy II devoid of manifestation of depression after application of apomorphine			○	

Note: ● positive value in test; evocation of depression
○ limited value in test; evocation of dysphory

Fig. 1. Results of the apomorphine test in neurotics and mentally healthy persons.

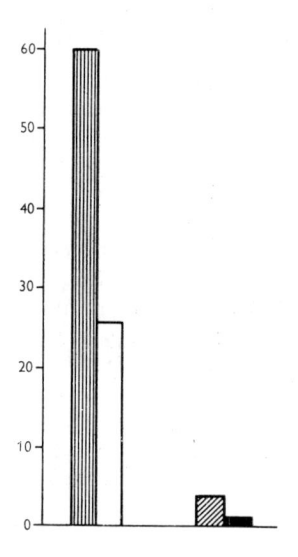

Fig. 2. Summary of appearance of latent signs of depressivity in psychodiagnostic tests.

Vertically hatched column indicates the appearance of latent signs of depressivity in neurotic group showing manifestation of depression in the course of application of apomorphine and phenoharmane.

Slanted hatched column indicates the appearance of latent signs in neurotic group devoid of manifestation of depression in the course of application of apomorphine and phenoharmane.

Empty column indicates the appearance of latent signs of depressivity in mentally healthy group showing depression in the course of application of apomorphine and phenoharmane.

Full column indicates the appearance of latent signs of depressivity in mentaly healthy group devoid of manifestation of depression in the course of application of apomorphine and phenoharmane.

TABLE 1
Group of patients showing symptoms of depression in the course of neuroleptic treatment

Patients	Age	Sex	Diagnosis	Therapy	Beck	M	Z
1. J. P.	24	M	Sch. simplex	Fluanxol	30 + +	+	AD ±
2. M. B.	27	W	Sch. simplex	Chlorpromazine, Perphenazine	24 +	+	AD +
3. E. K.	38	W	Sch. paranoides	Chlorprothixene, Eutumin	8 —	—	—
4. J. B.	23	W	Sch. simplex	Chlorpromazine	0	0	Ds +
5. M. K.	30	W	Sch. paranoides	Chlorprothixene	23 +	+	Dy +
6. J. K.	34	W	Sch. paranoid. defec.	Moditene depot, Chlorpromazine	13 ±	—	Dy ±
7. Š. K.	36	M	Sch. paranoid. defec.	Perphenazine	13 ±	—	—
8. J. J.	37	M	Sch. paranoides	Perphenazine, Chlorprothixene	5 —	—	—
9. M. L.	34	W	Sch. simplex	Fluanxol	0	—	AD +
10. L. F.	23	W	Sch. pseudoneurast. f.	Fluanxol	15 ±	—	D ±
11. M. S.	40	W	Sch. paranoides	Moditene depot, Chlorpromazine	3 —	+	—
12. D. S.	20	W	Sch. paranoides	Chlorprothixene	1 —	—	Dy +
13. K. K.	19	W	Hebefrenia	Fluanxol	0	+	—
14. J. D.	25	M	Sch. paranoid. defec.	Perphenazine	0	0	0
15. B. O.	37	M	Sch. defec.	Perphenazine	0	0	0
16. M. K.	50	W	Sch. defec.	Moditene depot	0	0	0
17. L. P.	41	W	Sch. paranoides	Chlorprothixene, Chlorpromazine	0	0	0
18. S. S.	46	W	Hy. neurosa	Thioridazine, Seduxene	0	0	AD +
19. M. H.	53	M	Neurastenia, Ab. et.	Thioridazine, Seduxene	21 +	—	AD +, AgD +
20. M. H.	39	M	Neurastenia	Thioridazine, Seduxene	21 +	+	AD +

Note

Qualitative variants of indicators of emotivity in Z-test:

D — latent depression,
Ds — latent depression mixed (emotive ambivalence in the sense of MD),
Dy — latent dysphory with significant latent depressive element,
AgD — symptoms of latent aggressivity and latent depression in test,
AD — latent anxious depressive symptomatology in test

Taking into consideration these results we wished to confirm that similar relations are also applicable to the development of depressive states accompanying psychopharmacotherapy. We randomly chose a group of 30 patients treated for a long time with neuroleptics (the majority of them being schizophrenic) who developed in the course of the treatment symptoms of depression. The patients underwent psychodiagnostic examinations by the above-metioned tests; at the time of the examination the patients did not show any clinically apparent depression. From this group of 30 patients only 20 patients were examined psychodiagnostically (2 are dead, 3 missing, 5 did not arrive), in 4 patients out of 20 the findings were not evaluable because they failed in the examination. From the remaining 16 patients, in two patients all three tests were negative when evaluating the presence of latent depressivity indicators. In both cases there were present signs of emotive disactivation, apathy in the test, which can be a sign of depression, but taking into consideration the fact that it was not able to differentiate if this sign in the test had not developed only on the basis of the effect of neuroleptics, we evaluated the Z-test as negative. The Beck-test was positive in 8 cases (50%), M-test in 6 cases (37,5%), Z-test in 11 cases (66.7%). In the global evaluation of all tests positivity was found in 87%. (20, 21) (Table 1 and Fig. 3).

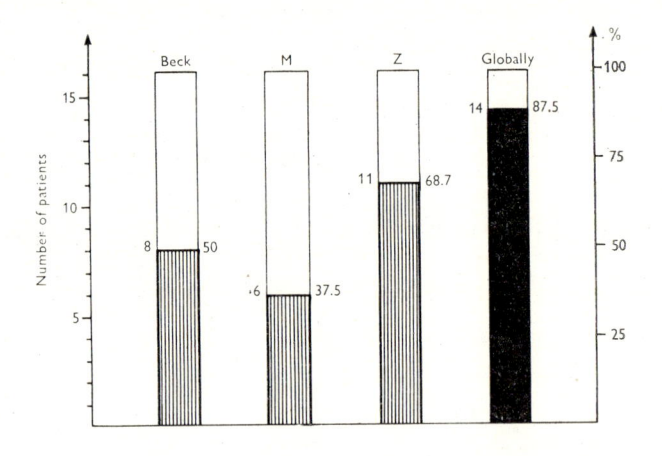

Fig. 3. Latent signs of depression globally in psychodiagnostic tests.

It may be concluded that in the total evaluation of this study the relations found in experimental depressions seem to be valid. The latent disposition of personality to depression seems to play a role even in the manifestation of accompanying depressive symptoms in the course of neuroleptic treatment. The results, however, only support hypothesis, as the small number of patients examined mean that it will be necessary to continue our observations with a larger group.

SUMMARY

When producing experimental apomorphine and phenoharmane depression we found that in the manifestation of the depressogene effect the matter itself does not play a role alone. The depresogene effect of both matters showed selectively only in persons with a latent disposition of the personality to react in a depressive way, which was proved by the statistically highly significant relationship between the presence of latent depressivity in psychodiagnostic tests (Beck, Zulliger and Mittenecker test), carried out before the experiment, and the following occurrence of experimental depression. On the basis of these experiences we wanted to make sure if similar relations are effective also in the occurrence of accompanying depressive conditions. We were aiming at investigating depressive conditions in the course of a long-term maintenance treatment by neuroleptics from the point of view of personality in their origin. 20 patients were examined by these tests. In 87.5% were the results of tests positive from the point of view of presence of latent depressivity marks.

REFERENCES

1. ANGST, J. (1960) Begleiterscheinungen und Nebenwirkungen moderner Psychofarmaka. Praxis, **49**, 546.
2. GRAHAM, H. and PETERS, U. (1962) Durch Psychofarmaka induzierte und provozierte Psychosen, ihre Psychopathologie und ihre therapeutische Bedeutung. Nervenarzt, **33**, 338.
3. HÄFFNER, H. and KUTSCHER, I. (1964) Komplikationen der klinischen Behandlung mit Psychofarmaka. Ärztl. Forsch. **18**, 18.
4. HELMCHEN, H. (1961) Delirante Abläufe unter psychiatrischer Pharmakotherapie. Arch. Psychiat. Nervenkr. **202**, 335.
5. HIPPIUS, H. (1960) Therapeutische unerwünschte Wirkungen der modernen Psychopharmaka. 1. Mitteilung. Internist, **1**, 453.
6. HIPPIUS, H. and SELBACH, H. (1961) Zur medikamentösen Dauertherapie bei Psychosen. Med. exp. **3**, 298.
7. HUBACH, H. and SCHILLING, R. (1965) Dämmerzustände durch Psychofarmaka. Psychopharmacologia (Berl.) **7**, 306.
8. JANZARIK, W. (1964) Die Wirkungsebene der Pharmakotherapie im Aufbau depressiver Syndrome. Arzneimittel-Forsch. **14**, 493.
9. KIELHOLZ, P. (1965) Psychiatrische Pharmakotherapie in Klinik und Praxis. Bern, Stuttgart, H. Huber.
10. KIELHOLZ, P. (1959) Differential diagnostik und Therapie der depressiven Zustandbilder. Acta psychosom. Basel, Geigy.
11. LEMIEUX, G., DAVIGNON, A. and GENEST, J. (1956) Depressive states during rauw. therapy for arterial hypertension. Canad. med. Ass. J. **74**, 522.
12. PETRILOWITSCH, N. (1968) Psychiatrische Krankheitslehre und psychiatrische Pharmakotherapie. Basel, New York, S. Karger.
13. TESAŘOVÁ, O. and MOLČAN, J. (1966) A contribution to the problem experimental depression. Activ. nerv. sup. **8**, 351.
14. TESAŘOVÁ, O. (1967) Experimental depression generating through apomorphine. Diss. (in Slovak) Bratislava.
15. TESAŘOVÁ, O. (1968) Mechanism of thymoleptic drug action studies on the model of apomorphine depression. Activ. nerv. sup. **10**, 287.
16. TESAŘOVÁ, O. (1968) On the feasibility of experimentally generating depression through apomorphine (in Czech). De psychiatria progrediente, Plzeň, 546.
17. TESAŘOVÁ, O. (1970) Experimental depression in people caused by apomorphine and phenoharmane. The paper appeared at the CINP congress, Prague.
18. TESAŘOVÁ, O. (1971) Pharmacogenous stated of depression (in Slovak). Folia Fac. med. Univ. Comenianae, Bratislava, **9**, 2.
19. TESAŘOVÁ, O. (1972) Experimental depression caused by apomorphine and phenoharmane. Pharmakopsychiat. **5**, 13.
20. TESAŘOVÁ, O. (1972) Psychopathological side effects of psychotropic drug therapy. Activ. nerv. sup. **14**, 91.
21. TESAŘOVÁ, O. (1972) To the problems of pharmacogenous pathomorphosis (in Slovak) Čs. Psychiat. **68**, 67.
22. ZULLIGER, H. (1948) Z - Test 1. Aufl. Bern, H. Huber, 72.

O.T., Department of Psychiatry, Institute of Postgraduate Medical and Pharmaceutical Studies, Bazová 8, Bratislava, Czechoslovakia

TOLERANCE TO THE NARCOTIC ANALGESICS
A LONG-TERM PHENOMENON

J. COCHIN

Department of Pharmacology, Boston University School of Medicine, Boston, Massachusetts

For many years the study of long-term effects of drugs concerned itself with problems of chronic, as opposed to acute, toxicity or with the effects of a single sensitizing dose of a drug followed by a challenging dose many days, months or even years later. But this kind of long-term effect is not the one to which I address myself today. For many years I, and others interested in the pharmacology of the narcotic analgesics and their mechanisms of action, have been intrigued by the phenomena of tolerance and dependence which accompany the repeated administration of this class of drugs. We have long known that the clinical use of these drugs induced long-term effects and that these effects are often profound and at times even difficult to believe. It is only relatively recently, however, that systematic studies of these phenomena have been undertaken, despite the fact that they have been described anecdotally for many centuries and more scientifically for almost a hundred years.

The tolerance that the narcotic analgesics induce is one which under certain circumstances is almost complete for some aspects of drug action and may be initiated even by a single dose of drug. We know somewhat less about dependence but we are convinced that a relatively small series of drug ingestions or injections will initiate significant physical dependence, that can be demonstrated and quantified, if not by abrupt termination of drug administration, then certainly by injection of a narcotic antagonist.

There have been many hypotheses proposed to explain tolerance and dependence to the narcotic analgesics. These include (a) altered metabolic disposition and distribution in the tolerant animal; (b) prevention of access of drugs to the site of action; (c) occupation and saturation of receptor sites; (d) cellular adaptation and finally (e) some sort of vague and ill-defined change at the cellular level that resembles an immune reaction or a reaction analogous to memory.

None of these hypotheses or explanations are completely satisfactory. For some, such as altered metabolic disposition or distribution, there is little or no evidence; for others, the experimental framework is firmer. Some of them, however, have succeeded in stimulating work in a little-researched field.

Because we believed that a phenomenon must be adequately described before the mechanism of its development could be investigated, KORNETSKY and I (1) initiated a series of experiments designed to elucidate in a more precise way the characteristics of the development and loss of tolerance to morphine. In designing the experiments we had to take into consideration something which had been overlooked in many previous studies of tolerance and dependence. In the very process of evaluating tolerance by giving animals a test dose of morphine, one initiated or hastened or made more profound the phenomenon one was measuring. Thus each test dose acted as a priming dose. We therefore designed an experiment with a large number of experimental and control groups. Fig. 1 is a complicated depiction of an even more complex experiment.

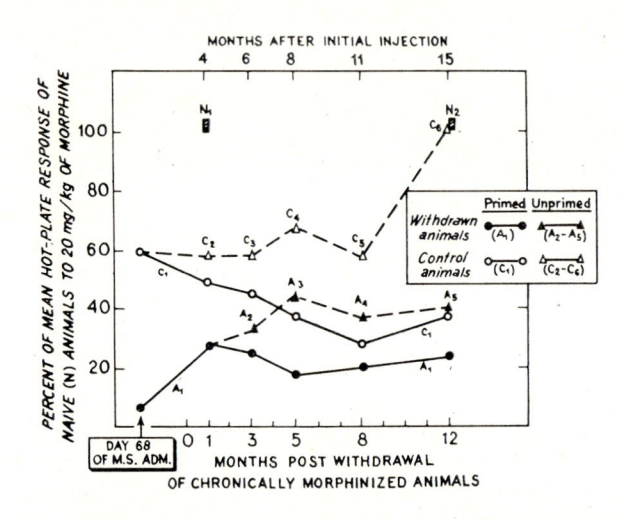

Fig. 1. A comparison of the response to 20 mg/kg of morphine sulfate of each of the animal groups on the hot-plate procedure at various intervals during the experiment. Animals in the primed group (closed or open circles) received injection at each point indicated. Each triangle (closed or open) represents a separate group of animals that were tested only once at the indicated interval. Groups N_1 and N_2 represent naive animals that were brought into the laboratory at the same time as the withdrawn and control animals but were never given morphine except at the indicated points (COCHIN and KORNETSKY [1]).

It is evident from this figure which shows the results obtained using an analgesic assay, the hot-plate technique, that a single injection of morphine given as long as twelve months previously significantly affected the response to a second injection of the same dose of morphine. Animals that had received a series of daily injections over a period of more than two months, still showed attenuation of the morphine effect some fifteen months after their last morphine injections. Our results indicated that what is important in maintaining tolerance to morphine is not necessarily the length of the previous period of chronic morphine administration or the amounts given, within certain limits, but rather a history of a few or even one, depending on the interval, previous injections of drug. The results were also consistent with those of WINTER (16) who reported a number of years ago that the same degree of tolerance was induced by daily doses of morphine given to rats for three weeks or by weekly injections for the same period of time. Similar findings have been reported in the mouse using the tail-flick response to heat as the measure of drug effect and several weeks as the elapsed time (11). FRASER and ISBELL (9), working with post-addicts at the Addiction Research Center in Lexington, Kentucky, reported tolerance to the nauseant and emetic effects of morphine and to the lowering of body temperature in man for as long as six months after termination of chronic morphine administration.

The comparisons were made with the effects of the drug on the same parameters in normal volunteers after a single injection.

EDDY (7) has noted that a second injection of morphine given to mice twenty four hours following an initial dose did not seem to initiate the development of tolerance to the analgesic effect of the drug. However, if there is a seventy-two or ninety-six hour interval between the first and second injection, the effect of the second injection is much reduced. Recent work in my laboratory (3), indicated quite clearly that the interval between injections is an extremely important factor in determining how much attenuation of effect results, another indication that a process is taking place that requires a finite amount of time for completion and once instituted is amazingly persistent.

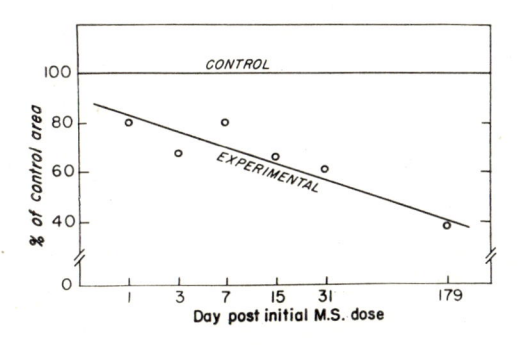

Fig. 2. Performance by rats on the voltage-attenuation apparatus after morphine. Animals in the control group received injections of 5 mg/kg on the designated days. Animals in the experimental groups received an injection of 10 mg/kg morphine sulfate on day 0 and an additional injection of 5 mg/kg morphine sulfate on one of the designated days. Each point represents eight control and eight experimental animals (Adapted from KORNETSKY and BAIN [12]).

In considering the types of changes that might account for the persistence of tolerance for periods of up to one year after the last exposure of an animal to a narcotic analgesic, most of the widely accepted explanations of tolerance involving receptor occupation or changes in drug-metabolizing enzymes have been found wanting. The possibility of the induction of a mechanism resembling an immune reaction is one that we have found most inviting. It has been observed by many workers in the fields of immunochemistry and immunology that the effects of a single previous dose of an antigen are most persistent and might even last for the lifetime of an individual animal or man. Drug-induced antigen-antibody reactions are unfortunately not an uncommon occurence in medicine—penicillin reactions being one of the best-known examples. These reactions are not only persistent but also take a finite time to develop. Since tolerance can be extremely persistent and since it does take a finite time to develop, it has been suggested that tolerance might be an immune-like phenomenon, a reaction to administration of a drug that was conditioned by the previous administration of that same drug or one closely related to it in structure or action.

KORNETSKY and I initiated a number of experiments that involved transfer of serum from tolerant donors to non-tolerant recipients to see whether or not there was a factor that could be transferred passively (2). Although our results and those of others indicate the possible presence of factors in the serum of tolerant animals that attenuate or potentiate the analgesic effects of morphine, the results are only suggestive and the presence of such factors has not been conclusively proven.

Recently KORNETSKY (12) undertook a study in which he was interested in delineating the onset of tolerance after a single injection and he used as a measure of drug effect a modification of the voltage-attenuation technique. Each rat in the experimental group received 10 mg/kg of morphine on day O and on one of the days indicated in Fig. 2 and the animals were again tested on the attenuator. No animal received more than two injections of morphine during the course of the experiment. The mean scores of eight experimental animals on each test day were compared with the mean scores of eight control rats that had never received morphine previously and that were given their first dose on the same test day. It is apparent even by day 3, certainly by days 15 and 31, that the effects of a second injection of morphine are significantly diminished. The time course of the tolerance induced by a single injection is also of interest. It is significantly greater at six months than at one month. On the other hand, a second injection has no attenuating effect when given twenty-four hours after the initial dose. These findings agree with those observed by EDDY and others and demonstrate anew that tolerance is a phenomenon that takes time to develop fully.

In order to understand better the characteristics of tolerance we undertook a series of studies in our laboratory to describe more fully various factors that affect the long-term persistence of drug effect and which may help explain why tolerance develops under some conditions more rapidly and more completely than under others. We decided to investigate the role of the interval between doses in the development of tolerance. We gave a number of rats 15 mg/kg of morphine sulphate and tested them for their response on the hot-plate. We then divided them into groups which were given drug at one week, two-week or three-week intervals (Fig. 3). Our results demonstrated that animals receiving morphine at seven-day intervals do not give responses significantly different from their initial reactions until the third injection, whereas animals receiving morphine at 14- and 21- day intervals have a significantly attenuated response after the second injection. There are significant differences in response between the groups until the fifth injection of morphine. Fig. 4 shows the effect of intervals shorter than seven days. It is almost as if the seven-day-period between doses was some sort of watershed — tolerance is induced more rapidly at longer and shorter intervals. Perhaps the seven-day interval marks the transition between long and short-term tolerance, both of which have been described for morphine.

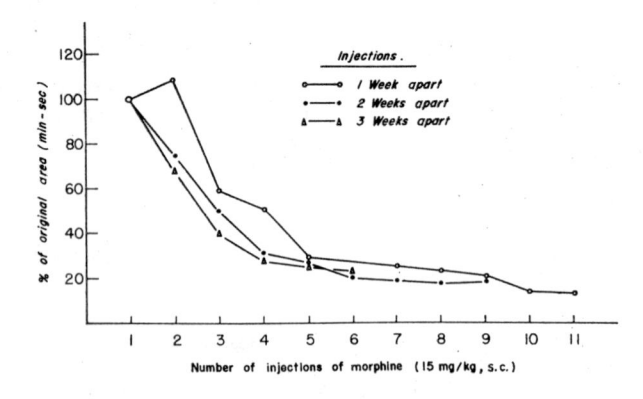

Fig. 3. The influence of intervals of one week or more on the development of tolerance to morphine. Injections of 15 mg/kg morphine sulfate were given at the indicated intervals. Animals were tested for their response to morphine using the hot-plate technique. The ordinate expresses per cent of their original response (presented in COCHIN and MUSHLIN [3]).

We have also studied the effects of simultaneous administration and pretreatment with Freund's adjuvant, a potent stimulator of immune responses. Both pretreatment and simultaneous administration alter the course of the long-term effect of morphine (4).

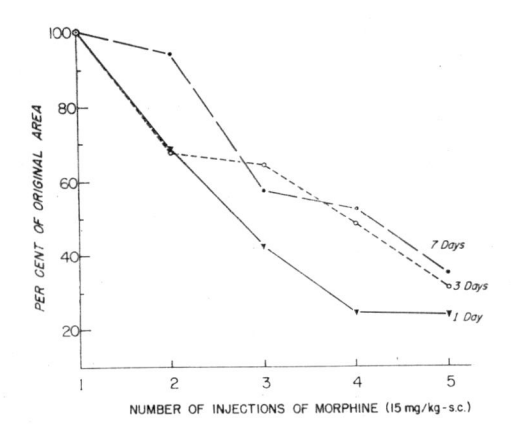

Fig. 4. The influence of intervals of one week or less on the development of tolerance to morphine. Injections of 15 mg/kg morphine sulfate were given at the indicated intervals. Animals were tested for their response to morphine using the hot-plate technique. The ordinate express per cent of their original response (COCHIN and MUSHLIN, unpublished observations).

One of my graduate students, DR. GLADY FRIEDLER, undertook a study of the effect of pretreatment of mothers with morphine on offspring (10). This was to search for additional evidence of a factor affecting morphine action that might be transferred across the placental barrier or via the mother's milk. Female rats were given relatively large doses of morphine for a number of days and then withdrawn from the drug for five to six days. They were then mated to drug-free males and the offspring resulting from their matings were studied for differences in sensitivity to drug and differences in growth pattern. We found significant differences in the weights of the offspring of drug-treated mothers compared with the weights of the offspring of controls despite the fact that neither group of offspring was exposed to drug either *in utero* or *post partum*. The greatest differences were found in the female young at 5-6 weeks of age. This experiment has now been repeated in mice and there seems to be no doubt that very profound changes take place in animals treated chronically with the narcotic analgesics that influence temporarily at least, the development pattern of the young born one to two months after the last exposure of the mother to drugs. In a continuation of this experiment we tested the offspring at eight weeks of age for their analgesic response to 10 mg/kg of morphine. The young born to previously treated mothers were significantly less sensitive to drug than those born to untreated mothers. We are now investigating how long after birth this tolerance lasts. We have also done a series of cross-fostering studies that have eliminated the possibility that the differences we have seen are due to either maternal neglect or something present in the milk of the mothers. We are not at all certain of the nature of this factor that affects the young, but we know that it crosses the placental barrier.

It seems obvious that effects so profound and long-lasting that they can affect succeeding generations must reflect long-lasting and profound cellular changes and at present a number of laboratories are attempting to modify these long-lasting cellular changes in various ways. One of the approaches is the investigation of the effects of compounds that disrupt either protein synthesis or short-term memory. A number of investigators have reported that suppressors of protein synthesis block the development of tolerance and they attribute their results to suppression of RNA synthesis (5, 6). However, it has been shown that actinomycin, the drug many of them used, alters the permeability of the

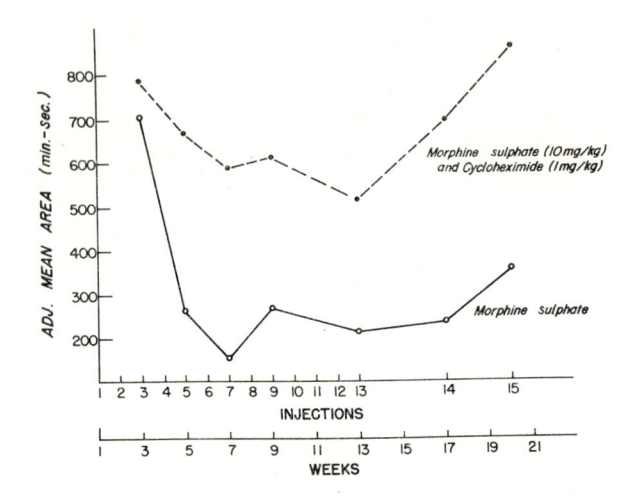

Fig. 5. The effect of the concomitant administration of morphine sulfate and cycloheximide on the development of tolerance as compared to the effect of morphine sulfate alone on the development of tolerance. Injections of 10 mg/kg of morphine sulfate were given one hour after the administration of 1 mg/kg of cycloheximide to those animals who received both agents. Injections of 10 mg/kg of morphine sulfate were given to those animals receiving only morphine sulfate. The animals were tested on the hot-plate for their response to morphine sulfate at each point indicated by either the closed or open circles. The ordinate indicates the adjusted mean area under the time-response curve. The abscissa indicates the schedule of injections and testing (FEINBERG and COCHIN, unpublished observations).

blood-brain barrier to morphine and facilitates its access to the central nervous system (13). Thus, what appears to be an inhibition of tolerance may actually be an enhancement of sensitivity to morphine. In our laboratory and in E. LEONG WAY's (14), studies of the effects of cycloheximide, a potent inhibitor of protein synthesis, have been underway for some time. One of my students, Mr. MICHAEL FEINBERG, has carried out a series of experiments in which one group of rats was given a single injection of 10 mg/kg of morphine every week for several weeks, while another group was given cycloheximide one hour before being injected with morphine. All the animals were then tested on the hot-plate. Fig. 5 shows the results obtained. There are striking differences between the two groups and the development of tolerance is inhibited in the animals treated with morphine plus cycloheximide. At week 13, the cycloheximide was discontinued for a period of 4 weeks and the animals were tested again for the persistence of tolerance in the 17th week. As would be expected, the animals that had received only morphine still showed an almost complete persistence of tolerance but the cycloheximide-treated animals showed a rapid loss of tolerance. By the 21st week, 8 weeks after the last dose of cycloheximide, they had recovered their sensitivity to morphine completely, whereas the morphine alone-group seemed to be as tolerant as at week 17 (8).

I have reviewed a number of examples of the special case of long-term effects of drugs that we call tolerance and have discussed how it can be modified and what some of the factors are upon which its development depends. Tolerance however is not a unitary phenomenon. Much of what I have discussed here might be different if one were to measure other actions of morphine such as respiratory depression, depression of swimming speed and so on. I thought it best, however, not to muddy the waters and limit my discussion to the one aspect of morphine action that has been most widely observed and studied.

REFERENCES

1. COCHIN, J. and KORNETSKY, C. (1964) Development and loss of tolerance to morphine in the rat after single and multiple injection. J. Pharmacol. exp. Ther. **145**, 1.
2. COCHIN, J. and KORNETSKY, C. (1968) Factors in blood of morphine-tolerant animals that attenuate or enhance effects of morphine in nontolerant animals. In: Proceedings of the Association for Research in Nervous and Mental Disease, Vol. 46. The Addictive States, edited by A. WIKLER, Baltimore: Williams and Wiklins, p. 268.
3. COCHIN, J. and MUSHLIN, B. E. (1970) The role of dose-interval in the development of tolerance to morphine. Fed. Proc. **29**, 685.
4. COCHIN, J. and MUSHLIN, B. E. (1972) The effects of Freund's adjuvant on morphine sensitivity and tolerance. Fed. Proc. **31**, 528.
5. COHEN, M., KEATS, A. S., KRIVOY, W. and UNGAR, G. (1965) Effect of Actinomycin D on morphine tolerance. Proc. Soc. exp. Biol. (N.Y.) **119**, 381.
6. COX, B. M. and OSMAN, O. H. (1970) Inhibition of the development of tolerance to morphine in rats by drugs which inhibit ribonucleic acid or protein synthesis. Brit. J. Pharmacol. **38**, 157.
7. EDDY, N. B. (1953) The hot-plate method for measuring analgesic effect in mice. Minutes of the 13th Meeting of the Committee on Problems of Drug Dependence, NAS-NRC, Appendix C, p. 603.
8. FEINBERG M. P. and COCHIN, J. (1972) Inhibition of development of tolerance to morphine by cycloheximide. Biochem. Pharmacol. **21**, 3082.
9. FRASER, H. F. and ISBELL, H. (1952) Comparative effects of 20 mgm of morphine sulfate on non-addicts and former morphine addicts, J. Pharmacol. exp. Ther. **105**, 498.
10. FRIEDLER, G. and COCHIN, J. (1972) Growth retardation in offspring of female rats treated with morphine prior to conception. Science, **175**, 654.
11. GREEN, A. F., YOUNG, P. A. and GODFREY, E. I. (1951) A comparison of heat and analgesiometric methods in rats. Brit. J. Pharmacol. **6**, 572.
12. KORNETSKY, C. and BAIN, G. (1972). Single dose tolerance to morphine. Pharmacologist, **9**, 219.
13. LOH, H. H., SHEN, F. S. and WAY, E. L. (1969) Inhibition of morphine tolerance and physical dependence and brain serotonin synthesis by cycloheximide. Biochem. Pharmacol. **18**, 2711.
14. LOH, H. H., SHEN, F. S. and WAY, E. L. (1971) Effect of d-actinomycin on the acute toxicity and brain uptake of morphine. J. Pharmacol. exp. Ther. **177**, 326.
15. WEISS, B. and LATIES, V. G. (1961) Changes in pain tolerance and other behavior produced by salicylates. J. Pharmacol. exp. Ther. **131**, 120.
16. WINTER, C. A. (1953) Measurement of analgesic effect: the tail-flick method. Minutes of the 12th Meeting of the Committee on Problems of Drug Dependence, NAS-NRC Appendix A, p. 577.

J.C., Department of Pharmacology, Boston University School of Medicine, Boston, Massachusetts, U.S.A.

TOLERANCE AND WITHDRAWAL EFFECTS AFTER ONE WEEK ADMINISTRATION OF PERPHENAZINE IN RABBITS

Z. VOTAVA

Research Institute for Pharmacy and Biochemistry, Prague

Since the discovery of the therapeutic effect of chlorpromazine in the treatment of schizophrenia in 1952, neuroleptics of the phenothiazine and other chemical types have been used all over the world. Generally it has been supposed that the pharmacological effect of these drugs does not change during long-term administration. Data on the pharmacological effect in animals have been obtained predominantely from the short-term experiments, however. Recently it has been found (2, 3, 6, 7) that the repeated administration of some neuroleptics in animals has led to decreasing effectiveness in several testing procedures. It has not been clear, however, whether a sudden interruption of the chronic administration of neuroleptics could evoke any withdrawal symptomps.

We decided therefore to examine the effect of neuroleptics not only during repeated administration, but also after its interruption. Perphenazine, one of the most effective neuroleptic drugs, used in the treatment of schizophrenia for more than fifteen years, was tested first.

METHODS

Ten New Zeeland male rabbits weighing 3.6—4.0 kg with deep electrodes implanted in their brains were used. Stainless steel screws contacting the dura mater served as monopolar cortical electrodes and ground reference. They were connected to the recording socket via coated wires. The deep bipolar electrodes were made from intertwined constantane wires 0.18 mm in diameter and Diamel coated except at the tips, and were implanted by standard stereotaxic techniques using the coordinates of FIFKOVÁ and MARŠALA (1) at the following sites: cortex frontalis, cortex parietalis, cortex occipitalis, hippocampus dorsalis, thalamus n. ven. med., formation reticularis mesencephali (Fig. 1). The electrodes were secured with acrylic resin and connected to a special socket which was then permanently mounted to the skull with acrylic resin. After cerebral electrode implantation under sodium pentobarbital and urethane anesthesia, the animals were given 300.000 I.U. of procaine penicillin and allowed to recover for fourteen days before control recordings were begun. After the last run, the position of the deep electrodes were verified by the histological techniques.

Rabbits were accustomed to the experimental procedure in several control trials, before

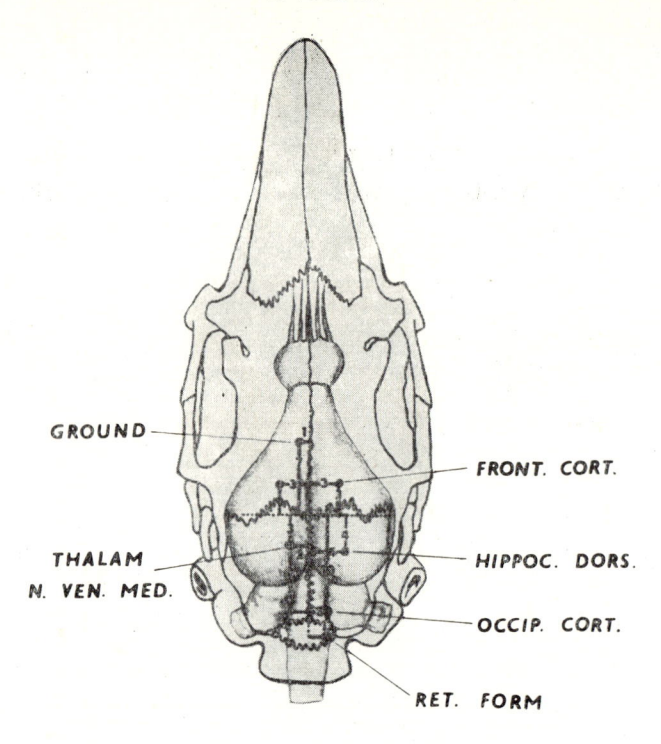

Fig. 1. Localization of brain electrodes in rabbit skull.

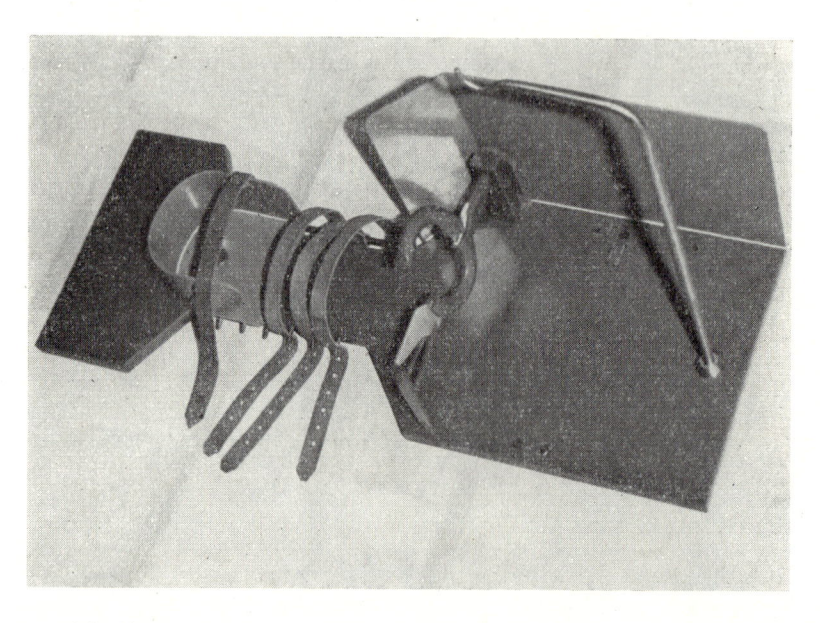

Fig. 2. Restraining box for rabbit, enabling the simultaneous registration of EEG, ECG, respiration and body movements.

the administration of test drug was started. During the experimental trial, each animal was placed into a quiet electrically screened room, and fixed in a special restraining box made in our laboratory (4). (Fig. 2). The rabbit's head was held in place by a neck yoke suspended on a rubber strip. This resulted in a convenient position of the rabbit during the EEG recording, and the simultaneous registration of respiration, heart rate and body movements were also performed. Polyphysiograph R 35f with eight channels for EEG and four channels for physiological registration was used.

The arousal reaction of animals was tested by sensory stimulation, with Photostimulator Model SL1b and Audiostimulator Model SA1a, using 5 and 50 cps frequency, and by electric stimulation of the reticular formation, using Electrostimulator Model SE1a, with 300 cps frequency and super-threshold voltage (2—4V). All devices were GALILEO origin.

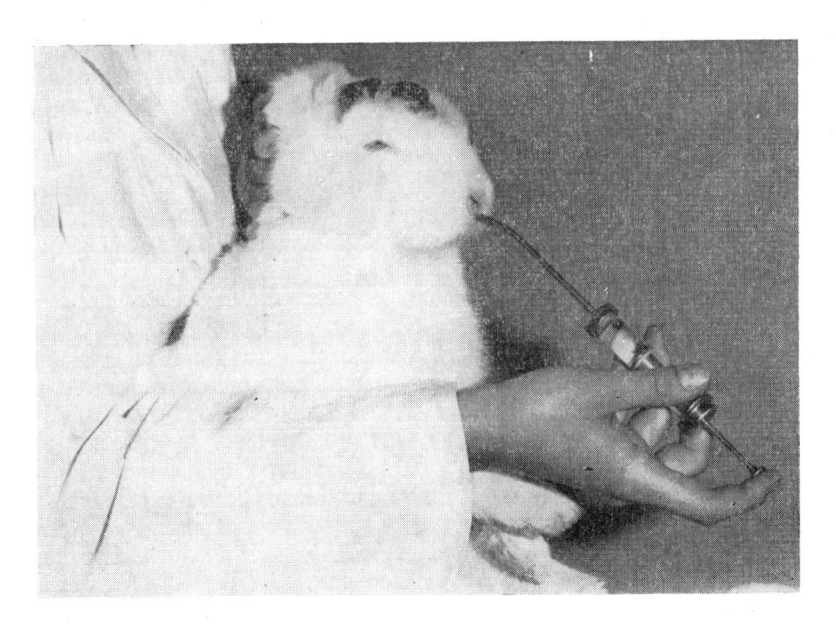

Fig. 3. Oral administration of drug solution using a special metal tube.

Perphenazine was administered orally, using a special metal tube of 80 mm length and 3 mm in diameter, bent in the oral end at an angle of 20° (Fig. 3). An aqueous suspension was given at the rate of 1 ml per kg body weight. Perphenazine was given daily for one week, starting with 10 mg/kg on the first two days, continuing with 15 mg/kg on the next two days, and finishing with 20 mg/kg during the last three days. Altogether 110 mg/kg of perphenazine was given during the one week period. Doses were expressed in terms of the free bases.

The EEG recordings were always tested 1 h after the administration of perphenazine, on the first day (10 mg/kg), third day (15 mg/kg), fifth day (20 mg/kg) and seventh day (20 mg/kg), and a further one day, two days and four days following the last perphenazine dose. Controls were given saline solution as a placebo.

All tracings from cortical and deep electrodes were evaluated page by page for frequency and voltage and characterized as "resting pattern" or "activated pattern". "Resting pattern" consisted of high voltage (100—250 μV), slow (2—7cps) waves in cortical leads with some high voltage "spindles", and irregular high voltage (50—150 μV) waves in leads from thalamus and hippocampus. "Activated pattern" consisted of low voltage (20—100 μV), fast (15—25 cps) waves in cortical leads and regular "theta" activity (30—50 μV, 6—7 cps) in leads from the thalamus and hippocampus and sometimes from the reticular formation.

Heart and respiration rates were calculated from the traces. Body weight and rectal body temperature were measured daily during all the experiment.

Results

In control trials, before the administration of perphenazine, the animals, habituated to the experimental procedure, were quietly sitting in the restraining box, with occasional body movements. "Resting pattern" traces were predominently present in the EEG, with some "spindles" (2.8 ± 0,15 in one page, that is in 20 s period) in the frontal cortex leads, and episodes of "activated pattern" (18.2 ± 3.0% of the total recording).

One hour after the first perphenazine dose (10 mg/kg), rabbits were sedated, without any movements in the restraining box. The "activated pattern" in EEG tracing almost disappeared (only 5.3 ± 1.2%), and the frequency of "spindles" increased to 3.2 ± 0.2 in one page.

The arousal reaction evoked by photic and acoustic stimulation was eliminated, the threshold of the reticular formation stimulation elevated of 3.1 ± 0.5 V. The respiration rate was lowered from 250 to 140 per/min, the heart rate was not changed significantly. Body temperature was lowered from 38.9 to 38.4°C. All these changes were statistically significant ($p < 0.05$).

After the third dose of perphenazine (15 mg/kg), the EEG recordings were rather "activated" (32 ± 5%), and the frequency of "spindles" in frontal cortex traces was low (0.3 per page). There were body movements of rabbits during the trial. The arousal reaction evoked by sensory as well as reticular formation stimulations was still eliminated. The rectal temperature was lowered about the same degree as after the first dose of perphenazine, the respiration rate returned to the control levels.

After the fifth (20 mg/kg) and seventh (20 mg/kg) doses of perphenazine, the results were almost the same as after the third dose, although the doses were rather high. The EEG traces and behaviour of the rabbits were very close to the control level before the administration of perphenazine. The appearance of "activated pattern" in EEG was somewhat higher then in controls (28.3 ± 5.5%) and the frequency of "spindles" was lower (1.8 ± 0.5). The arousal reactions evoked by sensory and reticular formation stimulation were still eliminatable. Body temperature, respiration and heart rates were not significantly changed.

One day after the last administration of perphenazine, a surprising change in EEG traces and behaviour of rabbits appeared. The animals were excited, the EEG traces highly "activated" (83.6 ± 12.3%), and no "spindles" were seen in cortical leads. The respiration rate was elevated to 283 per min, the heart rate and body temperature were not changed. The arousal reaction after sensory and reticular formation stimulations returned almost to the control level.

Forty-eight hours after the last perphenazine dose, rabbits were still excited and EEG traces very "activated", similarly to the previous day.

Ninety-six hours after the last perphenazine dose, the EEG traces and behaviour of rabbits returned almost to the control level. Body temperature, respiration and heart rates were also not significantly changed from the controls. The sensory (photic and acoustic) as well as reticular formation stimulations evoked the arousal reactions to about the same degree as in the control experiments.

Discussion

The results of our experiment showed that the daily oral administration of perphenazine caused a quick tolerance of rabbits to its behavioural (tranquillizing) and EEG ("resting pattern") effects. Nevertheless the inhibition of the arousal reaction evoked by photic, acoustic and reticular formation stimulation remained unchanged during repeated administration. Also Theobald et al. (7) have reported that the repeated administration of three neuroleptics, chlorpromazine, thioproperazine and thioridazine gave different results with regard to tolerance: either a tolerance developed or the activity remained constant. Similar results were also published by Metyšová (5).

Although the administration of perphenazine was limited in our experiment to only seven days, the relatively high and increasing doses caused the fast development of tolerance in animals to the tranquillizing properties of that neuroleptic. The interruption of the perphenazine administration provoked very peculiar withdrawal symptoms, characterized by the high behavioural excitation of animals and the appearance of the "activated pattern" in EEG traces. The respiration rate was also elevated. The duration of these "withdrawal symptoms" was short, lasting only about two days. Ninety-six hours after the last dose of perphenazine, the EEG traces and behavioural features showed almost the normal control patterns.

Summary

In ten rabbits with permanent indwelled brain electrodes, perphenazine was given in seven daily doses (2×10 mg, 2×15 mg, 3×20 mg/kg). EEG recording, photic, acoustic, and reticular formation stimulation were performed before, and 1 h after the first, third, fifth and seventh dose, and 24 h, 48 h and 96 h after the last perphenazine dose. Tolerance developed quickly to the tranquilizing perphenazine effect in EEG and behaviour. After perphenazine administration interruption, several withdrawal symptoms were observed, especially behavioural excitation, EEG "activated pattern" and acceleration of respiration rate. These "withdrawal symptoms" disappeared in about ninety-six hours.

References

1. Fifková, E. and Maršala J. (1962) Stereotaxic atlases for cat, rabbit and rat. In: Bureš J., Petráň, M. and Zachar J., Electrophysiological methods in biological research, 2nd Edition, p. 426, Academic Publish. House, Praha.
2. Irwin, S. (1961) Correlation in rats between the locomotor and avoidance suppressant potencies of eight phenothiazine tranquilizers. Arch. int. Pharmacodyn. 132, 279.
3. Julou, L., Bardone, M. C., Ducrot, R., Laffargue, B. and Loissea, G. (1967) Comparaison des effets des neuroleptiques dans divers tests, en administration unique et en administration répétées. Hypothèses sur la signification des tests utilisés et leur valeur prévisionelle. Neuropsychopharmacology, Proceedings of the Fifth Intern. Congress of the CINP, Washington 1966, Excerpta Medica Foundation, Amsterdam, p. 293.
4. Likovský, Z., Votava, Z., Formánek, J. and Menoušek S. (1973), Stolek pro vyšetřování králíků (The restraining box for the rabbit's experiments), Čs. Fysiol., 22, 152.
5. Metyšová, J. (1972) Changes in central effects of several neuroleptics after their repeated administration. Psychopharmacologia 26, (suppl.), 101.

6. MØLLER NIELSEN, I., FJALLAND, B., PEDERSEN, V., and NYMARK, M. (1972) Development of tolerance in animals by repeated administration of neuroleptics. Psychopharmacologia **26** (suppl.), 100.
7. THEOBALD, W., BÜCH, O., DELINI-STULA, A., EIGENMANN, R. and LEVIN, PH. (1968) Pharmakologische Untersuchungen zur Wirkung von Neuroleptika am Tier nach einmaliger und wiederholter Applikation. Arzneim.-Forsch. (Drug Res.) **18**, 1491.

Z. V., Research Institute for Pharmacy and Biochemistry,
Kouřimská 17, Prague 3, Czechoslovakia

DEVELOPMENT OF TOLERANCE IN ANIMALS BY REPEATED ADMINISTRATION OF NEUROLEPTICS

I. MØLLER NIELSEN, B. FJALLAND, V. PEDERSEN and M. NYMARK

Department of Pharmacology and Toxicology, H. Lundbeck & Co. A/S, Copenhagen

Clinical experience has not revealed any development of tolerance (decrease of potency with repeated dosage) to the antipsychotic effect of neuroleptics. On the contrary, the initial dosage may often be reduced to a lower maintenance level.

TABLE 1

Amphetamine-antagonism in rats after pretreatment with haloperidol and flupenthixol

Pretreatment	Daily dose mg/kg p.o.	Days of treatment	Flupenthixol ED 50 mg/kg s.c.	Tolerance factor
Haloperidol	20	5	0.42	2.2
Haloperidol	20	14	1.47	7.7
Haloperidol	10	12	0.98	5.2
Flupenthixol	10	12	0.38	2
No pretreatment			0.19	1

Test carried out 3 days after withdrawal of drug. Tolerance factor = ED 50 pretreated/ED 50 non-pretreated.

Tolerance and cross-tolerance to various neuroleptics were shown to develop with respect to amphetamine antagonism in rats (Table 1). Degree of tolerance increased with increasing dose and increasing days of pretreatment.

Fig. 1 shows the development, and duration after withdrawal, of homologous tolerance to various neuroleptics, using apomorphine antagonism in rats as a test model. The degree of tolerance varied between compounds. Tolerance was most pronounced the first week after withdrawal but persisted for several weeks. With the methylphenidate antagonism (2) in mice as test model (Fig. 2) tolerance was shown to develop after rather low doses of some neuroleptics. Although the degree of tolerance was considerable three days following withdrawal it was considerably reduced after seven days.

Apomorphine-induced stereotyped running in dogs is effectively antagonized by neuroleptics (1). Pretreatment with haloperidol induced marked cross-tolerance to the antagonistic effect of flupenthixol. The tolerance persisted for more than 45 days after withdrawal of haloperidol. Tolerance or cross-tolerance did not develop to the cataleptogenic

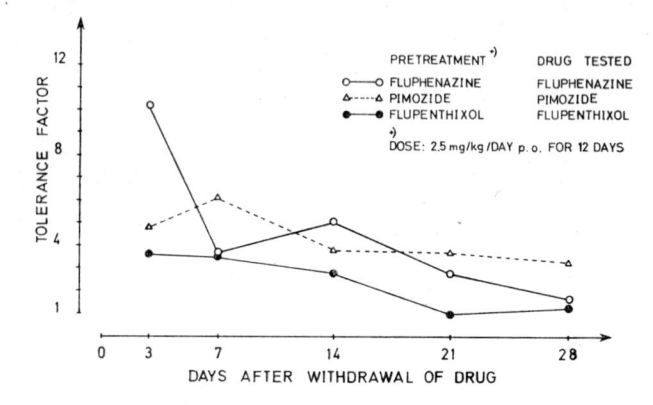

Fig. 1. Apomorphine antagonism in rats. Homologous tolerance.

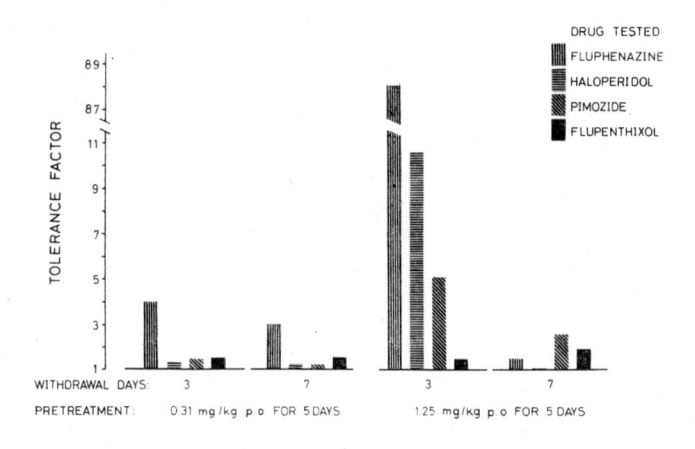

Fig. 2. Methylphenidate antagonism in mice. Homologous tolerance.

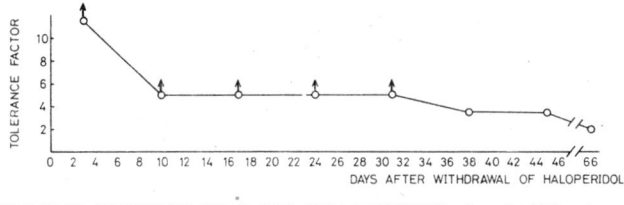

Fig. 3. Antagonism of apomorphine-induced stereotypy in the dog. Cross-tolerance from haloperidol to flupenthixol.

effect of haloperidol or flupenthixol. Similarly development of cross-tolerance was not demonstrated to the inhibition of conditioned avoidance reaction by flupenthixol in rats tested three days after withdrawal of haloperidol 10 mg/kg p.o. for 12 days. (Fig. 3).
A full report of the results will be published elsewhere.

References

1. Nymark, M. (1972) Apomorphine provoked stereotypy in the dog. Psychopharmacologia, (in press).
2. Pedersen, V. and Christensen, A. V. (1971) Methylphenidate antagonism in mice as a rapid screening test for neuroleptic drugs. Acta pharmacol. toxicol. 29, suppl. 4, 44.

I.M.N., Department of Pharmacology, and Toxicology,
H. Lundbeck & Co. A/S, Ottiliavej 7—9,
DK 2500 Copenhagen-Valby, Denmark

CHANGES IN CENTRAL EFFECTS OF SEVERAL NEUROLEPTICS AFTER THEIR REPEATED ADMINISTRATION

J. METYŠOVÁ

Research Institute for Pharmacy and Biochemistry, Prague

Neuroleptic drugs are being used in psychotic patients on a chronic dosage regimen. Compared with their initial clinical effects, their activity changes in the course of long-term administration. The intensive sedative action of many neuroleptics decreases gradually within a few days of the beginning of treatment, but in contrast, their full antipsychotic action is only achieved later.

Chronic or subacute administration of neuroleptics in animal experiments allows us to obtain data relevant to the clinical use of these drugs.

Experimental studies offer no simple answer; some data are even contradictory. Certainly, there are many variables involved, such as the experimental design, the chosen dosage of drugs, the period of administration, the animal species, sex and others.

Detailed pharmacological studies by THEOBALD et al. (5) allowed differentiation of effects of neuroleptics; either tolerance developed or the activity remained constant. These authors found no effects after repeated administration, that had not been seen after a single dose. HOROVITZ and BEER (2) recommended in their review that all standard and new psychotropic agents be tested for their major activities after chronic administration.

In our experiments in mice and rats, we concentrated on changes of sedative and cataleptic effects of subacutely administered perphenazine and two of our original neuroleptics of the 10,11–dihydrodibenzo (b, f) thiepin series, octoclothepin and oxyprothepin (Fig. 1).

We have studied the uncoordinating action of neuroleptics in the rota-rod test in mice and their cataleptic action in the test described by BOISSIER and SIMON (1) in rats. Drugs were given orally to groups of 40 female animals for 7 days in a daily dose corresponding approximately to the doubled ED_{50}, determined in preceding acute experiments (i.e. pretreatment with the daily dose of mostly 10 mg base per kg orally). In parallel experiments, control groups of 40 mice or rats were given distilled water. On the 8th day, the cataleptic action in rats and the uncoordinating action in mice were tested in both experimental and control groups, by giving suitable dose levels of the tested neuroleptics enabling the determination of ED_{50}'s.

In the test for uncoordinating action in mice, a statistically significant decrease of activity has been found for all neuroleptics after their subacute administration (Fig. 2). The lowest tolerance was observed with perphenazine, the highest with octoclothepin after the same dose of 10 mg (base) per kg.

The cataleptic potency of neuroleptics was also reduced after subacute treatment (Fig. 2); a pronounced and statistically significant reduction, however, was found only in perphenazine (as compared with the acute dosage).

The ptotic effect of the neuroleptics was usually also reduced; the doses required for induction of catalepsy were relatively high and disadvantageous as far as ptosis was concerned.

Our experimental results on subacute oral treatment with original neuroleptics of the 10,11-dihydrodibenzo (b, f) thiepin series and with perphenazine in mice are in agreement with published data on tolerance development as far as the sedative activity of neuroleptics is concerned.

Contrary to the data of JULOU et al. (3), THEOBALD et al. (5), and MØLLER NIELSEN et al., (4), we have found tolerance development or at least a clear trend to tolerance in the test for catalepsy in rats. Statistical significance, however, was found only using perphenazine.

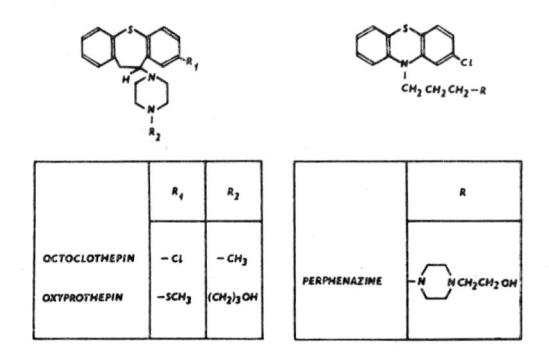

Fig. 1. Chemical structures of the tested neuroleptics.

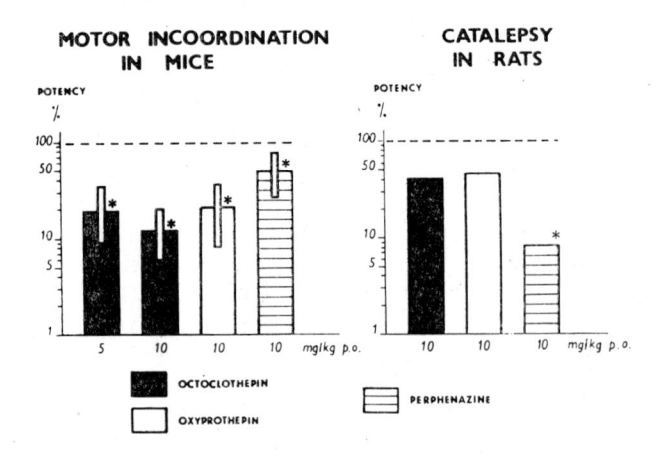

Fig. 2. Tolerance development to neuroleptic drugs after subacute treatment. Left side: rota rod test in mice; right side: catalepsy test in rats. The medium effective doses of single compounds in acute experiments represent 100%. The columns give the relative ED_{50}'s of neuroleptics after their subacute administration. Statistical significance at significance level 0.05 is indicated by an asterisk.

These differences between our findings and those reported in the literature may be due to the use of different neuroleptics, to the differences in experimental design, to the animals used as well as other factors.

On the basis of our preliminary data we cannot discuss possible mechanisms of tolerance development to the tested neuroleptics. We suppose that in our future work it will be necessary to extend our observations to other tests for central effects of neuroleptics, and to use several dose levels of neuroleptics.

REFERENCES

1. BOISSIER, J.-R. and SIMON, P. (1963) Un test simple pour l'étude quantitative de la catatonie provoquée chez le Rat par les neuroleptiques. Application à l'étude des anticatatoniques. Thérapie, 18, 1257.
2. HOROVITZ, Z. P. and BEER, B. (1971) Comparative effects of single and repeat dose administration of major tranquilizers. Psychopharmacol. Bull. 7, 24.
3. JULOU, L., BARDONE, M. C., DUCROT, R., LAFARGUE, B. and LOISEAU, G. (1967) Comparaison des effects des neuroleptiques dans divers tests, en administration unique et en administrations répétées. Hypothèses sur la signification des tests utilisés et leur valeur prévisionnelle. Neuropsychopharmacology (Eds. H. BRILL, J. O. COLE, P. DENIKER, H. HIPPIUS, P. B. BRADLEY), Excerpta Medica Foundation, Amsterdam, 293.
4. MØLLER NIELSEN, I., FJALLAND, B., PEDERSEN, V. and NYMARK, M. (1972) Development of tolerance in animals by repeated administration of neuroleptics. Psychopharmacologia, 26, Suppl. 100.
5. THEOBALD, W., BÜCH, O., DELINI-STULA, A., EIGENMANN, R. and LEVIN, PH. (1968) Pharmakologische Untersuchungen zur Wirkung von Neuroleptica am Tier nach einmaliger und wiederholter Applikation. Arzneim.-Forsch. 18, 1491.

J.M., Research Institute for Pharmacy and Biochemistry, Kouřimská 17, Prague, Czechoslovakia

LONG-TERM TREATMENT OF PSYCHIATRIC PATIENTS WITH CLOPENTHIXOL. ANALYSIS OF LABORATORY INVESTIGATIONS[*]

V. HANSEN, J. RAVN and C. RUD

Department K and the Laboratory, Mental Hospital, Middelfart and Research Department, Lundbeck & Co. A/S, Copenhagen

MATERIAL AND METHODS

There have been many reports on liver damage with phenothiazines (e.g. chlorpromazine) with or without jaundice. As a rule, the hepatic damage is transient. The thiaxanthenes have proved to cause fewer side effects than the phenothiazines. Clopenthixol (Ciatyl[R], Sordinol[R]) is a potent neuroleptic well suited for long-term therapy.

The data submitted here come from 57 patients, 49 of whom were in-patients and 8 out-patients on after-treatment. The age of the patients was between 20 to over 80 years, average 57.5 years. The diagnosis was mainly schizophrenia. The patients were treated with clopenthixol as the only neuroleptic, in varying doses for periods from 3 to 9 years. The doses were grouped into high dosage, i. e. 75 mg or more daily, and low dosage, i. e. below 75 mg daily.

The material falls into two groups, 26 patients, who had only mental diseases and 31 with co-existing somatic diseases.

Laboratory tests made were:

Hematology: ESR, Hbg, erythrocytes, differential count, thrombocytes.
Liver: Thymol, icterus index, alkaline phosphatases, GP-transaminases.
Kidney: Creatinine, urine protein, glucose, microscopy.
Other: Serum protein, electrophoresis, LE-cells.
      Antinuclear factor (ANF), EKG.

RESULTS

On analysis of the material the laboratory tests given above were found to be normal in the majority of cases. However, several slightly elevated values were registered, and in a few cases the values were definitely abnormal. But all abnormal results could naturally be explained by co-existent somatic disease.

---

[*] A preliminary study.

It was decided to investigate whether there might be any relationship between the recorded values, in particular the variations of the laboratory results within the normal range, and the treatment with clopenthixol. Using an IBM 1130 with standard programmes we investigated distribution (probit), two-way plotting, factor analysis, regression analysis and several correlation analyses. In particular the material was elucidated by the formation of Speaman's rank correlation coefficient (rho). Rho was chosen as a measure of the association between variables, regardless of type and distribution.

It was clearly confirmed that the material falls into two groups, patients with (26) and patients without (31) somatic disease. This applies to a number of parameters: ESR, ANF, alkaline phosphatases, albumin/globulin ratio, $alpha_1$, $alpha_2$, and gamma globulins. For these parameters the group of patients also suffering from somatic diseases show results tending towards more abnormal results than the „pure" psychiatric group. This group was also of a more advanced age and had a longer duration of disease than the „pure" group. Statistical analysis revealed some other interesting correlations. The explanation of a negative correlation between duration of treatment and creatinine in the „somatic" group is probably explained by the negative correlation between age and duration of treatment and the well-known positive correlation between age and creatinine.

In the "pure" psychiatric group thymol values appeared to increase with dosage. As the increase in thymol values is small (the average within normal limits) and the number of patients on high dose is only 5, we do not take this as an indication of a relationship between clopenthixol therapy and hepatic function. This is supported by the fact that there was no correlation between dose and gamma globulin concentration.

In the „pure" psychiatric patients there was a correlation (with a faintly rising regression line) between treatment and leucocyte number. The increase was within normal limits and continued for 3–9 years after the start of the treatment. The changes concern granulocytes and lymphocytes to the same extent.

Further correlations between any parameter and the two factors of special interest i. e. dose and duration of treatment, were not found. The granulocyte/lymphocyte ratio, platelet count, LE–cells, ANF, enzymes and their electrophoretic pattern were unaffected.

CONCLUSION

In conclusion we found nothing to indicate that long–term treatment with clopenthixol exerted a nephrotoxic, hepatoxic or haematotoxic effect. However, in connection with this treatment, mild changes seem to occur in certain parameters, predominantly within the normal range.

J.R., Ullerupdalvej 143^{II}, DK 7000 Fredericia, Denmark

STRIATUM AND NEUROLEPTICS

Chairman: J. R. Boissier

Associate chairman: T. Hallas – Møller

ANATOMIE ET PHYSIOLOGIE COMPARÉES DU SYSTÈME EXTRA-PYRAMIDAL.
ASPECT CHOLINERGIQUE

J. R. BOISSIER et E. BAUM

Unité de Neuropsychopharmacologie, Paris

On ne peut donner du système extra-pyramidal (SEP) qu'une définition par exclusion : le SEP est constitué par l'ensemble des centres moteurs et des voies motrices, à l'exclusion des centres et des voies relevant du système pyramidal. Défini ainsi, le SEP contient plusieurs systèmes: régulation motrice cérébelleuse, striée. Nous nous limiterons au système dit des noyaux de la base (basal ganglia) ou des corps striés.

Les noyaux de la base ou noyaux gris comprennent (Tableau 1):

TABLEAU 1
Les différents noyaux constituant les corps striés chez l'homme et chez le rat

Homme Primates supérieurs	Rat (ou chat)
Noyau lenticulaire { Noyau caudé, Putamen, Pallidum }	{ Neostriatum, Pallidum, Noyau entopédonculaire }

— le néostriatum, structure télencéphalique, que l'on divise en noyau caudé et putamen chez les mammifères supérieurs;
— le globus pallidus, qui forme une partie du noyau lenticulaire (l'autre partie étant constituée par le putamen). L'homologue chez le rat ou le chat, du globus pallidus des primates semble être constitué par l'ensemble globus pallidus — noyau ento-pédonculaire.

On rattache intimement à ce système divers éléments:
— les deux parties (compacte et réticulée) de la substance noire;
— le noyau subthalamique ou corps de Luys;
— le noyau rouge;
— divers noyaux thalamiques et les projections corticales de ces noyaux du thalamus, diffuses chez le mammifère inférieur, limitées aux aires 4 et 6 chez l'homme (Tableau 2).

TABLEAU 2

Structures cérébrales associées aux corps striés chez l'homme et chez le rat

Homme Primates supérieurs	Rat (ou chat)
Substance noire — p. compacte — p. réticulée	Substance noire — p. compacte — p. réticulée
Noyau subthalamique (corps de Luys)	Noyau subthalamique (corps de Luys)
Noyau rouge	Noyau rouge
Thalamus — n. ventral latéral — n. centre médian — n. parafasciculaire	Thalamus — n. ventral latéral — n. centre médian
Cortex — aires 4 et 6	Cortex

Que sait-on des connections qui unissent ces différents noyaux? (7, 8, 15, 16, 17, 19, 20, 21, 22, 23, 25, 26) (Fig. 1).

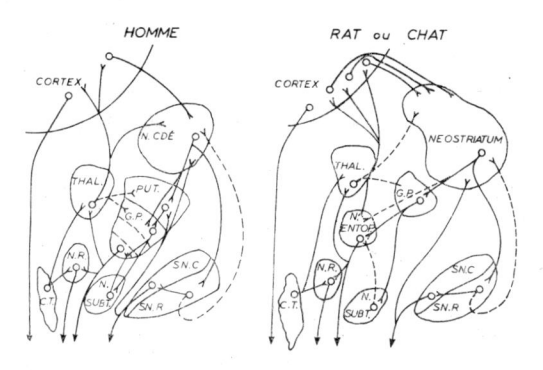

Fig. 1. Principales connections du système extrapyramidal chez l'homme et chez le rat.

Si l'on envisage les relations substance noire — néostriatum: il existe une voie dopaminergique nigrostriée, les corps cellulaires dont cette voie est issue sont situés dans la partie compacte de la substance noire; les axones rejoignent la portion la plus latérale du faisceau télencéphalique médian (ou MFB), ils gagnent ensuite la capsule interne et le striatum.

Il existe d'autre part une voie strio-nigrée; Szabo (25) a étudié l'organisation topographique de cette voie chez le rat. Elle se termine au niveau de la partie réticulée de la substance noire. La nature de la transmission est discutée: pour Olivier et coll. (22), cette voie serait cholinergique, pour Hassler (16), le médiateur serait le GABA.

En ce qui concerne les voies afférentes au thalamus: nous n'avons sur ces projections que des données encore parcellaires. Nous connaissons assez peu, chez les mammifères non primates, les équivalents des noyaux thalamiques affectés, chez l'homme, par les projections striées.

— Le noyau ventrolatéral (V.L.) reçoit entre autres projections, chez l'homme et les primates, une voie d'origine pallidale interne. Chez le chat, c'est le noyau entopédonculaire qui est à l'origine de la voie striée afférente au V.L.

— CARPENTER (7), METTLER (20), FAULL et CARMAN (15) ont mis en évidence une autre voie extra-pyramidale afférente au thalamus, ce serait une voie directe nigro-thalamique. L'existence de cette voie est encore discutée.

Il existe des différences notables entre le SEP des primates et le SEP des mammifères non primates (chat ou rat) aussi bien sur le plan anatomique que sur le plan physiologique. Nous n'envisagerons que deux très courts exemples illustrant ces différences.

Le tableau 3 nous montre la constitution du globus pallidus pour deux types de mammifères.

TABLEAU 3

Le pallidum chez l'homme et chez le rat

	Homme	Rat (ou chat)
Subdivisions	G. P. ext. G.P. méd. G.P. int.	G.P. non divisé + noyau entopédonculaire
Les projections vers le thalamus (VL) proviennent:	du G.P. int.	du noyau entopédonculaire
Electrophysiologiquement, la projection qui l'emporte sur le VL est d'origine (d'après DORMONT 1970)	plutôt lenticulaire	plutôt cérébelleuse

Le globus pallidus (G.P.) chez l'homme, est constitué de 3 parties, deux seulement chez les autres primates (G.P. interne et G.P. externe). Chez le rat ou chez le chat, le globus pallidus n'est pas divisé; il ne serait en fait l'homologue que du globus pallidus externe des primates.

Le pallidum est considéré comme étant le noyau efférent principal du striatum. C'est surtout à la partie interne qu'est dévolu ce rôle chez le primate, le globus pallidus externe ne projetant que sur le noyau subthalamique.

Chez les mammifères non primates: anatomiquement et électrophysiologiquement, c'est le noyau entopédonculaire qui projette vers le ventrolatéral du thalamus. C'est donc le noyau entopédonculaire (petit groupe cellulaire à l'intérieur de la capsule interne) qui serait l'homologue du globus pallidus interne.

Cette différence anatomique explique probablement les différences de comportement d'animaux d'espèces différentes porteurs de lésions du globus pallidus.

Autre exemple: d'après DORMONT (12), il existe un équilibre au niveau du V.L., entre les afférences cérébelleuses (par l'intermédiaire du brachium conjonctivum) et les afférences striées (par l'intermédiaire du noyau lenticulaire chez les primates, du noyau entopédonculaire chez le chat). L'équilibre entre ces deux influences semble à peu près réalisé chez les primates; par contre chez le chat les afférences cérébelleuses l'emportent largement sur les afférences striées.

Ces divergences, tant anatomiques que physiologiques, rendent difficilement exploitables les expériences de pathologie expérimentale. Les études pharmacologiques, en particulier, étant faites sur des mammifères non primates (le plus souvent le rat ou la souris) la connaissance de ces divergences et leurs implications fonctionnelles sont tout à fait essentielles.

Des réactifs pharmacologiques que l'on suppose agir sur le SEP provoquent chez des animaux tels que le rat, deux types de réaction motrice: catalepsie d'une part, stéréotypies d'autre part. La difficulté, bien entendu, est de déterminer si l'action du produit se situe bien au niveau du SEP, et si oui dans quelle structure?

Les principales substances entraînant de la catalepsie sont, d'une part les neuroleptiques, d'autre part les cholinergiques centraux. Le mécanisme d'action supposé pour ces deux types de produits dépend de l'existence d'une balance dopamine — acétylcholine (DA/ACh) au niveau du néostriatum; la catalepsie apparaît chaque fois qu'une action déséquilibre cette balance et tend à augmenter le fonctionnement du système cholinergique par rapport au système dopaminergique (Tableau 4).

TABLEAU 4

Principaux réactifs pharmacologiques provoquant un comportement cataleptique chez le rat

Reponse motrice du rat: catalepsie	
Produit	Mécanisme d'action supposé
Neuroleptiques	Bloquent les récepteurs DA striés.
Cholinergiques — Pilocarpine — Eserine	Stimulent les récepteurs ACh striés.
Histamine (chez le jeune)	„Oedème" au niveau du striatum.
Morphine	Action sur le thalamus?
Bulbocapnine	Action sur la boucle strio-thalamique.

L'action cataleptigène de l'histamine chez le jeune rat permet de penser que l'histamine pourrait posséder une activité au sein du SEP. Boissier et coll. (5), ont montré que l'histamine provoque au niveau du néostriatum une entrée massive d'eau dans le tissu cérébral, créant un véritable oedème. Cet oedème provoque une altération profonde du fonctionnement du noyau caudé visible à l'EEG (13). L'injection lente, bilatérale au niveau du néostriatum du rat de quelques microlitres d'eau provoque un comportement cataleptique. Le mécanisme de l'action cataleptigène de l'histamine passe probablement par la formation de cet oedème strié.

Afin de mieux connaître le versant cholinergique du système extrapyramidal, nous avons repris l'étude pharmacologique de deux cholinergiques centraux; un cholinergique direct: la pilocarpine, et un anti-cholinestérasique, le salicylate d'ésérine.

Qu'il s'agisse de la pilocarpine ou de l'ésérine, suivant la dose injectée et le temps qui sépare l'injection de l'observation, trois types de comportement sont susceptibles d'apparaître (Fig. 2):

1. Catalepsie seule, mesurée par le test du bouddha.
2. Stéréotypies de la sphère buccale, seules.
3. Les deux phénomènes précédents, simultanément.

ASPECT CHOLINERGIQUE DU SYSTÈME EXTRA-PYRAMIDAL

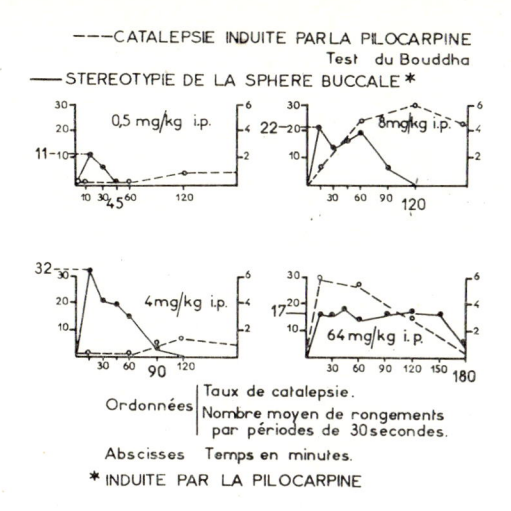

Fig. 2. Intensité du comportement cataleptique et stéréotypé du rat après injection intrapéritonéale de pilocarpine à différentes doses.

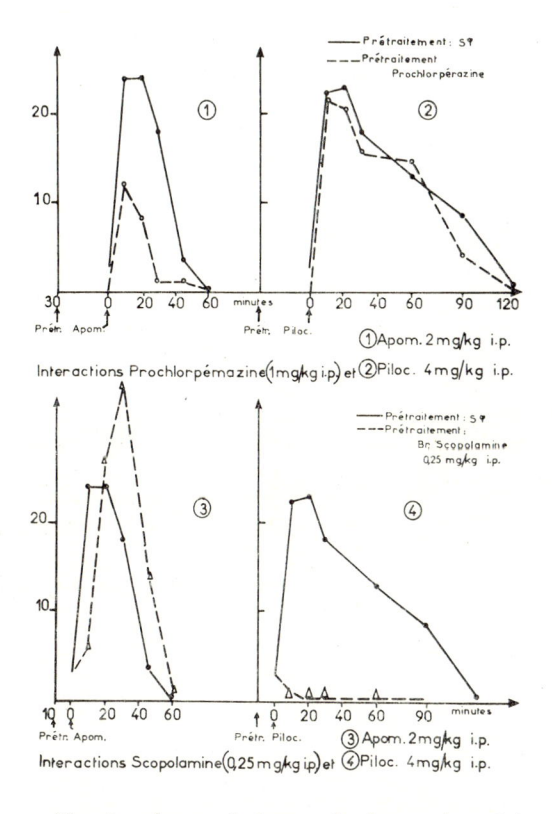

Fig. 3. Action de la prochlorpémazine ou de la scopolamine sur les stéréotypies provoquées par l'apomorphine ou la pilocarpine chez le rat.

Il existe une corrélation négative, à tout instant, entre les rongements et la catalepsie. Dans l'ordre des doses croissantes, les rongements apparaissent avant la catalepsie, et ils diminuent pour des doses nettement cataleptigènes. On retrouve les mêmes types de courbes avec l'ésérine. Rongements et catalepsie ont une origine centrale, car ils n'apparaissent pas après administration de néostigmine, anticholinestérasique qui ne pénètre pas au niveau du système nerveux central.

Les stéréotypies peuvent être induites par différents réactifs pharmacologiques (Tableau 5). Nous avons essayé de comparer les rongements induits par l'apomorphine et ceux induits par la pilocarpine.

Tableau 5

Principaux réactifs pharmacologiques provoquant un comportement stéréotypé chez le rat

Reponse motrice du rat: stéreotypies	
Produit	Mécanisme d'action supposé
Apomorphine Amphétamine	Stimule: — directement — indirectement les récepteurs DA striés
Cholinolytiques — Atropine — Scopolamine	Bloquent les récepteurs ACh (niveau strié?)
Cholinergiques — Pilocarpine — Esérine	Stimulent les récepteurs ACh (niveau?)

I. — A l'observation, ces rongements apparaissent différents: les stéréotypies de la sphère buccale induites par l'apomorphine sont dans nos conditions d'observation, des lèchements des parois de la cage; les rongements induits par la pilocarpine sont des mouvements "à vide" de la sphère buccale. D'autre part, les lèchements induits par l'apomorphine sont accompagnés d'autres stéréotypies (de la tête, des pattes antérieures...), ce qui ne se produit jamais avec la pilocarpine.

II. — La Figure 3 nous montre que la prochlorpérazine à la dose de 1 mg/kg i.p. antagonise les stéréotypies induites par l'apomorphine, alors qu'elle ne réduit pas les stéréotypies de la pilocarpine.

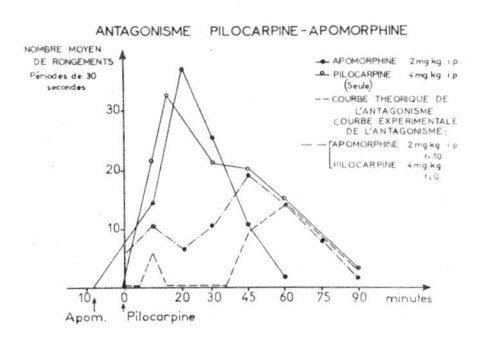

Fig. 4. Comportement stéréotypé du rat: antagonisme pilocarpine et l'apomorphine.

III. — La scopolamine (0,25 mg/kg i.p.) supprime totalement les stéréotypies induites par la pilocarpine; elle ne modifie pas, à cette dose, les stéréotypies induites par l'apomorphine; à plus forte dose, elle potentialise les stéréotypies apomorphiniques.

IV. — Il existe, pour les stéréotypies, un antagonisme entre la pilocarpine et l'apomorphine (Fig. 4).

Discussion

Que peut-on conclure sur ces stéréotypies cholinergiques ? Elles sont d'origine centrale comme le prouve la contre expérience de la néostigmine et elles sont liées à l'activité cholinergique de la molécule, puisqu'on les obtient aussi bien avec les cholinergiques directs qu'avec des anticholinestérasiques. Le lieu d'action ne peut être précisé actuellement.

Toujours en ce qui concerne le système cholinergique extrapyramidal, nous nous sommes efforcés de modifier son activité par différentes lésions.

Depuis quelques années, de très nombreuses études ont eu pour objet les relations entre la substance noire et le néostriatum.

L'existence de la voie nigro-striée dopaminergique n'est plus mise en doute (1). Les neurones constituant cette voie ont leur corps cellulaire dans la partie compacte de la substance noire et les axones, très fins, amyéliniques, gagnent le néostriatum en passant par la partie latérale de la MFB et la capsule interne. Les arguments en faveur de cette voie sont histochimiques, biochimiques, pharmacologiques.

Il existe une voie strio-nigrée dont les corps cellulaires sont situés dans l'ensemble noyau caudé-putamen. La terminaison au niveau de la substance noire serait dans la partie réticulée. Cette voie, dont le médiateur serait, suivant les auteurs, le GABA ou l'acétylcholine (16, 22), a été très bien étudiée par Szabo (25), chez le rat qui a montré que cette projection est topographiquement organisée.

Le néostriatum est la partie du système nerveux central la plus riche en deux transmetteurs: la dopamine d'une part, l'acétylcholine d'autre part. L'origine de la dopamine striée est pour la plus grande partie bien déterminée, il n'en est pas de même pour l'acétylcholine, et ceci essentiellement pour des raisons techniques. En effet, le dosage de l'acétylcholine se fait soit par des méthodes biochimiques, auquel cas il est très difficile à mettre au point, soit par des méthodes biologiques, peu rapides. La méthode très indirecte de visualisation histochimique des cholinestérases (ChE) de Koelle permet seulement d'apprécier qualitativement le fonctionnement cholinestérasique.

Très récemment, McGeer (18), a ainsi étudié le fonctionnement cholinestérasique du néostriatum du rat après diverses lésions. En fait, il a détruit tous les noyaux qui projettent ou pourraient éventuellement projeter sur le néostriatum; il a ainsi montré que des ablations très larges du cortex, du thalamus, du globus pallidus et de la substance noire compacte (par interruption de la MFB) ne modifient en rien le taux ou la répartition des ChE striées.

Rosegay (23), et Voneida (26), ont mis en évidence une voie nigro-striée, dont les corps cellulaires seraient situés dans la partie réticulée de la substance noire et dont les axones myélinisés gagnent ensuite le néostriatum. Ces caractéristiques indiquent qu'il ne peut, en aucun cas, s'agir de la voie nigro-striée à transmission dopaminergique.

Nous avons effectué des lésions sélectives de la partie réticulée de la substance noire et nous avons trouvé qu'en l'absence de toute atteinte de la partie compacte ou des pédoncules cérébraux, une lésion bilatérale de la partie réticulée de la substance noire provoque une diminution importante, dans quelques cas une disparition totale des ChE striées (Tableau 6).

Tableau 6

Mise en évidence des ChE du néostriatum du rat après lésion des différentes parties de la substance noire

	Lésion de la partie reticulée	Lésion de la partie compacte	ChE
Témoins (8 rats)	0	0	+
Groupe 1 (6 rats)	+	+ +	+
Groupe 2 (4 rats)	+ +	+ +	±
Groupe 3 (3 rats)	+ +	0	0

Lésion: 0   partie intacte
         +   atteinte partielle
         + + destruction importante bilatérale

ChE: + denses et uniformément réparties
     ± ne persistent qu'à la périphérie du néostriatum
     0 disparition totale

Les rats présentent tous après la lésion une phase importante de stéréotypies, une hyperkinésie marquée persiste très longtemps après la lésion; d'un point de vue biochimique, les taux de dopamine et de 5-HT striées sont identiques à ceux des témoins. Nous pensons donc que le comportement hyperkinétique, stéréotypé, de nos rats pourrait résulter d'un déficit cholinergique strié. L'administration, à ces rats lésés, de divers réactifs pharmacologiques a permis de confirmer cette hypothèse (4).

Il existe peut-être une certaine analogie entre les conséquences de cette lésion expérimentale et certains aspects de la chorée de Huntington. Outre la dégénérescence principale que l'on trouve chez tous les choréiques, c'est à dire la disparition des petites cellules du néostriatum, il existe très souvent des dégénérescences au niveau de la substance noire: c'est la partie réticulée qui est atteinte, la partie compacte étant toujours intacte. Le système dopaminergique strié n'est pas touché.

On sait d'autre part, que dans la maladie de Parkinson, les déficits moteurs observés seraient dus à un déséquilibre de la balance DA/ACh au niveau du striatum. Chez les choréiques, l'amélioration obtenue par les neuroleptiques alors que le système dopaminergique semble intact indique que le rétablissement d'un certain équilibre est réalisé par une diminution fonctionnelle du système cholinergique. On peut donc émettre l'hypothèse suivant laquelle, un déficit cholinergique strié pourrait être à l'origine de la chorée. Les bons résultats cliniques obtenus par Bonchut (6), en 1875 et beaucoup plus récemment par Aquilonius (2), en 1971, en traitant des choréiques par le salicylate d'ésérine, sont en faveur d'une telle hypothèse.

Il est donc possible que la chorée soit due à un déficit cholinergique strié et dans ce cas il existerait des phénomènes communs aux choréiques et à nos animaux lésés en partie réticulée de la substance noire. Il est bien évident que nous ne prétendons pas avoir obtenu un modèle de la chorée: il existe certes des analogies, mais aussi des divergences; après lésion les rats présentent une excitation motrice, des mouvements anormaux, mais ces mouvements sont stéréotypés, ce qui n'est pas du tout le cas des mouvements choréiques (encore que l'on puisse se demander si le rat est capable d'autre chose que de stéréotypies lors d'une importante excitation motrice).

D'autre part, Costall et coll. (9, 10, 11), ont montré que la présence du néostriatum n'est pas nécessaire pour qu'apparaisse l'action cataleptigène d'un cholinergique central, l'arécoline. Ils ont montré que cette action cataleptigène de l'arécoline n'était pas modifié après lésion du globus pallidus, alors que l'activité du halopéridol était considérablement diminuée. Nous avons retrouvé les résultats de Costall concernant la catalepsie après lésion du globus pallidus du rat.

En outre, les stéréotypies induites par de faibles doses de pilocarpine ne sont pas modifiées après lésion du pallidum alors que les stéréotypies apomorphiniques ou amphétaminiques sont diminuées. Après lésion du pallidum, on a donc une diminution fonctionelle du système dopaminergique (diminution de l'activité aussi bien des neuroleptiques que de l'apomorphine ou de l'amphétamine), et par contre aucune modification dans le fonctionnement du système cholinergique.

Une lésion du pallidum touche aussi bien la voie dopaminergique afférente au striatum que les voies efférentes des corps striés. En effet, une partie de la voie dopaminergique nigro-striée traverse la partie la plus latérale du pallidum; toutefois, nos lésions étaient situées dans une partie plus médiane et les dosages biochimiques ont montré que l'atteinte dopaminergique striée était faible. De plus, une atteinte bilatérale de la voie afférente nigro-striée dopaminergique, à un autre niveau, ne provoque pas de modification sensible dans l'activité pharmacologique des neuroleptiques ou de l'apomorphine.

La baisse d'activité de l'ensemble des produits agissant sur le système dopaminergique, ajoutée à un comportement cataleptique après la lésion indique que c'est la voie efférente striée transportant les informations qui résultent du fonctionnement du système dopaminergique qui est atteinte. L'intégrité du système cholinergique semble indiquer que les voies efférentes des systèmes dopaminergique et cholinergique soient distinctes, au moins chez le rat. Si ce résultat était retrouvé pour d'autres espèces animales, cela indiquerait que l'intégration entre les systèmes dopaminergique et cholinergique ne se fait pas entièrement au niveau du néostriatum.

Conclusion

L'antagonisme pharmacologique entre la dopamine et l'acétylcholine au niveau du système extrapyramidal est connu depuis longtemps: il est vrai que des cholinolytiques tels que l'atropine ou la scopolamine, provoquent des troubles moteurs, des stéréotypies, très semblables à celles que provoquent les stimulants du système dopaminergique tels que l'apomorphine ou l'amphétamine.

Mais ce seul antagonisme ne permet pas d'expliquer toutes les propriétés extrapyramidales des cholinergiques. Nous prendrons trois exemples:

1. — Si l'on compare différents tests de catalepsie, l'ordre de difficulté croissante que l'on peut établir, n'est pas le même pour les cholinergiques centraux et pour les bloquants des récepteurs dopaminergiques.

2. — Alors qu'avec les neuroleptiques, on rencontre un seul type de catalepsie: conservation des attitudes imposées et absence de mouvements spontanés (ou akinésie), après administration de pilocarpine (ou d'ésérine), la catalepsie induite peut être décomposée en deux phases:

— Une phase précoce, qui est la seule phase de catalepsie vraie pendant laquelle les animaux conservent les attitudes imposées et sont akinétiques.

— La deuxième phase ou phase tardive, particulièrement nette pour les doses moyennes est caractérisée par la seule conservation des attitudes imposées.

3. — Les modifications de l'équilibre DA/ACh strié ne peuvent pas expliquer l'existence de stéréotypies aussi bien après cholinergiques centraux qu'après cholinolytiques centraux.

Il ne faut donc pas ramener le système cholinergique extrapyramidal au seul antagonisme DA/ACh strié. D'autres mécanismes et d'autres sites d'action sont tout à fait probables et nécessitent une étude epprofondie en particulier dans le cadre d'un éventuel trouble cholinergique dans la chorée.

BIBLIOGRAPHIE

1. ANDEN, N., CARLSSON, A., DAHLSTRÖM, A., FUXE, K., HILLARP, N. A. et LARSSON, K. (1964) Demonstration and mapping out of nigroneostriatal dopamine neurons. Life Sci. **3**, 523.
2. AQUILONIUS, S. M. et SJÖSTRÖM, R. (1971) Cholinergic and dopaminergic mechanisms in Huntington's chorea. Life Sci. **10**, 405.
3. BAUM, E., ETEVENON, P., PIARROUX, M. C., SIMON, P. et BOISSIER, J. R. (1971) Modifications comportementales et pharmacologiques obtenues chez le rat après lésion bilatérale de la substance noire. J. Pharmacol. (Paris) **2**, 423.
4. BAUM, E., NORTH-DIEHL, A., PIARROUX, M. C., THENINT, F. et BOISSIER, J. R. (1972) Modifications biochimiques, histochimiques et pharmacologiques après lésion bilatérale des différentes parties de la substance noire chez le rat. J. Pharmacol. (Paris), sous presse.
5. BOISSIER, J. R., TILLEMENT, J. P., GUERNET, M., NORTH-DIEHL, A. et WINICKI J. (1972) Diffusion cérébrale des fortes doses d'histamine chez le rat. J. Pharmacol. (Paris), sous presse.
6. BONCHUT, E. (1875) Recherches thérapeutiques sur l'action de l'ésérine dans la chorée. Bull. Thér. **88**, 289.
7. CARPENTER, M. B. (1964) Lesions of the substantia nigra in the rhesus monkey. Amer. J. Anat. **144**, 293.
8. CARPENTER, M. B. et STROMINGER, N. L. (1967) Efferent fibers of the subthalamic nucleus in the monkey. Amer. J. Anat. **121**, 41.
9. COSTALL, B. et OLLEY, S. E. (1971) Cholinergic and neuroleptic-induced catalepsy: modification by lesions in the caudate-putamen. Neuropharmacology, **10**, 297.
10. COSTALL, B. et OLLEY, J. E. (1971) Cholinergic and neuroleptic-induced catalepsy: modification by lesions in the globus pallidus and substantia nigra. Neuropharmacology, **10**, 581.
11. COSTALL, B., NAYLOR, R. J. et OLLEY, J. E. (1972) On the involvement of the caudate-putamen, globus pallidus and substantia nigra with neuroleptic and cholinergic modification of locomotor activity. Neuropharmacology, **11**, 217.
12. DORMONT, J. F. et OHYE, C. (1971) Entopeduncular projection to the thalamic ventrolateral nucleus of the cat. Exp. Brain Res. **12**, 254.
13. DUMEUR, G. (1972) Communication personnelle.
14. ETEVENON, P., BOISSIER, J. R., SIMON, P. et PIARROUX, M. C. (1971) Pharmacological and biochemical changes in rats presenting a permanent catalepsy after bilateral mesencephalic ventral tegmentum lesions. J. Pharmacol. (Paris), sous presse.
15. FAUL, R. I. et CARMAN, J. B. (1969) Ascending projections of the substantia nigra in the rat. J. comp. Neurol. **132**, 73.
16. HASSLER, R. (1972) Corrélations entre les médiateurs chimiques (dopamine, sérotonine, acétylcholine et GABA), tonus musculaire et rapidité du mouvement. Rapport présenté à la XXIXème réunion neurologique internationale (Paris) 51.
17. JOHNSON, T. N. et CLEMENTE, C. D. (1959) An experimental study of the fiber connections between the putamen, globus pallidus, ventral thalamus and midbrain tegmentum in rat. J. comp. Neurol. **113**, 83.
18. MCGEER, P. L., MCGEER, E. G., FIBIGER, H. C. et WICKSON, V. (1791) Neostriatal choline acetylase and cholinesterase following selective brain lesions. Brain Res. **35**, 308.
19. METTLER, F. A. (1945) Fiber connections of the corpus striatum of the monkey and baboon. J. comp. Neurol. **82**, 169.
20. METTLER, M. A. (1970) Nigrofugal connections in the primate brain. J. comp. Neurol. **138**, 291.
21. NAUTA, W. J. N., MEHLER, W. R. (1966) Projections of the lentiform nucleus in the monkey. Brain Res. **1**, 1.
22. OLIVIER, A., PARENT, A., SIMARD, H. et POIRIER, L. J. (1970) Cholinesterasic striatopallidal and striatonigral efferents in the cat and the monkey. Brain Res. **18**, 273.
23. ROSEGAY, H. (1943) An experimental investigation of the connections between the corpus striatum and the substantia nigra in the cat. J. comp. Neurol. **80**, 293.
24. SHUTE, C. C. D. et LEWIS, P. R. (1963) Cholinesterase containing systems in the brain of the cat. Nature, **199**, 1160.

25. Szabo, J. (1970) Projections from the body of the caudate nucleus in the rhesus monkey. Exp. Neurol. **27**, 1.
26. Voneïda, T. S. (1960) An experimental study of the course and destination of fibers ending in the head of the caudate nucleus in the cat and the monkey. J. comp. Neurol. **115**, 75.

*J.R.B., Unité de Neuropsychopharmacologie, 2 rue d'Alésia,
Paris 14e, France*

ACTION OF NEUROLEPTICS
ON THE NIGRO-NEOSTRIATAL DOPAMINERGIC PATHWAY

N.-E. ANDÉN, H. CORRODI, K. FUXE and U. UNGERSTEDT

Department of Pharmacology, University of Göteborg, Astra Pharmaceuticals, Södertälje, and Department of Histology, Karolinska Institutet, Stockholm

We have during recent years analyzed the effects of neuroleptic drugs on the nigro-neostriatal dopaminergic (DA) pathway using biochemical, histochemical and behavioural techniques. The data suggest that neuroleptics of both the phenothiazine type (e.g. chlorpromazine) and of the butyrophenone type (e.g. haloperidol) can cause blockade of the DA receptors in the neostriatum as already suggested by CARLSSON and LINDQVIST in 1963 (15) (see also 2, 8, 9, 19). Other groups have also come to similar conclusions (24, 33, 37); for further references see the book on neuroleptics edited by BOBON et al. (12). New types of neuroleptics such as pimozide and fluspirilene (31, see also 12) are also able to block DA receptors (2, 36), but lack any blocking activity on NA receptors which make these drugs relatively specific in their action (2).

The present article will mainly review the evidence that neuroleptic drugs block neostriatal DA receptors and will in addition report results on dopaminergic and cholinergic interaction in the neostriatum.

FUNCTIONAL STUDIES ON DOPAMINERGIC-CHOLINERGIC MECHANISMS
IN THE NEOSTRIATUM AFTER NEUROLEPTICS

The degree of DA receptor activity in the neostriatum can be easily evaluated in rats with only one nigro-neostriatal DA neuron system. Such rats can be obtained in several ways. In our earlier work electrothermic lesions of the DA pathway to the neostriatum or removal of one corpus striatum was performed (8). Recently, this model has been refined by the use of stereotaxic injections of 6-OH-DA into the DA pathway causing much more specific lesions than previously was possible (46, 47). A specially built rotometer has also been designed to quantitatively record the number of turns (50). Based on pharmacological evidence with reserpine, DOPA, amphetamine and apomorphine, a DA receptor stimulating agent (10, 25), it could be shown that when the DA receptors in the neostriatum on one side are more active than those on the other side the rat will turn to the less activated side. This could be shown by injecting DA directly into the neostriatum after pretreatment with a MAO inhibitor (51). Thus, after the injection of DA the animals turned towards the non-injected side.

When chlorpromazine, haloperidol, pimozide or any of the other neuroleptics are injected into rats with electrocoagulation of the DA pathway or of the corpus striatum, a dose-dependent asymmetry and slow turning of the animals occurs towards the intact side. The mechanism for this behavioural effect is probably a DA receptor blockade, since it cannot be reversed by DOPA, apomorphine or by amphetamine. Nor can these drugs exert their normal action to turn the animals towards the operated side. The asymmetry itself is probably caused by a cholinergic dominance in the neostriatum of the non-operated side. Thus, the asymmetry can be counteracted by various types of anticholinergic drugs such as atropine, scopolamine, benzhexol and benztropine concomitant with a reduction of DA turnover (1, 20). Such effects are not found after treatment with apomorphine. The reason why asymmetry develops also in rats with a unilateral coagulation of the DA pathway is probably that this lesion also damages the antagonistic ascending cholinergic pathways to the neostriatum. In view of this cholinergic dominance can only develop on the intact side resulting in asymmetry towards the intact side.

In the case of the rats with a 6-OH-DA induced lesion of the DA pathway no asymmetry develops in many of the rats, whereas in some rats an asymmetry does occur that can be blocked by anticholinergic drugs (Fuxe and Ungerstedt, unpublished data). These findings can be explained on the basis that in the latter group of rats the 6-OH-DA injection has caused damage also to the ascending cholinergic pathway to the neostriatum. This interpretation is supported by the fact that these animals show less development of supersensitivity to the effects of DOPA and apomorphine on the denervated side (see 48). These results could be explained on the basis that also other pathways besides the DA pathway involved in the control of basal ganglia functions have been damaged by the injection, thus masking the behavioural expression of DA receptor overstimulation.

The asymmetrical posture obtained in the rats described above after neuroleptics are, thus, probably due to a cholinergic dominance in the neostriatum, since *inter alia* it can be counteracted by anticholinergics probably without changing the degree of DA receptor blockade (1, 20).

Another behavioural symptom found after treatment with neuroleptics that seems to be due to a cholinergic dominance in the basal ganglia is catalepsia. Thus, treatment with anticholinergic drugs will reduce the catalepsia induced by neuroleptics (13) an effect which is not mediated via the DA receptors, since apomorphine is ineffective in this respect (1, 20). The catalepsia seems to be caused by all neuroleptics with strong DA receptor blocking activity. However, it was recently suggested by Ungerstedt (49) on the basis of experiments with bilateral 6-OH-DA induced lesions of the DA pathway to the neostriatum that catalepsia was unrelated to low DA receptor activity. Thus, in these rats no catalepsia was found. However, the lack of catelepsia after these lesions could be explained in at least 3 different ways. Firstly, the lesion of the DA pathway by 6-OH-DA may not have been complete, resulting in maintenance of some DA receptor activity in the neostriatum. Secondly, in the postoperative period (1—8 weeks) some compensatory nervous mechanisms may gradually develop to take over the loss of function induced by the destruction of the DA system. Thirdly, the lack of catalepsia could have been due to simultaneous damage of a hypothetical ascending cholinergic pathway to the neostriatum (see above and 11). The group of Boissier (11) has in fact shown that the cataleptic action of neuroleptics is diminished after bilateral destruction of the substantia nigra. Similar results have been obtained after lesion of the neostriatum or the globus pallidus (35). Cholinergic drugs have also been shown to mimic the action of neuroleptics in the production of catalepsy (22, 23). It should be pointed out, however, that a recent report has failed to show any decrease of neostriatal cholineacetylase activity following lesions of the ventral tegmentum (34). — Cataleptic behaviour has been demonstrated after bilateral intrastriatal injections of neuroleptic drugs such as quaternary chlorpromazine

(28), illustrating the neostriatum as the site of action for this effect of neuroleptics.

It should be remembered, however, that the blockade of locomotion and akinesia found after treatment with neuroleptic drugs is *not* due to a cholinergic dominance but due to the DA receptor blockade in the neostriatum itself. Thus, the immobilization cannot be counteracted by anticholinergics but partly by pretreatment with a new type of DA receptor stimulating agent, ET 495 (17, 21), if sufficiently high doses are given. Also it should be remembered that many of the behavioural effects of anticholinergic drugs are dependent on DA receptor activity. Thus, there exists e.g. evidence that local injections of anticholinergics into one neostriatum will result in turning of the animals towards the non-injected side (29). In these rats neuroleptics given systemically will abolish the turning illustrating the importance of DA receptor activation for this turning behaviour. Similar results have been obtained after treatment with anticholinergic drugs of rats with a lesion of the DA pathway to the neostriatum (20).

In view of these results one of the main actions of the cholinergic pathway in the neostriatum seems to be to exert an inhibitory modulating influence on the effects of DA receptor activation in the neostriatum, probably by cholinergic synapses on the nerve cells of the neostriatum.

Studies on rats with supersensitive DA receptors (FUXE *and* UNGERSTEDT, *unpublished data*)

Many rats with a unilateral 6-OH-DA induced lesion of the nigro-neostriatal DA pathway do not show any asymmetries after treatment with neuroleptics such as chlorpromazine and haloperidol. Others do develop asymmetries after treatment with neuroleptics. This variation is probably related to the fact that in the latter case the lesion also involves other afferent and efferent pathways within the extrapyramidal motor system. This view is supported by the fact that in the latter group of rats the development of supersensitivity to apomorphine and DOPA is less easily demonstrated. Thus, after treatment with apomorphine and DOPA already in low doses the former group of rats will turn towards the innervated side due to the fact that the supersensitive DA receptors on the denervated side become more activated than those on the innervated side (48). Recently we have found that much higher (100—1000 times) doses of DA receptor blocking agents (spiroperidol, haloperidol) are needed to block the apomorphine-induced turning behaviour in these animals than in animals with a unilateral electrocoagulation of the neostriatum, the latter animals having only innervated DA receptors. On the other hand, the sensitivity of the rats in the different groups to neuroleptics was similar with regard to amphetamine-induced turning behaviour. This is to be expected, since amphetamine acts by releasing CA from the DA nerve terminals (14). Thus, the present findings (FUXE and UNGERSTEDT, unpublished) give evidence that supersensitive DA receptors are much less susceptible to the blocking action of neuroleptics. This may be due either to an increase in number of DA receptor sites and/or a conformational change in the receptor site itself. In agreement with this view it has recently been found that spiroperidol in normal rats can block both amphetamine and apomorphine-induced increases in holeboard behaviour in doses of 0.01 mg/kg (UNGERSTEDT, unpublished).

When treating patients having mental disease with neuroleptic drugs mainly two side-effects are observed. One is the parkinson-like side-effect which probably can be related to the DA receptor blocking activity of these drugs. The other is the dyskinesias involving involuntary choreo-athetoid movements. These are mainly observed in relation to interruption of the drug treatment and are similar to the dyskinesias found after DOPA treatment to parkinsonian patients. Since the latter probably are due to a powerful activation of supersensitive DA receptors it may be that a similar phenomenon can be present after treatment with neuroleptic drugs. Thus, the prolonged DA receptor blockade can result in a supersensitivity development in the DA receptors and in a compensatory activation of the DA neurons to overcome the receptor blockade (see below). Also a degeneration of some nigro-neostriatal DA neurons can occur. Thus, in view of the present discovery that neuroleptics only in very high doses block supersensitive DA receptors it seems possible to explain the dyskinesias on the basis mentioned above. The degree of DA receptor activity in various parts of the neostriatum will vary with the degree of supersensitivity development in the receptor.

Studies on a new neuroleptic compound, clozapine [8-chloro-11-(4-methyl-1-piperazinyl)-5H-dibenzo (b, e) (1,4) diazepine]

This compound is claimed to cause an anti-psychotic action without any extrapyramidal side-effects (30). In rats no catalepsia occurs (45) which is in agreement with the clinic. In a high dose of 25 mg/kg, however, we have found that this drug causes a marked asymmetry towards the intact side in rats with a unilateral electrocoagulation of the corpus striatum giving evidence that a DA receptor blockade is produced by this drug in the neostriatum. In agreement with this view clozapine has been found to increase DA turnover (unpublished data). Thus, it may be that a weak and not a strong DA receptor blocking activity may be a desirable property of neuroleptic compounds to avoid extrapyramidal side effects but still preventing overactivation of the DA neurons and in this way reducing psychosis.

Turnover studies on the nigro-neostriatal DA pathway after neuroleptics

The work of Carlsson and Lindqvist (15) on 3-0-methylated metabolites after chlorpromazine and haloperidol already suggested an increased release of DA in the forebrain after neuroleptic treatment in view of the increased amounts of 3-0-methylated metabolites found. Subsequent work showed that this was true also for the deaminated metabolites (9, 43). Later on varying degrees of increases in DA turnover in the neostriatum could be demonstrated after all known types of neuroleptics (such as pimozide and clozapine) with various techniques such as amine synthesis inhibition and labelled tyrosine (19, 24, 33, 37). Increases in central NA turnover were also found with most of the neuroleptics (5, 19). In many cases this effect is related to a NA receptor blockade, which seems to be partly responsible for the sedation found after this type of neuroleptics, the most potent ones being chlorpromazine, thioridazine, and clozapine (2, 3, 5, 19, 37, 42 and unpublished data). Pimozide and fluspirilene (31) also increase NA turnover but this effect seems to be unrelated to NA receptor blockade (2, 3). These compounds may therefore be considered relatively specific with regard to their ability to block DA receptors. Under all conditions a blockade of DA receptors in the neostriatum and the limbic forebrain seems to be a common property of neuroleptic compounds (2, 37, 12) and seems to be essential for their therapeutic action. The relative importance of DA receptor blockade in the neostriatum versus that in the limbic forebrain is as yet unknown.

The mechanism by which the DA receptor blockade causes increase in DA turnover is as yet not fully understood. However, it has recently been established that nervous impulse flow is essential for the increase in DA turnover to occur, since no increase occurs after interruption of the pathway (6, 36). Also Glowinski's group has demonstrated that not only does there occur an increase in turnover of the dopamine of the neostriatum after thioproperazine which is not present in the absence of impulse flow (16) but there occurs also an increase in the DA turnover in the substantia nigra, where the cell bodies are located (32), which supports the idea of a nervous feed-back from the neostriatum to the DA cell bodies. The increases in fluorescence intensity in the cell bodies are, however, only slight after prolonged treatment with neuroleptics in contrast to the case with the NA cell bodies (7).

There may also occur a transsynaptic feedback since increases in electrical field induced DA release have been found *in vitro* in neostriatal DA slices after incubation with DA receptor blocking agents (27). DA receptor sites on the DA nerve terminals themselves can also not be excluded. The influence of neuroleptic drugs on the rise in DA levels found after interruption of the DA pathway is currently being investigated to further understand the feedback by which neuroleptics exert their presynaptic actions.

The neuroleptic induced increase in DA turnover in the neostriatum is under the control of a cholinergic mechanism, since the increase in DA turnover is more or less counteracted by pretreatment with various types of anticholinergic drugs (1, 20, 40). There may be at least two cholinergic pathways that govern the activity in the DA pathway, one is a striato-nigral pathway (41) which appears to stimulate the DA system (26); the other one is the possible ascending cholinergic pathway to the neostriatum (44). The cholinergic dopaminergic interaction is further illustrated by the fact that anticholinergic drugs slightly to clearly reduce DA turnover (1, 4, 20), whereas cholinergic drugs increase DA turnover in the neostriatum (18).

SUMMARY

The present results illustrate the capacity of various types of neuroleptic drugs (chlorpromazine, haloperidol, pimozide, clozapine) used in the treatment of mental disease to cause blockade of DA receptors in the forebrain, *e.g.* in the neostriatum. This blockade results in a compensatory activation of the nigro-neostriatal DA pathway, which can be more or less blocked by anticholinergic drugs. These results illustrate that cholinergic pathways can govern the activity of the nigro-neostriatal DA pathway. Many of the pharmacological effects of neuroleptics are due to the DA receptor blockade itself (akinesia) or to the resulting disbalance between cholinergic-dopaminergic activity in the neostriatum (catalepsia).

ACKNOWLEDGEMENTS

This work has been supported by a grant (B73-04X-715-08A) from the Swedish Medical Research Council and by a grant from Magn. Bergvalls Stiftelse.

REFERENCES

1. ANDÉN, N.-E. and BÉDARD, P. (1971) Influences of cholinergic mechanisms on the function and turnover of brain dopamine. J. Pharm. Pharmacol. **23**, 460.
2. ANDÉN, N.-E., BUTCHER, S. G., CORRODI, H., FUXE, K. and UNGERSTEDT, U. (1970) Receptor activity and turnover of dopamine and noradrenaline after neuroleptics. Europ. J. Pharmacol. **11**, 303.
3. ANDÉN, N.-E., CORRODI, H. and FUXE, K. (1972) Effect of neuroleptic drugs on central catecholamine turnover assessed using tyrosine- and dopamine- β-hydroxylase inhibitors. J. Pharm. Pharmacol. **24**, 177.
4. ANDÉN, N.-E., CORRODI, H. and FUXE, K. (1972) The effect of psychotomimetic glycolate esters on central monoamine neurons. Europ. J. Pharmacol. **17**, 97.

5. ANDÉN, N.-E., CORRODI, H., FUXE, K. and HÖKFELT, T. (1967) Increased impulse flow in bulbospinal noradrenaline neurons produced by catecholamine receptor blocking agents. Europ. J. Pharmacol. 2, 59.
6. ANDÉN, N.-E., CORRODI, H., FUXE, K. and UNGERSTEDT, U. (1971) Importance of nervous impulse flow for the neuroleptic induced increase in amine turnover in central dopamine neurons. Europ. J. Pharmacol. 15, 193.
7. ANDÉN, N.-E., DAHLSTRÖM, A., FUXE, K. and HÖKFELT, T. (1966). The effect of haloperidol and chlorpromazine on the amine levels of central monoamine neurons. Acta physiol. scand. 68, 419.
8. ANDÉN, N.-E., DAHLSTRÖM, A., FUXE, K. and LARSSON, K. (1966). Functional role of the nigro-neostriatal dopamine neurons. Acta pharmacol. (Kbh.) 24, 263.
9. ANDÉN, N.-E., ROOS, B.-E. and WERDINIUS, B. (1964) Effects of chlorpromazine, haloperidol and reserpine on the levels of phenolic acids in rabbit corpus striatum. Life Sci. 3, 149.
10. ANDÉN, N.-E., RUBENSON, A., FUXE, K. and HÖKFELT, T. (1967) Evidence for dopamine receptor stimulation by apomorphine. J. Pharm. Pharmacol. 19, 627.
11. BAUM, E., ETEVENON, P., PIARROUX, M.-C., SIMON, P. and BOISSIER, J.-R. (1971). Modifications comportementales et pharmacologiques obtenues chez le rat après lésion bilatérale de la substance noire. J. Pharmacol. (Paris) 2, 423.
12. BOBON, D. P., JANSSEN, P. A. J. and BOBON, J. (Eds.) (1970) Modern Problems of Pharmacopsychiatry, Vol. 5, The Neuroleptics (Karger, Basel-München-Paris-New York).
13. BOISSIER, J. R. and SIMON, P. (1963) Un test simple pour l'étude quantitative de la catatonie provoquée chez le rat par les neuroleptiques. Thérapie, 18, 1257.
14. CARLSSON, A., FUXE, K., HAMBERGER, B. and LINDQVIST, M. (1966) Biochemical and histochemical studies on the effects of imipramine-like drugs and (+)-amphetamine on central and peripheral catecholamine neurons. Acta physiol. scand. 67, 481.
15. CARLSSON, A. and LINDQVIST, M. (1963) Effect of chlorpromazine or haloperidol on formation of 3-methoxy-tyramine and normetanephrine in mouse brain. Acta pharmacol. (Kbh.) 20, 140.
16. CHERAMY, A., BESSON, M. J. and GLOWINSKI, J. (1970) Increased release of dopamine from striatal dopaminergic terminals in the rat after treatment with a neuroleptic: thioproperazine. Europ. J. Pharmacol. 10, 206.
17. CORRODI, H., FARNEBO, L.-O., FUXE, K., HAMBERGER, B. and UNGERSTEDT, U. (1972). ET495 and brain catecholamine mechanisms: Evidence for stimulation of dopamine receptors. Europ. J. Pharmacol. 20, 195.
18. CORRODI, H., FUXE, K., HAMMER, W., SJÖQUIST, F. and UNGERSTEDT, U. (1967) Oxotremorine and central monoamine neurons. Life Sci. 6, 2557.
19. CORRODI, H., FUXE, K. and HÖKFELT, T. (1967) The effect of neuroleptics on the activity of central catecholamine neurones. Life Sci. 6, 767.
20. CORRODI, H., FUXE, K. and LIDBRINK, P. (1972) Interaction between cholinergic and catecholaminergic neurons in rat brain. Brain Res. 43, 397.
21. CORRODI, H., FUXE, K. and UNGERSTEDT, U. (1971) Evidence for a new type of dopamine receptor stimulating agent. J. Pharm. Pharmacol. 23, 989.
22. COSTALL, B. and OLLEY, J. E. (1971) Cholinergic and neuroleptic induced catalepsy: modification by lesions in the caudate-putamen. Neuropharmacology, 10, 297.
23. COSTALL, B. and OLLEY, J. E. (1971) Cholinergic and neuroleptic induced catalepsy: modification by lesions in the globus pallidus and substantia nigra. Neuropharmacology, 10, 581.
24. DA PRADA, M. and PLETSCHER, A. (1966) Acceleration of the cerebral dopamine turnover by chlorpromazine. Experientia, 22, 465.
25. ERNST, A. M. (1967) Mode of action of apomorphine and dexamphetamine on gnawing compulsion in rats. Psychopharmacologia (Berl.) 10, 316.
26. ERNST, A. M. and SMELIK, P. G. (1966). Site of action of dopamine and apomorphine on compulsive gnawing behaviour in rats. Experientia, 22, 837.
27. FARNEBO, L.-O. and HAMBERGER, B. (1971) Drug-induced changes in the release of ^{3}H-monoamines from field stimulated rat brain slices. Acta physiol. scand. Suppl., 371, 35.
28. FOG, R. L., RANDRUP, A. and PAKKENBERG, H. (1968) Neuroleptic action of quaternary chlorpromazine and related drugs injected into various brain areas in rats. Psychopharmacologia, 12, 428.
29. FUXE, K. and UNGERSTEDT, U. (1972) Studies on the cholinergic and dopaminergic projections to the neostriatum with the help of intraneostriatal injections. In "The Pharmacology of the Extrapyramidal System" (HORNYKIEWICZ, O., Ed.) in the series "International Encyclopedia of Pharmacology and Therapeutics", in press.
30. GROSS, H. and LANGNER, E. (1970) Das Neuroleptikum 100—129/HF-1854 (Clozapin) in der Psychiatrie. Int. Pharmacopsychiat. 4, 220.

31. Janssen, P. A. J., Niemegeers, C. J. E., Schellekens, K. H. L., Dresse, A., Lennaerts, F. M., Pinchard, A., Schaper, W. K. A., Van Nueten, J. M. and Verbruggen, F. J. (1968) Pimozide, a chemically novel, highly potent and orally long-acting neuroleptic drug. Arzneimittel-Forsch. (Drug Res.) 18, 261.
32. Javoy, F., Hamon, M. and Glowinski, J. (1970) Disposition of newly synthesized biogenic amines in cell bodies and terminals of central aminergic neurons. I. Effect of amphetamine and thioproperazine on the metabolism of catecholamines in the caudate nucleus, the substantia nigra and the ventromedial nucleus of the hypothalamus. Europ. J. Pharmacol. 10, 178.
33. Laverty, R. and Sharman, D. F. (1965) Modification by drugs of the metabolism of 3,4-dihydroxyphenylethylamine, noradrenaline and 5-hydroxytryptamine in brain. Brit. J. Pharmacol. 24, 759.
34. McGeer, P. L., McGeer, E. G., Fibiger, H. C. and Wickson, V. (1971) Neostriatal choline acetylase and cholinesterase following selective brain lesions. Brain Res. 35, 308.
35. Naylor, R. J. and Olley, J. E. (1972) Modification of the behavioural changes induced by haloperidol in the rat by lesions in the caudate nucleus, the caudate-putamen and globus pallidus. Neuropharmacology, 11, 81.
36. Nybäck, H. (1971). Effects of neuroleptic drugs on brain catecholamine neurons. An experimental study using ^{14}C-labelled tyrosine. M. D. Thesis, Stockholm.
37. Nybäck, H. and Sedvall, G. (1968) Effect of chlorpromazine on accumulation and disappearance of catecholamines formed from tyrosine-^{14}C in brain. J. Pharmacol. exp. Ther. 162, 294.
38. Nybäck, H. and Sedvall, G. (1970) Further studies on the accumulation and disappearance of catecholamines formed from tyrosine-^{14}C in mouse brain. Effect of some phenothiazine analogues. Europ. J. Pharmacol. 10, 193.
39. Nybäck, H., Schubert, J. and Sedvall, G. (1970) Effect of apomorphine and pimozide on synthesis and turnover of labelled catecholamines in mouse brain. J. Pharm. Pharmacol. 22, 622.
40. O'Keefe, R., Sharman, D. F. and Vogt, M. (1970) Effect of drugs used in psychoses on cerebral dopamine metabolism. Brit. J. Pharmacol. 38, 287.
41. Olivier, A., Parent, A., Simard, H. and Poirier, L. J. (1970) Cholinesterasic striato-pallidal and striatal nigral efferents in the cat and the monkey. Brain Res. 18, 273.
42. Persson, T. (1970) Catecholamine turnover in central nervous system. Thesis, Reports from the Psych. Res. Centre, St. Jörgens Hosp. Göteborg.
43. Roos, B.-E. (1965) Effects of certain tranquillizers on the level of homovanillic acid in the corpus striatum. J. Pharm. Pharmacol. 17, 820.
44. Shute, C. C. D. and Lewis, P. R. (1967) The ascending cholinergic reticular system: neocortical, olfactory and subcortical projections. Brain, 90, 497.
45. Stille, G., Lauener, H. and Eichenberger, E. (1971) The pharmacology of 8-chloro-11-(4-methyl-1-piperazinyl)-5H-dibenzo(b,e) (1,4)diazepine (clozapine). Il Farmaco, 26, 603.
46. Ungerstedt, U. (1968) 6-Hydroxydopamine induced degeneration of central monoamine neurons. Europ. J. Pharmacol. 5, 107.
47. Ungerstedt, U. (1971) Histochemical studies on the effect of intracerebral and intraventricular injections of 6-hydroxydopamine on monoamine neurons in the rat brain. In "6-Hydroxydopamine and Catecholamine Neurons" (Malmfors, T. and Thoenen, H., Eds.), p. 101. North-Holland Publ. Comp.
48. Ungerstedt, U. (1971) Postsynaptic supersensitivity after 6-hydroxydopamine induced degeneration of the nigro-striatal dopamine system. Acta physiol. scand. Suppl., 367, 69.
49. Ungerstedt, U. (1971) Adipsia and aphagia after 6-hydroxydopamine induced degeneration of the nigro-striatal dopamine system. Acta physiol. scand. Suppl., 367, 95.
50. Ungerstedt, U. and Arbuthnott, G. (1970) Quantitative recording of rotational behaviour in rats after 6-hydroxy-dopamine lesions of the nigrostriatal dopamine system. Brain Res. 24, 485.
51. Ungerstedt, U., Butcher, L. L., Butcher, S. G., Andén, N.-E. and Fuxe, K. (1969) Direct chemical stimulation of dopaminergic mechanism in the neostriatum of the rat. Brain Res. 14, 461.

N.-E.A., Department of Pharmacology of the University, Göteborg, Sweden

RELATION OF THE EFFECT OF NEUROLEPTICS IN ANIMALS TO PHARMACOLOGICAL PARKINSONISM AND ANTIPSYCHOTIC ACTION IN MAN

R. PAPESCHI*) and I. MUNKVAD

Research Laboratory, Sct. Hans Hospital, Dept. E, Roskilde

INTRODUCTION AND REVIEW OF THE LITERATURE

Neuroleptic drugs of interest to psychiatrists and neurologists include reserpine and congeners, the most commonly used phenothiazines, thioxanthines and butyrophenones and the more recently introduced diphenylbutylamines (pimozide, fluspirilene) and dibenzazepines (clothiapine, clozapine, etc.).

The psychoanalytical and the sociological schools (85) have questioned the validity of the use of these drugs in psychiatry. However, left aside any claim to etiological medication, neuroleptics have undoubtedly useful symptomatic effect. Nevertheless, two fact should make the administration of neuroleptics a cautious decision, to be taken only when and as long as strictly necessary: 1. neuroleptics do not completely antagonize all psychotic symptoms; it is well known that patients treated with neuroleptics may be ridden with cumbersome side-effects that make them easily recognizable from untreated patients, and may not freely interact in a social group. In the amphetamine model of psychosis (70) neuroleptics can only in part antagonize the social isolation induced by amphetamine in monkeys (45, 76), while they can themselves reduce social interactions (76). 2. The indiscriminate and prolonged use of neuroleptics is probably a questionable practice, because of the lack of an adequate documentation of the structural effects of these drugs (15, 17, 38). In a recent investigation by PAKKENBERG et al. (in press) the administration of perphenazine to rats over a period of one year was found to reduce by 18% the number of cells in the basal ganglia, even if no gross neurological abnormalities were detected.

Neuroleptics are provided of two main actions: the proper antipsychotic effect (or neuroleptic action) and the induction of side-effects, among which a state of general sedation and extrapyramidal side-effects (ESE) are especially standing out. It is not yet known whether the latter are a prerequisite of the former, at least in the form of "fine extrapyramidal hypokinesia" (34), or whether the two effects are only coincidental. This dilemma is not purely academic, because there is a demonstrated relationship between extrapyramidal hypokinesia and dopaminergic mechanisms in the brain (61); if the first alternative were true, then a correlation could be established between antagonism of dopaminergic mechanisms and antipsychotic action of neuroleptics (55).

---

*) Visiting scientist of the Danish Medical Research Council. Present address: Max-Planck-Institut für Psychiatrie, Kraepelinstrasse 2, 8 München, Deutschland.

Two points could help clarify this problem: 1. some of the phenothiazines, such as the piperidine substituted, induce few ESE while they are still provided of antipsychotic properties; however, it could be argued that piperidine phenothiazines have a strong sedative effect, which might be altogether different from the proper neuroleptic action (see below classification of neuroleptics). The induction of ESE is also a matter of dose for these compounds. The case of clozapine will be discussed separately. 2. The prevention of ESE by means of antiparkinsonian agents has been variously reported as not affecting neuroleptic activity (37), or as having an unfavourable influence on it, when fine hypokinesia was suppressed (34). However, reports of the induction of psychotic symptoms in pharmacological parkinsonism or in Parkinson's disease by L-DOPA (5, 16, 92), by benztropine, (77), or by biperiden (50), all well established antiparkinsonian agents, tend to favour the hypothesis of a correlation between antipsychotic action and appearance of ESE.

ESE can be classified in four main groups (4, 10, 19, 22, 28): acute dystonia, akathisia, parkinsonism and tardive dyskinesia, which bear some resemblance to corresponding extrapyramidal disease observed in spontaneous human pathology.

Little is known about the pathogenesis of acute dystonia and of tardive dyskinesia. The former is rapidly reversed by anticholinergics and by the dopamine receptor stimulating agent, apomorphine (33); thus, it would appear that an acute deficit of dopaminergic (nigrostriatal?) activity and a relative hyperactivity of cholinergic (striopallidal?) mechanisms is involved in it. In contrast, tardive dyskinesia is amenable to treatment with the dopamine depleting agents tetrabenazine (11), reserpine or alpha-methyl-DOPA (89), with the dopamine receptor blockers haloperidol and thiopropazate (43), or with a combination of tetrabenazine and pimozide (FOG, personal communication).

An anatomo-pathological study of tardive dyskinesia has indicated damage to the nigral and striatal areas of the brain (17); however, the pathological material investigated in this condition is still relatively scarce. The observed cell loss in the caudate nucleus after prolonged administration of neuroleptics (PAKKENBERG et al., in press) supports the hypothesis (61), that tardive dyskinesia is due to a destruction of the striatal cells which carry the receptors to dopamine, i.e. the receptors that in physiological conditions are supposed to inhibit caudate neurons and in acute experiments are blocked by neuroleptics. It is conceivable that the prolonged administration of a receptor blocker may have toxic consequences for the metabolism of the cells. Such a lesion of the caudate units would result in a hypoactivity of the striopallidal (cholinergic?) neurons relative to the inhibitory dopaminergic nigrostriatal pathway; as the striatum, in turn, exerts an inhibitory action on "purposeless" motor activity (61), its hypofunction may lead to the onset of purposeless, involuntary movements. It is understandable that, in order to block the predominance of dopaminergic activity on the remaining caudate neurons, more neuroleptics will be required, i.e. more of the same drugs which generated the dyskinesia.

This interpretation of tardive dyskinesia does not require to postulate a hypersensitivity of the dopaminergic receptors, as suggested by other authors (12, 46); nor a hyperactivity of dopaminergic neurons. Indeed, the concentration of homovanillic acid (HVA) in the ventricular CSF, which is an index of the dopaminergic activity of the nigrostriatal pathway (62), was found normal in patients with a similar type of dyskinetic movements, the choreo-athetoid type (65).

An apparently similar situation is represented by the dyskinesia observed in parkinsonian patients treated with large amounts of L-DOPA (perhaps favoured by a coexisting lesion in the striatum) or, in a broader sense, by the involuntary, stereotyped movements observed after amphetamine or apomorphine in animals (69): in both cases inhibition of striatal activity would be achieved via an excessive dopaminergic stimulation, which would amount to the same final result as a chronic anatomical lesion of the cholinergic neurons of the striatum. However, the stereotyped drug-induced movements may be a model of abnormal behaviour rather than a dyskinesia and it has not yet been established whether the amphetamine motor and behavioural compulsions observed in man can be inhibited by will (and therefore resemble more tics and obsessive compulsions) or not (and therefore can be alikened to choreo-athetoid movements).

Akathisia bears some resemblance to the paradoxical hyperactivity observed in animals after large doses of neuroleptics (9, 74). The mechanism of this phenomenon awaits further experimental work to be elucidated.

Much more is known on the pathogenesis of parkinsonian symptoms: some authors (67) consider a lesion of the dopaminergic nigrostriatal pathway directly responsible for all three main symptoms of Parkinson's disease; one of us (61) has discussed the reasons for which only akinesia should be considered directly dependent on this mechanism, whereas postural tremor and rigidity should not. Akinesia, but not tremor and rigidity, was found to be correlated with the decrease of HVA in the ventricular CSF of parkinsonian patients (65) (Table 1).

TABLE 1

Concentration of homovanillic acid (HVA) in ventricular CSF of parkinsonian patients according to the criterion of akinesia

Akinesia	N	HVA[1]	P[2]
Present	6	52 ± 24	< 0.001
Absent	41	169 ± 19	

[1] Mean ± SE, nanograms per milliliter
[2] t-test

Correlation coefficient between concentration of HVA and of 5-HIAA in ventricular CSF of parkinsonian patients and severity of tremor and rigidity

	N	Tremor (0—15)[1]	P	Rigidity (0—15)[1]	P
HVA (ng/ml)	53	− 0.060	NS	+ 0.141	NS
5-HIAA (ng/ml)	17	− 0.037	NS	+ 0.253	NS

[1] Severity of tremor and rigidity was scored on an conventional 0—3 scale for the muscles of each separate limb and neck, and the scores summed up to a total (maximum possible score = 15).
From: PAPESCHI et al. (65).

A similar correlation between akinesia and dopaminergic mechanisms exists in pharmacological parkinsonism as in idiopathic Parkinson's disease.

It has been postulated that phenothiazines and butyrophenones block two types of receptors in the brain: those to dopamine (DA) and those to noradrenaline (NA) (13); correspondingly, these drugs induce two main symptoms in man: hypokinesia and sedation. Hypokinesia is the most common, dose-dependent phenomenon, observed after neuroleptics in man (4, 22, 34); also pimozide and penfluridol, previously described as rarely attended by ESE, induce fine extrapyramidal hypokinesia as demonstrated by the handwriting technique (6, 48). Catalepsy can be considered the specific equivalent in experimental animals of hypokinesia in man, because, as a general rule, neuroleptics that induce hypokinesia induce catalepsy to the same extent. In contrast, sedation and drowsiness have no specific quantifiable behavioural equivalent in animals: reduction of exploratory activity in the open field and postural changes follow both neuroleptics that induce hypokinesia and those that induce a state of general sedation (39). Palpebral ptosis may be central or peripheral in origin (86). However, the combined evaluation of these phenomena may give an approximate estimate of sedation in rats.

On the basis of studies of animal pharmacology (2, 39—42, 57, 81—83); and their comparison with the clinical characteristics of neuroleptics, the following classification of these drugs can be proposed, which is based on four criteria: 1. biochemical property to deplete catecholamines from storage sites vs. property to block catecholamine receptors in the CNS; 2. biochemical and pharmacological antagonism of dopaminergic vs. noradrenergic mechanism in the brain; 3. induction of side-effects of the type of sedation vs. catalepsy/hypokinesia; 4. clinical indication in states of excitement with hallucinations and gross psychomotor hyperactivity vs. states characterized by flattening of affect, thought disorder and systematized delusions. Other properties of neuroleptics, viz. the interference with serotonergic or cholinergic mechanisms, should also be taken in account (75).

1. The reserpine type (reserpine, tetrabenazine and the like), which depletes both DA and NA from storage sites in the CNS to about the same extent, and induces both sedation and catalepsy. Although not currently used for schizophrenia, these drugs have been indicated for states of motor excitement (because of their sedative effect). Oxypertine which acts in part by a similar mechanism but depletes more NA than DA (31, 35), from a pharmacological point of view, induces more sedation than catalepsy (59) and has been used clinically in anxiety states; however, the indications for this drug are under discussion.

2. The chlorpromazine type (promazine, chlorpromazine, chlorprothixine etc., i.e. the aliphatic and piperidine phenothiazines and the thioxanthines), which induces more sedation than catalepsy/hypokinesia, possesses high antagonism to NA toxicity and low to amphetamine- and apomorphine-induced stereotypies in animals; biochemically this group appears to block more NA than DA receptors in the brain and clinically is better indicated in psychotic states with gross motor hyperactivity.

3. The pimozide-fluspirilene type (i.e. the diphenylbutylamines), which induces catalepsy/hypokinesia (although gross akinesia and rigidity are less evident than in group 4) but no sedation, has low antagonism to NA toxicity and high activity against amphetamine and apomorphine stereotypies in animals and blocks selectively (although less powerfully than group 4) DA receptors in the brain; clinically, this group is indicated in forms of schizophrenia with few productive symptoms.

4. The haloperidol type (haloperidol, fluphenazine, thioproperazine etc., i.e. the piperazine phenothiazines and the butyrophenones), which powerfully blocks DA but also to some extent NA receptors, induces maximal side-effects of the type of gross akinesia//catalepsy, rigidity and neurodysleptic reactions. Clinically it is a powerful remedy in states in which a specific neuroleptic effect is required.

Clozapine, a dibenzazepine derivative, appears at first sight to be an exception to the general rule that "incisive" neuroleptics possess dopaminergic antagonism; this drug is provided of powerful neuroleptic action (23, 82) (though this emerges only after a preliminary period of sedation of about two weeks), but does not induce ESE, catalepsy nor has it antagonism to apomorphine-stereotypies (83). However, the biochemical pharmacology of this drug is still largely incomplete, before one can claim that clozapine lacks antidopaminergic activity. For instance, its strong anticholinergic properties could very well mask the antidopaminergic effect, through antagonism of catalepsy (53) and potentiation of apomorphine stereotypies (73). As a specific antipsychotic action appears only after two weeks, investigations in animals should be carried out with chronic administration; it is conceivable that after some time a tolerance to the anticholinergic action may develop and the antidopaminergic activity become apparent.

From the above classification we can infer that a general relationship exists between property of neuroleptics to induce catalepsy and hypokinesia of the parkinsonian type, their effectiveness to antagonize dopaminergic mechanisms in the brain and their clinical application as specific remedies in schizophrenic forms with flattening of affect and thought disorder. On the other hand neuroleptics that induce general sedation appear to counteract noradrenergic activity in the CNS and are clinically more indicated in conditions characterized by gross psychomotor excitement or hallucinations. The apparent inconsistency that gross akinesia is more evident in the haloperidol than in the pimozide group is explained by the fact that group 4 has more potent, although less selective, cataleptogenic and antidopaminergic activity than group 3; besides, the more pronounced presence in group 4 of rigidity, which is not necessarily a sign of dopaminergic blockade, may result in an apparently higher clinical reduction of motor activity.

The site of dopaminergic and noradrenergic antagonism by neuroleptics in inducing motor changes is likely to be represented by the nigrostriatal pathway (1, 18, 30, 56, 58, 81); and by the arousal system of the medial forebrain bundle (60, 80, 81), respectively. Nothing is known on the site of action of neuroleptics in exerting their clinical sedative and their specific antipsychotic effect; however, the above two anatomical structures can be suggested for consideration to future investigations, although it is quite possible that other dopaminergic pathways, such as the mesolimbic system, be equally important.

If sedation and hypokinesia/catalepsy are clearly related to the interaction of neuroleptics with catecholamines in the CNS, a similar relationship is not at all clear for the tremor and rigidity observed in pharmacological parkinsonism. Rigidity is not a consistent finding after neuroleptics; hypotonia of the muscles can be observed in man (10, 21, 51, 54, 66) and in animals (40, 42, 87, 90). Although rigidity induced by reserpine in the rat can be reversed by L-DOPA, this effect is not specific because it was also obtained with 5-hydroxytryptophan and with i.v. serotonin but not dopamine (72). Besides, the possibility has to be considered that the antagonistic effect of L-DOPA on parkinsonian rigidity is not mediated by any central action, but by a direct inhibitory effect on the contractility of skeletal muscles (29). Furthermore, the changes of muscle tone following neuroleptics may reflect a lower brain stem or a spinal site of action rather than an effect on the nigrostriatal pathway, perhaps at the level of the monoaminergic fibres of the reticulospinal tract, in analogy to what may occur in rigidity of Parkinson's disease (61); indeed, chlorpromazine and clozapine were shown to inhibit decerebrate rigidity in the cat (36, 83), although apomorphine has the same effect (24).

On the other hand, tremor after neuroleptics is often of slight intensity (34) and not correlated to neuroleptic action; neuroleptic tremor in many instances is quite different from genuine parkinsonian tremor at rest (28) and resembles more the physiological tremor induced by emotions or shivering or attitudinal tremor (21). Insufficient attention in the description of ESE is usually paid to the frequency of tremor induced by neuroleptics, which is usually faster than that of parkinsonian tremor (78), and many case reports limit themselves to describe the presence of a not better identified "tremulousness". In experimental animals (dogs, monkeys) tremor induced by piperacetazine, reserpine and chlorpromazine was characterized as much faster than parkinsonian tremor or occurring during movement or effort (3, 26, 47), although reports have also appeared of resting tremor (25, 91). To support the hypothesis that neuroleptic-induced tremor is a non specific phenomenon or at least unrelated to the interaction of these drugs with dopaminergic neurons is the fact that tremor is quite a common finding after different types of drugs, such as imipramine (7), 5-hydroxytryptophan (88), harmaline (44), and tremorine (27). This might point to an interference of neuroleptics with serotonergic or cholinergic mechanisms in the brain underlying their tremorigenic action.

From the above analysis of the literature it appears that, among the effects of neuroleptics in man and in animals, the only safe, positive correlation that can be established is between specific neuroleptic action, parkinsonian hypokinesia (and its experimental model, catalepsy) and antagonism of dopaminergic mechanisms in the CNS, whereas resting tremor and rigidity are less consistently observed and may depend on other actions of these drugs. In addition, sedation and clinical indication in states of gross psychomotor hyperactivity appear correlated with antagonism of noradrenergic function.

If sedation and hypokinesia/catalepsy induced by neuroleptics are due to interference with catecholaminergic neurotransmission in the brain, it ought to be possible to reproduce them experimentally by blocking the synthesis of central catecholamines; conversely, if tremor and rigidity are not directly related to the activity of those neuronal systems, they should not appear under these conditions. It was reported that alpha-methyl-p-tyrosine (AMT), a compound that blocks the synthesis of both catecholamines (79), induces a state of "catatonia" in monkeys and, further, that this condition could be reversed by L-DOPA (8) or apomorphine (49).

However, in these studies of the behavioural effects of AMT a distinction was not made between: 1. the sedative and cataleptic components of "catatonia" and their respective dependence on the disruption of dopaminergic or noradrenergic mechanisms; 2. the specific effect of AMT in blocking tyrosine hydroxylase and the aspecific (toxic) action of this drug on the kidney or other organs (52); 3. the effect of blocking catecholamine synthesis centrally or peripherally in the nervous system. In the course of some experiments on the interaction between ECT and drugs affecting the metabolism of catecholamines (61, 63), it was observed that catalepsy and sedation could be induced by AMT also in rats. Because this observation provided a chance to test the pathogenetic mechanisms underlying catalepsy and sedation, which might be relevant to the interpretation of the similar phenomena induced by neuroleptics, the behavioural effects of AMT in the rat were investigated (PAPESCHI and RANDRUP, in press).

EXPERIMENTAL

The investigation was carried out by testing the rats for reduction of exploratory activity in an open field situation and for catalepsy by means of the vertical wire netting and four corks tests. It should be remembered that reduction of exploratory activity in the open field is not only indicative of a state of general sedation but may also be a consequence of hypokinesia.

AMT induced a dose-dependent decrease of exploratory activity and catalepsy, which started about 5—6 hours after the intraperitoneal injection, and followed the same temporal course as the decrease of concentration of DA and NA in the whole brain (Fig. 1 and 2). In contrast, these behavioural changes were not correlated with the temporal course of the inhibition of synthesis of catecholamines, as published by other authors (84); this inhibition is reported to be maximal 30 minutes after AMT and to have partly subsided by 8 hours, the time when sedation and catalepsy approached maximum intensity. Therefore, stored catecholamines appear to be more important in the maintenance of spontaneous behaviour than those "newly synthesized". This statement does not necessarily contradict the hypothesis that "newly synthesized" catecholamines are more important for drug-induced behaviour, such as that seen after amphetamine (68) or ethanol (14). The difference may be explained by postulating that drug-elicited behaviour depends on newly synthesized catecholamines because these are less protected in the vesicles or are in an unbound form and therefore more easily accessible to drugs, whereas behaviour under physiological conditions depends on all available catecholamines.

Twenty-four hours after two injections of 250 mg/kg, i.p., of AMT, three hours apart, the rats started to show signs of toxicity with hypotonia of the muscles, hypothermia and

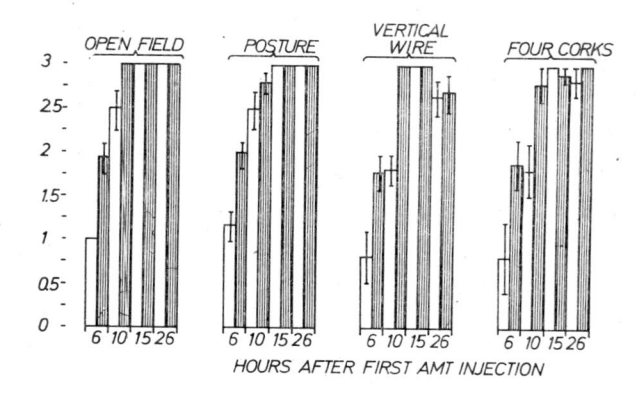

Fig. 1. Effect of AMT on various tests for sedation and catalepsy in the rat. Open bars: AMT, 250 mg/kg i.p., at 0 hr (n = 6). Stippled bars: AMT, 250 mg/kg, i.p., at 0 and 3 hr (n = 10). Vertical lines: ± SEM. Redrawn from Papeschi and Randrup, in press.

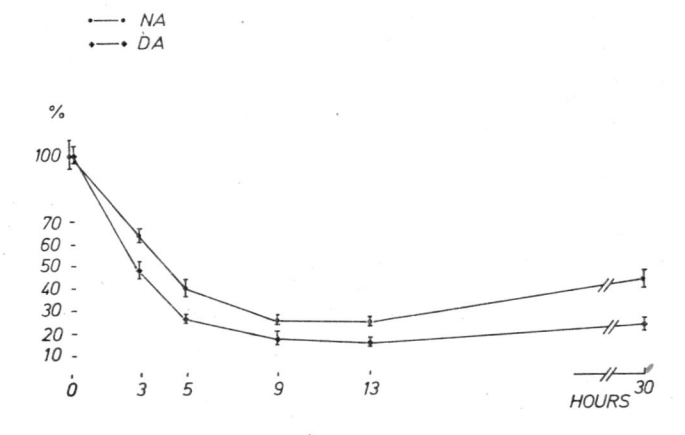

Fig. 2. Effect of AMT on the concentration of dopamine and noradrenaline in the brain of the rat. AMT was injected at the dose of 250 mg/kg, i.p., at 0 and 3 hr. Absolute values (mean ± SEM): NA = 440 ± 29; DA = 721 ± 28. Each point is the mean of 8 rats. Redrawn from: Papeschi and Randrup, in press.

bursts of fast intentional tremor; they all died in about 32 h. Slow, postural tremor and rigidity were never seen during the whole time the rats survived.

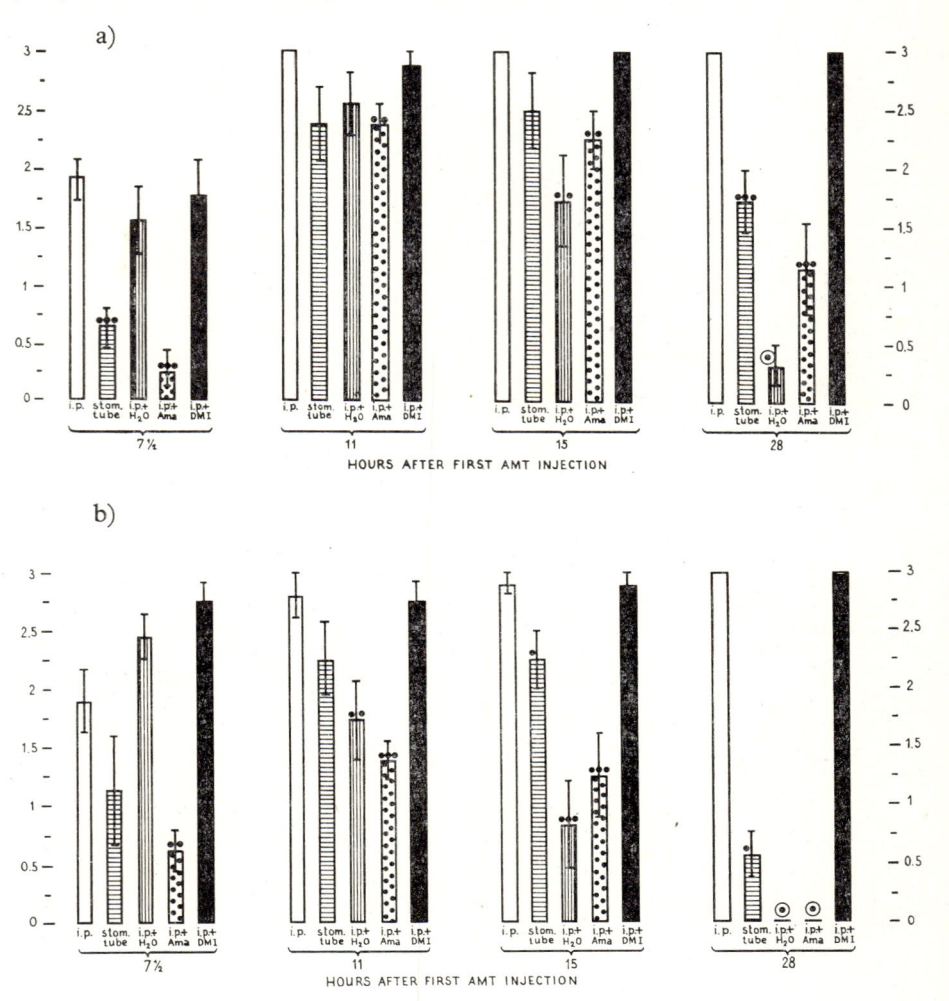

Fig. 3. Induction of sedation and catalepsy by AMT combined with various pretreatments or given by routes of administration that prevent AMT toxicity. a) Open field situation: b) four corks test. All groups received AMT, 250 mg/kg, at 0 and 3 hr; i.p. = AMT intraperitoneally; stom. tube = AMT by stomach tube; i.p. + H$_2$O = AMT intraperitoneally + 5% of body weight of a 0.8% solution of NH$_4$Cl in H$_2$O by stomach tube; i.p. + Ama = AMT intraperitoneally + + amantadine, 50 mg/kg, 15 minutes before each injection; i.p. + DMI = AMT intraperitoneally + desmethylimipramine, 10 mg/kg, 1 hr before each injection. Vertical lines: ± SEM; n = 10 for AMT i.p.; n = 8 for all other groups. Mann-Whitney U-test:

- • P less than 0.05 from the corresponding score of AMT i.p.
- •• P less than 0.02 from the corresponding score of AMT i.p.
- ••• P less than 0.01 from the corresponding score of AMT i.p.
- ⊙ P less than 0.001 from the corresponding score of AMT i.p.

Redraw from: PAPESCHI and RANDRUP, in press.

Sedation and catalepsy induced by AMT were not due to the toxicity of the drug, because it was possible to antagonize toxicity without preventing the onset of behavioural changes. AMT, given at the same dose as above, by stomach tube or intraperitoneally but together with an oral load of acidic aqueous solution, was not toxic for most of the rats (Table 2), but still induced a definite reduction of exploratory activity and catalepsy (Fig. 3).

Catalepsy was due to the block of synthesis of dopamine in the CNS, because L-DOPA, 200 mg/kg, 11 h after AMT and $\frac{1}{2}$ h after inhibition of peripheral decarboxylase with Ro4-4602, was able to completely antagonize it, and the antagonism was not affected when synthesis of noradrenaline from injected DOPA was prevented by an additional pretreatment with FLA-63, 20 mg/kg, at 4 and 7 h. Moreover, the dopamine receptor stimulating agent, apomorphine, 15 mg/kg, was also able to antagonize catalepsy (Fig. 4a).

Reduction of exploratory activity was mainly due to the block of synthesis of central NA, because the additional pretreatment with FLA-63 completely prevented the reversal by L-DOPA and in great part that by Ro4-4602 + L-DOPA; however the small but significant improvement observed under the last experimental conditions and after administration of apomorphine indicates that inhibition of synthesis of central dopamine is contributing to the reduction of exploratory activity induced by AMT (Fig. 4b), probably through its hypokinetic effect.

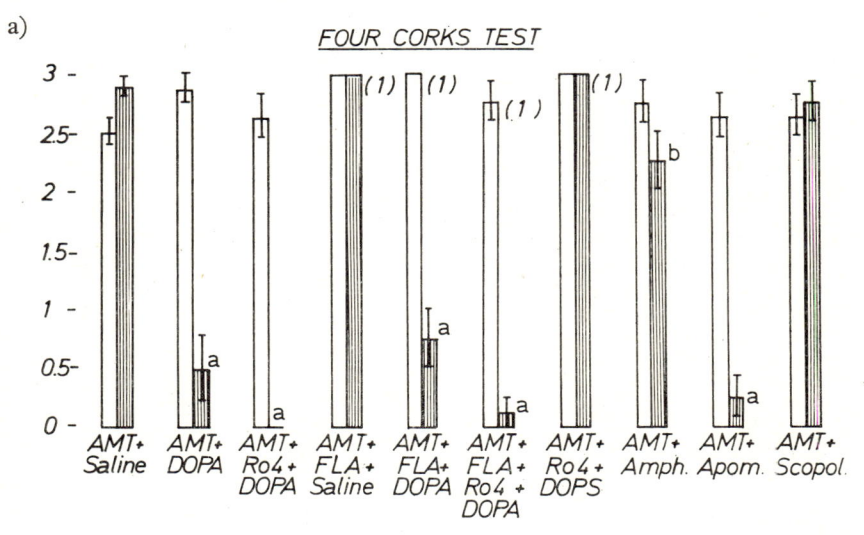

Fig. 4. Antagonism of AMT-induced catalepsy and sedation by various drugs that do not antagonize AMT toxicity. a) Four corks test; b) open field situation. All rats were injected with AMT 250 mg/kg i.p. at 0 and 3 hr. FLA-63 was given at 20 mg/kg, at 4 and 7 hr; Ro4-4602, 50 mg/kg, 1/2 hr before DOPA or DOPS; L-DOPA, 200 mg/kg, at 10—11 hr; DL-threo-DOPS, 400 mg/kg, at 10 hr; d-amphetamine, 15 mg/kg, at 9 1/2 hr; apomorphine, 15 mg/kg, at 9 1/2 hr; scopolamine, 5 mg/kg, at 10 1/2 hr; all drugs were injected intraperitoneally. The first test of each pair (open bars) was carried out at 7—8 hr, after AMT or AMT + FLA-63 and before the interaction drug(s); the second test (stippled bars) at 10—12 hr, after the interaction drug(s). Bars represent mean scores ± SEM; n = 20 for AMT + saline; n = 8 for all other groups.

(1) in Fig. 4a = hypotonia of the muscles;
(1) in Fig. 4b = sniffing and licking;
(2) in Fig. 4b = gnawing.

b) OPEN FIELD-TEST

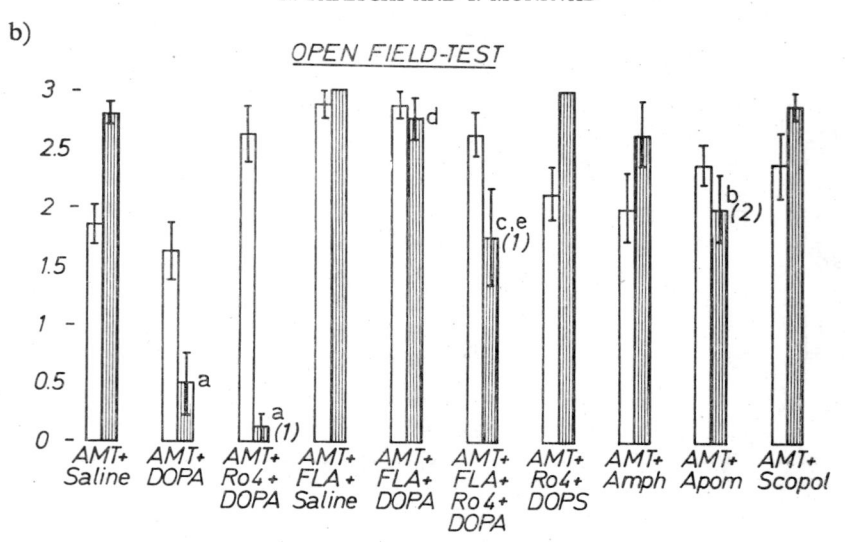

[Bar chart showing values for: AMT+Saline, AMT+DOPA, AMT+Ro4+DOPA, AMT+FLA+Saline, AMT+FLA+DOPA, AMT+FLA+Ro4+DOPA, AMT+Ro4+DOPS, AMT+Amph, AMT+Apom, AMT+Scopol]

Mann-Whitney U-test:

a = P less than 0.001 from AMT + saline on second test.
b = P less than 0.01 from AMT + saline on second test.
c = P less than 0.02 from AMT + saline on second test.
d = P less than 0.01 from AMT + DOPA on second test.
e = P less than 0.02 from AMT + Ro4-4602 + DOPA on second test.

Redrawn from: PAPESCHI and RANDRUP, in press.

TABLE 2

Antagonism of AMT toxicity by various treatment

Progr. number	Treatment[1]	N	Number of rats surviving indefinitely	P less than[2]
1	AMT, i.p., at 0 hr	6 } 16	0 } 0	—
	AMT, i.p., at 0 hr and 3 hr	10	0	—
2	AMT, by stomach tube at 0 and 3 hr	8	7	0.001
3	AMT, i.p. at 0 and 3 hr + water load	11	9	0.001
4	AMT, i.p. at 0 and 3 hr + amantadine	8	6	0.001

[1] AMT was always given at a dose of 250 mg/kg
[2] Compared to group 1, chi-square with Yate's correction for continuity

From: PAPESCHI and RANDRUP, in press.

CONCLUSIONS

From the above experimental evidence and from the review of the literature we can formulate the hypothesis that catalepsy, both after AMT or neuroleptics, is a specific phenomenon due to the interference with dopaminergic mechanisms in the CNS. On the other hand, sedation, both after neuroleptics of AMT, appears mainly related to the inhibition of synthesis of central NA. After neither drug treatment are postural tremor and rigidity a direct consequence of the disruption of catecholamine neurotransmission in the brain.

The evidence presented in this paper should not be interpreted to mean that all forms of catalepsy are due to a deficit of dopaminergic activity in the nigrostriatal pathway. It is known from the work of DE JONG and BARUK (20) that catalepsy can occur after a variety of treatments which may have nothing to do with dopaminergic neurons; however, some forms of catalepsy do bear a demonstrated relationship to central dopamine or to neuronal circuits that may be controlled by the nigrostriatal pathway (61) (Table 3); such a mechanism may be taken as a model to explain the pathogenesis of hypokinesia in pharmacological parkinsonism.

TABLE 3

Types of catalepsy experimentally obtained in lower mammals, primates and man

Treatments	Species	Proposed mechanism
A. *Catalepsy by hypofunction:*		
1. Large diencephalic lesions, interrupting all monoaminergic fiber systems	rat	interruption of NSP and of pallidotegmental pathway?
2. Pallidal lesions	monkey	interruption of pallidotegmental or of pallidothalamocortical circuit?
3. Parietal lesions	monkey	interruption of striopallido-thalamo-cortical circuit?
4. Neuroleptic drugs	rat, man	block of DA receptors in caudate, and/or block of NA receptors in spinal cord?
5. Bulbocapnine	cat, monkey, man	
6. Repeated doses of AMT	monkey, rat	block of synthesis of DA in NSP and of NA in RST?
B. *Catalepsy by hyperfunction:*		
1. Injections of AMT caudate nucleus	cat	stimulation of neostriatal inhibitory neurons
2. Cholinergic drugs	mouse	stimulation of (neostriatal?) cholinergic neurons

Abbreviations: NSP — nigrostriatal pathway; RST — reticulospinal tract; DA — dopamine; NA — noradrenaline.

From: PAPESCHI (61).

As hypokinesia/catalepsy and sedation are, on the other hand, correlated with the specific antipsychotic and the sedative action of neuroleptics, respectively, the interference with dopaminergic and noradrenergic mechanisms in the brain may form the anatomo-physiological substrate of these clinical effects.

AMT, being provided both with sedative and hypokinetic/cataleptic action and interrupting the synthesis of both catecholamines in the brain, should also be expected to possess antipsychotic activity; although this drug has already been tried in schizophrenic patients with not much success (32), a new trial should be undertaken with bigger doses; of course, the intrinsic toxicity of the drug, the development of tolerance and the peripheral effects of blocking catecholamine synthesis may represent complicating factors.

REFERENCES

1. ANDÉN, N. E., ROOS, B. E. and WERDINIUS, B. (1964) Effects of chlorpromazine, haloperidol and reserpine on the levels of phenolic acids in rabbit corpus striatum. Life Sci. **3**, 149.
2. ANDÉN, N. E., BUTCHER, S. G., CORRODI, H., FUXE, K. and UNGERSTEDT, U. (1970) Receptor activity and turnover of dopamine and noradrenaline after neuroleptics. Eur. J. Pharmacol. **11**, 303.
3. ARONSON, N. I., BECKER, B. E. and MCGOVERN, W. A. (1962) A study in experimental tremor. Confinia neurol. **22**, 397.
4. AYD, F. J. (1961) A survey of drug-induced extrapyramidal reactions. J. Amer. med. Ass. **175**, 1054.
5. BARBEAU, A. (1969) L-DOPA therapy in Parkinson's disease: a critical review of nine year's experience. Can. med. Ass. J., **101**, 791.
6. BARO, F., BRUGMANS, J., DOM, R. and VAN LOMMEL, R. (1970) Maintenance therapy of chronic psychotic patients with a weekly oral dose of R 16341. A controlled double-blind study. J. clin. Pharmacol. **10**, 330.
7. BARUK, H. and LAUNAY, J. (1961) La loi des stades et la psychopharmacologie expérimentale chez le singe. In: Neuropsychopharmacology, **2**, ed. by E. ROTHLIN, Elsevier Publ. Co., Amsterdam, p. 222.
8. BEDARD, P., LAROCHELLE, L., POIRIER, L. J. and SOURKES, T. L. (1970) Reversible effect of L-DOPA on tremor and catatonia induced by α-methyl-p-tyrosine. Can. J. Physiol. Pharmacol. **48**, 82.
9. BOISSIER, J. R. and SIMON, P. (1964) Equivalences expérimentales du syndrôme neurologique des neuroleptiques. L'Encephale, **53**, 109.
10. BORDELEAU, J. M. and TETREAULT, L. (1972) Étude des manifestations extrapyramidales induites par les neuroleptiques. Rev. can. Biol. **31**, suppl. printemps, 247.
11. BRANDRUP, E. (1961) Tetrabenazine treatment in persisting dyskinesia caused by psychopharmaca. Amer. J. Psychiat. **118**, 551.
12. CARLSSON, A. (1970) Biochemical implications of DOPA-induced action on the central nervous system with particular reference to abnormal movements. In: L-DOPA and parkinsonism, ed. by A. BARBEAU and F. H. MCDOWELL, Philadelphia, F. A. Davis Co., p. 205.
13. CARLSSON, A. and LINDQVIST, M. (1963) Effect of chlorpromazine and haloperidol on the formation of 3-methoxytyramine and normetanephrine in mouse brain. Acta pharmacol. toxicol. **20**, 140.
14. CARLSSON, A., ENGEL, J. and SVENSSON, T. H. (1972) Inhibition of ethanol-induced excitation in mice and rats by α-methyl-p-tyrosine. Psychopharmacologia, **26**, 307.
15. CAZZULLO, C. L. (1958) Biological aspects of pharmacodynamics in psychoses. 2nd Congr. Int. Psychiat., Zürich, 1957. In: Chemical concepts of psychosis, New York, McDowell Obolenski, p. 331.
16. CELESIA, G. G. and BARR, A. B. (1970) Psychosis and other psychotic manifestations of Levodopa therapy. Arch. Neurol. **23**, 193.
17. CHRISTENSEN, E., MØLLER, J. E. and FAURBYE, A. (1970) Neuropathological investigation of 28 brains from patients with dyskinesia. Acta psychiat. scand. **46**, 14.
18. COSTALL, B., NAYLOR, R. J. and OLLEY, J. E. (1972) Catalepsy and circling behavior after intracerebral injections of neuroleptic, cholinergic and anticholinergic agents into the caudate-putamen, globus pallidus and substantia nigra of rat brain. Neuropharmacology, **11**, 645.
19. CRANE, G. E. and NARANJO, E. R. (1971) Motor disorders induced by neuroleptics. Arch. gen. Psychiat. **24**, 179.
20. DE JONG, H. and BARUK, H. (1930) La catatonie expérimentale par le bulbocapnine. Étude physiologique et clinique. Paris, Masson.
21. DELAY, J. and DENIKER, P. (1961) Apport de la clinique à la connaissance de l'action des neuroleptiques. In: Système extrapyramidal et neuroleptiques, ed. by J. M. Bordeleau, Éditiones psychiatriques, Montreal, p. 301.
22. DELAY, J. and DENIKER, P. (1968) Drug-induced extrapyramidal syndromes. In: Hnd. Clin. Neurol., vol. **6**, ed. by P. J. Vinken and G. W. Bruyn, North-Holland Publ. Co., Amsterdam, p. 248.
23. DE MAIO, D. (1972) Clozapine, a novel major tranquilizer. Arzneim.-Forsch. **22**, 919.
24. DORDONI, F. (1948) Sugli effetti dell'associazione morfina-apomorfina nel cane. 1) Vomito,

depressione del sistema nervoso e ipotonia muscolare. 2) L'apomorfina e l'ipertono da decerebrazione. 3) La morfina e i centri rombencefalici del tono muscolare. Boll. Soc. ital. Biol. sper. **24**, 228.
25. DREYFUSS, J., BEER, B., DEVINE, D. D., ROBERTS, B. F. and SCHREIBER, E. C. (1972) Fluphenazine-induced parkinsonism in the baboon: pharmacological and metabolic studies. Neuropharmacology, **11**, 223.
26. ESSIG, C. F. and CARTER, W. W. (1957) Convulsions and bizarre behavior in monkeys receiving chlorpromazine. Proc. Soc. exp. Biol. Med. **95**, 726.
27. EVERETT, G. M. (1961) Tremorine. In: Extrapyramidal system and neuroleptics, ed. by J. M. BORDELEAU, Editions Psychiatriques, Montreal, p. 182.
28. FAURBYE, A. (1965) Discussion of clinical aspects of neuroleptic drugs. In: Neuropsychopharmacology, vol. **4**, ed. by D. Bente, P. B. Bradley. Elsevier Publ. Co., Amsterdam, p. 183.
29. FERKO, A. P. and CALESNICK, B. (1971) L-DOPA and dopamine on skeletal muscle. Res. Comm. Chem. path. Pharmacol. **2**, 146.
30. FOG, R., RANDRUP, A. and PAKKENBERG, H. (1971) Intrastriatal injection of quaternary butyrophenones and oxypertine: neuroleptic effect in rats. Psychopharmacologia, **19**, 224.
31. FUXE, K., GROBECKER, H., HÖKFELT, T., JÖNSSON, J. and MALMFORS, T. (1967) Some observations on the site of action of oxypertine. Naunyn-Schmiedeberg's Arch. exp. Path. Pharmak. **256**, 450.
32. GERSHON, S., HEKIMIAN, L. J., FLOYD, A. and HOLLISTER, L. E. (1967) Alphamethyl-p-tyrosine (AMT) in schizophrenia. Psychopharmacologia, **11**, 189.
33. GESSA, R., TAGLIAMONTE, A. and GESSA, G. L. (1973) Blockade by apomorphine of haloperidol-induced dyskinesia in schizophrenic patients. In press in Lancet.
34. HAASE, H. J. (1965) Clinical observations on the action of neuroleptics. In: The action of neuroleptic drugs, ed. by H. J. HAASE and P. A. J. JANSSEN. North-Holland Publ. Co., Amsterdam, part I, p. 3.
35. HASSLER, R., BAK, I. J. and KIM, J. S. (1970) Unterschiedliche Entleerung der Speicherorte für Noradrenalin, Dopamin und Serotonin als Wirkungsprinzip des Oxypertins. Nervenarzt, **41**, 105.
36. HENATSCH, H. D. and INGVAR, D. H.: Chlorpromazine und Spastizität. Eine experimentelle elektrophysiologische Untersuchung. Arch. Psychiat. Nervenkr. **195**, 77.
37. HIOB, J. and HIPPIUS, H. (1959) Avoidance of physical side-effects. In: Psychopharmacology Functions, ed. by N. S. KLINE, Boston, Little, Brown & Co.
38. HUNTER, R., BLACKWOOD, W., SMITH, M. C. and CUMINGS, J. N.: Neuropathological findings in three cases of persistent dyskinesia following phenothiazine medication. J. neurol. Sci. **7**, 263.
39. JANSSEN, P. A. J., NIEMEGEERS, C. J. E. and SCHELLEKENS, K. H. L. (1965) Is it possible to predict the clinical effects of neuroleptic drugs (major tranquillizers) from animal data? I. "Neuroleptic activity spectra" for rats. Arzneimittel-Forsch. **15**, 104.
40. JANSSEN, P. A. J., NIEMEGEERS, C. J. E., SCHELLEKENS, K. H. L., DRESSE, A., LENAERTS, F. M., PINCHARD, A., SCHAPER, W. K. A., VAN NUETEN, J. M. and VERBRUGGEN, F. J. (1968) Pimozide, a chemically novel, highly potent, and orally drug acting neuroleptic drug. Part I. The comparative pharmacology of pimozide, haloperidol and chlorpromazine. Arzneimittel-Forsch. **18**, 261.
41. JANSSEN, P. A. J., NIEMEGEERS, C. J. E., SCHELLEKENS, K. H. L., LENAERTS, F. M., VERBRUGGEN, F. J., VAN NUETEN, J. M., MARSBOOM, R. H. M., HERIN, V. V. and SCHAPER, W. K. A. (1970) The pharmacology of fluspirilene (R 6218), a potent, long-acting and injectable neuroleptic drug. Arzneimittel-Forsch. **11**, 1689.
42. JANSSEN, P. A. J., NIEMEGEERS, C. J. E., SCHELLEKENS, K. H. L., LENAERTS, F. M., VERBRUGGEN, Z. J., VAN NUETEN, J. M. and SCHAPER, W. K. A. (1970) The pharmacology of penfluridol (R16341) a new potent and orally long-acting neuroleptic drug. Europ. J. Pharmacol. **11**, 139.
43. KAZAMATSURI, H., CHIEN, C. P. and COLE, J. O. (1972) Treatment of tardive dyskinesia. II. Short-term efficacy of dopamine-blocking agents haloperidol and thiopropazate. Arch. gen. Psychiat. **27**, 100.
44. KIM, J. S., HASSLER, R., KUROKAWA, M. and BAK, I. J. (1970) Abnormal movements and rigidity induced by hamaline in relation to striatal acetylcholine, serotonine, and dopamine. Exp. Neurol. **29**, 189.
45. KJELLBERG, B. and RANDRUP, A. (1971) The effects of amphetamine and pimozide, a neuroleptic, on the social behaviour of vervet monkeys (cercopithecus sp.). In: Adv. Neuropharmacol. Proc. Symp. VII Congress CINP, Prague 1970, North-Holland Publ. Co. Amsterdam, p. 305.
46. KLAWANS, H. L. (1970) A pharmacologic analysis of Huntington's chorea. Europ. Neurol. **4**, 148.

47. KNAPP, D. L., STONE, G. C., HAMBOURGER, W. E. and DRILL, V. A. (1962) Behavioral and pharmacological studies of piperacetazine, a potent tranquilizing agent. Arch. int. Pharmacodyn. **135**, 152.
48. LA ROCHE, J. (1968) Klinische Prüfung eines neuen Neuroleptikums bei chronisch Schizophrenen, R 6238. Thesis for the degree of Medical Doctor, University of Düsseldorf.
49. LAROCHELLE, L., BEDARD, P., POIRIER, L. J. and SOURKES, T. L. (1971) Correlative neuroanatomical and neuropharmacological study of tremor and catatonia in the monkey. Neuropharmacology, **10**, 273.
50. MATIAR-VAHAR, H. (1961) Über eine durch Akineton ausgelöste Psychose schizophrener Prägung. Nervenarzt, **32**, 473.
51. MAY, R. H., SELYNES, P., WEEKLEY, R. D. and POTTS, A. M. (1960) Thioridazine therapy: results and complications. J. nerv. ment. Dis. **130**, 230.
52. MOORE, K. E., WRIGHT, P. F. and BERT, K. K. (1967) Toxicologic studies with α-methyltyrosine an inhibitor of tyrosine hydroxylase. J. Pharmacol. exp. Ther. **155**, 506.
53. MORPURGO, C. and THEOBALD, W. (1964) Influence of antiparkinson drugs and amphetamine on some pharmacological effect of phenothiazine derivatives used as neuroleptics. Psychopharmacologia, **6**, 178.
54. MÜLLER, D. (1961) Über ein neues Psychopharmakon (Chlorprothixen) in der Behandlung endogener Psychosen. Psychiat. Neurol. med. Psychol. (Leipzig) **13**, 184.
55. MUNKVAD, I. (1970) Neuroleptics in the treatment of schizophrenia. In: Modern Problems of Pharmacopsychiatry. The Neuroleptics, ed. by J. BOBON and P. A. J. JANSSEN. S. Karger, Basel, p. 44.
56. NYBÄCK, H. (1972) Effect of brain lesions and chlorpromazine on accumulation and disappearance of catecholamines formed *in vivo* from ^{14}C tyrosine. Acta physiol. scand. **84**, 54.
57. NYBÄCK, H. and SEDVALL, G. (1970) Further studies on the accumulation and disappearance of catecholamines formed from tyrosine-^{14}C in mouse brain. Effect of some phenothiazine analogues. Europ. J. Pharmacol. **10**, 193.
58. NYBÄCK, H. and SEDVALL, G. (1971) Effect of nigral lesion on chlorpromazine-induced acceleration of dopamine synthesis from ^{14}C-tyrosine. J. Pharm. Pharmacol. **23**, 322.
59. O'KEEFFE, R., SHARMAN, D. F. and VOGT, M. (1970) Effect of drugs used in psychoses on cerebral dopamine metabolism. Brit. J. Pharmacol. **38**, 287.
60. OLSON, L. and FUXE, K. (1971) On the projections from the locus coeruleus noradrenaline neurons: the cerebellar innervation. Brain Res. **28**, 165.
61. PAPESCHI, R. (1972) Dopamine, extrapyramidal system and psychomotor function. Psychiat. Neurol., Neurochir. **75**, 13.
62. PAPESCHI, R., SOURKES, T. L., POIRIER, L. J. and BOUCHER, R. (1971) On the intracerebral origin of homovanillic acid of the cerebrospinal fluid of experimental animals. Brain Res. **28**, 527.
63. PAPESCHI, R., LAL, S., SOURKES, T. L. and BOUCHER, R. (1971) The effect of ECT on the catalepsy induced by drugs interfering with brain monoamines. Proc. of the Meeting of Quebec Psychopharmacol. Soc., Joliette P. Q.
64. PAPESCHI, R. and RANDRUP, A. (1973) Catalepsy, sedation and hypothermia induced by alpha-methyl-p-tyrosine in the rat. An ideal tool for screening of drugs active on central catecholamine receptors. Submitted to Pharmakopsychiat. Neuro-Psychopharmak. (Stuttgart).
65. PAPESCHI, R., MOLINA-NEGRO, P., SOURKES, T. L. and ERBA, G. (1972) The concentration of homovanillic and 5-hydroxyindoleacetic acids in ventricular and lumbar CSF. Studies in patients with extrapyramidal disorders, epilepsy and other diseases. Neurology, **22**, 1151.
66. PENNINGTON, V. N. (1959) The phrenotropic action of Trilafon (perphenazine) in 323 neuropsychiatric patients. Amer. J. Psychiat. **116**, 65.
67. POIRIER, L. J. (1970) Le système striopallidal et ses mécanismes accessoires au regard de la physiopathologie extra-pyramidale. Presse méd. **78**, 1395.
68. RANDRUP, A. and MUNKVAD, I. (1966) Role of catecholamines in the amphetamine excitatory response. Nature, **211**, 540.
69. RANDRUP, A. and MUNKVAD, I. (1968) Behavicural stereotypies induced by pharmacological agents. Pharmakopsychiat. Neuro-Psychopharmak. (Stuttgart), **1**, 18.
70. RANDRUP, A. and MUNKVAD, I. (1972) Evidence indicating an association between schizophrenia and dopaminergic hyperactivity in the brain. Orthomolec. Psychiat. **1**, 2.
71. ROIZIN, L., TRUE, C. and KNIGHT, M. (1959) Structural effects of tranquillizers. Proc. Ass. Res. New. ment. Dis. **37**, 285.
72. ROOS, B. E. and STEG, G. (1964) The effect of L-DOPA and 5-HTP on rigidity and tremor induced by reserpine, chlorpromazine and phenoxybenzamine. Life Sci., **3**, 351.

73. Scheel-Krüger, J. (1970) Central effects of anticholinergic drugs measured by the apomorphine gnawing test in mice. Acta pharmacol. toxicol. **28**, 1.
74. Scheel-Krüger, J. and Randrup, A. (1968) Pharmacological evidence for a cholinergic mechanism in brain involved in a special stereotyped behaviour of reserpinized rats. Brit. J. Pharmacol. **34**, 217P.
75. Schelkunov, E. L. (1967) Integrated effect of psychotropic drugs on the balance of cholino-, adreno-, and serotoninergic processes in the brain as a basis of their gross behavioural and therapeutic actions. Activ. nerv. sup. **9**, 207.
76. Schiørring, E. and Randrup, A. (1971) Social isolation and changes in the formation of groups induced by amphetamine in an open-field test with rats. Pharmakopsychiat. Neuro-Psychopharmak. **4**, 1.
77. Singh, M. M. and Smith, J. M. (1973) Reversal of some therapeutic effects of an anti-psychotic agent by an anti-parkinsonism drug. Practical and theoretical implications. In press in J. nerv. ment. Dis.
78. Sloane, R. B. and Haden, P. (1961) Use of thioridazine (Melleril) in psychological disorders. Dis. nerv. Syst. **22**, 330.
79. Spector, S., Sjoerdsma, A. and Udenfriend, S. (1965) Blockade of endogenous norepinephrine synthesis by α-methyl-tyrosine, an inhibitor of tyrosine hydroxylase. J. Pharmacol. exp. Ther. **147**, 86.
80. Stille, G. (1966) Arousalhemmung und Katalepsie bei Neuroleptica. Arzneimittel-Forsch., **16**, 255.
81. Stille, G. (1971) Zur Pharmakologie Katatoniger Stoffe. Editio Cantor-Aulendorf i. Württ.
82. Stille, G. and Hippius, H. (1971) Kritische Stellungnahme zum Begriff der Neuroleptika. Pharmakopsych. Neuro-Psychopharm. **4**, 182.
83. Stille, G., Lawener, H. and Eichenberger, E. (1971) The pharmacology of 8-chloro-11-(4-methyl-1-piperazinyl)-5H-dibenzo [b, e] [1,4] diazepine (clozapine). Farmaco (ed. prat.) **26**, 603.
84. Svensson, T. H. and Waldeck, B. (1971) On the relation between motor activity and degree of enzyme inhibition following inhibition of tyrosine hydroxylase. Acta pharmacol. toxicol. **29**, 60.
85. Szasz, T. S. (1967) The myth of mental illness. New York, Harper and Row.
86. Tedeschi, D. H. (1970) Palpebral ptosis as an index of neuroleptic activity. In: The Neuroleptics, ed. by D. P. Bobon, P. A. J. Jansen and J. Bobon. Modern problems of pharmacopsychiatry. S. Karger, Basel, p. 55.
78. Tedeschi, D. H., Tedeschi, R. E., Cook, L., Mattis, P. A. and Fellows, E. J. (1959) The neuropharmacology of trifluoperazine: a potent psychotherapeutic agent. Arch. int. Pharmacodyn. **122**, 129.
88. Tedeschi, D. H., Tedeschi, R. E. and Fellows, E. J. (1959) The effects of tryptamine on the central neurons system, including a pharmacological procedure for the evaluation of iproniazide-like drugs. J. Pharmacol. exp. Ther. **126**, 223.
89. Villeneuve, A. and Böszörményi, Z. (1970) Treatment of drug-induced dyskinesias. Lancet, I, 353.
90. Weissman, A. (1969) A psychopharmacological comparison of thiothixine, chlorprothixine and clopenthixol in rats. In: Modern Problems of Pharmacopsychiatry, vol. 2. The Thioxanthines, ed. by H. E. Lehman and T. A. Ban, S. Karger, Basel, p. 15.
91. Windle, W. F., Cammermeyer, J., Feringa, E. R., Joralenon, J., Smart, J. O. and McQuillen, M. P. (1956) Tremor in African green monkeys. Fed. Proc. **15**, 202.
92. Yaryura-Tobias, J. A., Wolpert, A., Dana, L. and Merlis, S. (1970) Action of L-DOPA in drug-induced extrapyramidalism. Dis. nerv. Syst. **31**, 60.

R.P., Research Laboratory, Sct. Hans Hospital, Dept. E, DK-4000 Roskilde, Denmark

NEUROLEPTICS AND DYSKINESIAS

A. VILLENEUVE, K. JUS, A. JUS and J. GAUTIER

Research Division, Hôpital St. Michel-Archange and Department of Psychiatry, Faculty of Medicine, Laval University, Quebec

INTRODUCTION

Shortly after the introduction of neuroleptics, the extrapyramidal reactions were reported to constitute their most frequent side effects (10, 15, 33). A good proportion of the patients treated with these drugs experience indeed some type of extrapyramidal side effects (1, 14). The transitory, reversible, extrapyramidal symptoms are generally observed during the first days or weeks of treatment and are usually controlled by the antiparkinsonian agents, L–DOPA being ineffective (43). Later, a belated neurological complication associated with the use of neuroleptics was first described to affect the oral region (31,32) and this neurological syndrome became known as tardive dyskinesia (37) or terminal extrapyramidal insufficiency syndrome (16). Finally, a peculiar extrapyramidal reaction called „rabbit syndrome" has recently been described (39) and consists in its typical form of a fine parkinson–like tremor of the lips resembling the movements of a rabbit's mouth (frequency: 5—5.5 c/sec.).

Comprehensive reviews have dealt with the tardive dyskinesia syndrome from various aspects (6, 23–25) and its description will not be repeated. It is sufficient to say that this syndrome generally occurs after at least 6 months of treatment and that the administration of antiparkinsonian drugs not only does not improve it, but may even aggravate it (1, 6). After abrupt withdrawal of neuroleptics, tardive dyskinesia has been observed to appear more precociously in patients whose antiparkinsonian medication was pursued (41). Tardive dyskinesia does not always decrease in intensity with the cessation of neuroleptic therapy and can appear only upon its discontinuance. Paradoxically, the neuroleptics that block dopamine receptors and that induce these neurological symptoms can, administered at appropriate doses, attenuate them or even bring them under control (9). However, it cannot be excluded that this apparent clinical improvement is obtained at the expense of the aggravation of the underlying causal putative mechanism and that this type of treatment may render a tardive dyskinesia irreversible.

With regard to tardive dyskinesia and to certain extrapyramidal disorders, the beneficial effect of neuroleptics and of various other agents that can influence the metabolism of brain amines, such as tetrabenazine, reserpine, α–methyldopa and MAOI has been reported (Table 1) and the literature on this topic recently reviewed (2, 23). So far, among these agents, tetrabenazine and reserpine seem to be the most effective in reducing or abolishing tardive dyskinesia (2).

TABLE 1

Neuroleptics and extrapyramidal symptoms

Type	Acute dystonias	Parkinsonian-like syndrome	Rabbit syndrome	Tardive dyskinesia
Time of onset	Early	Early	Later	Late
	First days or weeks	Days — weeks	Months — years	Months — years
Response to antiparkinsonian agents	AP +	AP +	AP ±	AP 0 or W
	L-DOPA ?	L-DOPA 0	L-DOPA ?	L-DOPA 0 or W
Other drugs tested with some success	Phenobarbital Muscle relaxants (chlordiazepoxide, diazepam) Amitryptiline	Phenobarbital Methylphenidate Muscle relaxants	α-methyl-DOPA Amantadine Neuroleptics (thiopropazate, haloperidol) Pyridoxine L-tryptophan IMAO	Reserpine* Tetrabenazine*
Mechanisms	DA receptor blockade	DA receptor blockade	DA receptor blockade only?	Denervation hypersensitivity* Metabolic disturbance→lesional process
DA/Ach hypothesis	DA < Ach	DA < Ach	DA ? Ach	DA > Ach (5-HT ?)

Legend:
+ – effective
± – effective to various degrees
0 – ineffective
W – worse
? – unknown
* – believed the most effective
DA – Dopamine
Ach – Acetylcholine
5-HT – 5-Hydroxytryptamine
AP – Antiparkinsonian agents other than L-DOPA

The pathogenesis of tardive dyskinesia still remains obscure (27), but the brain dopaminergic system may play an important role in its etiology (28, 40–42).

Tardive dyskinesia can be modified by several physiological factors, disappearing for example during sleep and increasing with emotional tension or performance of a motor task (1, 8, 42). In a very detailed clinical description of the extrapyramidal motor disorders following long-term treatment with neuroleptics, attention has been drawn (7) to the phenomenon that voluntary movements involving the groups of muscles affected reduce abnormal involuntary activity in these muscles and that some dyskinesias become apparent only when patients are instructed to perform certain activities in remote groups of muscles. Voluntary movements would therefore seem to exert a fly-wheel effect in that they increase hyperkinesia in remote groups of muscles (7). Finally, it has been reported that in some patients oro-facial-lingual dyskinesias, apparently clinically similar to the neuroleptic-induced ones, either do not change with modifications of attention or appear during distraction or execution of voluntary movements (29).

With respect to the influence of sleep on the extrapyramidal movements, the clinical observation that tremor seldom persists during sleep has been made a long time ago (13). Later, with the advent of polygraphic techniques, the study of various extrapyramidal symptoms during different stages of sleep became possible, but in spite of this, there were few investigations in this field and the results are controversial. With these techniques, the clinical observation of the progressive diminution and disappearance of the tremor during sleep was confirmed (34, 35). The reappearance of parkinsonian and choreic symptoms during global movements when sleep is more superficial was also reported (34, 35). It was moreover noted that in Sydenham's chorea and in advanced cases of Huntington's chorea, the movements may reappear during the REM stage of sleep (34, 35). Finally, the disappearance of myoclonic jerks was observed during sleep, although in some cases (epileptic myoclonic jerks), they persisted during all phases of sleep (34). However, the small number of observations in these studies does not permit to draw any precise conclusions concerning the neurophysiological basis of these movements (35).

Owing to the limited number of physiological studies dealing with the influence of attention concentration and motor performance and that of sleep on various tardive drug-induced abnormal movements and in order to accumulate additional neurophysiological data on the mechanisms of tardive dyskinesia, polygraphic studies were undertaken by our group (20) and will be briefly summarized here.

Polygraphic studies

1. During wakefulness: Influence of attention concentration and motor performance

Polygraphic studies were performed in 29 schizophrenic patients on the influence of attention and voluntary movements on different types of tardive dyskinesia and on the rabbit syndrome. The utilization of polygraphic techniques during attention concentration and motor performance in patients with tardive dyskinesia constitutes a useful tool for investigating quantitative and qualitative changes. It may also be used for the objective measurement of such movements for comparative studies.

The bucco-lingual and the bucco-linguo-masticatory types of tardive dyskinesia are different from the rabbit syndrome in that the rabbit syndrome always increases in amplitude and EMG potential frequency during attention concentration and voluntary movements.

The modifications occurring in the bucco-lingual and bucco-linguo-masticatory types of dyskinesia during attention concentration and motor performance can either evolve in the same direction (increase or decrease in both experimental conditions) or in different directions (increase in one situation and decrease in the second or inversely).

The bucco-lingual and bucco-linguo-masticatory types of tardive dyskinesia and the rabbit syndrome are not mutually exclusive as evidenced by its superimposition on the bucco-lingual and bucco-linguo-masticatory types of tardive dyskinesia or their replacement by it under attention concentration and/or motor performance. In some cases of tardive dyskinesia, regularization and rhythmicity characterize the changes provoked by attention concentration and/or motor performance.

2. During sleep: Influence of different sleep stages

In 21 schizophrenic patients, polygraphic studies of the influence of sleep on different types of tardive dyskinesia and on the rabbit syndrome were executed.

The NREM stages of sleep and the REM state do not differ in their EEG characteristics, with the exception of drug-induced changes, from those found in a normal population of similar age. A certain degree of specific central nervous system activation is needed for the presence of these abnormal movements. There is however a difference in the degree of activation needed for the presence of tardive dyskinesia and that of the rabbit syndrome. The bucco–lingual and the bucco–linguo–masticatory types of tardive dyskinesia are absent during all NREM stages and during REM stage, whereas the rabbit syndrome usually persists during the NREM stage I and sometimes until the beginning of stage II. Tardive dyskinesia and the rabbit syndrome reappear during transition from REM stage to wakefulness. The rabbit syndrome can also reappear during transition from REM stage to NREM stage I. All types of tardive dyskinesia and the rabbit syndrome are present during the transitory stages from wakefulness to sleep and from sleep to wakefulness. In the mixed type of oral dyskinesia, the rhythmic movements of the rabbit syndrome are the last to disappear during transition from wakefulness to sleep and the first to reappear during passage from sleep to wakefulness. The tardive dyskinetic movements are the first to disappear during transition from wakefulness to sleep.

The changes in muscle tone seem to play an important role in the mechanism of tardive dyskinesia and of the the rabbit syndrome. A distinction must be established here between the changes in the tone of the muscles involved in these abnormal movements and those which are not, as well as between the phasic and tonic alterations in muscle tone. The increase of muscle tone in the sub-mental region represents an augmentation of tone of the muscles not primarily involved in the rabbit syndrome and the increase of tone of the muscles in the sub–mental region does not reflect necessarily the changes of tone in the muscles of the oral region. The phasic alterations of the muscle tone present during the REM state (muscle twitches) do not appear to play a role in triggering the dyskinetic movements, because they are not followed by their reappearance. On the contrary, the tonic changes seem to play an important role as can be seen during the transition from REM state into NREM stage I, when tardive dyskinesia and the rabbit syndrome reappear in relation with the tonic increase in muscle tone. The absence of muscle tone during the central nervous system activation in the REM state is one of the physiological features differentiating this kind of central nervous system activation from wakefulness. We could therefore assume that the absence of muscle tone in the REM state is one of the factors bound with the absence of extrapyramidal movements in this peculiar state of central nervous system activation.

During the waking state, tardive dyskinesia often decreased with the diminution of ocular activity (eyes closed, state of relaxation) and increased with the enhancement of ocular activity. On the contrary during the REM state, the disappearance or reappearance of eye movements did not influence tardive dyskinesia nor the rabbit syndrome which remained absent throughout this state. This could constitute additional evidence that the mechanisms of ocular activity during the REM period are different from the mechanisms of ocular activity during wakefulness.

Some difficulties do exist in distinguishing between physiological and pathological motor phenomena occurring during sleep. In normal persons, physiological masticatory movements may be present during sleep and particularly muscle twitching during the REM state. Some controversial results in the description of abnormal movements during sleep may possibly result from this fact. In our opinion, the rhythmicity of the oral movements seems to constitute an adequate criterion for differentiating physiological movements during sleep from the abnormal ones of tardive dyskinesia. A rhythmic oral motor phenomenon during sleep can with a very great probability be considered abnormal. The application of the criterion of rhythmicity, while being very useful, does not of course mean that quantitative criteria should be completely eliminated. Indeed, the unusually frequent appearance of masticatory movements can also indicate their abnormal character.

Theoretical Implications

The abnormal movements characterizing tardive dyskinesia appear to have a different pathogenesis than Parkinson's disease, early drug-induced extrapyramidal reactions and the rabbit syndrome, but do not seem to differ from them with respect to their presence or absence during sleep. In Parkinson's disease, there is principally a dopamine (DA) deficit (11, 17, 30) resulting from lesions in the pars compacta of the substantia nigra where DA-ergic cells are located and from where DA is transported to the receptor sites in the striatum. Even if the DA deficit is not restricted only to substantia nigra (3) in such cases exogenous L-DOPA represents a causal treatment by passing the blood-brain barrier to form DA. The early drug-induced parkinson-like symptoms are also likely the result of a DA deficit in the striatum, most probably caused by the blockage of receptor sites in the striatum by neuroleptics (38), the mechanism being thus different than in Parkinson's disease. L-DOPA is therefore ineffective in such cases because it cannot act on the DA receptor sites already blocked (26). In Parkinson's disease DA is not available in the striatum because of its absence or deficiency in the substantia nigra, whereas in early drug-induced parkinson-like syndrome it is delivered but cannot act probably because of a monolayer on water lipid interfaces in DA receptors in the striatum. To counteract the hypothetical dominance of the acetylcholinergic system provoked by the relative weakness of the DA-ergic system (4), anticholinergic drugs are administered in both cases. The pathogenesis of tardive drug-induced dyskinesia (choreoathetotic, bucco-lingual, bucco-linguo-masticatory types) is still unknown, but seems different from that of Parkinson's disease or of early extrapyramidal reactions. Neither L-DOPA nor anticholinergic drugs are effective here. However, anticholinergic agents may be beneficial to various degrees in the treatment of the rabbit syndrome (40, 41). A hypothesis has been proposed regarding the pathogenesis of tardive dyskinesia. The long-lasting blockage of receptor-sites in the striatum by neuroleptics (chemical denervation) might have provoked a hypersensitivity to DA and therefore these dyskinesias frequently appear only after drug withdrawal or diminution of dosage when the DA receptors are freed. A support for this hypothesis is given by the fact that L-DOPA may provoke an enhancement of such movements (28), whereas neuroleptic administration may be effective in some cases (2, 9, 24, 25) (Table 1).

From a neuropathological viewpoint, it has been suggested that persistent oral dyskinesias might be due to a degeneration of the substantia nigra in combination with other brain lesions, caused by an interference of the neuroleptics with cell membrane function and by an inhibition of the cell respiratory enzymes (5, 12).

Data from clinical research can form a basis for an approach to the neurophysiological and biochemical problems of tardive dyskinesia. An attempt is usually made to find correlations between the alterations in the brain amine metabolism of a given clinical syndrome and the changes in the pattern of sleep which is under the influence of the catechole- and of the indole-aminergic systems. Therefore, the sleep study of cases with possible alterations of brain amine metabolism such as in Parkinson's disease, parkinsonian drug-induced syndrome, tardive dyskinesia and rabbit syndrome seems especially attractive. An example of such conclusions made from sleep pattern observations is the inference of Kales et al. (22), that as the REM sleep pattern was normal in patients with Parkinson's disease, DA might not play the same role in the sleep of human subjects as in animals. The sleep difficulties in these patients were not influenced by short–term or chronic L–DOPA administration.

With respect to sleep theories or theories on the pathogenesis of tardive dyskinesia, some tentative inferences might be drawn from our studies. Insufficient data are at present available to explain why in the state of central nervous system activation constituted by the REM state where acetylcholine liberation from the surface of the cerebral cortex is increased significantly in comparison with the slow wave sleep (18, 19), those extrapyramidal movements presumably caused by a dominance of the cholinergic system do not reappear. There are also no sufficient data to explain why, with a similar rate of acetylcholine liberation from the surface of the cerebral cortex found during the REM state and during wakefulness that have a similar desynchronization EEG pattern, the dyskinetic movements are present in wakefulness and absent in the REM state.

It is rather difficult to assess the function of indole and catecholamine systems in connection to sleep on the sole fact that the NREM or REM sleep patterns are not altered in the sleep of patients with Parkinson's disease, in early drug-induced parkinson-like symptoms and in tardive dyskinesia. It would seem that hypotheses on the role of these brain amines would be more justified in cases where more dramatic changes in the sleep pattern such as for instance absence of REM sleep, absence in phasic phenomena in REM sleep etc. are present. To propose the reverse, that is hypotheses on the pathogenesis of tardive dyskinesia and of the rabbit syndrome on the only basis of their absence during REM state and NREM stages is also difficult. We can only state that a certain degree of a specific central nervous system activation characteristic of wakefulness, but not of the REM state, is necessary for the presence of tardive dyskinesia or of the rabbit syndrome and that this might be in relation with different biochemical mechanisms in both states of central nervous system activation. There is a difference in the degree of activation of CNS needed for presence of tardive dyskinesia and rabbit syndrome. More biochemical data are necessary to explain the mechanism of inhibition of the extrapyramidal movements during the REM sleep and their release with the central nervous system activation in wakefulness.

Conclusion

From our polygraphic studies conducted during sleep and wakefulness, tardive dyskinesia and the rabbit syndrome, both involving the oral region, and although not mutually exclusive, appear to possess different underlying mechanisms. Apart from its persistence during NREM stage I of sleep, the rabbit syndrome consistently increases in intensity during attention concentration and performance of a motor task. Finally, antiparkinsonian agents beneficial in various degrees in the treatment of the rabbit syndrome are not for the therapy of tardive dyskinesia. From the viewpoint of mechanisms, it might be helpful to attempt to develop some kind of classification of extrapyramidal symptoms taking into account the influence of pharmacological agents upon them.

Summary

Day and night polygraphic studies have been performed on a population of chronic schizophrenics with different types of tardive dyskinesia and with the rabbit syndrome. In 29 patients, we have analyzed the influence of attention concentration and motor performance on the pathology of these extrapyramidal movements. We have also investigated the influence of different stages of NREM sleep and REM sleep on these movements in 21 patients.

On the basis of the polygraphic studies in wakefulness, we can state that tardive dyskinesia differs from the rabbit syndrome, behaving differently under the influence of attention concentration and motor performance. On the basis of the night polygraphic studies, we can say that a certain degree of specific central nervous system activation is needed for the presence of tardive dyskinesia and of the rabbit syndrome. There is however a difference in the degree of activation needed for the presence of tardive dyskinesia or of the rabbit syndrome. All types of dyskinetic movements were absent during the NREM stages and during the REM stage, whereas the rabbit syndrome usually persisted during the NREM stage I. Both kinds of neuroleptic-induced movements were present during the transitory stages from wakefulness to sleep and from sleep to wakefulness.

The possible neurophysiological mechanisms on the influence of attention concentration and motor performance and of different stages of sleep on the neuroleptic-induced tardive dyskinesia and the rabbit syndrome are discussed.

References

1. Ayd, F. J. (1966) Persistent dyskinesias: A neurological complication of major tranquilizers. Int. Drug Therapy Newsletter, **1**: No. 5.
2. Ayd, J. F., Jr. (1972) Treatment of persistent dyskinesia. Int. Drug Therap. Newsletter, **7**, 9.
3. Barbeau, A. (1969) Parkinson's disease as a systemic disorder p. 66. In: Third Symposium on Parkinson's Disease (Gillingham, F. J. and Donaldson, I. M. L., Eds.). Livingstone Ltd. Edinburgh and London.
4. Barbeau, A., Sourkes, T. L. and Murphy, G. F. (1962) Les catécholamines dans la maladie de Parkinson. In: Monoamines et Système Nerveux Central (J. de Ajuriaguerra Ed.) Georg. Geneva and Masson, Paris, p. 247.
5. Christensen, E., Moller, J. E. and Faurbye, A. (1970) Neuropathological investigation of 28 brains from patients with dyskinesia. Acta psychiat. scand. **46**, 14.
6. Crane, G. E. (1968) Tardive dyskinesia in patients treated with major neuroleptics: a review of the literature. Amer. J. Psychiat. **124**, 40 (Supp.).
7. Degwitz, R. (1969) Extrapyramidal motor disorders following long-term treatment with neuroleptic drugs, p. 22. In: Psychotropic Drugs and Dysfunctions of the Basal Ganglia. (Eds. Crane, G. E. and Gardner, R. Jr.) Bethesda, NIMH, PHS Publication No. 1938.
8. Degkwitz, R. and Wenzel, W. (1967) Persistent extrapyramidal side effects after long term application of neuroleptics, p. 608. In: Neuro-Psycho-Pharmacology, (Brill, H., Cole, J. O., Deniker, P., Hippius, H., and Bradley, P. B., Eds.), Excerpta Medica Foundation, Publ., Amsterdam, International Congress Series No. 129.
9. Delay, J. and Deniker, P. (1969) Drug-induced extrapyramidal syndromes p. 248. In: Diseases of the Basal Ganglia (Vinken, P. J. and Bruyn, G. W., Eds.), Handbook of Clinical Neurology, Vol. 6, North-Holland Publ. Co., Amsterdam.
10. Delay, J., Deniker, P., Bourguignon, A. and Lempériére, T. (1956) Complications d'allure extrapyramidale au cours des traitements par la chlorpromazine et le serpasil. Coll. Intern. sur les Neuroleptiques, Paris, Octobre 1955. In: Encéphale, numéro spécial, 793.
11. Ehringer, H. and Hornykiewicz, O. (1960) Verteilung von Noradrenalin und Dopamin (3-Hydroxytyramin) im Gehirn des Menschen und ihr Verhalten bei Erkrankungen des extrapyramidalen Systems. Klin. Wschr. **38**, 1236.
12. Faurbye, A. (1970) The structural and biochemical basis of movement disorders in treatment with neuroleptic drugs and in extrapyramidal diseases. Comp. Psychiat. **11**, 205.
13. Gowers, W. R. A. (1901) Manual of Diseases of the Nervous System. Blakiston, Publ., Philadelphia.
14. Greenblatt, D. J., Shader, R. I. and Di Mascio, A. (1970) Extrapyramidal Effects. p. 92. In: Psychotropic Drug Effects (Shader, R. I. and Di Mascio, A., Eds.), Ch. II, Williams and Wilkins, Publ., Baltimore.

15. HAASE, H. J. (1954) Über Vorkommen und Deutung des psychomotorischen Parkinsonsyndroms bei Megaphen, bzw. Largactil-Dauerbehandlung. Nervenarzt, 25, 486.
16. HADDENBROCK, S. (1964) Hyperkinetische Dauersyndrome nach hochdosierter und Langstreckenbehandlung mit Neuroleptica. p. 54, In: Begleitwirkungen und Misserfolge der psychiatrischen Pharmakotherapie. (KRANZ, H. and HEINRICH, K., Eds.) Stuttgart: George Thieme.
17. HORNYKIEWICZ, O. (1966) Dopamine (3-hydroxytyramine) and brain function. Pharmacol. Rev. 18, 925.
18. JASPER, H. G. and TESSIER, J. (1971) Acetylcholine liberation from central cortex during paradoxial (REM) sleep. Science, 172, 601.
19. JOUVET, M. (1969) Neurophysiological and biochemical mechanisms of sleep. p. 89. In: Sleep Physiology and Pathology. (KALES, A. Ed.). Lippincott, Philadelphia.
20. JUS, K., JUS, A., VILLENEUVE, A. and VILLENEUVE, R. (1972) Etude polygraphique de l'influence de la concentration et de la motricité volontaire sur la dyskinésie tardive et le syndrome du lapin. Ann. med. Psychol. 2, 49.
21. JUS, K., VILLENEUVE, A. and JUS, A. (1972) Neuroleptic-induced tardive dyskinesia and the rabbit syndrome during different sleep stages (polygraphic studies). First Canadian International Symposium on Sleep, Montreal 14. IV. 1972 D. J. MCCLURE, Ed., Roche Scientific Service.
22. KALES, A. (1971) Sleep in patients with Parkinson's disease and normal subjects prior to and following levodopa administration. Clin. pharmacol. Ther. 12, 397.
23. KAZAMATSURI, H., CHING-PIAO CHIEN and COLE, J. O. (1972) Therapeutic approaches to tardive dyskinesia. A review of the literature. Arch. gen. Psychiat. 27, 491.
24. KAZAMATSURI, H., CHING-PIAO CHIEN and COLE, J. O. (1972) Treatment of tardive dyskinesia. I. Clinical efficacy of a dopamine-depleting agent, tetrabenazine. Arch. gen. Psychiat. 27, 95.
25. KAZAMATSURI, H., CHING-PIAO CHIEN and COLE, J. O. (1972) Treatment of tardive dyskinesia. II. Short-term efficacy of dopamine-blocking agents haloperidol and thiopropazate. Arch. gen. Psychiat. 27, 100.
26. KLAWANS, H. L. JR. (1968) The pharmacology of parkinsonism. Dis. nerv. Syst. 29, 805.
27. KLAWANS, H., JR., ILAHI, M. M. and SHENKER, D. (1970) Theoretical implications of the use of L-Dopa in Parkinsonism. Acta neutol. scand. 4, 409.
28. KLAWANS, H. L., JR. and MCKENDALL, R. R. (1971) Observations on the effect of levodopa on tardive lingual-facial-buccal-dyskinesia. J. neurol. Sci. 14, 189.
29. KURLAND, A. A. and TUREK, I. S. (1969) Persistent dyskinesias in chronically hospitalized mental patients. p. 4, In: Psychotropic Drugs and Dysfunctions of the Basal Ganglia. (Eds. CRANE, G. E. and GARDNER, R. JR.) Bethesda, NIMH., PHS Publication No. 1938.
30. POIRIER, L. J. and SOURKES, T. (1965) Influence of the substantia nigra on the catecholamine content of the striatum. Brain, 99, 181.
31. SCHÖNECKER, M. (1957) Ein eigentümliches Syndrom im oralem Bereich bei Megaphen Applikation. Nervenarzt, 28, 35.
32. SIGWALD, J., BOUTTIER, D., RAYMONDEAUD, C. and PIOT, C. (1959) Quatre cas de dyskinésie facio-bucco-linguo-masticatrice à évolution prolongée secondaires à un traitement par les neuroleptiques. Rev. Neurol. 100, 751.
33. STECK, H. (1954) Le syndrome extrapyramidal et diencéphalique au cours des traitements au Largactil et au Serpasil. Ann. Méd. Psychol. 112, 737.
34. TASSINARI, C. A., BROUGHTON, R., POIRÉ, R., ROGER, J. and GASTAUT, H. (1964) Etude électro-encéphalographique du sommeil nocturne chez les sujets présentant des mouvements anormaux. Rev. Neurol. 110, 313.
35. TASSINARI, C. A., BROUGHTON, R., POIRÉ, R., Roger, J. and GASTAUT, H. (1965) Sur l'évolution des mouvements anormaux au cours du sommeil. p. 314, In: Sommeil de Nuit Normal et Pathologique. FISCHGOLD, H. Ed., Masson Publ., Paris.
36. TASSINARI, C. A., BROUGHTON, R., ROGER, J. and GASTAUT, H. (1964) A polygraphic study of the evolution of abnormal movements during sleep. Electroenceph. clin. Neurophysiol. 17, 721.
37. UHRBRAND, L. and FAURBYE, A. (1960) Reversible and irreversible dyskinesia after treatment with perphenazine, chlorpromazine, reserpine and electroconvulsive therapy. Psychopharmacologia, 1, 408.
38. VAN ROSSUM, J. M. (1967) The significance of dopamine-receptor blockade for the action of neuroleptic drugs. p. 321, In: Neuro-Psycho-Pharmacology, (BRILL, H., COLE, J. O., DENIKER, P., HIPPIUS, H. and BRADLEY, B. P., Eds.), Amsterdam, Excerpta Medica Foundation Publ., I.C.S., No. 129.
39. VILLENEUVE, A. (1972) The rabbit syndrome. A peculiar extrapyramidal reaction. Canad. psychiat. Ass. J. 17, 69 (Suppl.).

40. VILLENEUVE, A. and BÖSZÖRMÉNYI, Z. (1970) Drug-induced dyskinesias and their treatment. Letter to the Editor. Lancet, I, 353.
41. VILLENEUVE, A., BÖSZÖRMÉNYI, Z., DESCHAMBAULT, M. and LACHANCE, R. (1970) Tentative de traitement de la dyskinésie post-neuroleptique de type permanent. Laval méd. **41**, 923.
42. VILLENEUVE, A., GAGNON, A. and DESCHAMBAULT, M. (1970) Les effets du sevrage des neuroleptiques chez les malades psychiatriques. Laval méd. **41**, 512.
43. YARYURA TOBIAS, J. A., WOLPERT, A., DANA, L. and MERLIS, S. (1970) Action of L-Dopa in drug induced extrapyramidalism. Dis. nerv. Syst. **31**, 60.

A.V., Research Division, Hôpital St-Michel-Archange,
Quebec 5, Quebec, Canada

EFFETS THÉRAPEUTIQUES ET EFFETS EXTRA-PYRAMIDAUX DES NEUROLEPTIQUES CHEZ L'HOMME

P. DENIKER et D. GINESTET

Service Hospitalo-Universitaire de Santé Mentale et de Thérapeutique, Centre Psychiatrique Ste Anne Paris

Si l'on fait un bref historique, on peut d'abord remarquer que les effets extra-pyramidaux décrits à partir de 1955 par STECK (32) sont associés à l'histoire de toutes les familles de neuroleptiques.

En 1957, J. DELAY et P. DENIKER (8) avaient inclus la détermination d'effets extrapyramidaux dans la définition même des neuroleptiques, conjointement avec l'action sur les psychoses aiguës et chroniques. Les classifications cliniques des neuroleptiques de LAMBERT (25), BOBON et coll. (4), DENIKER et GINESTET (12), introduisent également le syndrome extra-pyramidal à côté des diverses propriétés thérapeutiques ou en corrélation avec elles.

Les relations qui unissent ou qui opposent les effets thérapeutiques et les effets extra-pyramidaux chez les malades traités par les neuroleptiques ont pris le style d'une longue polémique depuis que FLÜGEL (15) eut affirmé en 1955 que les effets thérapeutiques étaient liés chez l'homme à l'importance des effets extra-pyramidaux.

Les positions doctrinales et pratiques ont oscillé de la production systématique des syndromes partinsoniens à la recherche actuelle de composés neuroleptiques qui soient le moins générateurs possible d'effets extra-pyramidaux. Il existe d'ailleurs des positions intermédiaires comme celle de HAASE (17) qui affirme que le tremblement, l'hypertonie et l'akathisie sont facultatifs, mais estime que l'hypokinésie ou l'akinésie, appréciées par l'altération de l'écriture, sont des symptômes obligatoires d'un traitement neuroleptique adéquat.

Des auteurs comme FREYHAN (16), COLE (6), BISHOP (3), TETRAULT et BORDELEAU (14) estiment qu'il n'est pas possible d'établir une corrélation entre les effets thérapeutiques et les effets neurologiques; certains comme SIMPSON (31) pensent que plus le syndrome extra-pyramidal est intense, moins il existe de chances d'améliorer le malade. 20 ans après l'introduction de la chlorpromazine, le débat est-il devenu purement académique et quelles sont les perspectives d'avenir dans la recherche de nouveaux composés neuroleptiques? Telles sont les questions que nous essayerons de discuter.

LES SYNDROMES EXTRA-PYRAMIDAUX

Les premiers signes extra-pyramidaux notés en France par THIEBAUX (34) mais systématisés par STECK (32), à propos de la chlorpromazine et de la réserpine, constituaient un tableau de parkinsonisme typique, avec akinésie, hypertonie, réalisant souvent un syndrome akinéto-hypertonique. *Remarquons cependant qu'akinésie et hypertonie ne sont pas nécessairement liées et l'akinésie est certainement le symptôme le plus remarquable*, ce manque d'initiative motrice pouvant rendre compte d'une certaine passivité des malades.

L'introduction des phénothiazines pipérazinées et des butyrophénones a permis d'individualiser un syndrome d'*hyperkinésies* et de *dyskinésies précoces* qui témoignent de l'action particulièrement puissante de certains composés neuroleptiques, phénothiazines pipérazinées ou butyrophénones. Tremblement, frissonnement, réactions de sursaut apparaissent avec les neuroleptiques puissants; parmi les dyskinésies précoces, les crises oculogyres et les contractions linguales, les torticolis évoquent la sémiologie des séquelles de l'encéphalite léthargique avec, d'ailleurs, la même sensibilité à la suggestion et aux émotions. Ces hyperkinésies peuvent être durables, semi-permanentes et caractérisées par l'akathisie (impossibilité de rester assis), la tasikinésie (tendance au mouvement), entraînant insomnie, impatiences et même sub-excitation anxieuse.

Plus particuliers aux butyrophénones, apparaissent les *syndromes dysesthésiques*, que Divry et Bobon (13) en 1959 avaient isolés sous le nom de „neuro-dyslepsie": cette sensibilité douloureuse était associée dans l'esprit des auteurs au syndrome excito-moteur.

Egalement à partir de 1959 ont été observées des *dyskinésies tardives*, mouvement chéiro-oraux, mouvements de type choréo-athétosique au niveau des extrémités: Sigwald et Bouttier (30) en France, Uhrband et Faurbye (35) au Danemark, Degwitz (7) en Allemagne, Hollister (19) aux U.S.A. ont étudié la fréquence et les caractéristiques sémiologiques de ces dyskinésies qui peuvent apparaître soit à la suppression du traitement, soit au cours de traitements prolongés avec la plupart des neuroleptiques. A. Vil-

Tableau 1

Les grands syndromes neurologiques créés par les neuroleptiques

Syndromes parkinsoniens	Steck	(1955)
Syndromes hyperkinétiques	Delay et Deniker	(1957)
Syndromes dysesthésiques	Divry et Bobon	(1959)
Dyskinésies tardives	Sigwald	(1959)
	Uhrband et Faurbye	(1960)

Tableau 2

Parallelisme entre les phenomènes neurologiques et les modifications psychiques induites par les neuroleptiques

Phenomènes somatiques	Phenomènes psychiques
Syndromes neurovégétatifs	Somnolence
Syndromes akinétiques	Indifférence, asthénie
Syndromes parkinsoniens	Tendance dépressive
Hyperkinésies paroxystiques	Suggestibilité, angoisse
Hyperkinésies permanentes	Insomnie, impatience, turbulence
Dyskinésies tardives	Souvent méconnues par le malade (anosognosie)

LENEUVE (36) a isolé récemment un syndrome du lapin ("rabbit-syndrom"), constitué par des mouvements rapides et incessants de la bouche rappelant ceux de ce rongeur. En dehors de la plus grande sensibilité des femmes aux neuroleptiques, le rôle des traitements antérieurs ou celui de la maladie n'est pas évident (18).

Nous avons présenté dans le Tableau 1 les principaux syndromes extra-pyramidaux et dans le Tableau 2 leurs corrélations psychologiques.

Enfin, nous mettrons à part les syndromes neurovégétatifs: non pas le syndrome neurovégétatif habituel simple fait d'hypotension et de tachycardie surtout avec les phénothiazines, mais le *syndrome neuro-végétatif malin* traduisant un dérèglement central, avec hyperthermie et sur le plan neurologique une aggravation de l'akinésie avec adynamie: l'issue peut-être mortelle si le traitement neuroleptique n'est pas arrêté.

L'APPORT THÉRAPEUTIQUE DES MANIFESTATIONS EXTRA-PYRAMIDALES

Le *syndrome akinétique*, sur le plan moteur, est un élément que l'on peut rechercher systématiquement dans les cas d'agitation: associé à sa corrélation psychologique, indifférence émotionnelle et neutralité affective, il est bénéfique dans ces cas où prédominent l'angoisse de dépersonnalisation ou l'exaltation maniaque. Ce syndrome akinétique, joint à l'hypertonie, se conjugue aux propriétés sédatives: il constitue l'un des avantages reconnu des neuroleptiques sur d'autres thérapeutiques, comme par exemple, le carbonate de lithium dans les états d'agitation (22). Les critiques n'ont pas manqué à l'encontre de cette „camisole chimique" qui aurait remplacé les camisoles de force, mais il faut bien remarquer que même les détracteurs de ces techniques chimiothérapiques ne dédaignent pas les utiliser en cas de nécessité.

Les phénomènes hyperkinétique, les dyskinésies précoces et les crises dysesthésiques sont souvent révélatrices de l'action originale d'un neuroleptique, action psycho-stimulante ou désinhibitrice, particulièrement intéressante dans les évolutions déficitaires, athymhormiques des schizophrénies. Il est certain que le malade éprouve une mise en question de son équilibre physique et psychique: nous avons insisté avec C. CONTE (11) sur la signification psychodynamique de ces modifications qui permettent d'entamer une relation psychothérapique au long cours.

A la faveur de ces crises spectaculaires de début de traitement qui se passent souvent en présence du personnel soignant, peuvent être réactivés des moments psychotiques anciens et des situations traumatisantes. Il n'est pas rare non plus que s'extériorisent alors des contenus hallucinatoires ou délirants jusqu'alors dissimulés par la réticence. DENBER (10) a bien étudié cette valeur symbolique de l'akathisie considérée comme une négation de la mort et une sorte de réassurance. Ces modifications motrices, associées aux troubles dysesthésiques, aboutissent à créer des moments féconds et des expériences plus ou moins brèves assez comparables à celles qui sont induites par des substances psycho-dysleptiques. Il nous semble que les hyperkinésies s'avèrent plus fréquentes lors d'une schizophrénie récente ou évolutive, alors que ce syndrome excito-moteur est plus rarement observé avec d'ailleurs des résultats thérapeutiques moins satisfaisants dans les schizophrénies chroniques. Cette relative valeur pronostique d'une sensibilité neurologique aux traitements est sans doute à rapprocher des constatations faites par ITIL (21) entre les corrélations électro-encéphalographiques, l'activité neuroleptique et l'évolution de la maladie.

Le bilan négatif des troubles extra-pyramidaux par rapport à l'activité thérapeutique

Nous commencerons par le problème difficile des *dyskinésies tardives*. Il faut constater que bien souvent elles sont méconnues par le malade, entraînant une véritable anosognosie du trouble, malgré l'éventuelle intensité du syndrome bucco-lingual ou de l'instabilité motrice produite par les mouvements choréiques. Les dyskinésies ne paraissent pas s'accompagner d'un état psychique particulier et elles peuvent survenir chez des malades souvent considérablement améliorés sur le plan psychique. Elles deviennent précisément gênantes au moment d'une reprise d'activité sociale entravée par la présentation grimaçante ou gesticulante de ces malades. Si ces dyskinésies ne paraissent pas avoir une incidence particulière quant à l'activité thérapeutique, elles n'en soulèvent pas moins la grave question de la création de lésions qui pourraient être définitives au niveau du névraxe, bien que les études conduites à ce sujet ne soient pas concluantes (20).

Le *syndrome malin* est une complication rare, sinon exceptionnelle, du traitement neuroleptique et il commande naturellement l'arrêt immédiat de la thérapeutique. Sa signification paraît liée à un désordre diencéphalique grave dont l'expression psychique est constituée par l'apparition d'un état d'hébétude et de torpeur. A l'autopsie, il a été observé des atelectasies pulmonaires que l'on peut rapprocher de celles qui avaient été décrites après les issues mortelles dues à l'encéphalite épidémique de 1918.

Nous nous attarderons davantage sur les manifestations du parkinsonisme dont la signification, comme nous l'avons remarqué plus haut, n'est pas univoque. Le *syndrome akinéto-hypertonique*, dont nous avons vu précédemment l'intérêt qu'il présentait dans les cas d'agitation, peut devenir à la longue un élément péjoratif, surtout dans les formes déficitaires de la schizophrénie, aggravant une athymie et enfermant davantage le malade dans son autisme. On a associé le syndrome akinéto-hypertonique au „*syndrome de passivité*", décrit par BALVET en 1959 (2): cet auteur faisait lui-même la part de ce qui revient à la maladie propre, dépouillée de ses manifestations productives hallucinatoires ou délirantes et de ce qui revient à l'action du neuroleptique.

On peut être également tenté de rapprocher le syndrome akinéto-hypertonique, entraîné par les neuroleptiques, du *syndrome dépressif* qui s'observe après quelques semaines ou quelques mois d'un traitement neuroleptique régulier: nous l'avions noté en 1958 avec l'emploi de la thiopropérazine. En 1959, AZIMA (1) avait insisté sur les modifications thymiques induites par les neuroleptiques et la transformation des structures schizophréniques en une structure d'allure maniaco-dépressive. Notre propre expérience avec PERON-MAGNAN, celle de SCHNETZLER, de LAMBERT et MIDENET, confirment ce point de vue. Nous savons que la pathogénie de cette dépression n'est pas univoque, soit liée directement à l'action pharmacologique neuroleptique (réserpine, halopéridol), soit témoignant d'un remaniement psychodynamique d'ailleurs souhaitable face aux réalités qui apparaissent au malade.

Bien que les neuroleptiques exercent une action favorable sur la *catatonie*, les rapports entre les poussées évolutives catatoniques et l'aptitude cataleptigène des neuroleptiques sont parfois difficiles à préciser (27).

Les *manifestations excito-motrices précoces*, le *syndrome akathisique* dont nous avons vu qu'il pouvait être un auxiliaire thérapeutique, constituent dans d'autres cas un obstacle à l'objectif thérapeutique: nous avons souligné le réveil de l'angoisse qu'il pouvait déterminer et l'aggravation d'un syndrome de dépersonnalisation. On devra conserver à l'esprit la surveillance nécessaire chez ces malades, surtout au début de la schizophrénie dont la propension suicidaire peut être stimulée. KAMMERER (23), en France, a étudié les correspondances phénoménologiques qui existent entre ces syndromes akathisiques et certaines évolutions hypochondriaques ou certaines évolutions d'allure maniaque avec hyperactivité stérile et angoissée.

Médicaments antiparkinsoniens et effet thérapeutique

Malgré plus de 20 ans de pratique et de recherche, à propos des neuroleptiques et des correcteurs des effets extra-pyramidaux, un certain nombre de points sont encore loins d'être éclaircis. Il existe en particulier peu de travaux qui aient étudié l'influence de médicaments antiparkinsoniens associés sur l'efficacité du traitement neuroleptique. Citons le travail de Kurland et Hallon (24) qui n'a pas observé une sensible différence dans les résultats thérapeutiques entre le groupe de malades traités par la perphénazine seule et un autre groupe de malades traités par l'association de perphénazine et de benztropine. Dans le même ordre d'idées, on peut remarquer que bien souvent les médicaments anti-parkinsoniens, prescrits au début d'un traitement, associés aux neuroleptiques, ne sont plus indispensables par la suite. Une étude de Orlov, Di Mascio et J. Cole (26) semble démontrer que, après trois mois de l'administration d'un médicament antiparkinsonien, celui-ci devient inutile et que 95% des patients à qui il était administré, n'en éprouvent plus le besoin.

Les études de Saint-Jean (29), de Cahan et de Parrish (5) vont dans le même sens. Ce fait est d'autant plus remarquable que l'action thérapeutique des neuroleptiques, contrairement aux effets secondaires, n'a pas tendance à s'épuiser comme le rappelait récemment Lambert.

Effets extra-pyramidaux et effets thérapeutiques dans les nouvelles familles de neuroleptiques

Une nouvelle présentation de neuroleptiques déjà connus, les neuroleptiques d'action prolongée, obtenus à partir de la fluphénazine (œnanthate et décanoate) permet de constater à la fois leurs propriétés thérapeutiques et la détermination d'effets neurologiques de fréquence au moins comparable à celle des produits standards. Il en va de même de neuroleptiques d'action prolongée plus récents, comme les sels de pipothiazine (19.551 RP et 19.552 RP). Cependant, l'ensemble des neuroleptiques proposés depuis dix ans possède une tolérance relativement bonne sur le plan extra-pyramidal sans toutefois une totale absence de syndromes neurologiques: c'est le cas notamment des phénothiazines comme la propériciazine (Neuleptil), de l'oxaflumazine (Oxaflumine) ou de dérivés de la dibenzothiazépine (Etumine).

Tableau 3

Nouveaux groupes de neuroleptiques reputés actifs, avec une faible incidence d'effets extra-pyramidaux

Dérivés des thioxanthènes	Thiothixène (Navane) Flupenthixol (Emergil)
Dérivés des benzamides	Sulpiride (Dogmatil)
Dérivés des di-phényl-butyl-pipéridines	Pimozide (Opiran — Orap 4)
Derivés des diazépines	Clozapine

Nous examinerons plus particulièrement le cas des formules nouvelles, réputées actives et ne provoquant que des effets extra-pyramidaux modérés, que nous avons réunies dans le Tableau 3.

Un dérivé des diphénylbutylpipéridines, le pimozide, est considéré plutôt comme un neuroleptique de relais pour un traitement au long cours, alors que ses indications dans les psychoses aiguës ou les phases évolutives des schizophrénies paraissent plus limitées.

Nous n'avons pas utilisé un dérivé du tryptophane, l'oxypertine (Equipertine) mais si les auteurs s'accordent pour reconnaître la rareté des effets extra-pyramidaux observés le choix des indications proposées rend compte de l'incertitude qui persiste sur le champ thérapeutique du produit.

Nos essais cliniques avec un dérivé récent des thioxanthènes, le thiothixène (Navane), nous ont montré qu'à côté d'une tolérance neurologique bonne, l'effet antipsychotique était aléatoire et s'épuisait rapidement.

Nous avons également utilisé des dérivés de la di-chloro-benzo-oxazépine (LW. 3170) ou des diazépines (LW. 1854 ou clozapine et LW. 2333). La clozapine est pour STILLE et HIPPIUS (33) un neuroleptique particulièrement intéressant. Notre expérience est restreinte ; l'action thérapeutique a été appréciable notamment sur le plan sédatif avec réduction de l'anxiété, voire euphorie, mais si les effets extra-pyramidaux n'ont pas été très importants, notre essai clinique a été interrompu par des complications d'allure centrale: deux cas de hypothermie, hyperthermie pouvant faire redouter un syndrome malin avec le LW. 3170; une crise convulsive et des malaises orthostatiques très marqués pour la clozapine. Le LW. 2333 qui ne détermine pas d'effets extra-pyramidaux, possède seulement une action sédative de type tranquillisant.

Le sulpiride (Dogmatil) dont on connaît le très large champ des indications, ne paraît pas non plus un neuroleptique dont la situation soit clairement définie sur la plan des actions thérapeutiques. Il semble s'agir essentiellement d'un neuroleptique psycho-stimulant et désinhibiteur assez voisin du thiothixène ou de phénothiazines pipérazinées et de butyrophénones comme le tripéridol, dans les schizophrénies déficitaires. De toute façon, le traitement par sulpiride s'accompagne d'une fréquence plus grande qu'on ne le dit de phénomènes extra-pyramidaux, en particulier de dyskinésies précoces, qui nous paraissent corrélées avec son action psycho-stimulante. D'autre part, comme la thioridazine, le sulpiride semble avoir un point d'impact neuro-endocrinien, ce dont rendent compte les nombreuses galactorrhées observées chez les sujets traités, hommes ou femmes, et les aménorrhées qui ont fait recommander par certains auteurs ce produit comme anti-conceptionnel.

On peut donc considérer que depuis 10 ans, les progrès en matière de neuroleptiques ont porté sur des produits stimulants mais leur action n'apparaît pas décisive par rapport à certaines phénothiazines pipérazinées connues depuis 1957 (prochlorpérazine, thiopropérazine) ou à certaines butyrophénones comme le triflupéridol. L'incidence des effets secondaires neurologiques a certes diminué mais, en contrepartie, des effets neuro-endocriniens ou diencéphaliques (dysrégulation des centres thermiques) apparaissent plus fréquents.

DISCUSSION ET CONCLUSION

Nous sommes frappés une fois encore du fait que des produits de structures chimiques très différentes, comme les phénothiazines, les butyrophénones, les réserpiniques, les dérivés des diazépines, les dérivés des benzamides, aient en commun, d'une part des propriétés thérapeutiques dans les psychoses aiguës et chroniques et, d'autre part, la production de syndromes parkinsoniens. Il faut bien reconnaître que, jusqu'à ce jour, tous les produits qui ont eu une action thérapeutique dans les psychoses, hormis le cas très particulier du lithium actif dans la seule psychose maniaco-dépressive, déterminent des effets extra-pyramidaux.

Nous avons souligné au passage que ces effets neurologiques: syndromes parkinsoniens, syndromes dyskinétiques, s'accompagnaient d'un état psychologique particulier et, d'autre part, permettaient sur le plan thérapeutique de prévoir le type d'action du neuroleptique: action prévalente dans les états d'agitation ou, au contraire, corrélation avec une action psycho-stimulante. Les médicaments qui possèdent des propriétés anti-délirantes ou anti-hallucinatoires majeures, comme l'halopéridol ou la fluphénazine, déterminent des syndromes neurologiques patents. Par contre, des neuroleptiques classiques comme la thioridazine ou des formes nouvelles comme les dérivés des thioxanthènes ou du benzamide, peu producteur d'effets extrapyramidaux, apparaissent moins puissants sur le plan thérapeutique; il faut remarquer, en outre, que parmi ces neuroleptiques beaucoup se signalent par une incidence d'effets diencéphaliques et neuro-endocriniens particulièrement nette.

Il n'est pas dans notre intention de soutenir que la recherche psychopharmacologique doive se cantonner dans la perspective de découvrir des produits anti-psychotiques, avec un obligatoire tropisme neurologique: on peut souhaiter au contraire qu'à puissance égale ou supérieure ces substances soient les moins perturbantes possible sur le plan extra-pyramidal, sans contrepartie endocrinienne ou végétative.

Sera-t-il possible de découvrir un jour le neuroleptique idéal à qui il manquera précisément un terme de sa définition, les déterminations neurologiques?

Pour l'instant, nous considérons que l'action des neuroleptiques engendre un processus thérapeutique global dont le clinicien doit tirer le meilleur parti possible grâce à une surveillance quotidienne des effets bénéfiques et adverses.

BIBLIOGRAPHIE

1. Azima, M. (1959) Changes in organisation of mood as a therapeutic and research problem in psychopharmacology. In: Neuropsychopharmacology, p. 491. Elsevier Edit., Amsterdam.
2. Balvet, P. (1959) Les comportements de passivité au cours de la chimiothérapie des psychoses (1959) J. Méd. Lyon, 129.
3. Bishop, M. P., Gallant, D. M. et Sykes, T. F. (1965) Extrapyramidal side effects and therapeutic response. Arch. gen. Psychiat., **13**, 155.
4. Bobon, J., Pinchard, A., Collard, J. et Bobon, D. P. (1972) Clinical classification of neuroleptics, with special reference to their antimanic, antiautistic and ataraxic properties. Comprehens. Psychiat. **13**, 123.
5. Cahan, R. B. et Parrish, D. D. (1960) Reversibility of drug induced parkinsonism. Amer. J. Psychiat. **116**, 1022.
6. Cole, J. O. et Clyde, D. J. (1961) Extrapyramidal side effects and clinical response to phenothiazines. In: Bordeleau (J. M.) réd. "Systéme extrapyramidal et neurcleptiques", p. 469. Edit. Psych. Montréal.
7. Degwitz, R. et Luxenburger, O. (1965) Das terminale extrapyramidale Insuffizienz bzw. Defekt Syndrom infolge chronischer Answendung von Neuroleptica. Nervenarzt, **36**, 173.
8. Delay, J. et Deniker, P. (1957) Caratéristiques psychophysiologiques des médicaments neuroleptiques. Psychotropic Drugs, p. 481. Elsevier Edit., Amsterdam.
9. Delay, J. et Deniker, P. (1968) Drug induced extrapyramidal syndromes. In: Handbook of Clinical Neurology, vol. 6, p. 248. North Holland Publish. Company, Amsterdam.
10. Denber, H. C. B. (1961) Psychodynamic effects of drug induced extrapyramidal reaction on ward social structure. In: Bordeleau, J. M. réd. "Système extrapyramidal et neuroleptiques". p. 535, Edit. Psych. Montréal.
11. Deniker, P. et Conte, C. (1967) Effets secondaires et processus thérapeutique. Proceedings of the Vth Congress of C.I.N.P., p. 650. Excerpta Med. Edit., Amsterdam.
12. Deniker, P. et Ginestet, D. (1971) Les neuroleptiques. p. 170. In: Psychopharmacologie — sous la direction de J. M. Sutter Litec Edit., Paris 1971.

13. DIVRY, P., BOBON, J., COLLARD, J., PINCHARD, A. et NOIS, E. (1959) Etude et expérimentation cliniques du R. 1625 ou halopéridol, nouveau neuroleptique et "neurodysleptique" Acta Neurol. Belg. **59**, 337.
14. FILOTTO, J., BORDELEAU, J. M. et TETRAULT, L. (1969) Corrélations entre les propriétés antipsychotiques et les propriétés extrapyramidales des neuroleptiques. Union Méd. du Canada, **98**, 562.
15. FLÜGEL, F. (1956) Thérapeutiques par médication neuroleptique obtenue en réalisant systématiquement des états parkinsoniens. Coll. Intern. sur les Neuroleptiques — Paris, oct. 1955. Encéphale, N° spécial, 720, Doin Edit.
16. FREYHAN, F. (1961) The relationship of drug induced neurological phenomena on therapeutic outcome. In: BORDELEAU (J. M.) réd. "Système extrapyramidal et neuroleptiques", p. 483. Edit. Psych., Montréal.
17. HAASE, H. J. (1954) Über Vorkommen und Deutung des psychomotorisches Parkinson Syndroms bei Megaphen — bzw. Largactil Dauerbehandlung. Nervenarzt, **25**, 486.
18. HEINRICH, K., WEGENER, J. et BENDER, H. J. (1968) Späte extrapyramidale Hyperkinesien bei neuroleptischer Langzeittherapie. Pharmakopsych. Neuro-Psychopharmakol. **3**, 169.
19. HOLLISTER, L. E. (1964) Adverse reactions to phenothiazines. J. Amer. med. Ass. **189**, 311.
20. HUNTER, R., BLACKWOOD, W., SMITH, M. L. and CUMINGS, J. N. (1968) Neuropathological findings in three cases of persistent dyskinesia following phenothiazine medication. J. Neurol. Sci. **7**, 263.
21. ITIL, T. M. (1968) Electroencepalography and pharmacology. Mod. Probl. Pharmacopsychiat., Vol. 1, p. 163. Karger Edit., Basel, New-York.
22. JOHNSSON, G., GERSHON, S. et HEKIMIAN, L. (1968) Controlled evaluation of lithium and chlorpromazine in the treatment of manic states. An interim report. Comp. Psychiat. **9**, 563.
23. KAMMERER, TH., EBTINGER, R. et BAUER, J. P. (1965) Approche phénoménologique et psychodynamiques des psychoses délirantes aiguës traitées par les neuroleptiques majeurs. In: La relation Médecin-Malade au cours des chimiothérapies psychiatriques, p. 17, Masson Edit., Paris.
24. KURLAND, A. A. et HANLON, T. E. (1971) The use of psychotropic drug combinations. Comments and observations. Pharmakopsych. Neuropsychopharmakologie, **4**, 297.
25. LAMBERT, P. A., PERRIN, J., REVOL, L., ACHAINTRE, A., BALVET, P., BEAUJARD, M., BERTHIER, C., BROUSSOLLE, P. et REQUET, A. (1959) Essai de classification des neuroleptiques d'après leurs activités psychopharmacologiques et cliniques. Réunion Intern. de Neuro-Psycho-Pharmacol., Rome 1958, p. 619, Elsevier Edit., 1959.
26. ORLOV, P., KASPARIAN, G., DI MASCIO, A. et COLE, J. O. (1971) Withdrawal of antiparkinsonian drugs. Arch. gen. Psychiat. **25**, 410.
27. OSTAPTZEFF, M. et OSTAPTZEFF-LAVOINE, M. (1970) Catatonie et syndrome extrapyramidal. Ann. méd. Psychol. **128**, 256.
28. PRIEN, R. F., CAFFEY, E. M. et KLETT, C. J. (1971) A comparison of lithium carbonate and chlorpromazine in the treatment of manic. Corporative studies in psychiatry. Report of the Veteran Administration NIMH.
29. SAINT-JEAN, A., DONALD, M. et BAN, J. A. (1964) Interchangeability of antiparkinson medication. Amer. J. Psychiat. **121**, 1189.
30. SIGWALD, J., BOUTTIER, D., RAYMONDEAU, C. et PIOT CL. (1959) Quatre cas de dyskinésies facio-bucco-linguo-masticatrices à évolution prolongée secondaire à un traitement par les neuroleptiques. Rev. Neurol. **100**, 751.
31. SIMPSON, G. M., AMUSO, D., BLAIR, J. et FARKER, T. (1964) Phenothiazine produced extrapyramidal system disturbance. Arch. gen. Psychiat. **10**, 199.
32. STECK, H. (1956) Le syndrome extrapyramidal dans les cures de chlorpromazine et Serpasil. Sa symptomatologie clinique et son rôle thérapeutique. Coll. Intern. sur les Neuroleptiques, Paris 1955. Encéphale, N° spécial, p. 777. Doin Edit.
33. STILLE, G. et HIPPIUS, H. (1971) Kritische Stellungnahme zum Begriff des Neuroleptica (Anhand von pharmakologischen und klinischen Befunden mit clozapin). Pharmakopsychiat. **4**, 182.
34. THIEBAUX, M., THIEBAUX, R., BOYER, R., LEBORGNE, F. et KIFFEL, M. (1954) Note sur l'apparition de troubles extrapyramidaux au cours du traitement par le 4560 RP. Ann. méd. Psychol. **112**, 732.
35. UHRBAND, L. et FAURBYE, A. (1960) Reversible and irreversible dyskinesia after treatment with perphenazine, chlorpromazine, reserpine and electro-convulsive-therapy. Psychopharmacologia, **1**, 408.
36. VILLENEUVE, A.: The rabbit syndrom, a peculiar extrapyramidal reaction. A paraître in Can. méd. Ass. J.

P.D., Service Hospitalo-Universitaire de Santé Mentale et de Thérapeutique, Centre Psychiatrique Ste Anne, 1 rue Cabanis, Paris 14e, France

DRUGS FOR TREATMENT OF SEXUAL DISORDERS

Chairmen: G. L. Gessa, U. Laschet and C. Kordon

Associate chairman: S. Rasmussen

ROLE OF BRAIN MONOAMINES IN CONTROLLING SEXUAL BEHAVIOR IN MALE ANIMALS

G. L. GESSA and A. TAGLIAMONTE

Institute of Pharmacology, University of Cagliari

Two recent findings, the aphrodisiac effect of *p*-chlorophenylalanine (PCPA) in animals and L-dihydroxyphenylalanine (L-DOPA) in humans, have stimulated a large number of studies concerning the possible role of brain monoamines in controlling the sexual behavior in male animals. In addition, the consideration that PCPA depletes rather selectively brain serotonin (5-HT) and that L-DOPA is the precursor of catecholamines supports the idea (58) that brain 5-HT inhibits and catecholamines stimulate the sexual activity in male animals.

In this article, we shall review the literature and report our more recent findings concerning the role of monoamines on the sexual behavior in male animals.

EFFECT OF RESERPINE AND TETRABENAZINE ON MALE SEXUAL BEHAVIOR

Indirect evidence that monoamines play a role in controlling sexual behavior of male animals is suggested by the experiments of SOULAIRAC et al. (56) and DEWSBURY (15, 16) showing that the administration of reserpine or tetrabenazine facilitates the copulatory behavior of male rats. This effect is interesting because this facilitation was found to be specific to one aspect of the total copulatory pattern: i.e. these drugs decrease the number of intromissions required to attain ejaculation.

These data led to the hypothesis that a partial reduction of brain monoamines produces facilitation of copulatory behavior. Reserpine, tetrabenazine and other benzoquinolizines deplete both brain serotonin and catecholamines; moreover, they do not reduce monoamine synthesis (25, 60). Therefore, it is difficult to relate their effect on the copulatory behavior to the depletion of one or another monoamine or even to the flow of a free, newly synthesized monoamine (serotonin) onto receptors (11). High doses of reserpine or tetrabenazine suppress copulatory behavior, but this inhibition might be the unspecific consequence of their sedative effect.

Effect of PCPA on male sexual behavior

PCPA inhibits rather selectively serotonin synthesis by blocking tryptophan hydroxylase (33). The finding that the depletion of brain serotonin causes hypersexuality indicates a possible physiological role of brain serotonin, that of inhibiting sexual behavior in male animals.

Since PCPA is the first drug known to induce hypersexuality in male animals, a definition of what we consider as PCPA-induced hypersexuality is needed.

The administration of PCPA to adult male rats produces:

1. Homosexual mounting behavior: i.e. male to male mounting behavior in conditions when this behavior does not occur in untreated animals and/or in a percentage of animals significantly greater than in controls (52, 53, 58).

2. Mounting behavior on non-receptive females: PCPA treated rats violently and persistently struggle to mount non-receptive females, indicating that PCPA increases the sexual drive (22).

3. PCPA increases heterosexual copulatory behavior: that is treatment with PCPA increases the percentage of animals copulating and ejaculating in respect to control animals (57).

These effects indicate that PCPA is a true aphrodisiac (23) and that 1. and 2. do not originate from the fact that PCPA alters the male's ability to adequately distinguish appropriate sexual partners (64).

A stimulatory effect of PCPA on heterosexual copulatory behavior can be observed provided the level of sexual activity of the animals is not already maximal prior to the administration of the drug (38, 57).

Thus, we have shown that PCPA increases the percentage of male rats copulating and ejaculating, when the experimental subjects were chosen among sexually sluggish animals (57). In addition, Meyerson could demonstrate a stimulatory effect of PCPA on the copulatory behavior of male rats by using castrated rats treated with subliminar doses of testosterone (38). Moreover, Mitler et al. showed that PCPA increases the number of ejaculations in rats of low baseline sexual activity (41). Finally, Singer (55) has observed that PCPA increases the male sexual behavior of testosterone injected female rats (i.e. anogenital explorations, mounts, thrusts and intromissive patterns), but did not affect the female sexual behavior (lordosis). Thus, the aphrodisiac effect of PCPA is not limited to males. The lack of increase in female behavior, however, also suggests that the increase in sexual arousal is limited only to the male behavior patterns.

Evidence that brain serotonin has an inhibitory role on male sexual behavior

Crucial importance is held by the question whether the effect of PCPA on sexual behavior is the consequence of the depletion of brain serotonin.

The principal arguments supporting such a mechanism are the following:

a) In rats and rabbits, there is a temporal correlation between the maximal depletion of brain serotonin by PCPA and the occurrence of hypersexuality (45, 58).

b) Selective destruction of serotoninergic nerve endings produced by 5,6-dihydroxytryptamine (5,6-DHT), administered in the lateral ventricle causes long lasting homosexual mounting behavior in male rats (14).

c) Homosexual behavior was observed in male rats with different serotonin antagonists such as methysergide, mesorgydine and WA-335-BS in combination with testosterone (4).

d) The homosexual behavior induced by PCPA or by 5,6-DHT is abolished by L-5-hydroxytryptophan (5-HTP), the direct precursor of serotonin (14, 53, 58).

The administration of 5-HTP not only abolishes PCPA-induced hypersexuality (53, 58), but also suppresses the copulatory behavior of normal rats exposed to receptive females. This effect is potentiated by Ro4-4602, a peripherally acting decarboxylase inhibitor (Table 1). Therefore, the blockade by 5-HTP has a central origin.

TABLE 1

Inhibition by L-5-hydroxytryptophan of homo- and heterosexual behavior in normal and in PCPA-treated male rats

	% males mounting other males			% males copulating with females		
	Controls	5-HTP	Ro4-4602 + 5-HTP	Controls	5-HTP	Ro4-4602 + 5-HTP
Normal rats	28	12	0	100	32	12
PCPA-rats	80	16	0	100	40	0

Groups of 25 male sexually experienced rats each.

Different monoamineoxidase inhibitors (MAOI) such as pargyline, phenelzin, iproniazide, suppress the copulatory behavior in normal rats with receptive females (17, 57). This effect is prevented by PCPA, indicating that the inhibition is secondary to the accumulation of brain 5-HT (57).

These latter results might provide a biochemical explanation to the frigidity and impotence produced by MAOI in male patients (50).

The above data strongly suggest that brain serotonin has an inhibitory role on sexual behavior in male animals. It was, therefore, surprising to find out that the administration of L-tryptophan, which increases brain serotonin synthesis, did not inhibit the copulatory behavior of normal male rats (Table 2).

TABLE 2

Failure of L-tryptophan (Try) to inhibit heterosexual behavior in male rats

Try mg/kg	hrs. before test	% males ejaculating
0	—	100
150	1	100
150 × 6	10, 8, 6, 4, 2, 1	100

Groups of 25 rats each which were male sexually experienced rats exposed to female rats in oestrus.

The data reported in Table 3 might provide an explanation for these apparently contradictory results. Following 5-HTP administration, serotonin and 5-HIAA accumulated in the rat brain to a much greater extent than after L-tryptophan, suggesting that the concentration of serotonin needed to inhibit heterosexual mounting behavior is very high.

This hypothesis might also explain the time-course of the inhibitory effect of MAOI on mounting behavior.

The inhibitory effect of pargyline and iproniazide is present from 8 to 24 hours after drug administration, when brain serotonin levels are maximally increased to about 197% the normal values. On the other hand, the inhibition is not present 72 hours after treatment, when brain serotonin levels are 72% above the normal values (Table 3).

TABLE 3

Effect of L-tryptophan, 5-HTP and pargyline on brain serotonin metabolism in male rats

Treatment	mg/kg i. p.	hrs. before sacrifice	Try $\mu g/g$	5-HT $\mu g/g$	5-HIAA $\mu g/g$	Inhibition of sexual behavior
None	—	—	5.48 ± .07	0.61 ± .03	0.54 ± .04	
5-HTP	50	0.5	4.81 ± .12	1.59 ± .08	2.36 ± .11	Yes
Ro4-4602 + 5-HTP	50 + 50	1 — 0.5	4.36 ± .09	1.36 ± .07	2.13 ± .08	Yes
Try	150	1	20.31 ± .89	0.73 ± .03	1.25 ± .06	No
Try	150 × 6	10-8-6-4-2-1	25.15 ± .65	0.78 ± .05	1.31 ± .06	No
Pargyline	80	18	5.21 ± .08	1.83 ± .06	0.09 ± .01	Yes
Pargyline	80	72	4.98 ± .05	1.05 ± .05	0.25 ± .02	No

Each value is the average ± S.E. of at least 6 determinations.

In conclusion, the data presented suggest that a depletion of brain 5-HT produces hypersexuality. However, this amine inhibits the heterosexual mounting behavior in normal male animals only when its concentration in brain is above a certain critical level.

Moreover, the results of the above mentioned studies of SINGER (55) imply that brain serotonin may also play an inhibitory role on the masculine sexual behavior of female rats, indicating that the biochemical process involved in this behavior is similar to that involved in the sexual behavior of male rats. On the other hand, in constrast to the hypothesis of MEYERSON (40) that brain serotonin inhibits receptivity in female rats, SEGAL and WHALEN (51) and SINGER (55) found no increase in female sexual behavior after PCPA.

SPECIES DIFFERENCES IN THE EFFECT OF PCPA

PCPA stimulates the homosexual mounting behavior not only in rats, but also in rabbits (45) and in cats (19, 28). However, ZITRIN et al. (67) failed to observe heightened sexual interest after PCPA in male cats, whose baseline sexual activity was already maximal before treatment. These results indicate that neither in cats does the drug enhance maximal performance.

The effect of PCPA in humans has been studied in low doses or in disease states (12, 13), which might have prevented adequate serotonin depletion or made the interpretation difficult.

We found (unpublished observations) no increase in homosexual mounting behavior in adult male mice treated with PCPA up to a dose of 300 mg/kg i.p. The lack of effect of

PCPA in mice might be due to the fact that the drug depletes in this species both brain serotonin and catecholamines to about the same extent (63).

In primates (Machaca speciosa), REDMOND et al. failed to observe increase in mountings, sexual presentations and copulations after PCPA (46). However, although great care was taken by these authors to keep "half of the observers in their experiments blind with respect to the behavioral hypothesis under investigation", their animals were housed in groups of mixed sex and observed for one hour daily, so that changes in social interactions might have occurred during the remaining 23 hours.

It is pertinent at this point to stress the importance of optimal conditions to observe the sexual stimulant effect of PCPA:

1. isolation of the animals during PCPA treatment;
2. a dosage of PCPA for depleting brain serotonin selectively (100 mg/kg body weight, intraperitoneally, daily for 3 to 5 days — too high a dosage may also affect chatecholamine stores);
3. testing for sexual stimulation should be done during the dark phase of the 24-hour cycle.

Pattern of copulatory behavior after PCPA

PCPA facilitates most aspects of the copulatory pattern. After PCPA ejaculations were attained sooner and after fewer mounts and intromissions and the refractory periods after ejaculations were shorter (48). A shortening of the ejaculation latency in male rats has been reported also by AHLENIUS et al. (1) and by MITLER et al. (41). It is interesting to note that reserpine in low doses also shortens the ejaculatory latency (15, 56), suggesting that this effect is mediated by the serotonin depletion.

It is striking that a single injection of reserpine or PCPA to the newborn male rat results in the same effect on the copulatory behavior in the adult animal as the acute administration of these drugs to the adult rat (29, 36): i.e. a reduction in the ejaculation latency. Although it is difficult to explain the delayed effect of reserpine and PCPA, rats presenting this ejaculatio precox might be a useful experimental model of the same defect occurring in man.

Role of hormones in the PCPA effect

Pineal gland — Several studies have suggested that indole hormones of the pineal gland exert an inhibitory effect on ovarian (66) and testicular (20, 59) growth and decrease estrus in female rats (39, 65). *p*-Chlorophenylalanine is known to inhibit serotonin synthesis in the pineal gland resulting in decreased formation of 5-methoxyindole hormones (44). We therefore carried out studies with PCPA in male pinealectomized rats (Sprague-Dawley rats weighing 250 to 300 g, 80 to 90 days of age, pinealectomized 1 to 4 weeks previously). No episodes of sexual stimulation occurred in untreated pinealectomized rats, but sexual excitement was observed with PCPA treatment at about the same frequency as in intact animals. These findings ruled out the possibility that the action of PCPA is mediated by inhibiting the formation of pineal indole hormones derived from serotonin (58).

Hypophysis — Twenty 8-month-old Sprague-Dawley male rats, hypophysectomized 4 months previously, were treated with PCPA. None of these animals exhibited homosexual mounting behavior. The failure of PCPA to produce its aphrodisiac effect was interpreted as secondary to the atrophy of the testicles (58). However, GAWIENOWSKI et al. (21) found that testosterone, given to hypophysectomized rats, did not restore the response to PCPA. These findings indicate that PCPA-induced hypersexuality is dependent not only on androgens, but also on some pituitary hormone.

It is pertinent at this point to mention that ACTH and MSH-peptides injected into the lateral ventricles of adult male animals produce a marked sexual stimulation which is also inhibited by 5-HTP (6) and abolished by castration and by cyproterone (7, 9). However, ACTH-induced sexual excitement is quite different from that induced by PCPA. In fact, it is probably not exact to define the former as "sexual excitement" at all, for the animal (rat, rabbit, cat) is not excited. It yawns and stretches, and its recurrent penile erections with copulatory movements and ejaculation occur almost as in a dream; the animal shows no interest for its partners (male or female) and seems surprised at what is happening in its body (5).

Rats treated with PCPA, on the other hand, are very excited; they move restlessly about the cage, mount the other rats, male and female, apparently without any preference. Occasionally, the PCPA-treated rats also exhibit penile erections with yawning and stretching (5), but the major activity consists of sexual interactions.

It seems likely, therefore, that ACTH and PCPA activate different neuronal mechanisms. The sexual activity induced by intraliquorally injected ACTH resembles masturbation or penile erections which occur during sleep; PCPA, on the other hand, greatly enhances interactions. There are, however, some common phenomena (stretching, yawning and penile erections, the antagonistic effect of 5-HTP and of castration) in the animals treated with PCPA and ACTH.

Adrenal gland — The adrenal gland does not seem to be involved in the PCPA effect since adrenalectomy does not prevent the PCPA induced heterosexual mounting behavior in male rats (38).

Testosterone — The theory that serotonin has an inhibitory role on sexual behavior in male animals raises a logical question: What is it that activates this behavior? Since sexual behavior is so specifically oriented, it seemed likely that testosterone was the stimulating agent.

We compared the sexual behavior of intact and castrated rats treated with PCPA or testosterone or both (24).

As with previous results, about 30% of the intact animals treated with PCPA alone displayed at least one mounting attempt on another rat during the 3-hour observation period. None of the castrated animals treated with PCPA exhibited such behavior. Treatment with testosterone alone did not cause sexual excitation in castrated rats, and only 5 of 40 intact rats receiving both drugs displayed mounting behavior that occurred repetitively at intervals of only 1 to 5 min. In fact, sometimes five to eight rats would line up and mount each other at the same time (Fig. 1). At the end of the 3rd hour, the various groups of animals were again isolated, treated at noon of the next day with the same drug or drug combination and retested for sexual activity at 6 p.m. Less than 10% of the rats treated with PCPA alone showed any further signs of sexual excitement. On the other hand, the animals treated daily with PCPA plus testosterone showed the same compulsive sexual behavior each day for 10 days or more.

In agreement with our findings, GAWIENOWSKI and HODGEN (21) reported that PCPA failed to produce homosexual mounting behavior in sexually immature male rats, but this behavior was produced if the animals were primed with testosterone.

The essential role of testosterone for the stimulatory effect of PCPA on male copulatory behavior has been confirmed also by MALMNÄS and MEYERSON (38).

The finding that sexual stimulation by PCPA is not only abolished by castration but is restored and greatly potentiated with testosterone indicates that testosterone plays an

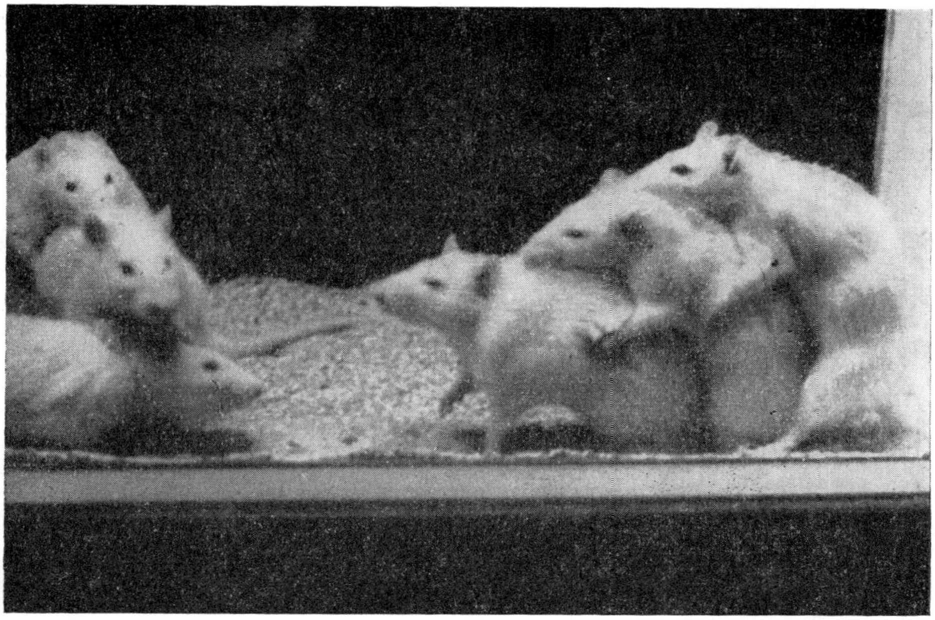

Fig. 1. Rats after the treatment with PCPA and testosterone, mounting each other at the same time.

essential role in this effect. It is clear that the depletion of serotonin is associated with sexual excitement only in the presence of testosterone. Conversely, testosterone produces little sexual stimulation in the presence of normal levels of serotonin in brain. These considerations and the fact that sexual stimulation is inhibited by 5-HTP indicate that brain serotonin plays an inhibitory role in sexual behavior in male animals and that sexual behavior is activated by an action of testosterone in the brain (24).

However, this theory has been recently challenged by BOND et al. (10) who reported that PCPA produces homosexual mounting behavior in male castrated rats. We cannot offer any convincing explanation for their discordant findings.

However, these authors have made their observations immediately following the change of the laboratory light from white to red, and refer that their most sexually active rats were the adrenalectomized-castrated-immature rats, which did not show any sign of exhaustion for the 3 days of the observation period.

We have observed that the sudden change of lights from white to red often triggers in normal or castrated male or female rats a pattern of social interactions which mimics the real male mounting behavior.

The latter is characterized as follows: "It is a requirement that the male mounts directly from the rear, clasps its partner firmly with the forelegs, palpates the subject's sides with the forelegs, and executes vigorous pelvic thrusts" (43). In our study mounts which were oriented in any other fashion or which are not accompanied by palpation and thrusting were not included.

It is possible that BOND et al. (10) did not follow in their study such strict criteria. Yet, full clarification of this problem is crucial for understanding the physiological role of testosterone and serotonin in brain. We are therefore presently engaged in studying the effect of PCPA on heterosexual copulatory behavior in male castrated rats.

It is interesting at this point to mention that a mutual interaction between serotonin and testosterone seems to be operating in the process of sexual differentiation. Thus LADOSKY and GAZIRI (35) and HABER and KAMANO (27) found that the concentration of serotonin in the brain of developing rats is comparable in males and females until the 8th day of age; at 12 days after birth, however, females show significantly higher values. LADOSKY and GAZIRI (35) demonstrated that testosterone is responsible for lowering serotonin concentration in the male's brain since its administration to females prevents the serotonin rise while this occurs in castrated males.

ROLE OF CATECHOLAMINES ON MALE SEXUAL BEHAVIOR

In the last few years, there have been increasing reports regarding the aphrodisiac effect of L-DOPA in parkinsonian patients. It is surprising that in previous controlled clinical trials with L-DOPA, no reports of its sexual stimulant effect have appeared. Literature on this matter was initially anecdotal, or the aphrodisiac effect was considered as a bizarre or toxic effect. Now when this neglecting attitude toward sexual problems has been abandoned, the aphrodisiac effect of L-DOPA is repeatedly reported to occur in a small percentage (2—4%) of the patients treated with L-DOPA (2, 3, 31, 42, 62). This effect has been referred to a lessening of the depression commonly present in Parkinson's disease, an increase in mobility, a "psychological factor"...etc.

However, the aphrodisiac effect of L-DOPA might find a biochemical explanation. This drug, in addition to being the precursor of catecholamines, depletes brain serotonin in animals (18) and reduces 5-hydroxyindoleacetic acid (5-HIAA) levels in the CSF of humans (26, 32, 61).

We initially suggested the possible stimulatory role of brain catecholamines in male sexual behavior (58). This conclusion originated from the observation that male rats treated with PCPA plus pargyline showed far more sexual excitation than those treated with PCPA alone.

Since this drug combination produced a selective accumulation of brain catecholamines, we postulated that both brain serotonin and catecholamines control sexual behavior in male animals, with serotonin inhibiting and catecholamines promoting this behavior.

However, the role of catecholamines on male sexual behavior is controversial. Thus, BERTOLINI and VERGONI (8) found that p-chloro-N-methylamphetamine, a compound which inhibits serotonin synthesis and also releases brain catecholamines (49) is more potent than PCPA in stimulating homosexual mounting behavior of male rats.

Moreover, BENKERT (3) observed an extremely active behavior when L-DOPA (in combination with the decarboxylase inhibitor Ro4-4602) was administered to rats treated with PCPA and reported that p-chloro-methyl-amphetamine has some beneficial effect in the treatment of impotence in male patients (see BENKERT's paper, at this symposium).

On the contrary, HYYPPÄ et al. (30) failed to observe an increase in heterosexual copulatory behavior in male adult rats treated with L-DOPA. Finally, we found that α-methyltyrosine does not inhibit heterosexual copulatory behavior in male rats (unpublished observations).

Therefore, the role of catecholamines in controlling sexual behavior is open to further investigations.

CHOLINERGIC SYSTEM

SHILLITO found that atropine (2.5 mg/kg) blocks the homosexual mounting behavior induced by PCPA in male rats (53). However, atropine inhibition was not specific for mounting behavior, since the drug blocked all social interactions (chasing, rolling over, lying on top of one another, social grooming) both in sexually immature and in adult male rats.

We confirmed her finding and, in addition, we found that atropine inhibits heterosexual copulatory behavior in normal and PCPA-treated male rats exposed to receptive females. On the contrary, no inhibitions were observed with homatropine methylbromide, a quaternary atropine derivative, indicating that atropine inhibition is central (Table 4).

TABLE 4

Effect of atropine and methylatropine on homo- and heterosexual behavior in normal and PCPA-treated male rats

	% rats with homosexual behavior			% rats with heterosexual behavior		
	controls	atropine	methyl-atropine	controls	atropine	methyl-atropine
Normal-rats	—	—	—	100	0	100
PCPA-rats	80	0	72	100	0	100

Groups of 25 rats each.
Atropine 2 mg/kg i.p. 30 min before test.
Methylatropine 2 mg/kg i.p. 30 min before test.

On the other hand, the central cholinergic system seems to exert an inhibitory role in female sexual behavior. Thus, LINDSTRÖM and MEYERSON (37) found that muscarinic compounds such as pilocarpine, oxotremorine and arecoline decrease the lordotic response in female rats and hamsters.

This inhibition was prevented by atropine (but not by methylatropine) and by PCPA, suggesting that the inhibitory effect of these muscarinic agents is central and has a serotoninergic link (51).

It is interesting to mention the finding of REID (47) that centrally acting muscarinic agents stimulate brain serotonin turnover. Apparently the cholinergic system has an inhibitory role in female and a stimulant one in male rodents. However, this problem is further complicated by the finding of SINGER (54) that atropine inhibits sexual behavior of female rats.

In conclusion, further experiments are needed to clarify whether the inhibitory effect of atropine for male copulatory sexual behavior is specific, i.e. if it reflects the existence of a cholinergic stimulatory mechanism for such behavior.

REFERENCES

1. AHLENIUS, S., ERIKSSON, H., LARSSON, K., MODIGH, K. and SÖDERSTEN, P. (1971) Mating behavior in the male rat treated with *p*-chlorophenylalanine methyl ester alone and in combination with pargyline. Psychopharmacologia, **20**, 383.
2. BARBEAU, A. (1969) L-dopa therapy in Parkinson's disease: a critical review of nine years' experience. Can. Med. Ass. J. **101**, 791.

3. BENKERT, O., CROMBACH, G. and KOCKOTT, G. (1972) Effect of L-dopa on sexually impotent patients. Psychopharmacologia, 23, 91.
4. BENKERT, O. and EVERSMANN, T. (1971) Importance of the anti-serotonin effect for mounting behavior in rats. Experientia, 28, 532.
5. BERTOLINI, A. (1971) Different type of sexual excitement produced in rats by intraliquoral ACTH and by intraperitoneal p-chlorophenylalanine. Riv. Farm. Ter. 2, 73.
6. BERTOLINI, A. and CASALGRANDI, L. (1970) Serotonin as the possible mediator of the sexual excitement produced in male animals by intraventricular ACTH. Riv. Farm. Ter. 1, 229.
7. BERTOLINI, A., GESSA, G. L., VERGONI, W. and FERRARI, W. (1968) Induction of sexual excitement with intraventricular ACTH; permissive role of testosterone in the male rabbit. Life Sci. 7, 1203.
8. BERTOLINI, A. and VERGONI, W. (1970) Effecto eccito-sessuale della p-chloro-N-metilamfetamina associata a testosterone, nel ratto maschio. Riv. Farm. Ter. 1, 423.
9. BERTOLINI, A., VERGONI, W., GESSA, G. L. and FERRARI, W. (1969) Induction of sexual excitement by the action of adrenocorticotrophic hormone in brain. Nature, 221, 667.
10. BOND, V. J., SHILLITO, E. E. and VOGT, M. (1972) Influence of age and of testosterone on the response of male rats to parachlorophenylalanine. Brit. J. Pharmacol. 46, 46.
11. BRODIE, B. B. and SHORE, P. A. (1957) A concept for a role of serotonin and norepinephrine as chemical mediators in the brain. Ann. N.Y. Acad. Sci. 66, 631.
12. CARPENTER, W., JR. (1970) Serotonin in affective disorders. Ann. int. Med. 73, 613.
13. CREMATA, V. Y., JR. and KOE, B. K. (1966) Clinical-pharmacological evaluation of p-chlorophenylalanine: a new serotonin-depleting agent. Clin. Pharmacol. Ther. 7, 768.
14. DA PRADA, M., CARRUBA, M., O'BRIEN, R. A., SANER, A. and PLETSCHER, A. (1972) The effect of 5,6-dihydroxytryptamine on sexual behavior of male rats. Eur. J. Pharmol., in press.
15. DEWSBURY, D. A. (1971) Copulatory behavior of male rats following reserpine administration. Psychon. Sci. 22, 177.
16. DEWSBURY, D. A. (1971) Effects of tetrabenazine on the copulatory behavior of male rats. Eur. J. Pharmol. 17, 221.
17. DEWSBURY, D. A., DAVIS, H. N., JR. and JANSEN, P. E. (1972) Effects of monoamine oxidase inhibitors on the copulatory behavior of male rats. Psychopharmacologia, 24, 209.
18. EVERETT, G. M. and BORCHERDING, J. W. (1970) L-dopa: effect on concentrations of dopamine, norepinephrine and serotonin in brains of mice. Science, 168, 849.
19. FERGUSON, J., HENRIKSEN, S., COHEN, H., MITCHELL, G., BARCHAS, J. and DEMENT, W. (1970) "Hypersexuality" and behavioral changes in cats caused by administration of p-chlorophenylalanine. Science, 168, 499.
20. GASTON, S. and MENAKER, M. (1967) Photoperiodic control of hamster testis. Science, 158, 925.
21. GAWIENOWSKI, A. M. and HODGEN, G. D. (1971) Homosexual activity in male rats after p-chlorophenylalanine: effects of hypophysectomy and testosterone. Physiol. Behav. 7, 551.
22. GESSA, G. L. (1970) Brain serotonin and sexual behavior in male animals. Ann. int. Med. 73, 622.
23. GESSA, G. L., TAGLIAMONTE, A. and TAGLIAMONTE, P. (1971) Aphrodisiac effect of p-chlorophenylalanine. Science, 171, 706.
24. GESSA, G. L., TAGLIAMONTE, A., TAGLIAMONTE, P. and BRODIE, B. B. (1970) Essential role of testosterone in the sexual stimulation induced by p-chlorophenylalanine in male animals. Nature, 227, 616.
25. GLOWINSKI, J., IVERSEN, L. L. and AXELROD, J. (1966) Storage and synthesis of norepinephrine in the reserpine-treated rat brain. J. Pharmacol. exp. Ther. 151, 385.
26. GOODWIN, F. K., DUNNER, D. L. and GERSHON, E. S. (1971) Effect of L-dopa treatment on brain serotonin metabolism in depressed patients. Life Sci. 10, 751.
27. HABER, B. and KAMANO, A. (1966): Sub-cellular distribution of serotonin in the developing rat brain. Nature, 209, 404.
28. HOYLAND, V. J., SHILLITO, E. E. and VOGT, M. (1970) The effect of parachlorophenylalanine on the behavior of cats. Brit. J. Pharmacol. 40, 659.
29. HYYPPÄ, M., LAMPINEN, P. and LEHTINEN, P. (1972) Alteration in the sexual behavior of male and female rats after neonatal administration of p-chlorophenylalanine. Psychopharmacologia, 25, 152.
30. HYYPPÄ, M., LEHTINEN, P. and RINNE, U. K. (1971) Effect of L-dopa on the hypothalamic, pineal and striatal monoamines and on the sexual behavior of the rat. Brain Res. 30, 265.
31. JENKINS, R. B. and GROH, R. H. (1970) Mental symptoms in Parkinsonian patients treated with L-dopa. Lancet II, 177.
32. JOHANSSON, B. and ROOS, B. E. (1971) 5-hydroxyindoleacetic acid in cerebrospinal fluid of patients with Parkinson's syndrome treated with L-dopa. Eur. J. clin. Pharmacol. 3, 232.

33. KOE, B. K. and WEISSMAN, A. (1966) p-Chlorophenylalanine: a specific depletor of brain serotonin. J. Pharmacol. exp. Ther. **154**, 499.
34. KORF, J. and VAN PRAAG, H. M. (1972) Action of p-chloroamphetamine on cerebral serotonin metabolism: an hypothesis. Neuropharm. **11**, 141.
35. LADOSKY, W. and GAZIRI, L. C. J. (1970) Brain serotonin and sexual differentiation of the nervous system. Neuroendocrin. **6**, 168.
36. LEHTINEN, P., HYYPPÄ, M. and LAMPINEN, P. (1972): Sexual behavior of adult rats after a single neonatal injection of reserpine. Psychopharm. **23**, 171.
37. LINDSTRÖM, L. H. and MEYERSON, B. J. (1967) The effect of pilocarpine, oxotremorine and arecoline in combination with methyl-atropine or atropine on hormone activated oestrous behavior in ovariectomized rats. Psychopharm. **11**, 405.
38. MALMNÄS, C. and MEYERSON, B. J. (1971) p-Chlorophenylalanine and copulatory behavior in the male rat. Nature, **232**, 398.
39. MEYER, C. J., WURTMAN, R. J., ALTSCHULE, M. D. et al. (1961) The arrest of prolonged estrus in "middle aged" rats by pineal gland extract. Endocrinology, **68**, 795.
40. MEYERSON, B. J. and LEWANDER, T. (1970) Serotonin synthesis inhibition and estrous behavior in female rats. Life Sci. **9**, 661.
41. MITLER, M. M., MORDEN, B., LEVINE, S. and DEMENT, W. (1972) The effects of parachlorophenylalanine on the mating behavior of male rats. Physiology and Behavior, **8**, 1147.
42. MONES, R. J., ELIZAN, T. S. and SIEGEL, G. J. (1970) Evaluation of L-dopa therapy in Parkinson's disease. N.Y. State J. Med. **70**, 2309.
43. MONEY, J. and EHRHARDT, A. A. (1971) Fetal hormones and the brain: effect on sexual dimorphism of behavior, — review. Arch. sex. Behav. **1**, 241.
44. NEFF, N. H., BARRETT, R. E. and COSTA, E. (1969) Kinetic and fluorescence histochemical analysis of the serotonin compartments in rat pineal gland. Eur. J. Pharmacol. **5**, 348.
45. PEREZ-CRUET, J., TAGLIAMONTE, A., TAGLIAMONTE, P. and GESSA, G. L. (1971) Differential effect of p-chlorophenylalanine (PCPA) on sexual behavior and on sleep patterns of male rabbits. Riv. Farm. Ter. **2**, 27.
46. REDMOND, D. E., JR., MAAS, J. W., KLING, A., GRAHAM, C. W. and DEKIRMENJIAN, H. (1971) Social behavior of monkeys selectively depleted of monoamines. Science, **174**, 428.
47. REID, W. D. (1970) Turnover rate of brain 5-hydroxytryptamine increased by D-amphetamine. Brit. J. Pharmacol. **40**, 483.
48. SALIS, P. J. and DEWSBURY, D. A. (1971) p-Chlorophenylalanine facilitates copulatory behavior in male rats. Nature, **232**, 400.
49. SANDERS-BUSH, E. and SULSER, F. (1970) p-Chloroamphetamine: *in vivo* investigations on the mechanism of action of the selective depletion of cerebral serotonin. J. Pharmacol. exp. Ther. **175**, 419.
50. SCHNETZLER, J. P. (1967) Effets des chimiothérapies psychiatriques sur le comportement sexuel. Actualités de Thérapeutique Psychiatrique. Ed: Masson et Cie; published by P.-A. Lambert II, 267.
51. SEGAL, D. and WHALEN, R. (1970) Effect of chronic administration of p-chlorophenylalanine on sexual receptivity of the female rat. Psychopharmacologia, **16**, 434.
52. SHEARD, M. H. (1969) The effect of p-chlorophenylalanine on the behavior in rats: relation to 5-hydroxytryptamine (5-HT) and 5-hydroxyindoleacetic acid. Brain Res. **15**, 524.
53. SHILLITO, E. E. (1970) The effect of parachlorophenylalanine on social interaction of male rats. Brit. J. Pharmacol. **38**, 305.
54. SINGER, J. (1968) The effects of atropine upon the female and male sexual behavior of female rats. Psychol. Behav. **3**, 377.
55. SINGER, J. (1972) Effects of p-chlorophenylalanine on the male and female sexual behavior of female rats. Psychol. Rep. **30**, 891.
56. SOULAIRAC, A. and SOULAIRAC, M. L. (1961) Action de la reserpine sur le comportment sexuel du rat male. C. r. Soc. Biol. **155**, 1010.
57. TAGLIAMONTE, A., TAGLIAMONTE, P. and GESSA, G. L. (1971) Reversal of pargyline-induced inhibition of sexual behavior in male rats by p-chlorophenylalanine. Nature, **230**, 244.
58. TAGLIAMONTE, A., TAGLIAMONTE, P., GESSA, G. L. and BRODIE, B. B. (1969) Compulsive sexual activity induced by p-chlorophenylalanine in normal and pinealectomized male rats. Science, **166**, 1433.
59. TAIT, G. R., BARFUSS, D. W. and ELLIS, L. C. (1969) Pineal gland, melatonin synthesis, and testicular development in the rat. Life Sci. **8**, 717.
60. TOZER, T. N., NEFF, N. H. and BRODIE, B. B. (1966) Application of steady state kinetics to the synthesis rate and turnover time of serotonin in the brain of normal and reserpine-treated rats. J. Pharmacol. exp. Ther. **153**, 177.

61. VAN WOERT, M. H. and BOWERS, M. B., JR. (1970) The effect of L-dopa on monoamine metabolites in Parkinson's disease. Experimentia, **26**, 4.
62. VAN WOERT, M. H., HENINGER, G., RATHEY, U. and BOWERS, M. B., JR. (1970) L-dopa in senile dementia. Lancet, I, 573.
63. WELCH, A. S. and WELCH, B. L. (1968) Effect of stress and parachlorophenylalanine upon brain serotonin, 5-hydroxyindoleacetic acid and catecholamines in grouped and isolated mice. Biochem. Pharmacol. **17**, 699.
64. WHALEN, R. E. and LUTTGE, W. G. (1970) p-Chlorophenylalanine methyl ester: an aphrodisiac? Science, **169**, 1000.
65. WURTMAN, R. J., ALTSCHULE, M. D. and HOLMGREN, U. (1959) Effects of pinealectomy and of bovine pineal extract in rats. Amer. J. Physiol. **197**, 108.
66. WURTMAN, R. J., AXELROD, J. and CHU, E. W. (1963) Melatonin, a pineal substance: effect on the rat ovary. Science, **141**, 277.
67. ZITRIN, A. (1970) Sexual behavior of male cats after administration of parachlorophenylalanine. Science, **170**, 868.

G.L.G., Pharmacological Institute of the University, via Porcell 4, Cagliari, Italy

MONOAMINES AND FEMALE SEXUAL BEHAVIOUR[*]

B. J. MEYERSON, M. ELIASSON, L. LINDSTRÖM, A. MICHANEK
and A. CH. SÖDERLUND

Department of Pharmacology, University of Uppsala

The general term sexual behaviour in fact comprises a number of discrete behaviour components. It is unlikely that all components are governed by identical neuroendocrine functions having the same neuropharmacology. Most investigations in animals have focused on the sex-characteristic performance displayed during the copulatory act. It is well established that copulatory behaviour in female mammals is dependent on ovarian hormones, in some species oestrogens (cat, rabbit) in others oestrogens + progesterone (rat, hamster, guinea-pig, mouse) (32). Labelled oestrogens are taken up and retained in certain cerebral neuron systems (3, 6, 8, 26, 30, 33). Implantation of minute amounts of oestrogens into hypothalamic areas produces copulatory behaviour in ovariectomized animals, without detectable activation of peripheral oestrogen target tissue (7, 15, 27, 29), suggesting a local functional significance of the hormone in the brain. The neuroendocrinology of sexual motivation, i.e. the urge of the female animal to seek sexual contact has been studied less. Recently three methods have been employed in our laboratory which differ in respect to the behaviour required by an ovariectomized rat to enable it to make contact with a sexually active male (17, 18). It was a consistent finding that oestradiol treatment induced a specific urge in the female to seek contact with a vigorous male. Progesterone did not have the same significance in the production of sexual motivation in the female rat as it has in the activation of copulatory behaviour.

Drugs might interfere with hormone activated behaviour either through an effect on neuronal functions directly involved in the establishment of the behaviour or indirectly by an effect on neuroendocrine functions with an action on endogenous hormone production or peripheral tissues involved in the sexual behaviour. To exclude effects on endogenous gonadal hormone production, the effect of different compounds on hormone activated sexual behaviour has been studied in castrated females given exogenous hormone treatment. The hormone treatment has been adjusted to induce a certain submaximal response in order to see a stimulatory or inhibitory effect of the drugs given.

---

[*] The investigation was supported by grants from National Institute of Child Health and Development HD 4108 and the Swedish Medical Research Council 7204 × 64.

Copulatory behaviour

Methods

Details of the testing procedures and environmental conditions are described elsewhere (21, 25). Ovariectomized rats (Sprague-Dawley 250—300 g), hamsters (inbred at this institute 90—130 g), mice (Naval Medical Research Institute, U.S.A., 30—40 g) and

TABLE 1

The effects of monoamine oxidase inhibitors on hormone activated copulatory behavior (lordosis response) in ovariectomized rats, hamsters, mice and rabbits

Species	Compound	Treatment mg/kg s.c.	Hours after treatment	Lordosis response Controls %	Exptls %	N
Rat[1])	Nialamide	135	19—23	73	45**	40
		250	6	71	67	24
			7	79	71	
	Pargyline	25	4	62	50	32
			5	82	60**	
		50	4		21**	59
			5		18**	
Hamster[1])	Nialamide	200	2	68	64	33
			6	77	33**	
			21—23		36**	31
	Pargyline	150	2	60	38	39
			4	73	28**	
Mouse	Nialamide	200	2	86	38**	21
Rabbit	Nialamide	50	16	67	67	9
			22	67	78	
		100	16	78	30**	13
			22	78	46**	
		250	16	78	0	9
			22	78	0	
		250	2	67	56	9
			8	89	44**	

Copulatory behaviour was activated by oestradiol benzoate (rat 10 µg/kg, hamster 25 µg/kg, mouse 25 µg/animal, rabbit 0.5 µg/kg) followed by progesterone 48 hours later (mg/animal: rat 0.4, hamster 0.2, mouse 1.0, rabbit none). Tests for copulatory behaviour were performed 52—58 hours and in the rabbit 26—32 hours after the oestradiol injection. Significant difference between controls and experimentals.

** $p < 0.01$.
[1]) Data partially taken from ref. 21, 25.

rabbits (dwarf-rabbits local breader 1000—2000 g) were kept under reversed light regime (light 9 p.m.—9 a.m.) and tests for mating behaviour performed during the dark period of the cycle. The female was transferred to an observation cage which held a sexually active male (the male hamster was transferred to the female cage) and tested for copulatory behaviour (lordosis response) on mounting by the male. The estimate of the percentage of lordosis response is based on the number of animals showing a clearcut lordosis reflex after at least 2 out of 5—6 mounts. The copulatory behaviour was, if not otherwise stated, induced by a single subcutaneous injection of oestradiol benzoate, followed 48 hours later by progesterone. Rabbits had oestradiol benzoate alone. The hormones were dissolved in olive oil.

The effect of monoamine oxidase inhibitors

To investigate the effect on copulatory behaviour of a decreased monoamine metabolism, the monoamine oxidase inhibitors nialamide and pargyline were used (Table 1). Nialamide, 100—250 mg/kg s.c. significantly reduced the copulatory behaviour in all four species tested. The effect was present within 8 hours except in the rat where a longer time was required until the effect was seen. The effect of pargyline was tested in rats and hamsters. A significant decrease of the copulatory response was obtained in both groups, however, the dose necessary to inhibit the response was higher in the hamster than in the

TABLE 2

The effect on oestradiol benzoate + progesterone activated copulatory behaviour in ovariectomized rats and hamsters of DL-5-HTP or DL-DOPA in combination with the monoamine oxidase inhibitor pargyline

Treatment		Hours after precursor treatment	Lordosis response Controls %	Exptls %	N
Rat					
Pargyline, 50 mg/kg and 1 hr later:	5-HTP 5 mg/kg	1	58	0	24
		2.5	16	0	
	DOPA 5 mg/kg	1	50	31	48
		2.5	44	42	
Hamster					
Pargyline, 100 mg/kg and 1 hr later:	5-HTP 5 mg/kg	1	70	6**	41
		3	74	6**	
	DOPA 10 mg/kg	1	68	36*	25
		3	68	72	

Data are taken from ref. 21, 25. Progesterone (0.4 mg/rat, 0.2 mg/hamster) was given 48 hours after the oestrogen injection. Pargyline was administered 2—3 hours after the progesterone injection. All injections were s.c. Controls had the same amount of pargyline as exptls. The response to hormones alone was 65—75 % in both species.
Significant difference between controls and experiments: *$p < 0.05$ **$p < 0.01$.

rat. The monoamine oxidase inhibitors clearly inhibited the hormone activated copulatory behaviour, although there are differences in time and dose response relationships between the species tested.

The effect of selective increase in serotonin and catecholamines

Pargyline followed one hour later by the serotonin precursor 5-hydroxytryptophane (5-HTP) totally or almost completely inhibited the lordosis response in the rat as well as in the hamster (Table 2). The same or a higher dose of DOPA in an otherwise analogous

TABLE 3

The effects of pargyline in combination with p-chlorophenylalanine methyl ester (PCPA) or α-methyl-p-tyrosine methyl ester (mTyr) on oestradiol benzoate (10 μg/kg) + progesterone (0,4 mg/rat) activated copulatory behaviour in ovariectomized rats

Treatment	Hours after pargyline treatment	Lordosis response %	N
Pargyline, 50 mg/kg s.c. and 2 hrs earlier:			
1. PCPA, 350 mg/kg i.p.	2	75	24
	4	83**	
2. α–mTyr, 350 mg/kg i.p.	2	75	36
	4	50	
3. saline, 0.2 ml i.p.	2	70	22
	4	50	

Progesterone was given 48 hours after the oestrogen treatment, pargyline was given 4 hours after the progesterone treatment. Significant difference between treatment 1 and 2 ** $p < 0.01$. The effect of pargyline + PCPA was not significantly different from only hormone treated animals (see controls Table 1).

experiment slightly reduced the response one hour after the DOPA-treatment but the animals had completely recovered 3 hours after the precursor treatment. In Table 3 is shown the effect of pargyline 50 mg/kg after pretreatment with the serotonin synthesis inhibitor p-chlorophenylalanine (PCPA) (350 mg/kg i.p.) or the catecholamine synthesis inhibitor α-methyl-p-tyrosine (α-mTyr) (350 mg/kg i.p.). It is obvious that the inhibitory effect of pargyline is prevented by pretreatment with the serotonin synthesis inhibitor whereas the inhibitory effect is still obvious when the α-mTyr was given before pargyline.

Accumulating evidence suggests that the copulatory behaviour in the female rat is inhibited by increased central serotoninergic tone. The specificity of this antagonistic relationship between serotonin and female copulatory behaviour has been demonstrated by the use of neuropharmacological agents which in different ways exert an influence on monoaminergic mechanisms, such as LSD (0.10—0.50 mg/kg i.p.) which recently was shown to inhibit the lordosis response (4). The evidence is scattered among several papers and is summarized for convenience in Table 4. Taken together these results clearly indicate that serotoninergic pathways exist which mediate inhibition of the copulatory behaviour in the female rat.

TABLE 4

Neuropharmacological compounds and copulatory behaviour in the female rat

Main effect achieved on central nervous monoaminergic tone	Compounds used	Effect on copulatory behaviour	Reference
General increase by:			
A. Decreased monoamine metabolism	MAO inhibitors: pargyline, nialamide, pheniprazine	Inhibition	20, 21
B. Decreased axonal "pump back" elimination	Tricyclic antidepressants: imipramine and others (see below)	Inhibition	23
Predominant increase of monoaminergic tone by:			
C. Decreased monoamine metabolism + precursor treatment:	MAO inhibitor: precursor:		20, 21
serotoninergic	pargyline 5-HTP	Inhibition	
dopaminergic* } noradrenergic }	pargyline DOPA	None	
noradrenergic	pargyline DOPS	None	
D. Decreased monoamine metabolism + serotonin synthesis inhibition dopaminergic + noradrenergic	MAO inhibitor: tryptophan hydroxylase inhibitor: pargyline H 22/54, PCPA	Pargyline-induced inhibition was prevented	20 and present paper
E. Decreased monoamine metabolism + catecholamine synthesis inhibition	MAO inhibitor: tyrosine hydroxylase inhibitor:	Pargyline-induced inhibition was not prevented	Present paper
serotoninergic	pargyline α-m-tyrosine		
F. Predominant decrease of serotonin or catecholamine axonal "pump back" elimination	Tricyclic antidepressants: imipramine, desmethylimipramine, amitryptyline, trimeprimine, nortriptyline, protriptyline	No correlation between effectiveness on copulatory behaviour and on catecholamine dependent behaviour patterns	23
G. Stimulation of serotonin receptors	LSD	Inhibition	4
General descrease by:			
H. Depletion of storage	Amine depletors: reserpine, tetrabenazine	Copulatory behavior effectively activated even in the absence of progesterone which is otherwise necessary to get a response	19, 28

TABLE 4 (Cont.)

Main effect achieved on central nervous monoaminergic tone	Compounds used	Effect on copulatory behaviour	Reference
Selective descrease by:			
I. Receptor blockage catecholaminergic	Receptor blocker: chlorpromazine	Could not replace progesterone treatment	22
J. The combined effect of serotonin synthesis inhibition and serotonin release	Tryptophan hydroxylase inhibitor: PCPA	Copulatory behaviour activated even in the absence of progesterone	16

5-HTP (DL-5-hydroxytryptophane), H22/54 (α-propyldopacetamid), PCPA (DL-*p*-chlorophenylalanine methyl ester HCl), LSD (lysergic acid diethylamide).

The effect of decreased monoaminergic tone on female copulatory behaviour

It is well established that oestrogens followed after a certain time by progesterone more effectively activate copulatory behaviour in ovariectomized rats, hamsters and mice than oestrogens alone (32). In ovariectomized oestrogen treated rats progesterone could be replaced by the amine depletors reserpine and tetrabenazine (19) and by the serotonin synthesis inhibitor PCPA (16). Chlorpromazine which is considered to block catecholamine receptors was not effective in replacing progesterone (22). The reserpine effect was not obtained in the hamster (25). In the mouse, the effect of reserpine to produce oestrous behaviour was not seen after adrenalectomy (31). The implication of the adrenals in the activation of lordosis in the oestrogen treated female rat is suggested by PARIS et al. (28). They found that reserpine treatment increased the concentration of progesterone in plasma in spayed female rats, presumably by ACTH release (see also FEDER and RUF — 5). The oestrogen+reserpine activated lordosis response was inhibited by dexamethasone (500 μg/kg of the free steroid). However, in contrast to the data of PARIS et al., LINDSTRÖM (13) recently reported that also the oestrogen+progesterone activated lordosis response was almost completely inhibited by dexamethasone (100 μg/kg of the water soluble ester 21-phosphate). The reason for the discrepancy between the data of PARIS et al. and LINDSTRÖM is not clear. Experiments are in progress in this laboratory to further elucidate the effect of dexamethasone on the reserpine-activated lordosis response.

Lordotic behaviour is infrequently seen in the male rat castrated as adult, unless very large doses of oestrogen are given. The facilitatory effect of progesterone is absent (1, 2, 24). Reserpine and tetrabenazine facilitated, however, the occurrence of lordotic behaviour in male rats castrated as adults and treated with relatively low doses of oestradiol benzoate (25 μg/kg s.c.). This effect was confirmed by LARSSON et al. (9), who also showed that the effect of tetrabenazine was antagonized by the monoamine oxidase inhibitor nialamide.

It is likely that the facilitatory effect on the lordotic behaviour achieved by amine depletion at least in the female involves secretion from the adrenals of steroids effective in augmenting the oestrogen activated behaviour. However, considering all evidence of inhibition of the copulatory response by increased monoaminergic tone it seems justified to suggest that also other mechanisms than adrenal activation are involved which are more directly related to the central nervous production of the lordosis response. Further experiments to clarify this point are obviously necessary.

The effect of muscarinic compounds on female copulatory behaviour

Muscarinic compounds also decrease female copulatory behaviour. This has been shown by LINDSTRÖM et al. in the rat (10, 11, 14) as well as in the hamster (12). The effect of pilocarpine is inhibited by atropine but not by methylatropine indicating that the effect of pilocarpine is exerted beyond the blood brain barrier. Table 5 shows the effect on the

TABLE 5

The effect of pilocarpine alone and in combination with pargyline, *p*-chlorophenylalanine methyl ester (PCPA) or α-methyl-*p*-tyrosine methyl ester (α-mTyr) on oestradiol benzoate (10μg/kg) + + progesterone (0.4 mg/rat) activated copulatory behaviour in ovariectomized rats.

Treatment	Lordosis response % Hours after last treatment ½	1½	N
A. 1. Pilocarpine, 25 mg/kg	39**	70	46
2. Saline	68	83	45
B. 1. Pargyline, 25 mg/kg and 4 hrs later pilocarpine, 25 mg/kg	20**	30**	46
2. Pargyline, 25 mg/kg	59	61	46
C. 1. PCPA, 400 mg/kg and 8 hrs later pilocarpine, 25 mg/kg	71	71	34
2. PCPA, 400 mg/kg + saline	63	66	35
D. 1. α-mTyr, 200 mg/kg 22 and 8 hrs before pilocarpine, 25 mg/kg	38**	86	21
2. α-mTyr, 2 × 200 mg/kg + saline	86	90	21

Oestradiol benzoate was given at 0 hour, progesterone at 48 hours and pilocarpine at 52.5 (A) or 56 (B, C, D) hours. Significant difference between treatment 1 and 2** p <0.01

oestrogen+progesterone activated lordosis response in the ovariectomized rat by pilocarpine 25 mg/kg s.c. Analogous effects were obtained by oxotremorine and arecoline. The inhibitory effect of pilocarpine was prolonged by pretreatment with pargyline. When pilocarpine was given 8 hours after PCPA, 400 mg/kg s.c., no inhibitory effect was seen. This lack of inhibition was not seen after pretreatment with the catecholamine synthesis inhibitor α-mTyr. It seems as if the effect of pilocarpine depends on the presence of serotonin and that the inhibitory effect of pilocarpine on hormone activated oestrous behaviour in the rat is mediated by serotoninergic mechanisms.

MONOAMINES AND SEXUAL MOTIVATION

Most investigations on the influence of hormonal and neuropharmacological agents on female sexual behaviour have been focused on the performance intimately related to the copulatory act. The urge to seek sexual contact, sexual motivation, has been considered less but might be of more clinical relevance. Different methods of studying sexual motivation have recently been employed in our laboratory (12, 13). Oestrogens were shown to induce a clearcut urge to seek sexual contact in the female rat. In the present study we have used one of these methods to investigate the effect on the oestrogen activated sexual motivation in the ovariectomized female rat of the serotonin synthesis inhibitor PCPA. The increasing barrier method was used. The method is described in Fig. 1. The subject has to pass a grid in order to reach contact with a sexually active male. Every second time the female passes the electric grid, the grid current increases. When the subject spends more than 5 min in the starting cage the run is ended. The number of grid crossings the female is willing to make to reach contact with the male is the estimate of her motivation. The animals were kept under the same laboratory conditions as the animals used in the study of the lordosis response. Fig. 2 shows the effect of PCPA on oestrogen induced sexual motivation. Oestradiol benzoate 10 µg/kg was given in a single dose at day 0 and PCPA was given 100 mg/kg on day 0 and 50 mg/kg on days 1, 2 and 3. Controls had saline instead of PCPA, the injections were done 4 hours before the animals were tested. Tests

INCREASING BARRIER

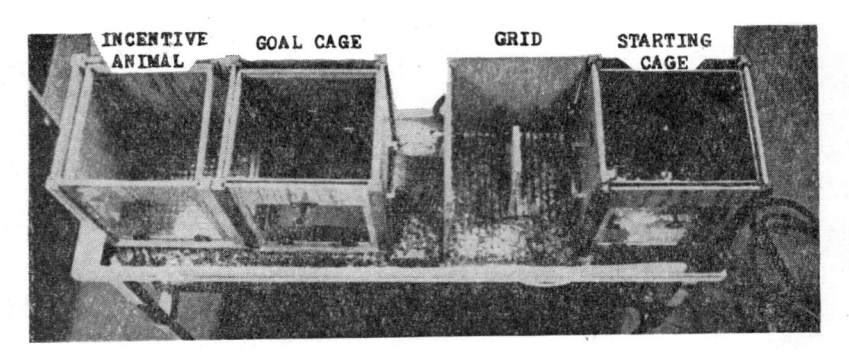

Fig. 1. The increasing barrier technique.

Recorded: No. of grid crossings.
Program: Grid current increases every 2nd time subject crosses the grid. 15 sec. allowed in goal cage. Inter-trial time = 0. If subject hesitates > 5 min. run is ended.

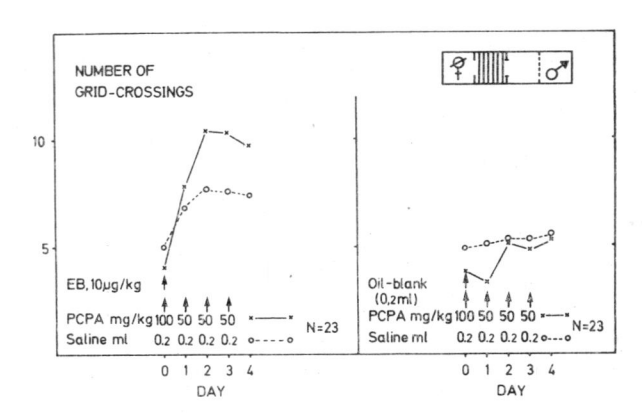

Fig. 2. The effect of p-chlorophenylalanine (PCPA) on the urge to seak contact with a sexually active male in the ovariectomized rat. EB — oestradiol benzoate. Treatments were given 4—6 hours before test.

were performed once daily for 5 days starting the day of oestrogen treatment. PCPA treated females crossed the grid significantly more on days 2, 3 and 4 (Wilcoxon matched pairs signed ranks test p < 0.01). An analogous experiment was performed but an oil blank solution was given instead of oestradiol treatment. This experiment shows that in the first 2 days of PCPA treatment there was a slight decline in the number of grid crossings compared to the saline treated controls. On days 2, 3 and 4 no difference was seen between the two treatments. When these data are taken together they suggest that PCPA increased the motivation of the female to cross the grid to reach contact with the sexually active male only if the female had been treated with oestradiol benzoate which indicates that the effect of PCPA is specifically related to the oestrogen-induced sexual motivation.

SUMMARY AND CONCLUSIONS

Studies in which agents have been used to influence monoaminergic mechanisms in different ways suggest that serotoninergic pathways exist which mediate inhibition of hormone activated copulatory behaviour in the female rat. There is also evidence that copulatory behaviour is inhibited by increased monoaminergic tone in other species such as hamster, mouse and rabbit. The role of serotonin in these species has to be further investigated. The implication of monoaminergic mechanisms in sexual motivation has also to be further investigated. However, preliminary data indicate that decreased serotoninergic tone might also facilitate this hormone activated response.

REFERENCES

1. BARÉN ENGELBREKTSSON, LARSSON, K., SÖDERSTEN, P. and WILHELMSSON, M. (1970) The female lordosis pattern induced in male rats by estrogen. Horm. Behav. 1, 181.
2. DAVIDSON, J. M. (1969) Effects of estrogen on the sexual behavior of male rats. Endocrinology, 84, 1365.
3. EISENFELD, A. J. and AXELROD, J. (1967) Evidence for estradiol binding sites in the hypothalamus effect of drugs. Biochem. Pharmacol. 16, 1781.
4. ELIASSON, M., MICHANEK, A. and MEYERSON, B. J. (1972) A differential inhibitory action of LSD and amphetamine on copulatory behavior in the female rat. Acta pharmacol. toxicol. 31, suppl. 1.
5. FEDER, H. H. and RUF, K. B. (1969) Stimulation of progesterone release and estrous behavior by ACTH in ovariectomized rodents. Endocrinology, 84, 171.
6. GLASCOCK, R. F. and HOEKSTRA, W. G. (1959) Selective accumulation of tritium-labeled hexoestrol by the reproductive organs of immature female sheep and goats. Biochem. J. 72, 673.
7. HARRIS, G. W. and MICHAEL, R. P. (1964) The activation of sexual behavior by hypothalamic implants of oestrogen. J. Physiol. 171, 275.
8. KATO, J. and VILLEE, C. A. (1967) Preferential uptake of estradiol by the anterior hypothalamus of the rat. Endocrinology, 80, 567.
9. LARSSON, K. and SÖDERSTEN, P. (1971) Lordosis behavior in male rats treated with estrogen in combination with tetrabenazine and nialamide. Psychopharmacologia, 21, 13.
10. LINDSTRÖM, L. H. (1970) The effect of pilocarpine in combination with monoamine oxidase inhibitors, imipramine or desmethylimipramine on oestrous behaviour in female rats. Psychopharmacologia, 17, 160.
11. LINDSTRÖM, L. H. (1971) The effect of pilocarpine and oxotremorine in oestrous behaviour in female rats after treatment with monoamine depletors or monoamine synthesis inhibitors. Europ. J. Pharmacol. 15, 60.
12. LINDSTRÖM, L. H. (1972) The effect of pilocarpine and oxotremorine on hormone activated copulatory behavior in the ovariectomized hamster. Naunyn.-Schmiedeberg's Arch. Pharmakol. 275, 333.
13. LINDSTRÖM, L. H. (1972). Further studies on cholinergic mechanism and hormone activated copulatory behaviour in the female rat. J. Endocrin. 56, 275.
14. LINDSTRÖM, L. H. and MEYERSON, B. J. (1967) The effect of pilocarpine, oxotremorine and

arecoline in combination with methylatropine or atropine on hormone-activated oestrous behaviour in ovariectomized rats. Psychopharmacologia, **11**, 405.
15. LISK, R. D. (1962). Diencephalic placement of estradiol and sexual receptivity in the female rat. Amer. J. Physiol. **203**, 493.
16. MEYERSON, B. J. and LEWANDER, T. (1970), Serotonin synthesis inhibition and estrous behavior in female rats. Life Sci. **9**, 661.
17. MEYERSON, B. J. and LINDSTRÖM, L. (1971) Sexual motivation in the estrogen treated ovariectomized rat. In: Hormonal Steroids, Excerpta med. Internat. Congr. Ser. No. 219.
18. MEYERSON, B. J. and LINDSTRÖM, L. (1973) Sexual motivation in the female rat. A methodological study applied to the investigation of the effect of ovarian hormones. Acta physiol. scand. suppl. 389.
19. MEYERSON, B. J. (1964) Estrous behaviour in spayed rats after estrogen or progesterone treatment in combination with reserpine or tetrabenazine. Psychopharmacologia, **6**, 210.
20. MEYERSON, B. J. (1964) Central nervous monoamines and hormone-induced estrous behaviour in the spayed rat. Acta physiol. scand. **53**, suppl. 241.
21. MEYERSON, B. J. (1964) The effect of neuropharmacological agents on hormone-activated estrous behaviour in ovariectomized rats. Arch. int. Pharmacodyn. **150**, 4.
22. MEYERSON, B. J. (1966) Oestrous behaviour in oestrogen treated ovariectomized rats after chlorpromazine alone or in combination with progesterone, tetrabenazine or reserpine. Acta pharmacol. toxicol. **24**, 363.
23. MEYERSON, B. J. (1966) The effect of imipramine and related antidepressive drugs on estrous behaviour in ovariectomized rats activated by progesterone, reserpine or tetrabenazine in combination with estrogen. Acta physiol. scand. **67**, 411.
24. MEYERSON, B. J. (1968) Female copulatory behavior in male and androgenized female rats after estrogen and amine depletor treatment. Nature (Lond.) **217**, 683.
25. MEYERSON, B. J. (1970) Monoamines and hormone activated oestrous behaviour in the ovariectomized hamster. Psychopharmacologia, **18**, 50.
26. MICHAEL, R. P. (1955) Oestrogens in the central nervous system. Brit. med. Bull. **21**, 87.
27. PALKA, Y. S. and SAWYER, C. H. (1966) The effects of hypothalamic implants of ovarian steroids on oestrous behaviour in rabbits. J. Physiol. (Lond.) **185**, 251.
28. PARIS, C. A., RESKO, J. A. and GOY, R. W. (1971) A possible mechanism for the induction of lordosis by reserpine in spayed rats. Biol. of Reprod. **4**, 23.
29. SAYWER, C. H. (1963) Induction of estrus in the ovariectomized cat by local hypothalamic treatment with estrogen. Anat. Rec. **145**, 280.
30. STUMPF, W. E. (1968) Estradiol-concentrating neurons: topography in the hypothalamus by dry mount autoradiography. Science, **162**, 1001.
31. UPHOUSE, L. L. (1970) Induction of estrus in mice: possible role of adrenal progesterone. Horm. Behav. **1**, 255.
32. YOUNG, W. C. (1961) The hormones and mating behavior. In: Sex and Internal Secretions, vol. 2, 1173. Ed: W. C. Young, Williams and Wilkins Co., Baltimore.
33. ZIGMOND, R. E. and MCEWEN, B. S. (1970) Selective retention of estradiol by cell nuclei in specific brain regions of the ovariectomized rat. J. Neurochem. **17**, 889.

B.J.M., Department of Pharmacology of the University, Biomedicum, Box 573, Uppsala, Sweden

INTERACTIONS BETWEEN TUBERO-INFUNDIBULAR DOPAMINE NEURONS AND THE PITUITARY-GONADAL AXIS[*]

W. LICHTENSTEIGER

Department of Pharmacology, University of Zürich

Monoamine-containing neurons are involved in a great variety of neurophysiological processes; it is therefore not surprising that they should also participate in neuroendocrine regulations. By their control of both behavioral manifestations and hormonal changes, they could help to establish the coordinate pattern of responses which is typical of neuroendocrine reactions. Since many brain regions which are important for neuroendocrine regulations, receive projections of monoamine neurons, a rather complex interplay of the various monoamine systems is to be expected. This is especially true for the mediobasal tuberal region, where it is essential to distinguish between the long projecting systems of the noradrenaline (NA) and serotonin (5-HT) neurons and the short tubero-infundibular dopamine (DA) neurons. If one looks for coordinative influences on the behavioral and hormonal state of the animal, the NA and 5-HT systems seem to be the better candidates from a structural point of view. Yet, I would like to discuss some evidence which indicates that the activity of the local DA neurons is also influenced from higher-order integrative centers.

With regard to the pituitary-gonadal axis, that part of the tubero-infundibular DA system which originates mainly in the arcuate nucleus of the hypothalamus and terminates in the external layer of the median eminence in proximity to the primary capillary plexus of the hypophysial portal system, is of main importance (3, 8, 9, 29). It should be remembered, however, that in addition the intermediary and neural lobes of the pituitary receive a direct innervation by central catecholamine neurons (2, 6). We have studied the functional involvement of the tubero-infundibular DA system by combining morphological identification and quantitation of intracellular catecholamines by means of a microfluorimetric approach, which makes use of the histochemical fluorescence method of FALCK and HILLARP (24, 25, 27). This method yields relative intensities of individual DA or NA nerve cell bodies as fractions of a NA standard. Since we have found that in cell populations from various central catecholamine neuron groups, the individual intensity values are distributed according to the lognormal type of frequency distribution (27), it is most convenient to use the mean of logarithmically transformed frequency distributions

---

[*] Supported by the Swiss National Foundation for Scientific Research (grant No. 3.258.69), the Barell-Stiftung, the Hartmann-Müller Stiftung and the Jubiläumsspende of the University of Zürich.

of relative fluorescence intensity for the comparison of different functional states. As the amine concentration of nerve cells is usually below the limit of concentration quenching, these values are a measure for intraneuronal amine concentrations. Yet, additional physico-chemical effects cannot always be completely ruled out (27, 28), and therefore, I shall use the more precise term "fluorescence intensity".

With this technique, changes in the fluorescence intensity of the tuberal DA nerve cell group were seen in female rats during the oestrous cycle (25), after ovariectomy and oestrogen treatment (27) as well as after acute exposure to cold (4°C) and thyroxine treatment (26). Not all of these reactions show the same degree of specificity: whereas the variations during the oestrous cycle were not observed in another DA nerve cell group, that of the substantia nigra, and thus are probably linked with certain events of the cycle, acute exposure to cold also provoked intensity changes in the cell bodies of the nigro-neostriatal system, at least in the mouse (LIENHART and LICHTENSTEIGER, unpublished observations). The interpretation of these various observations is hampered by the fact that the gap between the function studied and the intraneuronal process is rather large. We were therefore looking for conditions where there should exist a closer correlation between some neurophysiological event and the cellular changes. Short-term electrical stimulation in various central loci appeared to offer such a condition. Most of these experiments were done on ovariectomized rats pretreated for one day with oestradiol-dipropionate and progesterone. In such animals, the DA nerve cell population of the arcuate nucleus of the hypothalamus is very stable and the hormonal situation well defined.

Effect of electrical stimulation on DA neurons and gonadotropins

If unilateral intermittent stimulation is applied directly to the arcuate nucleus, where the bulk of the tuberal DA nerve cells is situated, a marked increase in fluorescence intensity occurs in these cells within 10 min (28). The response resembles that seen after acute exposure to cold and the reaction produced in midbrain DA nerve cell groups by a single injection of morphine, i.e., during an acute increase in catecholamine turnover (13), with the restriction that the latter effect was more pronounced in mice. Both the response to local electrical stimulation and that to morphine have been shown to depend on an intact amine synthesis. This intensity response, which at present we believe to be characteristic for an acute increase in neuronal activity, was also induced, after 5 and 10 min, in the arcuate nucleus of both sides by unilateral stimulation of the medial preoptic area, i.e., through one or more synapses (Fig. 1). Both arcuate und preoptic stimulation were accompanied by an increase in LH secretion (20; Fig. 1). The coincidence suggests a relation between the DA neurons and hormone secretion. In this respect, the result of arcuate stimulation is obviously less conclusive, since neurons containing releasing factors were probably also stimulated directly (20). Therefore, I would rather insist on the effect of preoptic stimulation when relating the enhanced release of LH to the activation of the tuberal DA neurons. Since in this case the cellular response preceded the hormonal one, the former does not appear to be the consequence, but rather the cause, of the latter. An early counter-regulation on a neuronal basis can, of course, not be excluded. The concept of a facilitating action of these DA neurons on LRF release is in keeping with the results of injection and incubation studies (16, 17, 38, 39). It also agrees with pharmacological experiments (21, 22), but is at variance with the histochemical results of FUXE and his coworkers (1, 10—12). These discrepancies are most probably due to differences in the experimental parameters which may easily lead to contrasting results in a complex system.

BLOCKADE OF THE STIMULATORY RESPONSE OF THE DA NEURONS BY ATROPINE

We have subsequently tried to get further insight in the position occupied by the tuberal DA neurons within neuroendocrine systems. For this purpose, the initial part of the acute stimulatory response of cellular fluorescence intensity (Fig. 1) appeared to be especially

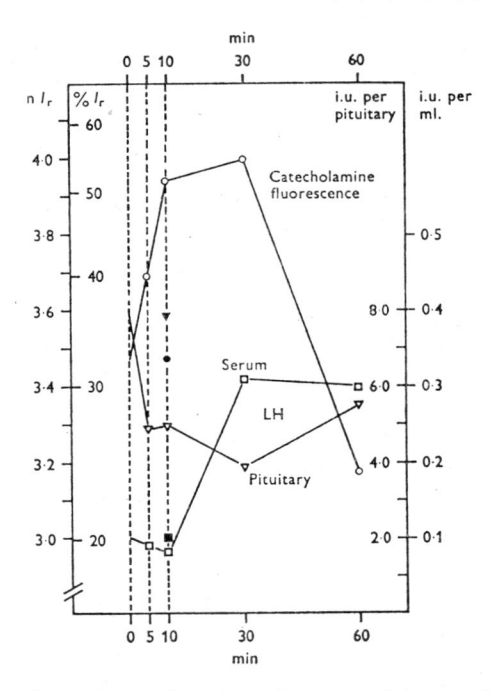

Fig. 1. Effect of preoptic stimulation on the relative intensity of the catecholamine fluorescence of the tuberal nerve cell group (means of lognormal distributions in natural logarithms and as percentage of the NA standard, left) and on concentrations of luteinizing hormone (LH, i.u. referring to the 2nd International Reference Preparation for human menopausal gonadotropin). Electrical stimulation of the medial preoptic area resulted in a biphasic change in fluorescence intensity with a marked initial increase. The response was accompanied by a drop in pituitary LH and preceded a rise in serum LH (from KELLER and LICHTENSTEIGER, 1971).

suitable because it is almost linear and can be used as an evoked response in a way similar to procedures in electrophysiology. In a first step, we tried to obtain a pharmacological characterization of synapses interposed between the medial preoptic area and the tuberal DA neurons. It has long been known that in addition to adrenergic blockers, also atropine blocks ovulation, although in the spontaneously ovulating rat very high doses are required (35, 36). In our studies, atropine was injected s.c. 15 min before the onset of electrical stimulation in considerably lower doses which, however, are known to be centrally active. Again ovariectomized rats pretreated with oestrogen and progesterone were used in most cases. While atropine did not affect the intensity level of the sham-operated controls (Fig. 2), 10 mg/kg of the drug completely blocked the increase in fluorescence intensity of the tuberal DA neuron group which is produced by electrical stimulation (10 or 30 min) of the medial preoptic area in untreated animals. I believe this to be a specific effect due to an antagonistic action of atropine at a cholinergic synapse somewhere between the preoptic area and the DA neurones, for the following reasons: 1. Local electrical stimulation within the arcuate nucleus elicited a stimulatory response of the tuberal DA nerve cells also in atropine-treated rats (Fig. 2). 2. The blockade of the stimulation-induced increase in fluorescence intensity was found to be dose-dependent

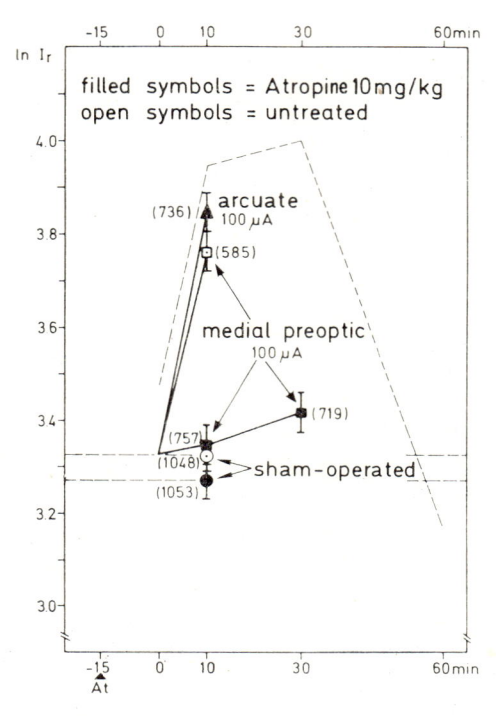

Fig. 2. Effect of atropine (ordinate: relative fluorescence intensity in natural logarithms, mean values with 99 % confidence limits and number of investigated cells in brackets; abscissa: time in min). Whereas local electrical stimulation in the arcuate nucleus was effective despite administration of atropine 15 min before the onset of stimulation, the response of the DA neurons to medial preoptic stimulation was completely blocked at 10 and 30 min. Stimulation was performed in ovariectomized rats pretreated for one day with oestradiol-dipropionate (5 μg) and progesterone (2 mg). In the sham-operated animals, atropine did not affect the fluorescence intensity. The biphasic broken line indicates the course of fluorescence intensity as observed in a previous study (cf. Fig. 1).

(Fig. 3). In this and the other experiments, only animals with electrode positions in the ventromedial corner of the medial preoptic area and in the adjacent suprachiasmatic preoptic area were used, in order to avoid differences in the magnitude of the reaction that might have been caused by different electrode positions within the medial preoptic area. 3. Methylatropine, which is more potent than atropine in the periphery, was practically unable to block the stimulatory response in a dose that was equimolar to the highest atropine dose administered (Fig. 3). I would assume then that there exists a cholinergic link between the medial preoptic area and the tubero-infundibular DA neurons.

Influence of Higher-Order Neuroendocrine "Centers"

The demonstration of a cholinergic link between the medial preoptic area and the tuberal DA neurons raises some questions: Thus, Shute and Lewis (37) in their extensive studies on acetylcholinesterase-containing pathways do not describe a connection of

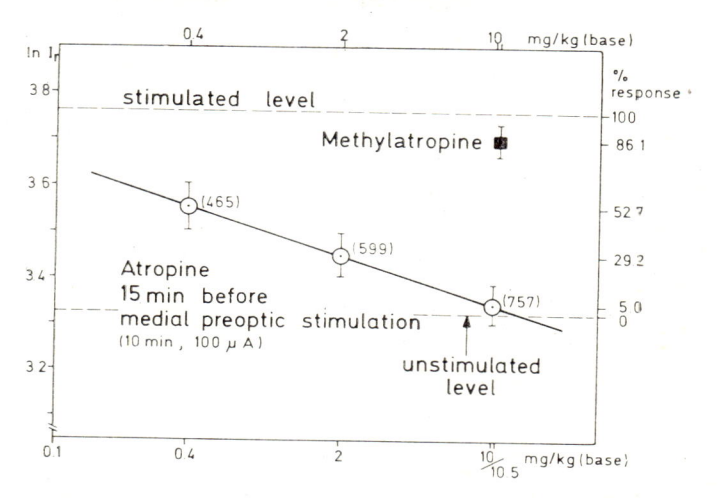

Fig. 3. Log dose-response relationship of atropine blockade of the stimulatory response, and effect of methylatropine (ordinate as in Fig. 2; abscissa: dose in logarithms). The increase in fluorescence intensity elicited in the DA nerve cells by 10 min electrical stimulation in the medial preoptic area, is reduced in a linear relation with the log dose. "Stimulated level" = mean of untreated stimulated group (cf. Fig. 2), "unstimulated level" = mean of untreated, sham-operated group (Fig. 2). — Methylatropine (10.5 mg/kg s.c.; cell count = 963) is almost without blocking effect.

some importance that would descend from the *medial* preoptic area to the arcuate nucleus. There appear to be two possible solutions to the problem: Either the pathway quantitatively is only a minor one — the DA nerve cells of the arcuate and periventricular nuclei likewise represent a minority — or else, a more complex system of relays may be intercalated between the medial preoptic area and the DA neurons.

In a search for additional areas influencing the DA neurons, we have first looked at the amygdala, also since some of the projections it receives from the preoptic region, appear to be cholinergic (37). A rapid increase in the fluorescence intensity of the tuberal DA nerve cells was seen after unilateral electrical stimulation (10 min) of either the ventral part of the *bed nucleus of the stria terminalis* (mean fluorescence intensities (2 rats) m = 3.778 and 3.733; cf. control level in Fig. 2) or the *medial amygdaloid nucleus*. Stimulation in the latter nucleus was effective in two different functional situations, namely, in ovariectomized, oestrogen-progesterone-pretreated rats (m = 3.748; cf. control level in Fig. 2) and in cycling rats during the afternoon of the first day of dioestrus (sham-operated controls m = 3.338; after 10 min of stimulation m = 3.666 and 3.625 in 2 rats). Atropine (10 mg/kg) did not block the cellular response to amygdaloid stimulation (m = 3.665 in one rat; cf. dioestrus 1 — control level). With regard to stimulation in the bed nucleus, the effect of the drug is as yet not quite clear, possibly because stimulation in this site may affect both afferent and efferent projections of the amygdala.

It may be assumed on these grounds that the medial amygdala — stria terminalis system can exert stimulatory effects on the tuberal DA neurons, whereby the projection from the medial amygdaloid nucleus probably is non-cholinergic. It seems noteworthy that VELASCO and TALEISNIK (41) also were unable to block ovulation elicited by stimulation of the medial amygdaloid region with atropine. — While these results so far do not yet allow to localize the cholinergic link, their main interest appears to reside in the fact that they place the tubero-infundibular DA neurons under the influence of components of the limbic system, and thus extend considerably the possibilities of functional interactions. The problem of sex differences may be raised in this context. RAISMAN and FIELD (32) recently described sex differences in the neuropile of projection areas of the stria terminalis (preoptic area and ventromedial nucleus) which were due partly to stria fibres and partly to fibres of unknown origin. On the other hand, RELKIN (33) reported differential effects of lesions in the mediobasal amygdala on the onset of puberty in male and female rats. We have in turn regularly observed a lower number of visibly fluorescent DA nerve cells in the tuberal region of male rats, as compared to females in various functional states (unpublished observations). This finding may indicate qualitative and/or quantitative differences in the input to the tuberal DA neurons.

In a few preliminary experiments, we have been looking for effects from the hippocampal system. A stimulatory response was elicited in two rats from one of its relay nuclei, the *nucleus of the diagonal tract* (m = 3.668; cf. control level in Fig. 2). On the other hand, stimulation in the ventral hippocampus, close to the subiculum, did not provoke a clearcut stimulatory response but rather, after pretreatment with α-methyl-tyrosine, yielded some indications for a reduction of cellular amine turnover.

Besides limbic forebrain structures, *ascending systems* of the lower brain stem deserve consideration, especially in reflex ovulators but also in spontaneous ovulators. Our experience is as yet limited, but it may nevertheless be mentioned that marked stimulatory reactions were provoked in two rats by stimulation in the *ventral tegmental area* of Tsai at the anterior border of the midbrain (m = 3.751 and 3.617), i.e., from a region which may exert positive or negative influences on gonadotropin secretion (4, 5, yet cf. 31).

CONCLUSION

In conclusion, I would like to point out that the tubero-infundibular DA neurons appear to be placed under the influence of *limbic structures* and possibly also of *ascending brainstem systems*. One or more *cholinergic synapses* occur in part of the circuits that impinge on the DA neurons; their precise location is as yet unknown. This cholinergic involvement seems noteworthy also because acetylcholinesterase-containing neuron groups have been related, on structural grounds, to ascending and limbic systems (23, 37). The various relays allow for many modulatory inputs such as hormonal feedback effects, sensory modalities or emotional cues. In this context, it would be interesting to know whether some of the neuroendocrine effects attributable to NA or 5-HT neurons (7, 15) might have been achieved through modifications of the input to the DA neurons. — We have earlier suggested that the tubero-infundibular DA neurons might be considered as an amplifying or (positive and/or negative) reinforcing system, especially for phasic events (20, 27). This assumption seems to be compatible with our recent findings. Reinforcing effects, such as the increase in the ovulatory response of a spontaneous ovulator after copulation (34), might well be mediated by the tubero-infundibular DA neurons. Inherent in this concept is the view that the action of these DA neurons need not be restricted to the control of one single hormone. This assumption is supported by the results of other investigators (7, 14, 18, 19, 30, 40, 42), although in some of these studies the possible role of NA systems is difficult to assess. As a further consequence of the concept presented above, one should consider the possibility that the changes in hormone levels initiated by the DA neurons might also depend upon the actual neuroendocrine situation. Some differential effects might be brought about in this way.

REFERENCES

1. AHRÉN, K., FUXE, K., HAMBERGER, L. and HÖKFELT, T. (1971) Turnover changes in the tuberoinfundibular dopamine neurons during the ovarian cycle of the rat. Endocrinology, **88**, 1415.
2. BJÖRKLUND, A. (1968) Monoamine-containing fibres in the neurointermediate lobe of the pig and rat. Z. Zellforsch. **89**, 573.
3. BJÖRKLUND, A., HROMEK, F., OWMAN, C. and WEST, K. A. (1970) Identification and terminal distribution of the tubero-hypophyseal monoamine fibre systems in the rat by means of stereotaxic and microspectrofluorimetric techniques. Brain Res. **17**, 1.
4. CARRER, H. F. and TALEISNIK, S. (1970) Effect of mesencephalic stimulation on the release of gonadotrophins. J. Endocr. **48**, 527.
5. CRITCHLOW, V. (1958) Blockade of ovulation in the rat by mesencephalic lesions. Endocrinology, **63**, 596.
6. DAHLSTRÖM, A. and FUXE, K. (1966) Monoamines in the pituitary gland. Acta endocr. **51**, 301.
7. DONOSO, A. O., BISHOP, W., FAWCETT, C. P., KRULICH, L. and MCCANN, S. M. (1971) Effects of drugs that modify brain monoamine concentrations on plasma gonadotropin and prolactin levels in the rat. Endocrinology, **89**, 774.
8. FUXE, K. (1964) Cellular localization of monoamines in the median eminence and the infundibular stem of some mammals. Z. Zellforsch. **61**, 710.
9. FUXE, K. and HÖKFELT, T. (1966) Further evidence for the existence of tubero-infundibular dopamine neurons. Acta physiol. scand. **66**, 245.
10. FUXE, K., HÖKFELT, T. and NILSSON, O. (1967) Activity changes in the tubero-infundibular dopamine neurons of the rat during various states of the reproductive cycle. Life Sci. Oxford **6**, 2057.
11. FUXE, K., HÖKFELT, T. and NILSSON, O. (1969) Castration, sex hormones, and the tuberoinfundibular dopamine neurons. Neuroendocrinology, **5**, 107.
12. FUXE, K., HÖKFELT, T. and NILSSON, O. (1972) Effect of constant light and androgen sterilization on the amine turnover of the tubero-infundibular dopamine neurons: Blockade of cyclic activity and induction of a persistent high dopamine turnover in the median eminence. Acta endocr. **69**, 625.
13. HEINRICH, U., LICHTENSTEIGER, W. and LANGEMANN, H. (1971) Effect of morphine on the catecholamine content of midbrain nerve cell groups in rat and house. J. Pharmacol. exp. Ther. **179**, 259.
14. HÖKFELT, T. and FUXE, K. (1972) Effects of prolactin and ergot alkaloids on the tubero-infundibular dopamine (DA) neurons. Neuroendocrinology, **9**, 100.
15. KALRA, S. P. and MCCANN, S. M. (1972) Modification of brain catecholamine levels and LH release by preoptic stimulation. IV Intern. Congr. of Endocrinology, Abstract no. 508, Excerpta Medica Intern. Congr. Series No. 256.
16. KAMBERI, I. A., MICAL, R. S. and PORTER, J. C. (1969) Luteinizing hormone-releasing activity in hypophysial stalk blood and elevation by dopamine. Science, **166**, 388.
17. KAMBERI, I. A., MICAL, R. S. and PORTER, J. C. (1970) Effect of anterior pituitary perfusion and intraventricular injection of catecholamines and indoleamines on LH release. Endocrinology, **87**, 1.
18. KAMBERI, I. A., MICAL, R. S. and PORTER, J. C. (1971) Effect of anterior pituitary perfusion and intraventricular injection of catecholamines on FSH release. Endocrinology, **88**, 1003.
19. KAMBERI, I. A., MICAL, R. S. and PORTER, J. C. (1971) Effect of anterior pituitary perfusion and intraventricular injection of catecholamines on prolactin release. Endocrinology, **88**, 1012.
20. KELLER, P. J. and LICHTENSTEIGER, W. (1971) Stimulation of tubero-infundibular dopamine neurons and gonadotrophin secretion. J. Physiol. (London) **219**, 385.
21. KORDON, C. (1971) Blockade of ovulation in the immature rat by local microinjection of α-methyl-dopa into the arcuate region of the hypothalamus. Neuroendocrinology, **7**, 202.
22. KORDON, C. and GLOWINSKI, J. (1969) Selective inhibition of superovulation by blockade of dopamine synthesis during the 'critical period' in the immature rat. Endocrinology, **85**, 924.
23. LEWIS, P. R. and SHUTE, C. C. D. (1967) The cholinergic limbic system: Projections to hippo-

campal formation, medial cortex, nuclei of the ascending cholinergic reticular system, and the subfornical organ and supra-optic crest. Brain, **90**, 521.
24. LICHTENSTEIGER, W. (1967) Mikrofluorimetrische Studien an katecholaminhaltigen hypothalamischen Nervenzellen der Ratte in den verschiedenen Phasen des viertägigen Oestruszyklus. Helv. physiol. pharmacol. Acta **25**, CR 423.
25. LICHTENSTEIGER, W. (1969) Cyclic variations of catecholamine content in hypothalamic nerve cells during the estreus cycle of the rat, with a concomitant study of the substantia nigra. J. Pharmacol. exp. Ther. **165**, 204.
26. LICHTENSTEIGER, W. (1969) The catecholamine content of hypothalamic nerve cells after acute exposure to cold and thyroxine administration. J. Physiol. (London) **203**, 675.
27. LICHTENSTEIGER, W. (1970) Katecholaminhaltige Neurone in der neuroendokrinen Steuerung. Prinzip und Anwendung der Mikrofluorimetrie. Prog. Histochem. Cytochem. **1** (No. 4), 185. G. Fischer, Stuttgart.
28. LICHTENSTEIGER, W. (1971) Effect of electrical stimulation on the fluorescence intensity of catecholamine-containing tuberal nerve cells. J. Physiol. (London) **218**, 63.
29. LICHTENSTEIGER, W. and LANGEMANN, H. (1966) Uptake of exogenous catecholamines by monoamine-containing neurons of the central nervous system: Uptake of catecholamines by arcuato-infundibular neurons. J. Pharmacol. exp. Ther. **151**, 400.
30. MÜLLER, E. E., DAL PRA, P. and PECILE, A. (1968) Influence of brain neurohumors injected into the lateral ventricle of the rat on growth hormone release. Endocrinology, **83**, 893.
31. PEKARY, A. E., DAVIDSON, J. M. and ZONDEK, B. (1967) Failure to demonstrate a role of midbrain-hypothalamic afferents in reproductive processes. Endocrinology, **80**, 365.
32. RAISMAN, G. and FIELD, P. M. (1971): Sexual dimorphism in the preoptic area of the rat. Science, **173**, 731.
33. RELKIN, R. (1971) Absence of alteration in puberal onset in male rats following amygdaloid lesioning. Endocrinology, **88**, 1272.
34. Rodgers, C. H. (1971) Influence of copulation on ovulation in the cycling rat. Endocrinology, **88**, 433.
35. SAWYER, C. H., EVERETT, J. W. and MARKEE, J. E. (1949) A neural factor in the mechanism by which estrogen induces the release of luteinizing hormone in the rat. Endocrinology, **44**, 218.
36. SAWYER, C. H., MARKEE, J. E. and TOWNSEND, B. F. (1949) Cholinergic and adrenergic components in the neurohumoral control of the release of LH in the rabbit. Endocrinology, **44**, 18.
37. SHUTE, C. C. D. and LEWIS, P. R. (1967) The ascending cholinergic reticular system: Neocortical, olfactory and subcortical projections. Brain, **90**, 497.
38. SCHNEIDER, H. P. G. and MCCANN, S. M. (1969) Possible role of dopamine as transmitter to promote discharge of LH-releasing factor. Endocrinology, **85**, 121.
39. SCHNEIDER, H. P. G. and MCCANN, S. M. (1970) Release of LH-releasing factor (LRF) into the peripheral circulation of hypophysectomized rats by dopamine and its blockage by estradiol. Endocrinology, **87**, 249.
40. VAN MAANEN, J. H. and SMELIK, P. G. (1968) Induction of pseudopregnancy in rats following local depletion of monoamines in the median eminence of the hypothalamus. Neuroendocrinology, **3**, 177.
41. VELASCO, M. E. and TALEISNIK, S. (1969) Release of gonadotropins induced by amygdaloid stimulation in the rat. Endocrinology, **84**, 132.
42. WUTTKE, W., CASSELL, E. and MEITES, J. (1971) Effects of ergocornine on serum prolactin and LH, and on hypothalamic content of PIF and LRF. Endocrinology **88**, 737.

W. L., Department of Pharmacology of the University, Zürich, Switzerland

EFFECT OF DRUGS INTERFERING WITH CENTRAL NEUROTRANSMITTERS ON PITUITARY GONADOTROPIC REGULATION

C. KORDON

Neurobiological Unit, National Institute of Health and Medical Research, Paris

INTRODUCTION

Various hypothalamic structures participate in the regulation of pituitary functions. Schematically, one may classify them in three groups (15):

1. *Integrating* structures, that is a level where neurons receive extrahypothalamic inputs conveying "environmental" information (as for instance sensory or somesthetic information). These neurons integrate such inputs and transform them into "orders" delivered to neurosecretory neurons.

2. A *neurosecretory* level, where polypeptidic neurohormones are elaborated by specialized neurons.

3. Finally, a *neurovascular* level, where neurosecretory axons and the capillary loops of the hypothalamo-hypophyseal portal system are in close association; each neurohormone is released into the portal blood, reaches the adenohypophysis and triggers the secretion of the corresponding pituitary hormone. This organization pattern is schematized on Fig. 1.

All these "levels" are richly innervated by fibers containing monoamines, particularly serotonin (5-HT), dopamine (DA) and noradrenaline (NA). Most of these fibers originate in discrete areas of the mesencephalon (2). This highly centralised pattern of distribution suggests that monoaminergic systems do not transfer a specific information from one area of the brain to the other — like, for instance, fiber systems involved in specific sensory pathways —, but that they rather act as a general "dispatching" system for regulating the threshold sensivity of synaptic relays included in such pathways.

Little is known as yet on the precise role of aminergic fibers innervating directly the two first levels described above — integrating structures and neurosecretory cell bodies —, though some biochemical data suggest that they also play a role in neuroendocrine regulations: for instance, important changes in the turn-over rates of catecholamines at the integrating level (preoptic area) have been observed after castration (7); recent results show that monoamines can affect *in vitro* the rate of biosynthesis of hypothalamic neurohormones (11). However, aminergic involvement at the last control level — neurovascular junctions — has been more extensively investigated. We will thus mainly summarize the present knowledge on this point and review recent data concerning the effect of drugs interfering with the metabolism of endogenous transmitters on gonadotropic regulations.

Such studies are of growing *clinical* importance, in view of the wide use of drugs in neurology or psychiatry and of the necessity to understand better possible endocrine side effects of these treatments. But this type of investigation is also of great *theoretical* importance, since drugs acting specifically on the biosynthesis or the release of monoamines are still the best available tool for investigating the mechanisms by which aminergic fibers can affect neuroendocrine control systems.

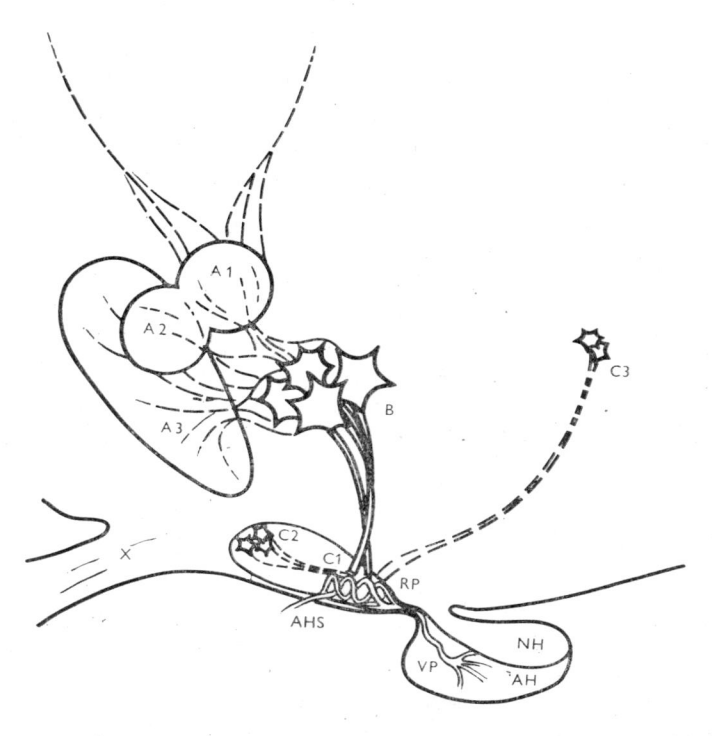

Fig. 1. Schematic representation of the various neuronal levels involved in the hypothalamic hormonostat. A_1, A_2, A_3 — "integration" centers; B — neurosecretory cell bodies; C — monoaminergic tuning fibers (C_1 and C_2 — cell bodies and endings of the dopaminergic tubero-infundibular tract; C_3 — 5-HT containing neurons). AH — adenohypophysis, AHS — superior hypophyseal artery; NH — neurohypophysis; RP — primary portal plexus; VP — portal vessels.

EFFECT OF DRUGS ON TONIC LEVELS OF GONADOTROPINS

Drugs interfering with monoamine metabolism do not seem to have important effects on the "tonic" or "steady state" secretion of gonadotropins. Blockade of CA synthesis has little or no effect on the average plasma levels of LH in castrated female rats (19). For instance, LH levels are unaffected for a period of 8 hours following the injection of α-methyl-DOPA, a "false transmitter" forming precursor which displaces DA for about 6 hours and NA for over 24 hours in the brain (32). It therefore seems that CA are not essential for the release of LH in the castrate; this conclusion is in agreement with results reported by DONOSO et al. (8) after administration of other CA inhibitors. It is possible, however, that blockade of CA receptors may suppress the high frequency surges of LH observed in castrated animals (5) and thus interfere with the so-called "circhoral" secretion pattern of LH reported in some species.

Inhibition of 5-HT synthesis does not either affect LH levels in the castrate (8, 19), or prolactin secretion in lactating rats (KORDON, BLAKE and SAWYER, unpublished observations) as well as in castrated females or in intact males (8).

EFFECT OF DRUGS ON NEURALLY INDUCED SURGES OF GONADOTROPINS

The picture is different when one studies the involvement of monoamine-containing neurons in *induced* endocrine responses, for instance by blocking biosynthesis of either CA or 5-HT at various intervals in advance of a neural stimulus affecting hormone release. In studies of prolactin regulation, the suckling stimulus in lactating rats was used as the neural input; in the case of LH control, the endogenous input triggering the cyclic ovulatory surge of LH was taken as stimulus. We then measured parallely changes in the hormone response and changes in the hypothalamic monoamine content resulting from treatment. In order to check that the treatment-induced endocrine changes were due to the modulation of amine levels, and not merely to possible pharmacological effects of the drugs used, we performed restoration experiments, repleting experimentally amine levels and looking for correlative restoration of hormone concentrations.

The pharmacological tools used in these experiments are summarized in Fig. 2.

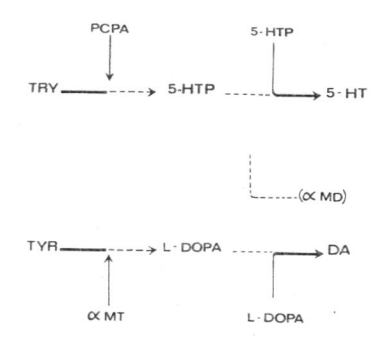

Fig. 2. Diagram of the pharmacological tools used in the "depletion" and "restoration" experiments (see text). PCPA, p-chlorphenylalanine (5-HT synthesis inhibitor); α-MT, -α-methyl-p-tyrosine (catecholamine synthesis inhibitor); TRY — tryptophan; TYR — tyrosine; α-MD — α-methyl-DOPA. Solid line — normal or restored synthesis; dotted line — interrupted synthesis.

Inhibition of CA biosynthesis blocks ovulation (6, 21, 27). Depletion of intracellular storage sites of the amines by reserpine (3, 29) or blockade of α-adrenergic receptors (31) has the same effect. Restoration of normal amine levels by administration of a precursor restores also the ability of the animals to ovulate (21). The receptor blocking experiments by SCHNEIDER and McCANN (31), as well as data obtained after elective restoration of DA or NA following inhibition of CA synthesis, suggest that DA is the most important catecholamine involved in the regulation of the ovulatory surge of LH (21). This is in good agreement with histochemical observations showing that the DA-containing tubero-infundibular system undergoes fluorescence changes which are correlated to the gonadotropic activity of the pituitary (4, 9, 26).

An increase in central levels of 5-HT induced either by administration of the immediate precursor of the amine, 5-hydroxy-tryptamine (5-HTP) (30) or by inhibition of monoamine oxidase (MAO) activity (1, 25, 27) also blocks ovulation. In the latter case, a specific involvement of 5-HT neurons is suggested by the observation that this effect is prevented by simultaneous administration of drugs which block the increase in 5-HT due to MAO inhibition (25). A converse situation exists in the case of induced changes in prolactin secretion: the suckling-induced rise in plasma prolactin, which has been shown to occur within minutes after the beginning of suckling (12, 33) is completely inhibited when the 5-HT synthesis inhibitor *p*-chlorophenylalanin (PCPA) is administered 0 to 96 hours before the suckling stimulus (20). The ability of lactating rats to release pituitary prolactin only reappears after 120 hours, an interval which corresponds well to that reported for full repletion of central 5-HT stores (28). The corresponding restoration experiment confirms that the effect of the drug involves a specific 5-HT mechanism, since repletion of central levels of the amine by 5-HTP results in a parallel restoration of the pituitary response (20).

An increase in brain CA induced by administration of L-DOPA is also able to block the prolactin response to suckling (Kordon, Blake and Sawyer, unpublished observations).

The response of hypothalamic structures responsible for triggering LH and prolactin release to specific neural inputs is thus modulated by antagonistic DA and 5-HT containing neurons. Surges in LH and prolactin are blocked respectively by drug-induced *decreases* or *increases* in hypothalamic levels of DA; restoration of normal levels of the amine parallely restores the capacity of the hypothalamo-hypophyseal system to release the hormones. The same responses are also inhibited by *converse* manipulations of hypothalamic 5-HT levels. In addition, micropharmacological experiments have shown that CA and 5-HT containing nerve endings involved in short time regulation of gonadotropic secretion are located in the medio-basal hypothalamus (16, 18).

Recent experiments suggest that a partial recovery of the neuroendocrine regulating mechanisms may occur in certain instances after modulatory or tuning influences delivered by aminergic neurons are permanently switched off. For instance, ovulation is blocked by 6-hydroxy-dopamine, a drug known to induce an irreversible destruction of DA containing neurons; but irregular estrous cycles have been shown to resume between 2 and 3 weeks after treatment (23). This observation raises the possibility that CA neurons may merely *sensitize* hypothalamic structures to neural inputs triggering ovulation; LH secretion regulating structures may however still be able to function in the absence of this modulatory influence.

"Long-term" versus "Short-term" Effects of Drugs on Hormonal Regulation

When suckling-induced release of prolactin is prevented by PCPA, the duration of the drug effect on hormonal and neurotransmitter levels are in good correspondence, as stated before. The situation is more complex, however, in the case of the interference of drugs affecting 5-HT metabolism with LH release.

An increase in 5-HT induced shortly before the "critical period" of ovulation control blocks the release of LH (25, 30). The converse manipulation, i.e. central 5-HT depletion, has no effect in the same time conditons (Fig. 3). However, if PCPA is given earlier, in the evening of diestrous day 2 (18 to 24 hours before the "critical period"), it blocks the ability of the pituitary to respond to the cyclic LH trigger input (Fig. 3). That 5-HT is also specifically involved in this delayed effect is shown by the ability of increasing doses of 5-HTP, when given together with PCPA, to induce a graded restoration of LH release (Fig. 4) (14).

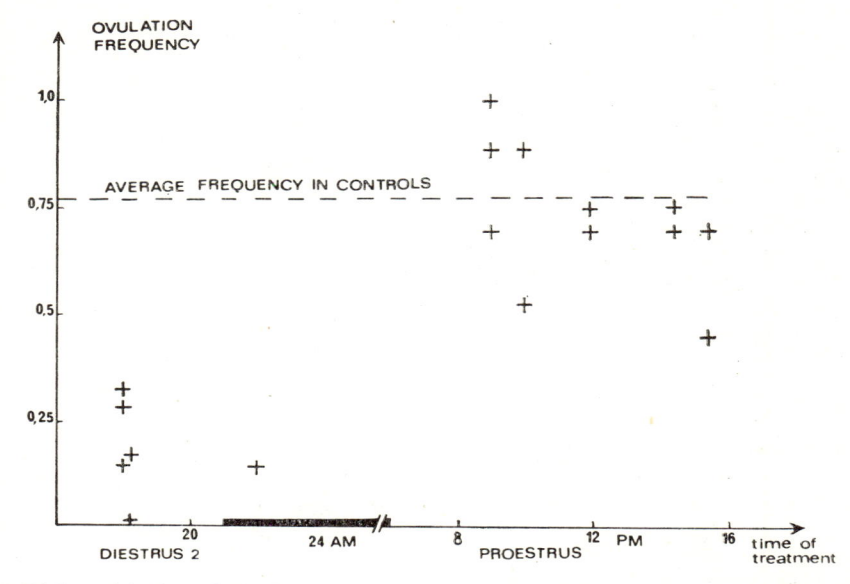

Fig. 3. Differential effect of 5-HT synthesis inhibition at various intervals in advance of the "critical period" of hypothalamic triggering of ovulation. Each dot represents the average ovulation frequency from groups of 8 to 10 experimental animals treated at the indicated time (from 14).

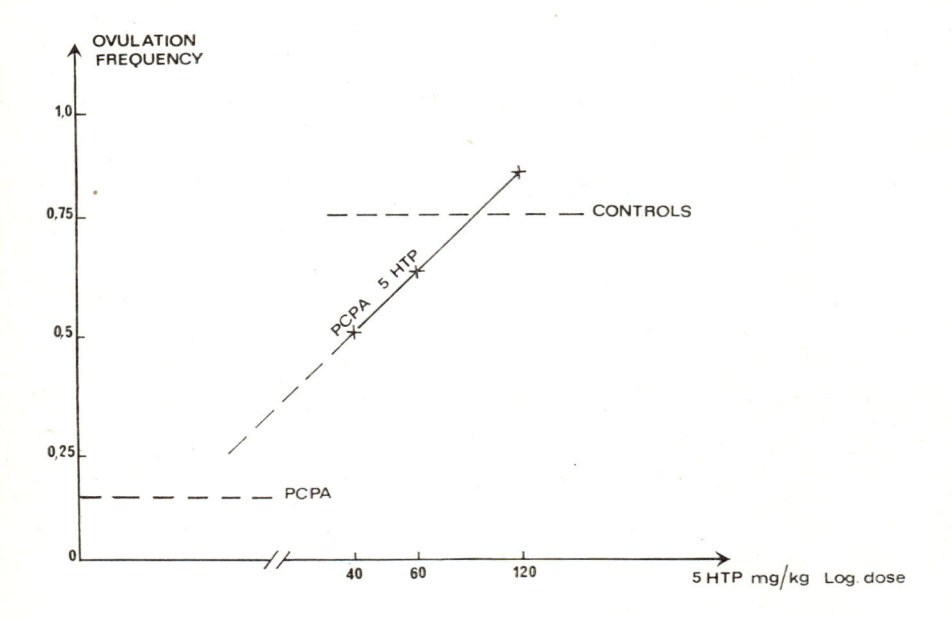

Fig. 4. Graded restoration of ovulation by increasing doses of 5-HTP given simultaneously with PCPA (treatment time: 20 hours in advance of the "critical period") (from 14).

This paradoxical effect of 5-HT depletion is hard to interpret at present. It may be connected with the sensitivity of the hypothalamus to estrogens: the endogenous rise in estrogens levels has been shown to play an important role in triggering the ovulatory surge of LH, and it has recently been suggested that 5-HT containing neurons may interfere with the uptake of ^{3}H-estradiol by the hypothalamus (10, 24). But it also seems that this paradoxical effect is related to the position of the treatment period in the circadian cycle of 5-HT metabolism. Incorporation of ^{3}H-tryptophan into ^{3}H-5-HT and ^{3}H-5-hydroxyindole-acetic acid (an extraneuronal metabolite of 5-HT which can be taken as an index of amine release) is subject to important circadian variations; synthesis of 5-HT is high during the light period and low during the night period, whereas 5-HT release follows a reverse pattern and appears to be more important during the night than in the daytime (13). Administration of PCPA, besides blocking the biosynthesis of 5-HT, also results in a rapid inhibition of the release of the amine (HAMON and GLOWINSKI, unpublished observations). Thus, everything happens as if an experimental modulation of 5-HT activity were only effective in blocking ovulation when it disrupts the rhythmical pattern of release of the amine: treatment with PCPA inhibits LH release whenever it *precedes* the period of high 5-HT release, but not when it follows it; the same explanation holds in the case of treatment with the precursor of the amine: 5-HTP has no effect *per se* at the beginning of the night, when 5-HT neurons are already active spontaneously, but blocks ovulation in the morning of proestrous, when 5-HT release is at its nadir.

CONCLUSIONS

We have reviewed here some of the multiple elements involved in the processing of neuroendocrine information, such as: a complex network of hypothalamic afferences and circuits and in particular important limbico-hypothalamic connexions; specialized neurons exhibiting the property of synthetizing specific steroid receptors; neurosecretory neurons elaborating hypothalamic neurohormones; and, finally, monoamine containing neurons supplying fibers to all above mentioned levels of the system.

Most available data suggest the monoaminergic component of the system mainly sensitizes the other neuronal elements towards afferent inputs. It thus behaves like an overall tuning system — in the acception often referred to in the case of the classical "sympathetic — parasympathetic" antagonism. Tuning variations are not by themselves highly specific, and can have parallel effects on several neuroendocrine functions (as well as on other autonomous regulations): we have seen for instance that an increased dopamine release within the median eminence simultaneously inhibits prolactin and stimulates the secretion of LH, but it also facilitates the release of other pituitary hormones, like TSH.

In order to understand how more elective endocrine regulations can be achieved, the notion of a monoaminergic "coding system" has been postulated (17). If we take the example of ovulation control, we have seen that the cyclic LH release is paralleled by an increased NA turnover within the preoptic area (22), but that it also depends upon a dopaminergic facilitation and upon the absence of a 5-HT inhibition at the neurovascular level. The sequential message for ovulation may therefore be written "NA $\nearrow$ (preoptic) + +(DA $\nearrow$ + 5-HT $\searrow$)(median eminence)"; taken as a whole, this message is more specific than any of its isolated components (other coding "bits", such as an additional involvement of acetylcholine, will probably also have to be added into the picture).

Complex interactions between neurons, hormone receptors and tuning systems involved in hormonostatic control account for the wide variety of factors which may affect or disturb it. It also calls for the development of new, more selective functional tests permitting to determine more accurately the primary impact of neuroendocrine syndromes.

REFERENCES

1. ALLEVA, J. J. and UMBERGER, E. J. (1966) Evidence for neural control of the release of pituitary ovulating hormone in the golden syrian hamster. Endocrinology, 78, 1125.
2. ANDEN, N. E., DAHLSTROM, A., FUXE, K., LARSSON, K., OLSON, L. and UNGERSTEDT, U. (1966) Ascending monoamine neurons to the telencephalon and diencephalon. Acta physiol. scand. 67, 313.
3. BARRACLOUGH, C. A. and SAWYER, C. H. (1957) Blockade of release of pituitary ovulating hormone in the rat by chlorpromazine and reserpine. Endocrinology, 61, 341.
4. BARRY, J. and LEONARDELLI, J. (1968) Etude comparée des neurones et des fibres monoaminergiques de la région tubero-infundibulaire chez le Cobaye male normal et castré. C. R. Acad. Sci. (Paris) 266, 15.
5. BHATTACHARYA, A. N., DIERSCHE, D. J., YAMAJI, Z. and KNOBIL, E. (1972) The pharmacological blockade of the circhoral mode of LH secretion in the ovariectomized Rhesus monkey. Endocrinology, 90, 778.
6. BROWN, P. S. (1967) Antigonadotropic effects of α-methyl tyrosine, methysergide and reserpine. Nature, 214, 1268.
7. DONOSO, A. D., GUTTIEREZ-MOVANO, M. B. and SANTOLAYA, R. L. (1969) Metabolism of noradrenalin in the hypothalamus of castrated rats. Neuroendocrinology, 4, 12.
8. DONOSO, A. O., BISHOP, W., FAWCETT, C. KRULICH, L. and MCCANN, S. M. (1971) Effects of drugs that modify brain monoamine concentrations on plasma gonadotropin and prolactin levels in the rat. Endocrinology, 89, 774.
9. FUXE, K. and HÖKFELT, T. (1967) The influence of central catecholamines neurons on the hormone secretion from the anterior and posterior pituitary. In: Neurosecretion, p. 227, Springer, Berlin.
10. GOGAN, F., MESS, B. and KORDON, C. (1971) Effet de drogues affectant la libération des monoamines centrales sur la captation d'oestradiol-³H dans l'hypothalamus. J. Endocrinol. 37, 225.
11. GRIMM, Y. and REICHLIN, S. (1972) Neurotransmitter and ionic control of thyrotropin releasing hormone release from mouse hypothalamic fragments in vitro. Excerpta Med. intern. Congr. Ser. 256, 84.
12. GROSVENOR, C. E. and TURNER, C. W. (1958) Assay of lactogenic hormone. Endocrinology, 63, 530.
13. HERY, F., ROUER, E. and GLOWINSKI, J. (1972) Daily variations of serotonin metabolism in the rat brain. Brain Res. 43, 445.
14. HERY, M. and KORDON, C. (1972) Effets rapides et différés de l'inhibition de la biosynthèse de sérotonine sur l'ovulation chez la ratte. C.R. Soc. Biol. (Paris), in press.
15. KORDON, C. (1967) Contrôle nerveux du cycle ovarien. Arch. Anat. micr. morphol. exp. 56, suppl. 34, 458.
16. KORDON, C. (1969) Effects of selective experimental changes in regional hypothalamic monoamine levels on superovulation in the immature rat. Neuroendocrinology, 4, 129.
17. KORDON, C. (1970) Rôle des monoamines dans les régulations adénohypophysaires. In: Neuroendocrinologie. Ed. by J. BENOIT and C. KORDON, CNRS, Paris, p. 73.
18. KORDON, C. (1971) Blockade of ovulation in the immature rat by local dopamine release inhibition in the arcuate region of the hypothalamus. Neuroendocrinology, 6, 202.
19. KORDON, C. (1972) Effect of drugs acting on brain monoamines and control of gonadotropic secretion. Excerpta Med. intern. Congr. Series, in press.
20. KORDON, C., BLAKE, C. A., TERKEL, J. and SAWYER, C. H. (1973) Participation of serotonin containing neurons in the suckling induced rise in plasma prolactin levels in lactating rats. Neuroendocrinology, in press.
21. KORDON, C. and GLOWINSKI, J. (1969) Selective inhibition of superovulation by blockade of dopamine synthesis during the critical period in the immature rat. Endocrinology, 85, 924.
22. KORDON, C. and GLOWINSKI, J. (1970) Role of brain catecholamines in the control of anterior pituitary functions. In: Neurochemistry of the hypothalamus, Academic Press, New York, p. 85.
23. KORDON, C. and HERY, M. (1971) Effects of destruction of central catecholaminergic neurons by 6-hydroxy-dopamine and of L-DOPA on ovulation in the rat. Physiologist, 95, 338.
24. KORDON, C., HERY, M., ROTSZTEJN, W. and GOGAN, F. (1972) Interactions between hypothala-

mic serotoninergic neurons and the regulation of gonadotropic secretion. Gynec. Invest. **2**, 116.
25. KORDON, C., JAVOY, F., VASSENT, G. and GLOWINSKI, J. (1968) Blockade of superovulation in the immature rat by increased brain serotonin. Europ. J. Pharmacol. **4**, 169.
26. LICHTENSTEIGER, W. (1969) Cyclic variations of catecholamine content in hypothalamic nerve cells during the estrous cycle of the rat, with a concomitant study of the substantia nigra. J. Pharmacol. exp. Ther. **165**, 204.
27. LIPPMANN, W. (1968) Relationship between norepinephrine and serotonin and gonadotropic secretion in the hamster. Nature, **218**, 173.
28. LOVENBERG, W., JEQUIER, E. and SJOERDSMA, A. (1968) Tryptophan hydroxylation in mammalian systems. In: Advances in pharmacology, Vol. **6,** p. 21, Academic Press, New York.
29. MEYERSON, B. and SAWYER, C. H. (1968) Monoamines and ovulation in the rat. Endocrinology, **83**, 170.
30. PSYCHOYOS, A. (1966). Effet de la photopériodicité et de diverses substances sur la réponse de l'ovaire à l'hormone lutéinisante hypophysaire. C.R. Acad. Sci. (Paris), **263**, 986.
31. SCHNEIDER, H. P. G. and MCCANN, S. M. (1969) Possible role of dopamine as a transmitter to promote discharge of LH-releasing factor. Endocrinology, **85**, 121.
32. SOURKES, T. L. (1965) The action of α-methyl-dopa in the brain. Brit. med. Bull. **21**, 68.
33. TERKEL, J., BLAKE, C. A. and SAWYER, C. H. (1972). Differential effects of suckling and of stress to release prolactin in the lactating rat. Endocrinology, in press.

C.K.,Neurobiological Unit, National Institute of Health and Medical Research, 2 rue d'Alésia, 75014 Paris, France

PHARMACOLOGICAL EXPERIMENTS TO STIMULATE HUMAN SEXUAL BEHAVIOUR

O. BENKERT

Psychiatric Clinic of the University, Munich

Sexual impotence represents a difficult clinical task for the psychiatrist as it occurs quite frequently and is hardly affected by therapy. The psychiatrist engaged in biological research faces problems of the same magnitude when dealing with sexual disorders. Our knowledge of the biology of sexual behaviour is scanty, in addition we lack the suitable psychometric scales necessary for the objectification of sexual behaviour, a prerequisite indispensable in evaluating the effect on therapy of the substance in question.

By sexual impotence, we understand diminished or non-existent capacity of erection together with a retained, diminished or non-existent sexual drive in intercourse. Occasionally, the capacity of orgasm and ejaculation may be obstructed.

Diseases accompanied by sexual impotence are manifold. But sexual impotence also occurs as an exclusive symptom lacking any discernible accompanying disease. It is customary to distinguish its causes as being either organic or psychic. *Organic* sexual impotence is classified according to its accompanying disease. Impotence may occur above all with the following diseases, as a concomitant symptom: in endocrinological disorders, in metabolic disorders and in disorders of the central nervous system. *Psychic* sexual impotence is accounted for either reactively, or by means of psychodynamics. Classification of sexual impotence as a concomitant symptom of psychosis varies as being either of psychic or organic origin.

Medicamentous therapy of impotence is essentially based on substitution of the male sexual hormones. But a substantial increase in sexual activity through this substitution is only possible for hypogonadism and castrates. Some authors have registered a decrease in testosterone-plasma concentration in the case of impotence. Nonetheless, in view of the pertinent studies up to date, a correlation between the production of testosterone and sexual activity is not warranted (15).

It is therefore hardly surprising that the therapy of impotence by administration of male sexual hormones with e.g. vitamine A, vitamin E, yohimbine or strychnine turn out to be unsatisfactory for therapy as well. Doses of opiates or of derivatives of amphetamine are not feasible for therapy as they induce addiction. On the other hand, of course, there is agreement on male sexual hormones being indispensable for the sexual drive.

One reason for the hitherto unsuccessful medicamentous therapy has been obsoleteness of the pharmacotherapy of impotence even when its determinants were only partly of psychic origin. In pharmacotherapy, however, in the first stage of scientific examination, it would be more expedient to abandon the customary frame of reference to classic therapy and its nosological classification in favour of one less prone to presuppositions, such as the target-symptom (7). The example of the pharmacotherapy of depression illustrates the practical significance of this approach. Antidepressives are not only able to exert an influence in case of an "endogenous" genesis but also when "exogenous" or "neurotic" origin is given. This ought to induce us not to assign every depression, as a first step, to its nosological category. It seems justifiable, at least during the initial stage of therapy, to reverse the usual procedure and to do without distinguishing between somatogenic and psychogenic components.

This perspective offers the advantage of abandoning the nosological approach in other psychopathological syndromes as well. Thus, a new field of study will be launched for pharmacotherapy in the treatment of sexual disorders as well, precisely omitting the customary first step of distinguishing between somatogenic and psychogenic factors. Just as anti-depressives are applied in depression "sexually stimulating substances" may be given for sexual impotence (Fig. 1).

This approach has become conceivable solely on the basis of the results of experimental research with animals. For a long time, investigation of sexual behaviour had been predominant. Information on the site of the centers of sexual behaviour in the brain had delivered decisive support to this orientation (18). Side by side with the clarification of the influence of sexual hormones on the sexual behaviour of animals (15), the effect of neurohormones on sexual behaviour has now been placed into the foreground. The results of the latter have been discussed at length at this symposium.

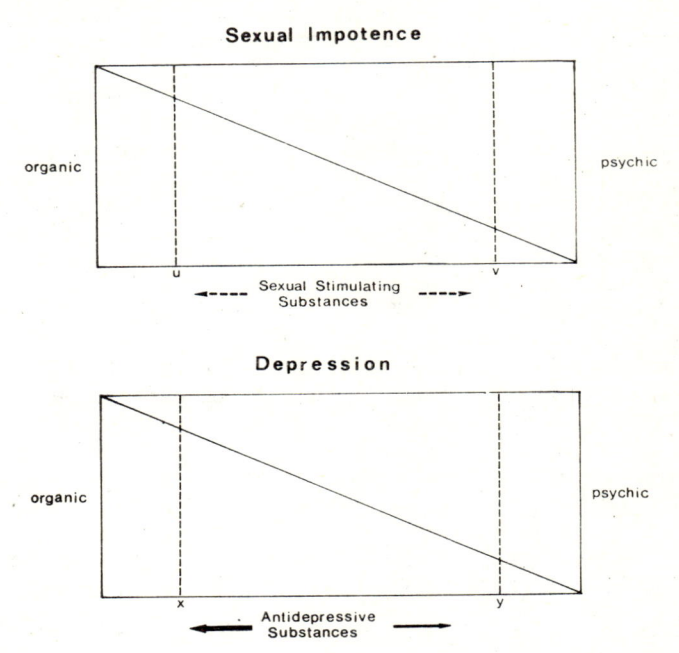

Fig. 1. Comparison of the organic and psychic origin of depression and sexual impotence, as well as the treatments possible.
For explanation see text. x, y and u, v characterize 4 patients with organic resp. psychic component of disease.

The extent to which these results may signify a point of departure for pharmacotherapy will be stated in the following.

The starting-point of the study had been two observations:

1. A higher dose of L-DOPA, administered to patients with Parkinson's disease, brings about increased sexuality for some patients (6, 8, 9).

2. After *p*-chlorophenylalanine (PCPA), mounting behaviour is increased in animals (20).

In treating Parkinson's disease with L-DOPA, there remained the question whether the increase in sexual activity had been in fact due to L-DOPA or whether an unspecific effect had evolved on the strength of general improvement. In order to inquire into this question 10 male out-patients were chosen for this pilot-study (2). All patients complained of insufficient penile erection; in addition, some complained of a decrease in libido. The complaints had persisted for at least one year; all had a permanent female partner, and there were no aversions against these partners. The patients filled out a daily questionnaire specifying the most important data on sexual activity. There were no pathological findings in the spermiograms.

The patients received 3 g L-DOPA for 12 weeks. Two patients experienced severe side-effects and were excluded from the experiment. A slight increase in the degree of penile erection ensued in 6 out of 8 patients; in no case, however, was the degree of erection attained sufficient for sexual intercourse to be performed successfully as it had been in the past. Increased frequency of spontaneous erections during the night was noted by the patients as the most conspicuous symptom after more prolonged L-DOPA treatment. An increase of libido was registered in only 2 patients. Also worth mentioning is the increase of working capacity. The frequency of the other symptoms is listed in Table 1.

TABLE 1

Effect of L-DOPA on sexually impotent patients

	L-DOPA vs no medication n = 8	Mesterolone vs (mest.) placebo n = 10	Mesterolone + L-DOPA vs mesterolone n = 8
Increase in degree of penile erection (2)	6	1	3
Increase in degree of penile erection (3)	0	0	0
Increased frequency of spontaneous erection during the night	5	1	1
Change in ejaculation consistency	2	0	1
Increase of ejaculation volume	2	1	0
Retarded ejaculation	0	0	0
Scrotal discomfort and pain	1	0	2
Increase of libido	2	1	1
Increased frequency of sexual dreams during the night	2	1	1
Increase of working capacity	5	0	3

Dosages: mesterolone 150 mg/daily, L-DOPA 3 g/daily.

Furthermore, mesterolone only (10, 13) at a dosage of 50 mg 3× daily, was given for 8 weeks. Essentially, no effect in stimulating sexual potency or libido was observed (for the small changes see Table 1). Eight of these patients were after 8 weeks given 3 g L-DOPA daily for 4 to 8 weeks in addition to the basic therapy of mesterolone. Thus a comparison between L-DOPA alone and mesterolone plus L-DOPA was possible. But the combination treatment with mesterolone plus L-DOPA proved to be no more effective than L-DOPA applied alone; its effect was even smaller than the slight increase in sexual behaviour observed after treatment with L-DOPA alone.

It is indubitable that L-DOPA had a positive influence on sexual behaviour. This influence does not, however, suffice for an effective therapy of impotence. Furthermore, in establishing the cause of this effect, it should be noted that in animal experiments L-DOPA exerts an influence on the gonadotropic hormones and that there is a decrease of the serotonin brain-level.

Before the human experiments on the stimulation of sexual activity were continued, the influence of a decrease of the serotonin concentration in the brain with simultaneous maximum increase in dopamine (DA) concentration in the brain was tested regarding the mounting behaviour of the rat (4). TAGLIAMONTE et al. have shown the combination of PCPA and the monoaminoxidase inhibitor pargyline to induce a further increase in mounting behaviour in contrast to an exclusive PCPA dosage (19).

We tested first the combination of the decarboxylaseinhibitor Ro 4-4602 (17) plus L-DOPA to induce mounting behaviour. This combination leads to a high and significant increase in dopamine; to a slight and insignificant increase of 7% in norepinephrine and a significant decrease of 41.1% in the serotonin level of the rat brain (Table 2, for methods see legend). Only one of forty rats showed mounting behaviour. A further increase of the DA-level and a further decrease of the serotonin level of the brain to 34.2% by pre-treatment with reserpine caused mounting behaviour in one of four rats ($1/4$) in almost every cage. When PCPA pre-treatment was given instead of reserpine, a considerable increase in mounting behaviour occurred. In almost every cage, two of four rats showed

TABLE 2

Correlation between brain amine level and behaviour

Substance, i.p. (mg/kg)					Brain levels (%)			Behaviour
Reserpine	PCPA	Ro 4-4602	L-DOPA	DA	NE	5-HT	Mountings
—	—	50	200	740.0±23	107.0±7	41.1±3	0
2	—	50	200	1,050.0±40	60.9±5	34.2±2	*
—	3×100	50	200	532.0±15	105.5±6	38.5±2	**

The amine level of the whole brain was listed in % of controls. The controls were injected with saline. DA = 1.07±0.116 mg/kg; NE = 0.45±0.046 mg/kg; 5-HT = 0.83±0.098. For methods see (1,11). Each value refers to 4 to 10 rats. Reserpine was injected 16 hr, and Ro 4-4602 45 min before L-DOPA. PCPA was injected three times at 24-hr intervals; 24 hr after the last PCPA injection, Ro 4-4602 plus L-DOPA was given. The time of observation follows 1 hr after the L-DOPA injection for 4 rats in each cage (4 to 10 cages).

The note 1/4—4/4 refers to the number of active animals in a cage (max. 4/4); the symbols often, very often) relate to the number of cages in which the respective behaviour was observed.

Mountings: *: often 1/4; 3 to 40 mountings
 **: very often 2/4; 3 to 40 mountings

mountings. The relationship between a high DA-level and the serotonin level remains (Table 2). It should be added that these trials took place in the morning under normal lighting conditions and not, as usually, in the evening. Testosterone was not administered. These experiments indicate that under these conditions of simultaneously lowering the serotonin level and raising the DA-level mounting behaviour increases.

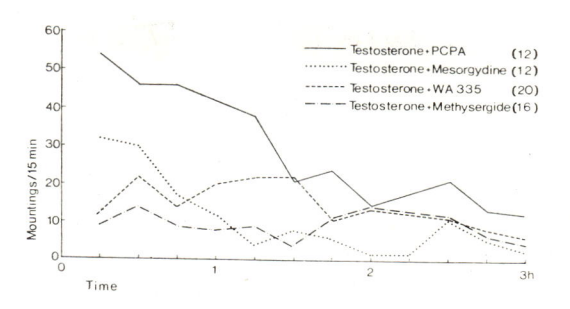

Fig. 2. Mounting behaviour after substances with anti-serotonergic effect.
The number of mountings over 3 hr were added in periods of 15 minutes. Number of rats in brackets. There were 4 rats in each cage. After testosterone alone (12 rats) 2 rats exhibited mountings only very occasionally — on an average of once every 1/4 hr. Testosterone-proprionate (10 mg/kg) was given s.c. 4 times in periods of 24 hr, the last dosage being 5 1/2 h before the beginning of the observation. PCPA-ester (100 mg/kg) was injected i.p. twice in periods of 24 hr. The last dosage being 24 hr before the beginning of the observation. Methysergide (1 mg/kg; i.p.) was injected 2 h, mesorgydine (0,5 mg/kg; i.p.) 2 h and WA 335-BS (0.1 mg/kg; i.p.) 2 hr before the beginning of the observation. The observation started at 18.30.

On the basis of these experiments and the publication of relevant findings the attempt was undertaken to solve the question whether mounting behaviour induced by PCPA is prompted specifically by this substance or non-specifically by lowering the serotonin level of the brain. Thus, the effect of the serotonin antagonists, mesorgydine (12), methysergide (14) and WA 335-BS (21) was observed on mounting behaviour in rats compared with PCPA (3). It was shown that testosterone plus PCPA determine the highest increase in mounting behaviour (Fig. 2). Mountings are especially frequent in the first 1½ hr. After doses of mesorgydine, WA 335-BS and methysergide in combination with testosterone, mountings were less frequent in the first 1½ hr when compared with PCPA. During the last period of observation mountings decreased slowly for all tested substances. Minimally increased sexual excitation was also noted after mesorgydine by PODVALOVÁ and DLABAČ (16) and after p-chloromethylamphetamine (PCMA) (5) which has been shown to decrease the serotonin level of the brain in the rat. These observations consequently lead to the conclusion that the anti-serotonin effect in combination with testosterone could have a causative effect on the activation of mounting behaviour in male rats.

The next step was to utilize the anti-serotonergic effect for stimulating sexual activity in the human male. In the following experiment the patients had to observe identical conditions as in the experiment with L-DOPA described above. First, the patients were given placebos for a period of 8 weeks. One patient observed an increased capacity of erection as a result of the placebo medication. Thereafter, PCMA (90 mg/daily) and methysergide resp. (6 mg/daily) in combination with mesterolone (150 mg/daily) were administered to 8 impotent patients. Two patients out of 10 had to be excluded from the experiment because of initial side-effects. PCMA and methysergide resp. was administered for 5 weeks while the dosage of mesterolone was maintained. The ultimate dosage of PCMA and methysergide resp. was reached at the end of the first week through gradual increase. Subsequent to the dosage of PCMA an increase in the erective capacity of 5 patients became conspicuous; 2 of the patients felt to have regained their former full sexual capacity. Two patients displayed retarded ejaculation under the influence of PCMA, 2 others a rise in libido. Two patients manifested no changes in sexual behaviour, in fact, they suffered severest side-effects: headaches, vertigo, irritability. After treatment with methysergide, a completely normal capacity of erection was noted in 2 patients while 2 others showed an increase in libido (Table 3).

TABLE 3

Effect of anti-serotonergic substances on sexually impotent patients

	Placebo vs no medication n = 10	Mesterolone + PCMA vs mesterolone n = 8	Mesterolone + methysergide vs mesterolone n = 8
Increase in degree of penile erection (2)	1	3	0
Increase in degree of penile erection (3)	0	2	2
Increased frequency of spontaneous erection during the night	0	0	0
Change in ejaculation consistency	0	1	0
Increase of ejaculation volume	0	0	0
Retarded ejaculation	0	2	1
Scrotal discomfort and pain	0	1	0
Increase of libido	0	2	2
Increased frequency of sexual dreams during the night	0	0	0
Increase of working capacity	0	1	1

Dosages: mesterolone 150 mg/daily, PCMA 90 mg/daily, methysergide 6 mg/daily.

In contrast to the treatment with L-DOPA, the dosage of the serotonin antagonists induced in 2 patients complete normalization of a previously diminished capacity of erection. The patients pleaded strongly to be allowed to continue with the medicamentation.

The dosage of PCPA in combination with mesterolone was also tried with some impotent patients. The experiment, however, encountered difficulties as a high dosage of this combination produces considerable side-effects with out-patients. Inspite of these side-effects, 3 out of 5 patients liked to continue the combination of mesterolone plus PCPA because of the increase in the degree of penile erection.

These results show that the dosage of the serotonin antagonists — possibly in combination with L-DOPA — suggest a new method of increasing sexual activity in humans. Together with the development of adequate psychometric scales making it possible to objectivize sexual disorders, further attempts at neuro-hormonal alteration must be made in animal and human experiments with the aim to activate sexual activity.

References

1. ANTON, A. H. and SAYRE, D. F. (1964) The distribution of dopamine and Dopa in various animals and a method for their determination in diverse biological material. J. Pharmacol. exp. Ther. 145, 326.
2. BENKERT, O., CROMBACH, G. and KOCKOTT, G. (1972) Effect of L-Dopa on sexually impotent patients. Psychopharmacologia, 23, 91.
3. BENKERT, O. and EVERSMANN, T. (1972) Importance of the anti-serotonin effect for mounting behaviour in rats. Experientia, 28, 532.
4. BENKERT, O., GLUBA, H. and MATUSSEK, N. (1973) Dopamine, Norepinephrine and 5-Hydromine in relation to motor activity, fighting and mounting behaviour; part II. Neuropharmacology, 12, 187.
5. BERTOLINI, A. and VERGONI, W. (1970) Effecto eccito-sessuale della P-Cloro-N-Metilamfetamina associata a testosterone, nel ratto maschio. Riv. Farmacol. Ter. 1, 423.
6. CALNE, D. B. and SANDLER, M. (1970) L-Dopa and parkinsonism. Nature, 226, 21.
7. FREYHAN, F. A. (1957) Psychomotilität, extrapyramidale Syndrome und Wirkungsweisen neuroleptischer Therapien. Nervenarzt, 28, 504.
8. HYYPPÄ, M., RINNE, V. K. and SONNINEN, V. (1970) The activating effect of L-Dopa treatment on sexual function and its experimental background. Acta neurol. scand., 46 Suppl. 43, 223.
9. JENKINS, R. B. and GROH, R. H. (1970) Mental symptoms in parkinsonian patients treated with L-Dopa. Lancet, II, 177.
10. LASCHET, U., LASCHET, L. and PAARMAN, H. F. (1966) Die Gonadotropin- und Steroidhormon-Ausscheidung während der Behandlung mit Mesterolon. Arzneimittel. Forsch. 16, 469.
11. MAICKEL, R. P., COX., R. H. JR., SAILLANT, J. and MILLER, F. P. (1968) A method for the determination of serotonin and norepinephrine in discrete areas of rat brain. Int. J. Neuropharmacol. 7, 275.
12. Mesorgydine = N-(D-6-methyl-8-isoergolenyl)-N',N'-diethylurea (Lysenyl Spofa, Prague).
13. Mesterolone = 1α-methyl-5α-androstan-17ß-ol-3-on, Schering AG, Berlin.
14. Methysergide = Deseril, Sandoz AG, Basel.
15. NEUMANN, F. and STEINBECK, H. (1971) Hormonale Beeinflussung des Verhaltens. Klin. Wschr. 49, 790.
16. PODVALOVÁ, I. and DLABAČ, A. (1970) Aggressive behaviour of rats induced by mesorgydine. Act. nerv. Sup. 12, 81.
17. Ro 4-4602 = N (DL-Seryl)-N'-(2, 3, 4-trihydroxy-benzyl) hydrazine, Hoffmann-La Roche AG, Basel.
18. SPATZ, H. (1951) Neues über die Verknüpfung von Hypophyse und Hypothalamus. Mit besonderer Berücksichtigung der Regulation sexueller Leistungen. Acta neuroveg. 3, 5.
19. TAGLIAMONTE, A., TAGLIAMONTE, P., GESSA, G. L. (1971) Reversal of pargyline-induced inhibition of sexual behaviour in male rats by parachlorophenylanine. Nature, 230, 244.
20. TAGLIAMONTE, A. (1972) Control of male sexual behaviour by monoaminergic and cholinergic mechanisms. This symposium.
21. WA 335-BS = 9, 10-Dihydro-10 (1-methyl-4-piperidyliden)-9-anthrol. Thomae AG, Biberach.

O.B., Psychiatric Clinic of the University, 8 München 2, Nussbaumstr. 7, B.R.D.

ANTIANDROGENS IN SEXUAL DISORDERS: INFLUENCE OF CYPROTERONE ACETATE ON THE HUMAN NEURO-ENDOCRINE SYSTEM

URSULA LASCHET and L. LASCHET

Department of Psychoendocrinology, Psychiatric Clinic, Landeck

Antiandrogens inhibit competitively the action of endogenous and exogenous androgens at all androgen target organs.

The competitive blocking of the central nervous target organs through the antiandrogen cyproterone acetate is being used therapeutically for the dose-dependent temporary and therefore reversible reduction or inhibition of sexuality in the human male (1—6; 8—14). We reported on these results at the last CINP Congress in Prague and are overlooking now the results in more than 200 treated men.

Apart from the competitive inhibition of the diencephalic receptors which are dependent on androgen stimulation and responsible for the release of sexual reactions such as libido, erection and orgasm, the hypothalamic target areas which are responsible for the positive and negative feedback between androgen blood level and gonadotropin releasers are also influenced.

Pharmacologically, cyproterone acetate belongs first and foremost to the group of antiandrogens. Although its progestogenic partial action plays no role whatsoever in the reversible reduction of sexuality, it is precisely this which permits long-term therapy via the cybernetic regulatory mechanisms in the endocrine system with an antiandrogen.

Figure 1 gives a schematic representation of the regulatory mechanisms which operate in the circle of function gonadotropin releaser (gonadotropin release) androgen production and secretion of the testes during treatment with a pure antiandrogen (free unesterified cyproterone), with cyproterone acetate (antiandrogen with progestogenic partial action) and with a steroid with an antigonadotropic action without antiandrogenic activity (e.g. oestrogens). A comparison is made with the influence on the neuroendocrine regulatory mechanisms of surgical castration and of optimal stereotactical neutralization of the central-nervous androgen target areas (mating centers). Physiologically, there is a cybernetically regulated equilibrium between the production and secretion of gonadotropin releasers and hence the release of gonadotropins from the anterior lobe of the pituitary and the testicular production and secretion of testosterone.

The absence of the testosterone feedback regulation following surgical castration results in an increased production and secretion of gonadotropin releasers and hence an above-normal release of gonadotropins.

Following optimal stereotactical neutralization of the hypothalamic androgen target areas the production of gonadotropin releasers ceases. Consequently, the release of gonadotropins from the pituitary also comes to a stand-still. The testes atrophy and the Leydig cells cease the production and secretion of testosterone.

Exogenous steroids with an antigonadotropic action reduce the production and secretion of gonadotropin releasers dose and time dependently; with optimal antigonadotropic action the production of releasers is completely suppressed and gonadotropin release is brought to a complete halt. The testes atrophy here, too, and the secretion of testosterone by the Leydig cells also ceases. Suppression is not always reversible.

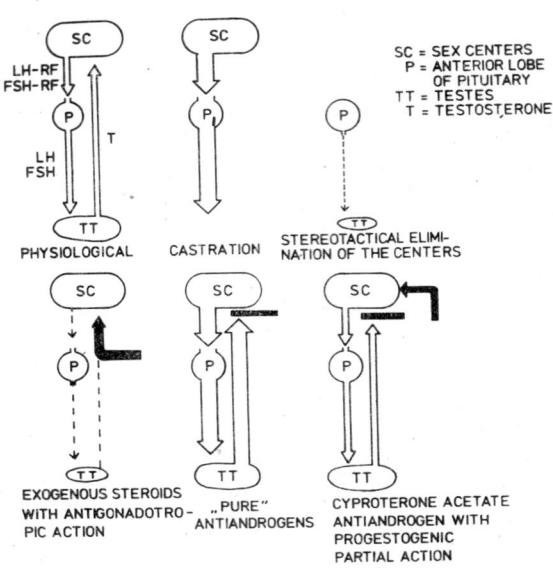

Fig. 1. Schematic representation of the regulatory mechanisms in gonadotropin releaser function.

The competitive inhibition of the hypothalamic androgen target areas by a "pure" antiandrogen, i.e. by an antiandrogen without an antigonadotropic partial action (free unesterified cyproterone) has the same effect on the production and secretion of gonadotropin releasers and gonadotropin release from the pituitary as surgical castration. The resulting above-normal gonadotropin blood level stimulates testicular Leydig cell function and hence testosterone production and secretion to beyond the physiological and, because of the elevated testosterone blood level, makes an increase in the dosage necessary during the antiandrogen therapy — a measure which is still not capable of preventing the continued disequilibrium of the system. A protracted hypergonadotropic condition, however, leads to irreversible testicular damage.

With cyproterone acetate, the increase in gonadotropin release resulting from the antiandrogen action is to a great extent counterbalanced by the antigonadotropic action of the progestogenic partial function, as assays of gonadotropin excretion in 24-hour urine, spermatogenetic findings and clinical findings during long-term therapy with cyproterone acetate have demonstrated. Checks were also made to establish whether the circle of function corticotropin releaser (CRF)/ACTH release of the pituitary/ adrenal cortex is disturbed by long-term cyproterone acetate treatment.

Methods

We studied 120 men between the ages of 16 and 67, who had been treated orally with cyproterone acetate at daily doses of 50—200 mg for at least 8 months and a maximum of 5 years.

We assayed the gonadotropins in 24-hour urine following fractionated alcohol precipitation (7). ICSH, the total gonadotropic activity and FSH were assayed using the same extract. ICSH was determined immunologically in the quantitative, standardized, modified Pregnosticon-test against the II. international reference preparation for HMG, the total gonadotropic activity in the mouse uterus test, FSH in the Steelman-Pohley test. Results are in IU (II. international reference preparation for HMG).

The ACTH capacity of the pituitary was checked: in the oral metopirone test, 4 g/day for two days, 8 g/day for two days; the adrenocortical capacity in the ACTH loading test; 4 examination days following 2 mg synthetic Zn-ACTH i.m. and ACTH suppression test with 2 and 8 mg dexamethasone/day orally for two days. 17-Ketosteroid assay was performed according to Zimmermann; 17-ketogenic steroids after Norymberski; cortisol after Mattingly. Glucose tolerance test was done following a single administration of 50 g orally.

Results

In the first months of treatment in all cases examined the antigonadotropic action from the progestogenic partial action was clearly superior to the increase in gonadotropin production and secretion rate resulting from the antiandrogen partial action. During the first months we were able to detect in every single case a decrease of gonadotropin excretion in the 24-hours urine. An example of this is given in Tables 1 and 2.

Table 1

Gonadotropins during 100 mg/day cyproterone acetate treatment (IU 2nd IRP for HMG)

		ICSH	TGA
Pretreatment values (Schäf.)		22	21
		35	18
		24	10
Weeks	1	24	9
	2	8	4
	3	10	<2
	6	<5	4
	9	5	6
	12	<4	<2
	20	<2	3
	30	2	5
	52	4	8

In Table 1 are the values of a 57-year-old exhibitionist, who was treated with 100 mg cyproterone acetate orally per day; ICSH and TGA excretion was under the lower limits of detection at the end of the 12th week of treatment. At the end of the 20th week of treatment TGA excretion had recovered to 3 IU/24 hrs, and at the end of the 30th week of treatment 2 IU ICSH and 5 IU TGA were again demonstrable.

The equalization of the initially dominant antigonadotropic action occurs at different times depending on the individual and also on the daily dose; when 100 mg orally/day are administered, this usually occurs between the 8th and the 15th month of treatment.

TABLE 2

Gonadotropins during 100 mg/day cyproterone acetate treatment (IU 2nd IRP for HMG)

	ICSH	TGA
Pretreatment	19	3
values (Schn.)	4	3
	3	3
Months: 2	<4	<4
4	<3	<2
6	<3	2
7	3	3
15	4	5
23	3	3
30	4	4
40	20	6
51	17	6

Table 2 shows the gonadotropin excretion values of a 47-year-old heterosexual paedophilic poriomaniac, in whom the maximum antigonadotropic effect was registered at the end of the 4th month of treatment. Between the 7th and the 15th month ICSH and TGA excretion recover to the pre-treatment values. From about the 40th month of treatment there is a noticeable tendency for the values to increase to above the pre-treatment control values in the sense of a developing preponderance of the increase in releaser production and gonadotropin release resulting from the antiandrogen action. This does not, however, affect the inhibition of sexuality.

If 200 mg cyproterone acetate orally/day are administered, the equalization of the initially dominant antigonadotropic action seems to take a bit longer. In most cases it occurs between the 15th and the 20th month of treatment (Table 3).

This exhibitionist, 16 years old at the start of treatment, with hypergonadotropic values (a genetic defect had been excluded) excreted upto the 14th month of treatment ICSH, TGA and FSH amounts which lay below the limits of detection. From the 15th month of treatment onwards, gonadotropin excretion rose again and reached the pre-treatment values in the 23rd month; after this and upto the end of five years of treatment there was no further rise.

As long as an antigonadotropic effect is demonstrable, one must expect suppression of spermatogenesis from its presence alone; the occupation of the androgen-sensitive

TABLE 3
Gonadotropins during 200 mg/day cyproterone acetate treatment (IU 2nd IRP for HMG)

	ICSH	TGA	FSH
Pretreatment	32	18	61
values (Mar.)	36	14	24
Months: 2	<7	11	<15
5	<2.5	9	<12
8	<3	<4	<20
15	5	11	<15
18	20	13	18
23	37	17	31
30	33	31	33
34	43	22	61
48	31	13	72
58	38	34	45

testicular receptors is of only secondary importance for the inhibition of fertility during this therapy period.

With the normalization of gonadotropin production and secretion, Leydig cell function and hence testosterone production and secretion must also normalize. Whilst an antiandrogen is still active, however, a normalization of spermatogenesis or of the ejaculate need not necessarily result. For the decisive factor for spermatogenesis is the intratesticular testosterone level, but for the ejaculate the androgen-dependent excretory function of the accessory sex glands.

The intratesticular testosterone level should normalize with the return of gonadotropin excretion values to the individual pre-treatment norm. If the daily administered dose of cyproterone acetate allows an adequate excretory function of the accessory sex glands, one can theoretically expect a fertile ejaculate from the moment gonadotropin secretion normalizes.

When we administered 100 or 200 mg cyproterone acetate orally per day, after a time which varied from case to case — usually after 2—3 months of treatment — no ejaculate or at the most a total amount of upto 0.5 ml per masturbation could be obtained. This situation remained unchanged right upto the end of 5 years of treatment with 200 mg/day. With 100 mg/day, however, a gradual increase in the volume of the ejaculate to about 1 ml towards the end of the 2nd year of treatment was recorded in some cases. This was variable, however, and occurred in the presence of continuing, severely suppressed sexuality. In no case was the ejaculate fertile.

Two men, who were initially treated with 100 mg orally per day, followed by a maintenance dose of 50 mg/day, produced offspring during the supervised, uninterrupted treatment.

A 33-year-old, married teacher with heterosexual paedophilic and exhibitionistic drive variant, father of two children (no criminal record), was given 100 mg the day for the first month of treatment followed by 50 mg the day for a total of 21 months. Under 50 mg/day cohabitation was possible at the most once a week. During the first year of treatment no ejaculate worth studying could be obtained. In the 17th month of treatment a pregnancy mens II was diagnosed in his wife. At this time 1.9 ml ejaculate with 29 million sperms/ml was obtained after 2 days of abstinence.

A 41-year old, married exhibitionist with a long criminal record but nothing outstanding at the moment, father of one child, who requested treatment because of pressure of emotion, was given 100 mg/day for the first 10 months of treatment, followed by 50 mg the day for 19 months. During the first year of treatment cohabitation was possible only rarely; there was a condition of anorgasm. In the 21st month of treatment a pregnancy mens II was diagnosed in his wife. At this time 2 ml ejaculate with 37.8 million sperms/ml was obtained after 5 days of abstinence. A healthy girl was born at term.

The test for the reactivity of the adrenal cortex against ACTH, for the ACTH reserve in the oral Metopirone test and ACTH suppression through Dexamethasone showed no deviations from the norm in 10 men studied, who had been treated with 100 or 200 mg cyproterone acetate orally/day. The treatment periods upto the test varied between 1 and 4 years. Glucose-tolerance was not disturbed.

Clinical observation in more than 200 men treated in our department brought no evidence for an effect on thyroid function in the sense of an inhibition or stimulation of function. An effect on the thyrotropin releasers is therefore improbable.

There were also no indications that the function of the posterior lobe of the pituitary or the melatonin level are affected by long-term treatment with cyproterone acetate.

As far as we know, no studies have yet been carried out into LTH changes in man under treatment with cyproterone acetate. In about 20% of the men treated without interruption for more than 8 months we observed mild gynaecomastia, which proved to be reversible in some cases even during the further course of the treatment. It is questionable whether LTH plays a role in this; further studies will probably bring clarification. We would rather conclude that it is caused by a relative hyperoestrogenaemia brought about by the fact that oestrogen target organs naturally remain unaffected by cyproterone acetate and the endogenous oestrogens are thus free to exert their full influence on the receptors of the mammae.

ACKNOWLEDGEMENT

We are grateful to Schering AG, Berlin, for the benevolent support of our studies and for supplying the large amounts of cyproterone acetate required for our work.

REFERENCES

1. HOFFET, H. (1968) Praxis **57**, 221.
2. HOFFET, H. (1968) Schweiz. Z. Strafr. **84**, 378.
3. LASCHET, U. (1971) Kriminologische Gegenwartsfragen, **9**, 174.
4. LASCHET, U. and LASCHET, L. (1967) Klin. Wschr. **45**, 324.
5. LASCHET, U. and LASCHET, L. (1968) 13. Symp. Dtsch. Ges. Endokrin., Springer 116.
6. LASCHET, U. and LASCHET, L. (1969) In: Simposio Esteroides Sexuales, Fundaction para Investigaciones Hormonales, Bogota 1968, Berlin: Sala-Druck p. 194.
7. LASCHET, U. and LASCHET, L. (1966) Excerpta Medica Internat. Congr. Ser. No. 133, p. 138.
8. LASCHET, U. and LASCHET, L. (1970) Excerpta Medica Internat. Congr. Ser. No. 210, p. 196.
9. LASCHET, U. and LASCHET, L. (1971) Pharmakopsychiatrie, Neuro-Psychopharmakologie **4**, 99.
10. OTT, F. and HOFFET, H. (1968) Schweiz. med. Wschr. **98**, 1812.
11. PETRI, H. (1969) Nervenarzt, **40**, 220.
12. ROTHSCHILD, B. (1970) Schweiz. med. Wschr. **100**, 1918.
13. SEEBANDT, G. (1968) Öff. Gesundh.-Wesen, **30**, 66.
14. SEEBANDT, G. (1969) Bewährungshilfe, **16**.

U.L., Department of Psychoendocrinology, Psychiatric Clinic, D 6749 Landeck, F.R.G.

REGULATION OF SEXUAL BEHAVIOR

H. STEINBECK and F. NEUMANN

Department of Endocrinepharmacology, Research Laboratories of Schering AG, Berlin/Bergkamen

The title of this paper does not mean that we are reviewing all factors that are involved in sexual performance. Rather, we restrict our manuscript to the hormonal control of sexual behavior or, in other words, to the mutual relationship between gonads and brain.

This relationship is already existent in the fetus. During distinct periods of fetal development, the neural substrate for behavioral responses of the adult animal to gonadal hormones is irreversibly determined. In most mammalian species, this first step of hormonal regulation of sex behavior is completed before birth; in a few, e.g. rats, the differentiation period of later behavioral patterns lasts for a short time after birth. The species that have been investigated until now have in common that psychosexual differentiation is the last step of fetal development (Fig. 1) which opens up interesting possibilities for hormonal manipulation.

Basically, the undeveloped brain in either genetic sex is capable of acquiring both directions of sexual orientation and eventually any intermediate state. At least in a number of laboratory animal species, gonadal hormones exert a profound influence on the permanent impression of masculine or feminine psychosexual orientation. In contrast to somatic sexual differentiation, however, a great number of conflicting results have been obtained. Therefore, the hormonal regulation of the organizational phase of sex behavior is still not fully understood. One can only try to draw a general outline of what has been done experimentally.

The fetal ovary does not contribute to psychosexual differentiation. Neonatal ovariectomy of rats does not have any influence on the development of normal feminine receptivity, such animals behave essentially like unmanipulated females upon appropriate hormonal stimulation later in life (53, 55).

In contrast, removal of the testes from newborn male rats seriously interferes with the development of normal masculine copulatory behavior (23, 52), and enhances the animals' ability to display feminine receptivity (2, 15, 23, 53). These effects of gonadectomy in both genetic sexes show again the principle of "basic femaleness" that is found throughout somatic sex differentiation, i.e. femininity results regardless of the genetic sex if a developing substrate is deprived of any hormonal (testicular) influence.

Experimental interference with normal masculine development of psycho-orientation has also been achieved by temporary chemical castration of fetal male rats (38, 39, 40), guinea-pigs (19, 43) and dogs (47) which is possible when androgen-antagonists are administered during the appropriate period of brain development.

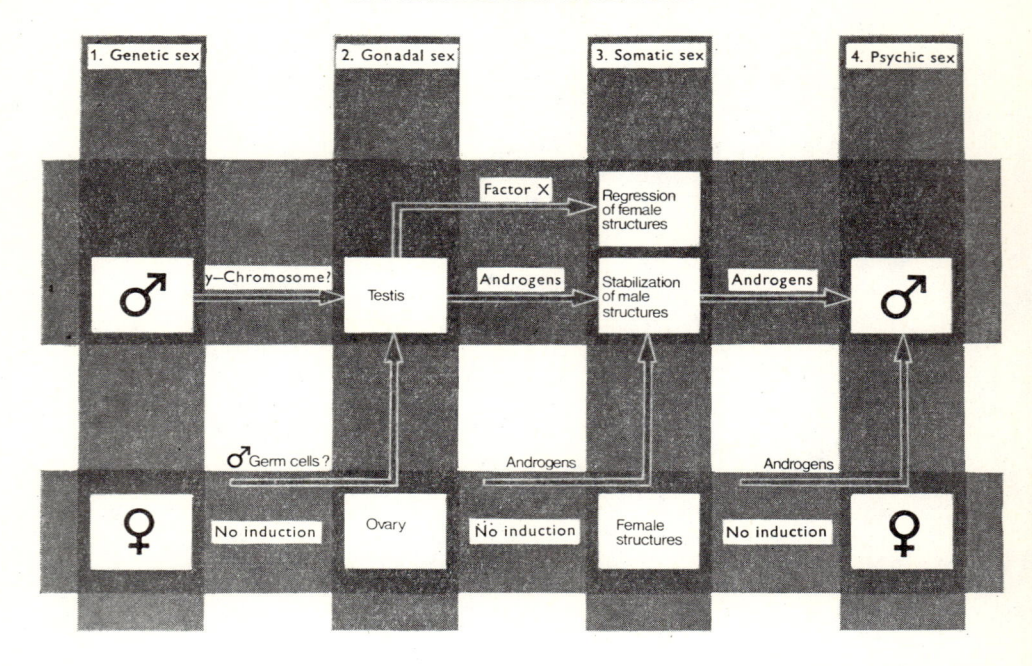

Fig. 1. Schematic presentation of successive steps of sexual differentiation including possibilities for natural or experimental hormonal interference with female development.

Androgen treatment of female fetuses has, of course, the opposite effect than has castration of males. In fact, from experiments on guinea-pigs it has been reported more than three decades ago that testosterone injections into the amniotic cavity made the female offspring to behave like males in response to testosterone treatment in adulthood (10). Much later, the early findings in this species were confirmed and extended (21, 42).

When the female offspring of testosterone-treated pregnant guinea-pigs were spayed in adulthood and subjected to either testicular or ovarian hormone treatment, striking deviations from normal feminine behavioral response became apparent. Their capacity to display feminine receptivity in response to ovarian hormones was greatly reduced as compared to normal ovariectomized females whereas testosterone propionate treatment evoked more frequent, intense and complete male-like copulatory responses than could be elicited in female controls.

The afore-mentioned studies on guinea-pigs have partly been done in order to find out whether there is a period of fetal differentiation in which the developing central nervous system is especially sensitive to masculinizing effects of testosterone. Such a period exists indeed during the 30th through 50th day of intrauterine development in this species (20, 21).

When testosterone propionate was administered from birth to 80 days of life, no enduring effect on normal female behavior was found.

The critical time for androgen alteration of the developing brain in monkeys is also prior to birth, it extends from about the 39th to the 90th day of pregnancy in rhesus monkeys since genetic females exposed to testosterone propionate via maternal injection during this time displayed typical masculine behavioral patterns of social interaction (20).

The human fetus seems also to be susceptible to hormonally induced psychic orientation. In the early days of synthetic progestins, pregnant women have been treated in cases of threatened abortion with progestins that are structurally closely related to testosterone. A number of these women have given birth to partially masculinized female babies. A group of these children has later been psychologically investigated at the Johns Hopkins Hospital in Baltimore. Thorough examinations revealed that nine out of ten girls showed unmistakable signs of psychological masculinization, they were classified as typical tomboys (13). Psychological studies on female patients with congenital adrenogenital syndrome who were presumably under excess androgen influence during brain differentiation point also in this direction (30). Finally, psychosexual orientation is invariably female in genetic males lacking androgenic stimulation in cases of testicular feminization.

In rats, the sensitive period for androgenic modification of psychosexual differentiation extends from birth to at least five days of age. Males castrated at this age or earlier display much more female characteristics of sex behavior in response to various estrogen doses in adulthood than rats castrated at day 10 or later (23). However, the ability of such animals to respond in a masculine fashion to testosterone injection when adult is not completely abolished by neonatal castration. Although they do not exactly behave like normal males in that several characteristics of the copulatory pattern are missing, they display both vigorous mounting when given testosterone and feminine receptivity when substituted with ovarian hormones (52, 53).

The situation is even more complicated when newborn female rats are treated with testosterone. After puberty, these animals develop persistent vaginal estrus but female receptivity is virtually absent. There is also no behavioral response to the administration of ovarian hormones (3, 27). In analogy to the above-mentioned species, one should expect that androgen-manipulated rats display more male behavior than normal females upon testosterone stimulation in adulthood. There are several reports which describe an increase in masculine behavior of neonatally androgenized rats, either females or males castrated shortly after birth (27, 37). Facilitation of masculine behavior was particularly pronounced when androgenic treatment commenced before birth (17, 38, 51).

Other authors, however, did not find that neonatal androgen treatment greatly facilitated the incidence of masculine behavioral traits, especially not in genetic females (35, 53).

Differences between genetic males and females in the degree of behavioral masculinization produced by neonatal androgen treatment have simply been ascribed to differences in genital development (5). The male's penis is differentiated before birth, neonatal castration does only impair its growth and response to later androgenic stimulation to a certain extent, depending on the age at castration.

In the female rat, however, only a clitoris develops before birth. Although this structure can be stimulated after birth to exhibit considerable growth, it will never become a male-like penis. Pre- and postnatal androgen treatment, however, eventually results in the formation of a complete penis, depending on the dose of androgen and the time at which treatment starts.

Not only testosterone but also other gonadal hormones are capable of exerting profound enduring effects on the developing brain. Besides testosterone, a second mayor androgen, androstenedione, is produced by the fetal rat testis (41, 44). When androstenedione was injected into newborn castrated rats, these animals responded later with the complete male copulatory pattern to androgenic stimulation. However, upon treatment with ovarian hormones, the same rats displayed feminine receptivity indistinguishable from normal females (18, 48). Thus, androstenedione during the critical period of psychic differentiation induced extreme bisexuality.

Neonatally administered estrogens, on the other hand, have no feminizing effect. On the contrary, they suppress the capacity for feminine performance in females or castrated males to the same extent as androgens do (33, 54) (Fig. 2).

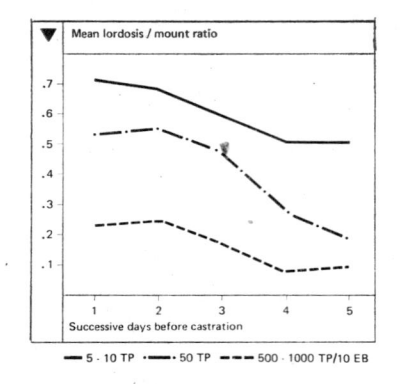

Fig. 2. Mean lordosis-to-mount ratio for female rats given 5, 10, 50, 500, or 1000 micrograms of testosterone propionate (TP) or 10 micrograms of estradiol benzoate (EB) either 96 or 120 hours after birth. Tests with a sexually vigorous male took place when the animals were 90 days old [after (33)].

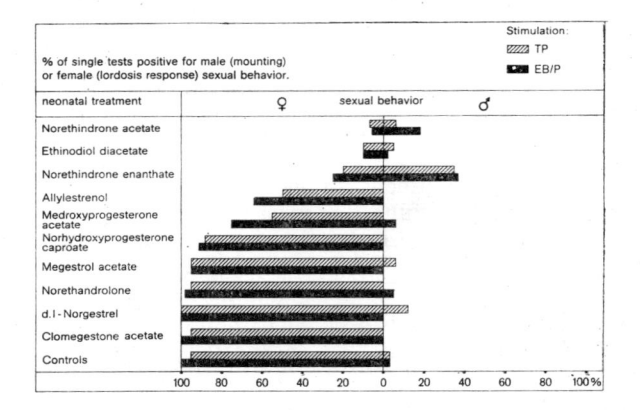

Fig. 3. Behavioral response of female rats, neonatally steroid treated and castrated in adulthood, to steroidal stimulation in adulthood [after (46)].

Although a certain degree of facilitation of masculinity has been reported (33, 36), neonatally estrogenized rats do not execute normal coital responses to adult androgen stimulation. It seems therefore that estrogens acting on the developing brain of either genetic sex induce a tendency towards permanent sexual neutrality.

Similar trends have been described when synthetic gestagens with inherent estrogenic side activity were administered to one day old female rats (46) (Fig. 3).

Which type of behavioral response to hormonal stimulation in adulthood is likely to occur in rats of either genetic sex who have been differently manipulated shortly after birth is summarized on Fig. 4.

It seems that, at least in animal experiments, androgens are not specific for the impairment of feminine gender orientation establishment but that the developing brain is sensitive to gonadal hormone influence in general.

Genetic sex, neonatal manipulation	Adult stimulation, type of response			
	TP male	TP female	E/P male	E/P female
♂	+	–	–	–
♂ castr.	+1	+	–	+
♂ castr. + TP	+	–	–	–
♂ castr. + E	+	–	–	–
♀	–	+	–	+
♀ castr.	–	(+)2	–	+
♀ castr. + TP	+1	–	–	–
♀ castr. + E	+1	–	–	–

1 = frequent but incomplete or not in all cases
2 = theoretical, no data available
TP = testosterone propionate
E = estrogen (mostly estradiol benzoate)
P = progesterone
♂/♀ castr. = castration

Fig. 4. Types of behavioral response to different hormonal stimulation of adult rats who have been manipulated shortly after birth. This model is based on experimental evidence and theoretical considerations.

On the other hand, there can be no doubt that androgens secreted by the fetal testis are of crucial importance for the development of masculine psychic orientation.

The currently held concept of gender orientation development is that androgens do not so much imprint male psychosexuality but rather act to alter the potential to display feminine behavior so that finally, since the brain is inherently bisexual, masculinity becomes predominant (14, 22, 53). This concept was developed since:

1. Early ablation of the testes or pre- and postnatal antiandrogen treatment (39, 40), does not extinguish masculine sexual motivation in males.
2. A certain amount of the capacity to display both types of behavior persists throughout life in both sexes, in manipulated as well as in normal animals.

This leads to the second stage of hormonal regulation of sex behavior, i.e. the activational phase. There are two fundamental differences between the two phases:

1. The organizational phase in all mammalian species that have been investigated in this respect is restricted to a very limited period of development whereas the activational phase, once initiated, lasts for a very long and probably unrestricted time.
2. Although several traits of social interaction that are closely linked to organizational hormone influence occur already in the prepubertal animal or infant, all consequences of the organizational phase become not fully overt until considerable time after hormonal action has elapsed. In contrast, the consequences of activational hormonal action are almost immediately visible.

Upon onset of puberty, increasing hormone levels act on the predisposed brain to elicit the predetermined pattern of behavior in response to a stimulant sex partner. Under normal conditions, androgenic hormones from the testis induce the masculine pattern of sex behavior in males and ovarian hormones catalyze feminine receptivity in the female.

However, if an adult male is castrated and thereby deprived of the hormonal activator of behavior, sexual motivation or libido is not immediately lost as one would expect. Rather, there is a slow decline of sexual arousability and even potency. In most rats, it takes about 4—10 weeks until sexual desire is extinguished (Fig. 5).

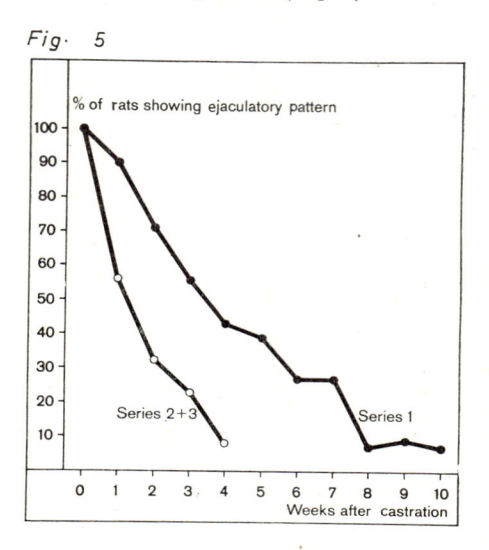

Fig. 5. Extinction of ejaculatory behavior following castration [after (11)].

In the dog (and also in man), this time is considerably longer. Individual variation may even exceed variation between species. Almost undisturbed sexual behavior after castration has been observed in some rats for 5 months (11) and in dogs after 5 years (4), rhesus monkeys were normally potent after 4 years (43).

The behavior of male animals consists of a rather complicated pattern of sexual activities directed towards the female. Most species have their own stereotypically performed characteristics. A male rat mounts the receptive female repeatedly with or without insertion of the penis before he eventually achieves ejaculation which is followed by an inactive pause of fairly constant length before he resumes his efforts. Following castration, decline of sexual activity proceeds in several steps. First, the capacity to ejaculate is lost followed later by the ability to achieve intromission. Extinction of libido, hence any sexual behavior, is complete much later when he no longer attempts at mounting.

Since the changes following castration are nothing but hormone deficiency, administration of testicular hormone will correct this deficiency at any time. If androgen treatment begins shortly after castration, the full pattern of sexual behavior can be maintained (Fig. 6).

Behavior can also be restored in long-term castrates. In this case, the first component of the pattern to reappear is the one that is last lost, e.g. mounts without intromission in rats. Restoration is complete when the behavioral component that was first lost (ejaculation) is re-established. It is now understandable that castrates have to be treated for a while until the typical pattern of behavior is restored.

It is important to note that the intensity of sexual performance does not depend on the amount of androgen administered. Precastrational individual differences in vigor and frequency disappear after castration since mating reactions decline to low levels in most animals. When equal amounts of testosterone propionate are then administered to all males, the individual differences observed prior to castration reappear despite the fact that all animals receive the same hormonal dose. This effect has been described for guinea-pigs (24) and rats (6).

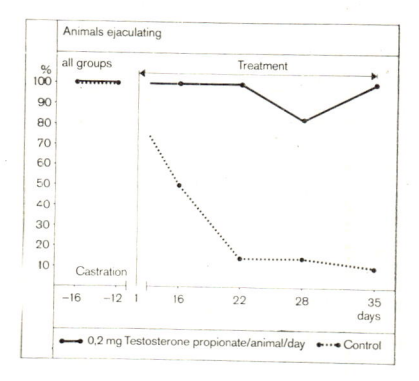

Fig. 6. Maintenance of ejaculatory behavior in castrate rats by testosterone propionate treatment.

To activate masculine behavior in the male, testicular hormones (androgens) seem to be specific since no report is available describing any such effect induced by ovarian hormones. On the contrary, it has been demonstrated that normally differentiated, castrated male rats displayed typical feminine sexual behavior when treated with estrogens (2, 12).

In the male, both testicular and ovarian hormones seem to exert a directional activation of the tissues mediating sexual behavior since androgens induce nothing but masculine behavior and estrogens, if anything, trigger feminine responses.

In this connection it might be noteworthy how genetic males who have been manipulated during development respond to androgenic stimulation.

We treated beagle bitches from the second trimester of pregnancy to term with the antiandrogen cyproterone acetate, the male newborn were also treated for the first 2 weeks of life. Morphologically, the male puppies looked like females since they had no penis but a well-developed vagina instead. When adult, the surviving three feminized dogs were tested for male sex behavior with receptive bitches. It must be noted that all three were uncastrated and untreated. Since their clitoris was greatly enlarged, it must be assumed that their testes were functional, therefore the dogs were endogenously androgen-stimulated.

In general, all three dogs displayed components of masculine coital behavior including extensive exploration and licking of the females' genitals. They all mounted the bitches from the rear, clasped their flanks with the forepaws and initiated vigorous pelvic thrusting. These activities are all typical components of normal male mating behavior. The feminized dogs would probably have shown even intromission and ejaculation if they had been able anatomically to do so.

However, there were individual differences between them indicating that at least in two dogs masculine behavioral traits were disturbed (Fig. 7).

One dog (0542) had only poor interest in the estrous bitch. In spite of her continous presentations, it took an unusual long time before he investigated her genitals. He mounted her only in two out of twelve test sessions. Another feminized dog (0537) explored the female's genitals extensively but he also mounted her only in two test sessions out of twelve. The third dog (0536) behaved like a normal male although his sex-orientated interactions were short and hasty.

Variations in mating behavior become also overt through the total time of sexual interactions. Dog No. 0542 devoted very little of his time to the bitch because he was not interested in her. No. 0537 spent more time with the bitch but his sexual interactions were incomplete since in most instances they did not further proceed than to exploration. Interactions of the third dog (0536) with the bitch were frequent and complete but of short duration (Fig. 8).

It would be more interesting to investigate the female-type response of these dogs to stimulation with ovarian hormones since, as mentioned above, the effect of androgens on the developing brain is rather the elimination of feminine traits. Prevention of androgen influence by antiandrogen treatment might thus result in permanent retention of feminine characteristics. We have indeed evidence that some feminine behavior is not eliminated in our feminized dogs.

Normal dogs attain a sex-specific position of the body when urinating. Bitches squat down on the floor while males stand upright with one leg lifted. One of the dogs (0542) is

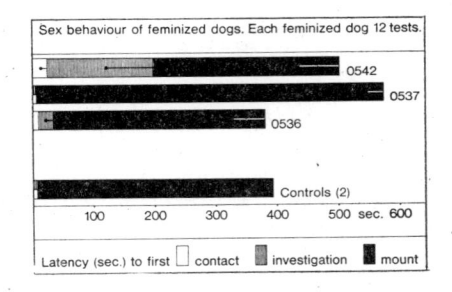

Fig. 7. Masculine sex behavior of feminized dogs. Latencies (sec.) from the onset of test sessions to the first contact with the bitch, first exploration of her genitals and first rear mount.

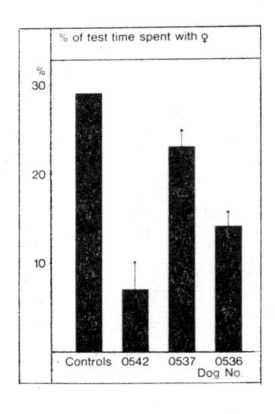

Fig. 8. Mean percentage of test time each dog spent in sex-orientated interactions with the bitch.

almost exclusively squatting like a bitch when he urinates. Since normal males urinate in an entirely different posture, the urinating performance of this dog is clearly evidence of psychologic femaleness (Fig. 9).

In contrast to male animals who are, according to their acyclic secretion of activating hormones, permanently ready to engage in sexual activities, females do not respond to the partner's efforts if they are not under the influence of specific hormonal constellations. Normally, properly timed sequences of estrogen and progesterone influence evoke the

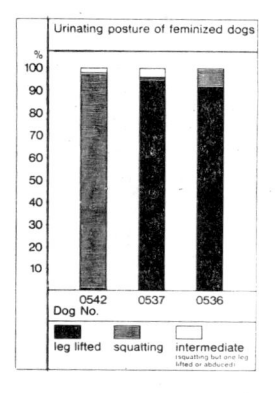

Fig. 9. Frequencies of male or female urination postures of feminized dogs.

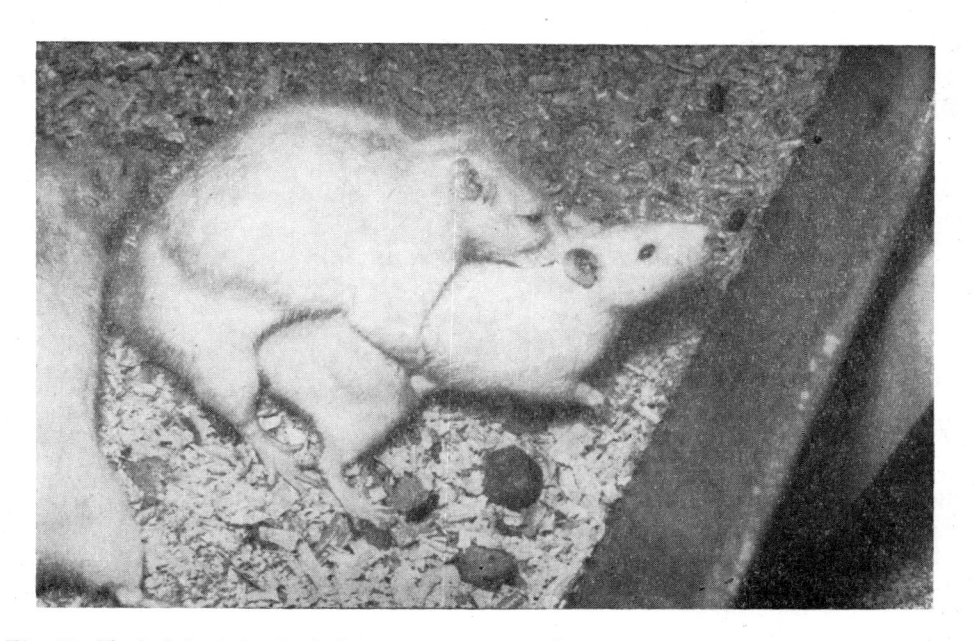

Fig. 10. Typical feminine lordosis response to mounting by a vigorous male rat. The animal showing lordosis is a genetic male who has been feminized by pre- and postnatal antiandrogen treatment. It bears cyclic ovary transplants.

cycle of feminine sex behavior, consisting of alternating periods of receptivity and sexual neutrality.

Timing and nature of the hormones that will induce full receptivity are known from substitution experiments on spayed but otherwise normal females of many species. They all have in common that female sex behavior is aimed at enabling the male to mount from the rear. The common copulatory reflex of fully receptive or aroused females is the lordosis posture, i.e. arching the back ventrally and raising thereby the hindquarters upon being mounted by the male (Fig. 10).

This kind of passive behavior has been termed "receptivity", since it is triggered only by the sexual activity of the partner. The full pattern of sexual arousal, however, has also actively performed constituents, like ear wiggling and darting. Most important, from the phylogenetic point of view, is that in many species mounting the partner by the female is a frequently displayed component of normal feminine behavior.

Any sexual responsiveness of infrahuman females is immediately terminated following castration. It can be completely restored by hormone treatment. In some species, e.g. rabbits and cats, estrogen alone is sufficient for complete restoration. In others, additional progesterone is essential. A certain degree of responsiveness can be induced in most species by estrogen alone but to evoke full arousability progesterone is also required. However, it is not sufficient merely to inject both hormones together. Rather, they have to act in a distinctly timed sequence (Table 1).

TABLE 1

Induction of receptivity with estradiol benzoate (EB) and progesterone (P) in spayed rats [after (9)]

EB (μg)	P (I. U.)	hours between injections	% animals responding	duration of estrus (hours)
5	—	—	0	—
10	—	—	13	52
20	—	—	20	49.5
100	—	—	90	50
5	0.4	48	91	10.5
5	0.3	48	68	9.6
10	0.4	72	100	11.5
10	0.3	72	100	9.6

In rats, progesterone has to be administered after estrogen priming whereas in ewes progesterone must precede estrogen. The dosage relation is also of crucial importance. If the dose of progesterone is too low in relation to estrogen, receptivity is not optimal. On the other hand, too high doses of progesterone suppress female sex behavior (Fig. 11).

These responses to experimentally created hormonal conditions remind strongly the changes in sexual activity that have been observed during the cycle of primates. In rhesus monkeys, the copulatory activity is positively correlated with ovarian estrogen secretion but progesterone dominance is accompanied by a decrease of sexual interaction (Fig. 12).

Inhowfar animal findings can be applied to women, remains open to discussion. It has been reported that sexual arousability of women is also subject to cyclic alterations which follow about the same pattern observed in infrahuman primates (26, 50). On the other hand, women with a feminine predisposed brain but deprived of hormonal activation (after castration or, in genetic males, in cases of gonadal aplasia or testicular feminization) usually have a normal female sex drive.

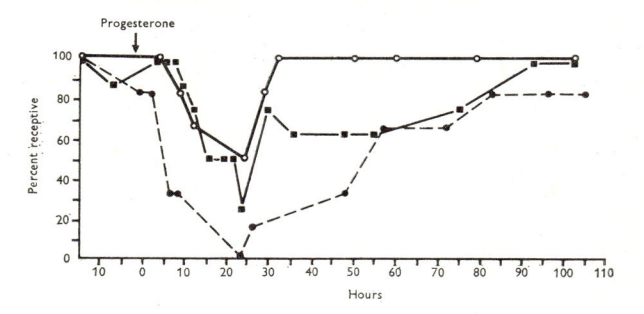

Fig. 11. Inhibition of estrogen-induced receptivity by various amounts of progesterone in spayed rabbits [after (8)].

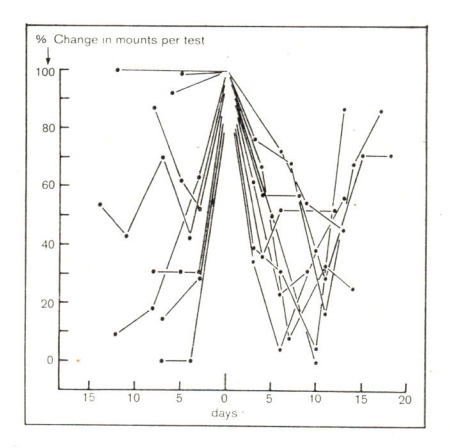

Fig. 12. Rhythms of mounting activity that occur in relation to the menstrual cycles of female rhesus monkeys [after (34)].

The importance of hormones as activators of sexual behavior seems not to be the same in all mammalian species. In rodents, equal receptivity of a female to any male can be induced by simple hormone treatment. In higher mammals, although necessary, the ovarian hormones may not be sufficient to produce receptivity in every instance. Some dogs (7) and monkeys (34) resist to engage in sexual relationship with a particular partner but promptly do so with another mate. Thus, individual preferences (some would call it love) act in higher species as an additive to hormones.

Even in lower mammals, ovarian hormones are not the only activators of feminine performance. Female animals as well as women are readily stimulated by androgens to display the full pattern of normal female excitability. It is important to note that masculine elements of sex behavior are not augmented by androgens in the normal female, she responds invariably according to her predisposed female gender orientation. Therefore, sexual desire and erotic functioning of both males and females are stimulated by the same hormone — androgens. In the female, androgens act nondirectionally, only activationally. The direction of sexual behavior comes from another source which is in all probability an irreversibly predisposed neural substrate.

A recent discovery is that not only gonadal hormones are involved in the regulation of sexual behavior but that hormonal secretion is also stimulated by sexual activity. In rabbit bucks (25, 45) and bulls (32), sexual stimulation was found to increase plasma testosterone levels within a few minutes. Sexual activity was also reported to increase testosterone secretion in men (16, 31); which in turn stimulated beard growth and sebum excretion (1). The latter effects were observed even in anticipation of the resumption of sexual activity after periods of abstinence.

We are not aware of any data from women showing hormonal fluctuations in response to sexual activity. It cannot be excluded that women are also subject to changes in blood levels of hypophyseal and ovarian hormones upon sexual relations. Elevation of plasma levels of these hormones have been reported to occur shortly after mating in rabbits (28, 29), and rats (49). This is surprising insofar as rabbits are known to ovulate in response to mating but rats are spontaneous ovulators, as are women. Uterine contractions and milk release in pregnant women associated with orgasm suggests that at least oxytocin is released. The high incidence of pregnancies resulting from rape could also mean that under certain conditions reflex ovulation can be induced in women.

REFERENCES

1. Anon (1970) Effects of sexual activity on beard growth in man. Nature (Lond.) **226**, 869.
2. Aren-Engelbrektsson, B., Larsson, K., Sodersten, P. and Wilhelmsson, M. (1970) The female lordosis pattern induced in male rats by estrogen. Horm. Behav. **1**, 181.
3. Barraclough, C. A. and Gorski, R. A. (1962) Studies on mating behaviour in the androgen-sterilized female rat in relation to the hypothalamic regulation of sexual behaviour. J. Endocrin. **25**, 175.
4. Beach, F. A. (1970) Coital behavior in dogs. VI. Long-term effects of castration upon mating in the male. J. comp. Physiol. Psychol. **70**, 1.
5. Beach, F. A. (1971) Hormonal factors controlling the differentiation, development, and display of copulatory behavior in the ramstergig and related species. In: The Biopsychology of Development (Tobach, E., Aronson, L. R. and Shaw, E., Eds.), p. 249. Academic Press, New York and London.
6. Beach, F. A. and Fowler, H. (1959) Individual differences in the response of male rats to androgen. J. comp. Physiol. Psychol. **52**, 50.
7. Beach, F. A. and Leboeuf, B. J. (1967) Coital behavior in dogs. I. Preferential mating in the bitch. Anim. Behav. **15**, 546.
8. Beyer, C., Vidal, N. and McDonald, P. G. (1969) Interaction of gonadal steroids and their effect on sexual behaviour in the rabbit. J. Endocrin. **45**, 407.
9. Boling, J. L. and Blandau, R. J. (1939) The estrogen-progesterone induction of mating responses in the spayed female rat. Endocrinology, **25**, 359.
10. Dantchakoff, V. (1938) Rôle des hormones dans la manifestation des instincts sexuel. C.R. Acad. Sci. (Paris) **206**, 945.
11. Davidson, J. M. (1969) Hormonal control of sexual behavior in adult rats. Advan. Biosci. **1**, 119.
12. Davidson, J. M. (1969) Effects of estrogen on the sexual behavior of male rats. Endocrinology, **84**, 1365.
13. Ehrhardt, A. E. and Money, J. (1967) Progestin-induced hermaphroditism: IQ and psychosexual identity in a study of ten girls. J. Sex Res. **3**, 83.
14. Feder, H. H. (1967) Specifity of testosterone and estradiol in the differentiating neonatal rat. Anat. Rec. **157**, 79.
15. Feder, H. H. and Whalen, R. E. (1965) Feminine behavior in neonatally castrated and estrogen-treated male rats. Science, **147**, 306.

16. Fox, C. A., Ismail, A. A. A., Love, D. N., Kirkham, K. E. and Loraine, J. A. (1972) Studies on the relationship between plasma testosterone levels and human sexual activity. J. Endocr. **52**, 51.
17. Gerall, A. A. and Ward, I. L. (1966) Effects of prenatal exogenous androgen on the sexual behavior of the female albino rat. J. comp. Physiol. Psychol. **62**, 370.
18. Goldfoot, D. A., Feder, H. H. and Goy, R. W. (1969) Development of bisexuality in the male rat treated neonatally with androstenedione. J. comp. Physiol. Psychol. **67**, 41.
19. Goldfoot, D. A., Resko, J. A. and Goy, R. W. (1971) Induction of target organ intensitivity to testosterone in the male guinea-pig with cyproterone. J. Endocrin. **50**, 423.
20. Goy, R. W. (1966) Role of androgens in the establishment and regulation of behavioral differences in mammals. J. Anim. Sci. **25** (Suppl.), 21.
21. Goy, R. W., Bridson, W. E. and Young, W. C. (1964) Period of maximal susceptibility of the prenatal female guinea pig to masculinizing effects of testosterone propionate. J. comp. Physiol. Psychol. **57**, 166.
22. Goy, R. W., Phoenix, C. H. and Meidinger, R. (1967) Postnatal development of sensitivity to estrogen and androgen in male, female and pseudohermaphroditic guinea pigs. Anat. Rec. **157**, 87.
23. Grady, K. L., Phoenix, C. H. and Young, W. C. (1965) Role of the developing rat testis in differentiation of the neural tissues mediating mating behavior. J. comp. Physiol. Psychol. **59**, 176.
24. Grunt, J. A. and Young, W. C. (1952) Differential reactivity of individuals and the response of the male guinea pig to testosterone propionate. Endocrinology, **51**, 237.
25. Haltmeyer, G. C. and Eik-Nes, K. B. (1969) Plasma levels of testosterone in male rabbits following copulation. J. Reprod. Fertil. **19**, 273.
26. Hamburg, D. A., Moos, R. M. and Yalom, I. D. (1968) Studies of distress in the menstrual cycle and the postpartum period. In: Endocrinology and Human Behavior (Michael, R. P., Ed.), p. 94, chapt. 6. Oxford University Press, London - New York - Toronto.
27. Harris, G. W. and Levine, S. (1965) Sexual differentiation of the brain and its experimental control. J. Physiol. (Lond.) **181**, 379.
28. Hilliard, J., Archibald, D. and Sawyer, C. H. (1963) Gonadotropic activation of preovulatory synthesis and release of progestin in the rabbit. Endocrinology, **72**, 59.
29. Hilliard, J., Hayward, J. N. and Sawyer, C. H. (1964) Postcoital patterns of secretion of pituitary gonadotropin and ovarian progestin in the rabbit. Endocrinology, **75**, 957.
30. Hinman, F. (1951) Sexual trends in female pseudohermaphroditism. J. clin. Endocr. **11**, 477.
31. Ismail, A. A. A. and Harkness, R. A. (1967) Urinary testosterone excretion in men in normal and pathological conditions. Acta endocrin. (Kbh.) **56**, 469.
32. Katongole, C. B., Naftolin, F. and Short, R. V. (1971) Relationship between blood levels of luteinizing hormone and testosterone in bulls, and the effects of sexual stimulation. J. Endocrin. **50**, 457.
33. Levine, S. and Mullins, R. F. (1964) Estrogen administered neonatally affects adult sexual behavior in male and female rats. Science, **144**, 185.
34. Michael, R. P. (1968) Gonadal hormone and the control of primate behaviour. In: Endocrinology and Human Behavior (Michael, R. P., Ed.), p. 69, chapt. 5. Oxford University Press, London — New York — Toronto.
35. Mullins, R. F. and Levine, S. (1968) Hormonal determinants during infancy of adult sexual behavior in the female rat. Physiol. Behav. **3**, 333.
36. Mullins, R. F. and Levine, S. (1968) Hormonal determinants during infancy of adult sexual behavior in the male rat. Physiol. Behav. **3**, 339.
37. Nadler, R. D. (1968) Masculinization of female rats by intracranial implantation of androgen in infancy. J. comp. Physiol. Psychol. **66**, 157.
38. Nadler, R. D. (1969) Differentiation of the capacity for male sexual behavior in the rat. Horm. Behav. **1**, 53.
39. Neumann, F. and Elger, W. (1965) Physiological and psychical intersexuality of male rats by early treatment with an anti-androgenic agent (1,2 α-methylene-6-chloro-Δ^6-hydroxy-progesterone-acetate). Acta endocrin. (Kbh.) Suppl. **100**, 174.
40. Neumann, F. and Elger, W. (1966) Permanent changes in gonadal function and sexual behavior as a result of early feminization of male rats by treatment with an antiandrogenic steroid. Endokrinologie, **50**, 209.
41. Noumura, T., Weisz, J. and Lloyd, C. W. (1966) In vitro conversion of 7-^{3}H-progesterone to androgens by the rat testis during the second half of fetal life. Endocrinology, **78**, 245.
42. Phoenix, C. H., Goy, R. W., Gerall, A. A. and Young, W. C. (1959) Organizing action of

prenatally administered testosterone propionate on the tissues mediating mating behavior in the female guinea pig. Endocrinology, **65**, 369.
43. PHOENIX, C. H., GOY, R. W. and YOUNG, W. C. (1967) Sexual behavior: General aspects. In: Neuroendocrinology (MARTINI, L. and GANONG, W. F., Eds.), p. 163. Academic Press, New York and London.
44. RESKO, J. A., FEDER, H. H. and GOY, R. W. (1968) Androgen concentrations in plasma and testis of developing rats. J. Endocr. **40**, 485.
45. SAGINOR, M. and HORTON, R. (1968) Reflex release of gonadotropin and increased plasma testosterone concentration in male rabbits during copulation. Endocrinology, **82**, 627.
46. STEINBECK, H., CUPCEANCU, B., MEHRING, M. and NEUMANN, F. (1971) Influence of neonatal gestagen injection on the differentiation of psychosexuality in female rats. Acta endocr. (Kbh.) **67**, 544.
47. STEINBECK, H. and NEUMANN, F. (1971) Aspects of steroidal influence on fetal development. International Symposium on the Effect of Prolonged Drug Usage on Fetal Development, Beit-Berl, Israel. Advanc. exp. Med. Biol. 27, in press.
48. STERN, J. J. (1969) The neonatal castration, androstenedione, and mating behavior of the male rat. J. comp. Physiol. Psychol. **69**, 608.
49. TALEISNIK, S., CALIGARIS, L. and ASTRADA, J. J. (1966) Effect of copulation on the release of pituitary gonadotropins in male and female rats. Endocrinology, **79**, 49.
50. UDRY, R. J. and MORRIS, N. M. (1968) Distribution of coitus in the menstrual cycle. Nature (Lond.) **220**, 593.
51. WARD, I. L. (1969) Differential effect of pre- and postnatal androgen on the sexual behavior of intact and spayed female rats. Horm. Behav. **1**, 25.
52. WHALEN, R. E. and EDWARDS, D. A. (1966) Sexual reversibility in neonatally castrated male rats. J. comp. Physiol. Psychol. **62**, 307.
53. WHALEN, R. E. and EDWARDS, D. A. (1967) Hormonal determinants of the development of masculine and feminine behavior in male and female rats. Anat. Rec. **157**, 173.
54. WHALEN, R. E. and NADLER, R. D. (1963) Suppression of the development of female mating behavior by estrogen administered in infancy. Science, **141**, 273.
55. WILSON, J. G. and YOUNG, W. C. (1941) Sensitivity to estrogen studied by means of experimentally induced mating responses in the female guinea pig and rat. Endocrinology, **29**, 779.

H.S., Department of Endocrinepharmacology, Research Laboratories of Schering AG, 1 Berlin 65, Müllerstrasse 170—172, West Berlin

THE ACTION OF 5,6-DIHYDROXYTRYPTAMINE AND L-DOPA ON SEXUAL BEHAVIOUR OF MALE RATS

M. DA PRADA, M. CARRUBA, A. SANER, R. A. O'BRIEN and A. PLETSCHER

Research Division, F. Hoffmann-La Roche & Co. Ltd., Basel

The evidence that cerebral 5-hydroxytryptamine (5-HT) is involved in the regulation of sexual behaviour has been supported by experiments with drugs interfering with the 5HT metabolism in the brain. For instance, *p*-chlorophenylalanine, a long-acting inhibitor of tryptophan hydroxylase, causes a relatively selective decrease of brain 5-HT (18) and markedly stimulates sexual behaviour (14, 20, 21).

In this work, the effect of two other compounds, i.e. 5,6-dihydroxytryptamine (5,6-DHT) and L-3,4-dihydroxyphenylalanine (L-DOPA), on sexual behaviour will be presented. Both of these substances decrease the 5-HT content of the brain (3, 5, 9, 11).

5,6-DHT

5,6-DHT, injected into the lateral cerebral ventricles of rats, has been reported to cause a relatively selective diminution of 5-HT in the central nervous system and, subsequently, also in the spinal cord (5, 9, 11). The mechanism of action of 5,6-DHT is probably different from that of *p*-chlorophenylalanine, since 5,6-DHT seems to selectively destroy the 5-hydroxytryptaminergic nerve terminals in the central nervous system (6, 7). Simultaneously with the 5-HT decrease in the brain, the rats show marked sexual stimulation (11). In fact, when male rats, kept in isolation, were put together 9 hours after an intraventricular injection of 50 μg 5,6-DHT, over 35% of the animals mounted more than 10 times and 63% mounted at least once within 3 hours (Table 1). The mounts were characterized by the typical coital position followed by pelvic thrusts. Furthermore, other signs of sexual stimulation (e.g. penile erection, grooming, licking and scratching the genitals) and excessive irritability to external stimuli and increased aggressivity were observed. Male rats not treated with 5,6-DHT, but kept under the same experimental conditions showed no mounting behaviour and no other signs of sexual excitation.

Nine hours after the 5,6-DHT administration, concomitantly with the sexual stimulation, the 5-HT level in the brain was lowered to about half the normal level, while at this same time the 5-HT content in the spinal cord had not decreased significantly. Brain norepinephrine and dopamine were practically unaffected by 5,6-DHT. Intraperitoneal administration of L-5-hydroxytryptophan, the immediate precursor of 5-HT, normalized the brain 5-HT levels and also abolished the enhanced mounting behaviour and the other signs of sexual stimulation induced by 5,6-DHT (Table 1) (11).

TABLE 1

Effect of 5,6-dihydroxytryptamine (5,6-DHT) alone and in combination with L-5-hydroxytryptophan (L-5HTP) on brain amines and sexual behaviour of male rats

Experiment	Cerebral amines (%)			Mounting animals (number in %)	
	5-HT	DA	NE	$\geq 1 \times$	$> 10 \times$
Controls	100 ± 2	100 ± 2	100 ± 4	0	0
5,6-DHT	49 ± 4	93 ± 1	92 ± 3	63	36
5,6-DHT + 5-HTP	104 ± 9	106 ± 3	83 ± 3	0	0

Rats were kept isolated for 48 hours. 5,6-DHT (50 µg) was injected into the cerebral ventricles, and 9 hours later the animals were put together and their behaviour was watched for 3 hours. L-5HTP (100 mg/kg) was administered i.p. before the start of the observation period. At the end of the observation period, the animals were sacrificed to measure brain amines by spectrophotofluorimetric methods. The experiments with 5,6-DHT were carried out on 70 animals, those with 5,6-DHT + 5-HTP and controls on 30 animals each. The brain amines are indicated in percent of controls (= 100) and represent averages with SEM (11). 5-HT — 5-hydroxytryptamine; DA — dopamine; NE — noradrenaline. The 5-HTP was administered as ethyl ester. The doses refer to the free amino acid.

L-DOPA

In patients with Parkinson's syndrome, treated with L-DOPA, increased libido has been reported to occur in rare instances (1, 8, 15, 17, 19). Therefore, it was of interest to investigate whether the L-DOPA, which is known to lower the cerebral 5-HT content in animals (3, 13), induces sexual stimulation in rats (12).

1. L-DOPA alone

Two successive i.p. doses, each of 100 mg/kg or 200 mg/kg L-DOPA (time interval 45 minutes), failed to enhance mounting behaviour, although a decrease of cerebral 5-HT was observed. This lack of response might be the consequence of cardiovascular and other side effects due to formation of catecholamines in extracerebral tissues (15). In fact, the animals appeared apathetic, exhibited little exploratory behaviour and showed marked tachyarrhythmia.

In animals pretreated with 8 repeated injections each of 50 or 100 mg/kg L-DOPA i.p. (at intervals of 4 hours), a subsequent administration (4 hours after the last pretreatment dose) of L-DOPA i.p. markedly enhanced the percentage of animals mounting and the number of mounts per animal (Table 2). In addition, the other signs of sexual stimulation described for 5,6-DHT were observed. Pretreatment with repeated doses of L-DOPA may have caused tachyphylaxis (10, 15, 22), so that the extracerebral side effects of L-DOPA were less pronounced and sexual stimulation became apparent.

In animals with and without L-DOPA pretreatment, 200 mg/kg L-DOPA (in two successive doses with an interval of 45 minutes) induced a drop of the cerebral 5-HT content to about 75% of controls 75 minutes after the first L-DOPA injection. The amine level was restored to normal after 225 minutes (Fig. 1). The 5-HT content of the spinal cord behaved similarly to that of brain. 100 mg/kg L-DOPA also caused a drop of the cerebral 5-HT content, though to only about 90% of controls.

2. L-DOPA combined with Ro 4-4602

Ro 4-4602*), an inhibitor of extracerebral decarboxylase, markedly inhibits the formation of catecholamines from L-DOPA in extracerebral tissues, but not in brain (2, 4). After pretreatment of rats with Ro 4-4602, 100 mg/kg L-DOPA increased mounting

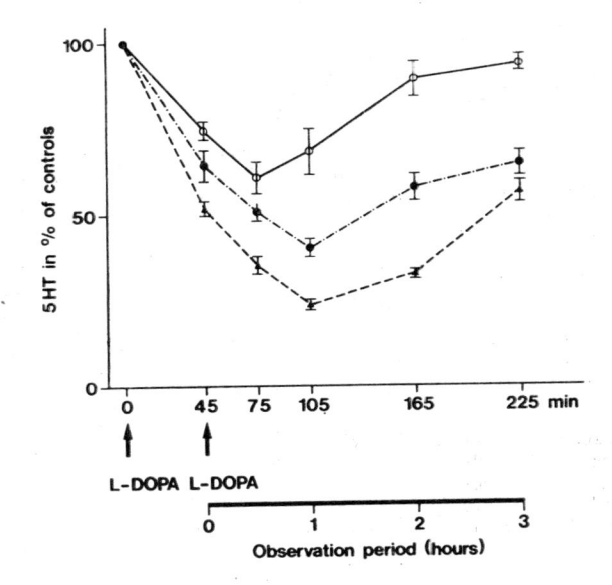

Fig. 1. Effect of L-DOPA alone and in combination with Ro 4-4602 on the cerebral 5-hydroxytryptamine (5-HT) content of male rats kept isolated for 48 hours.

o————o 2 successive doses each of 100 mg/kg L-DOPA were injected i.p. (arrows). The first dose was given 4 hours after the last injection of the pretreatment period. The rats were pretreated with 8 × 100 mg/kg L-DOPA i.p. given at intervals of 4 hours. The cerebral 5-HT levels 4 hours after the last pretreatment dose of L-DOPA were not significantly different ($p > 0.1$) from those of untreated controls.

●–·–·–● 2 successive doses each of 50 mg/kg L-DOPA were injected i.p. (arrows). The first L-DOPA dose was administered 30 minutes after 50 mg/kg Ro 4-4602 i.p.

▲-----▲ 2 successive doses each of 100 mg/kg L-DOPA were injected i.p. (arrows). The first L-DOPA dose was administered 30 minutes after 50 mg/kg Ro 4-4602 i.p.
The points indicate averages with SE of 3 experiments. (12).

behaviour (Table 2) and also induced other signs of sexual stimulation (see above). 200 mg/kg L-DOPA was approximately as active in causing sexual stimulation as 100 mg/kg of the amino acid. 400 mg/kg L-DOPA caused less pronounced sexual stimulation than 100 mg/kg L-DOPA, but the animals showed marked fighting behaviour. Ro 4-4602 alone had no effect on mounting activity (Table 2).

In rats pretreated with Ro 4-4602, the 5-HT diminution in the brain induced by 100 mg/kg or 200 mg/kg L-DOPA was more pronounced than that induced by 200 mg/kg

---

*) 1-DL-seryl-2-(2, 3, 4-trihydroxybenzyl) hydrazine hydrochloride

L-DOPA alone, but 100 mg/kg L-DOPA were less effective than 200 mg/kg of the amino acid (Fig. 1).

Administration of 30 mg/kg 5-hydroxytryptophan (30 minutes after the second L-DOPA dose) to animals pretreated with Ro 4-4602 plus 100 mg/kg L-DOPA raised the decreased cerebral 5-HT content to values somewhat above normal and simultaneously reduced the enhanced mounting frequency to control levels.

TABLE 2

Effect of L-DOPA alone and in combination with Ro 4-4602 on sexual activity of male rats

Experiment	Mounting animals (number in %) $\geq 1 \times$	Mounting animals (number in %) $> 10 \times$	Number of mountings per animal
Controls	20	2	1
L-DOPA	87	33	13
Ro 4-4602	20	0	1
Ro 4-4602 + L-DOPA	61	38	16

Rats were kept isolated for 48 hours. They were put together after the last injection of L-DOPA (see below) and observed for behavioural changes for 3 hours. The observations were made using a total of 30—90 rats per experiment.

L-DOPA alone: Two doses of L-DOPA (each of 50 mg/kg) were administered i.p. at an interval of 45 minutes. The first dose was injected 4 hours after the last injection of the pretreatment period. The rats were pretreated with 8 i.p. injections, each of 50 mg/kg L-DOPA at intervals of 4 hours.

L-DOPA in combination with Ro 4-4602: Two doses of L-DOPA (each of 50 mg/kg) were injected i.p. at intervals of 45 minutes. The first dose of L-DOPA was administered 30 minutes after Ro 4-4602. Dose of Ro 4-4602: 50 mg/kg i.p. (12).

L-DOPA was administered as methyl ester. The doses refer to the free amino acid.

Conclusion

The present experiments indicate that sexual stimulation induced by 5,6-DHT and L-DOPA correlates more with a decrease of brain 5-HT than with changes of the cerebral catecholamines. Thus, in the central nervous system, L-DOPA has been shown to increase the catecholamine content (4, 15), whereas 5,6-DHT did not alter or at best slightly decreased the catecholamine levels (5, 9, 11). However, both 5,6-DHT and L-DOPA caused marked sexual stimulation, concomitantly with the 5-HT decrease. The importance of the cerebral 5-HT levels for sexual behaviour is also supported by results with 5-hydroxytryptophan, the immediate precursor of 5-HT. This amino acid elevated the cerebral 5-HT levels decreased by 5,6-DHT or L-DOPA and simultaneously normalized sexual behaviour.

It remains to be elucidated whether the enhanced sexual activity due to 5,6-DHT and L-DOPA is the consequence of a 5-HT decrease in specific areas of the brain, e.g. of the limbic system. The increased aggressivity of rats seen after Ro 4-4602 plus L-DOPA (400 mg/kg) may be due to an accumulation of catecholamines in the brain (4).

The role of cerebral 5-HT in the regulation of sexual behaviour of man is not yet clear. A diminution of the cerebral 5-HT may be responsible for the hypersexuality occasionally seen in some patients with Parkinson's syndrome during chronic treatment with L-DOPA. There is, however, a marked difference between rats and man. Thus in rats L-DOPA in doses similar to those administered in humans produces hypersexuality in a high percentage of animals, whereas in man the L-DOPA-induced sexual overstimulation is rather rare.

SUMMARY

Nine hours after injection of 5,6-dihydroxytryptamine (5,6-DHT) into the lateral cerebral ventricles of male rats, the animals showed markedly increased copulatory behaviour. Simultaneously, the 5-hydroxytryptamine (5-HT) content of the brain, but not of the spinal cord, was decreased. The cerebral content of dopamine and noradrenaline remained practically unaffected.

Intraperitoneal injection of L-3,4-dihydroxyphenylalanine (L-DOPA) alone (i.e. after a pretreatment period with L-DOPA) and in combination with Ro 4-4602, an inhibitor of extracerebral decarboxylase, also caused sexual stimulation in male rats together with a decrease of the 5-HT content in brain and spinal cord.

The 5,6-DHT and L-DOPA-induced sexual stimulation and decrease of cerebral 5-HT were normalized by intraperitoneal injection of 5-hydroxytryptophan, the immediate precursor of 5-HT.

It is concluded that in male rats a causal connection exists between enhanced copulatory behaviour and decrease of cerebral 5-HT due to administration of 5,6-DHT or L-DOPA.

REFERENCES

1. BARBEAU, A. (1969) L-DOPA therapy in Parkinson's disease: a critical review of nine years experience. Can. med. Ass. J. **101**, 791.
2. BARTHOLINI, G., BURKARD, W. P., PLETSCHER, A. and BATES, H. M. (1967) Increase of cerebral catecholamines caused by 3,4-dihydroxyphenylalanine after inhibition of peripheral decarboxylase. Nature (Lond.) **215**, 852.
3. BARTHOLINI, G., DA PRADA, M. and PLETSCHER, A. (1968) Decrease of cerebral 5-hydroxytryptamine by 3,4-dihydroxyphenylalanine after inhibition of extracerebral decarboxylase. J. Pharm. Pharmacol. **20**, 228.
4. BARTHOLINI, G. and PLETSCHER, A. (1968) Cerebral accumulation and metabolism of ^{14}C-DOPA after selective inhibition of peripheral decarboxylase. J. Pharmacol. exp. Ther. **161**, 14.
5. BAUMGARTEN, H. G., BJÖRKLUND, A., LACHENMAYER, L., NOBIN, A. and STENEVI, U. (1971) Long-lasting selective depletion of brain serotonin by 5,6-dihydroxytryptamine. Acta Physiol. scand., Suppl. **373**, 1.
6. BAUMGARTEN, H. G., BJÖRKLUND, A., HOLSTEIN, A. F. and NOBIN, A. (1972) Chemical degeneration of indolamine axons in rat brain by 5,6-dihydroxytryptamine. Z. Zellforsch. **129**, 256.
7. BAUMGARTEN, H. G. and LACHENMAYER, L. (1972) Chemically induced degeneration of indoleamine-containing nerve terminals in rat brain. Brain Res. **38**, 228.
8. CALNE, D. B. and SANDLER, M. (1970) L-DOPA and Parkinsonism. Nature (Lond.) **226**, 21.
9. COSTA, E., LEFEVRE, H., MEEK, J., REVUELTA, A., SPANO, P., STRADA, S. and DALY, J. (1972) Serotonin and catecholamine concentrations in brain of rats injected intracerebrally with 5,6-dihydroxytryptamine. Brain Res. **44**, 304.
10. DAIRMAN, V., CHRISTENSON, J. G. and UDENFRIEND, S. (1971) Decrease in liver aromatic L-amino-acid decarboxylase produced by chronic administration of L-DOPA. Proc. nat. Acad. Sci. U.S. **68**, 2117.
11. DA PRADA, M., CARRUBA, M., O'BRIEN, R. A., SANER, A. and PLETSCHER, A. (1972) The effect of 5,6-dihydroxytryptamine on sexual behaviour of male rats. Europ. J. Pharmacol. **19**, 288.
12. DA PRADA, M., CARRUBA, M., SANER, A., O'BRIEN, R. A. and PLETSCHER, A. (1973) The action of L-DOPA on sexual behaviour of male rats. Brain Res. in press.

13. EVERETT, G. M. and BORCHERDING, J. W. (1970) L-DOPA: Effect on concentration of dopamine, norepinephrine and serotonin in brains of mice. Science, **168**, 849.
14. GESSA, G. L. (1970) Brain serotonin and sexual behaviour in male animals. Ann. intern. Med. **73**, 622.
15. HORNYKIEWICZ, O. (1971) Dopamine: its physiology, pharmacology and pathological neurochemistry. In: Biogenic Amines and Physiological Membranes in Drug Therapy, Part B, p. 173. Dekker, New York.
16. HYYPPÄ, M., RINNE, U. K. and SONNINEN, V. (1970) The activating effect of L-DOPA treatment on sexual functions and its experimental background. Acta neurol. scand. **46**, Suppl. 43, 223.
17. JENKINS, R. B. and GROK, R. H. (1970) Psychic effects from levodopa. J. Amer. med. Ass. **212**, 2265.
18. KOE, B. K. and WEISSMAN, A. (1966) p-Chlorophenylalanine: a specific depletor of brain serotonin. J. Pharmacol. exp. Ther. **154**, 499.
19. SANDLER, M. (1972) Catecholamine synthesis and metabolism in man: Clinical implications (with special reference to parkinsonism). In: Handbook of Experimental Pharmacology, vol. **23**, p. 845. Springer, Berlin.
20. SHEARD, M. H. (1969) The effect of p-chlorophenylalanine on behaviour of rats: relation to brain serotonin and 5-hydroxyindoleacetic acid. Brain Res. **15**, 524.
21. TAGLIAMONTE, A., TAGLIAMONTE, P., GESSA, G. L. and BRODIE, B. B. (1969) Compulsive sexual activity induced by p-chlorophenylalanine in normal and pinealectomized rats. Science, **166**, 1433.
22. TATE, S. S., SWEET, R., MCDOWELL, F. H. and MEISTER, A. (1971) Decrease of the 3,4-dihydroxyphenylalanine (DOPA) decarboxylase activities in human erythrocytes and mouse tissues after administration of DOPA. Proc. nat. Acad. Sci. U. S. **68**, 2121.

M.D.P., Research Division, F. Hoffmann-La Roche & Co. Ltd., Basel Switzerland

CHOLINERGIC MECHANISMS
IN THE CENTRAL NERVOUS SYSTEM

Chairman: A. SUNDWALL

Associate chairman: B. CHRISTENSEN

ION PAIR EXTRACTION IN COMBINATION WITH GAS PHASE ANYLYSIS OF ACETYLCHOLINE*)

B. KARLÉN, G. LUNDGREN, I. NORDGREN and B. HOLMSTEDT

Department of Toxicology, Swedish Medical Research Council, Karolinska Institutet and Division of Pharmacy, Department of Drugs, National Board of Health and Welfare, Stockholm

Bioassays were until recently the only methods available for estimation of acetylcholine (ACh) in the small amounts normally occurring in biological tissues. These assays are sensitive but their lack of specificity has repeatedly been pointed out. Traces of pharmacological agents used in a given experiment might sensitize or alter the response to acetylcholine. This and other factors, e.g. residues of organic solvents, may affect the intensity of the biological response and thus question the reliability of acetylcholine bioassay. For this reason there has been a constant search for chemical methods of sufficient sensitivity. Several have by now been devised including radioisotopic, fluorimetric and gas chromatographic techniques.

Since 1968 at least three such methods have been developed for estimation of both choline esters and choline. Two of them are based on gas chromatography while the third is radiometric, based on an enzymatic reaction (2). The gas chromatographic techniques undoubtedly offer the best advantages, especially if a mass spectrometer, which supplies further sensitivity and specificity, can be used as a detector. To be able to gas chromatograph these quaternary ammonium compounds they must first be converted to volatile derivatives. This is achieved either with sodium benzenethiolate by chemical demethylation (5) or by controlled pyrolysis (11). These methods are excellent for separation and quantitation of ACh. However, the isolation of endogenous ACh is carried out by precipitation, as reineckate (5) or enneaiodide (10). The precipitation step in these methods is not quantitative and the recovery may vary, but this has been compensated for by the use of internal standards, chemically similar to ACh. When one works with diluted extracts containing ACh in low concentrations (nanogram amounts) the isolation step must be nearly quantitative. To meet this demand in the isolation of ACh, we have adopted a method (1) which is based on ion pair extraction.

The results of this extraction technique together with analysis of ACh by flame ionisation detection or mass fragmentography after chemical demethylation or pyrolysis are presented in this paper.

---

*) This project has been supported by grants from the Swedish Medical Research Council B70-13X-2827, B70-19P-2905, B71-40X-199-07, B72-40Y- 2375-05 and B73-14-3902-01; The Tri-Centennial Fund of the Bank of Sweden; the National Institute of Mental Health (MH 12007); the Wallenberg Foundation and by funds from the Karolinska Institutet.

Methods

Preparation of rat brain extracts

Sprague-Dawley rats weighing 200—300 grams were killed by a blow on the head. The brains were rapidly removed (within one minute) and homogenized in 0.15 M ice-cooled sodium chloride (200 mg tissue/ml) by means of an Ultra-Turrax homogenizer. Eserine (10^{-5} M) was added to the homogenate for protection of "free" ACh.

ACh was extracted by ice-cooled 1.2 M perchloric acid added to a final concentration of 0.4 M. Propionyl choline iodide (PCh) was added as internal standard (20 nmoles to each brain) and the extracts were left for 30 minutes at about 8°C in a refrigerator. The samples were then centrifuged for 20 minutes at 100,000 × g and 4°C.

Isolation of ACh by ion pair extraction. The supernatant (about 10 ml) was diluted with 0.5 M disodium hydrogenphosphate buffer (15.0 ml) and extracted once for 5 minutes with a 1.2×10^{-3} M solution of hexanitrodiphenylamine in dichloromethane (10 ml) according to EKSBORG and PERSSON (1). The organic phase was evaporated to 1 ml under a stream of nitrogen and washed with 1 ml ice-cooled sodium carbonate buffer (15.5 ml 0.5 M Na_2CO_3 + + 77 ml 1 M $NaHCO_3$ per 1000 ml; pH 9.0) for one minute to remove excess hexanitrodiphenylamine. The washed organic phase was then transferred to another centrifuge tube and evaporated to dryness. ACh and internal standard in the residue were estimated gas chromatographically either by pyrolysis or after demethylation with sodium benzenethiolate. For estimation of low amounts of ACh mass fragmentography was used in combination with chemical demethylation.

Estimation of ACh

1. By pyrolysis

The technique used is essentially that described by SZILAGYI et al. (10). A capillary glass tube (50 mm, 0.9 mm i.d.) fitted at both ends with polyethylene tubings was filled with a slurry of Amberlite IRA 400 (5 mm) and Amberlite CG-4B type 1 ion exchange resins in distilled water, both in chloride form. Before use the columns were rinsed with about 100 μl acetonitrile-water (1 : 1).

The evaporated residue was dissolved in 75 μl of acetonitrile-water (1 : 1). This solution was slowly sucked through the capillary tube followed by 10 μl of the solvent. About 50 μl of the combined eluate and washing was placed on the pyrolyzing ribbon and evaporated to dryness at about 100°C. Pyrolysis was carried out for 15 seconds at 550°C. The pyrolysis products were separated on an aluminum column (3.5 m × 4 mm i.d.) packed with 4% polyethylenimine (PE1 1800) (Dow. Chem. Co., Michigan) on acid washed Chromosorb G 80/100 mesh, which had been conditioned at 140°C in a stream of nitrogen for 3 days. An Aerograph 1200 gas chromatograph equipped with hydrogen flame ionization detector and connected with a Barber-Coleman Model 5180 pyrolyzer with a platinum ribbon was used. Oxygen and hydrogen flow was adjusted to give maximum detector sensitivity. Column temperature was maintained at 80°C with a nitrogen flow of 70 ml/min.

2. After chemical demethylation

a) By flame ionisation detection

The evaporated ion pair residue was dried in a vacuum desiccator for 5 minutes. Extracted ACh and internal standard were demethylated according to HANIN and JENDEN (5) with the following modifications: The demethylation reagent was prepared to contain

9.91 mg sodium benzenethiolate and 1.5 mg glacial acetic acid per ml butanone. One ml of this reagent was added to the reaction vessel. After demethylation the content was washed with 5 × 2 ml pentane. An Aerograph 1200 gas chromatograph equipped with a hydrogen flame ionization detector was used. The demethylation products were separated on an aluminum column (2.5 m × 4 mm i.d.) packed with 4% Amine 220, 6% THEED (Wilkens Instr. and Res., Inc., California) on acid washed hexamethyldisilazane treated Chromosorb W, 80/100 mesh, which had been conditioned at 120°C in a stream of nitrogen for 48 hours. Column temperature was kept at 80°C and nitrogen flow at 25 ml/min. Oxygen and hydrogen flow was adjusted to give maximal detector response.

b) *By mass fragmentography*

An LKB 9000 combined gas chromatograph — mass spectrometer was used. The instrument was equipped with a mass marker and the recently described (4) multiple ion detector (MID) and connected to a PDP 12 computer (Digital Equipment Corporation) over an interface developed in this department. Two different accelerating voltages were used on separate channels of the MID. Alternation between the two channels allows continuous monitoring of two different masses on a UV-recorder. The equipment also includes a bucking unit, which allows separate bucking out on each channel of signals originating from bleeding of the column.

An aluminum column (4.5 m × 1.9 mm i.d.) packed with 1% DDTS (4-dodecyldiethylenetriamine succinamide polymer; 7) on Poropak P was used. Column temperature was 165°C and carrier gas flow (He) was at 30 ml/min. The ionization potential and trap current were 50 eV and 60 μA, respectively. The temperature of the flash heater was 200°C and the ion source was kept at 250°C. Multiplier voltage, 3.5 kV.

Chemical identification of the pyrolysis products

An LKB 9000 gas chromatograph — mass spectrometer was connected with a Barber-Coleman Model 5180 pyrolyzer. An aluminum column (2 m × 4 mm i.d.) packed with 4% PEI 1800 on acid washed Chromosorb G, 80/100 mesh was used. Column temperature was 70°C and carrier gas flow (He) 35 ml per minute. The pyrolysis conditions were the same as described earlier. Mass spectrometric conditions: separator temperature, 200°C; ion source temperature, 290°C; ionization potential, 70 eV; multiplier voltage, 3.5 kV. Mass spectra of the pyrolysis products were recorded at the summit of the gas chromatographic peaks.

Recovery of ACh in the ion pair extraction step

a) 25 ml of a buffer solution (HClO$_4$, 0.15 M; Na$_2$HPO$_4$, 0.3 M; NaCl, 0.04 M) containing 20 nmole ACh was extracted once with 10 ml of a 1.2×10^{-3} M solution of hexanitrodiphenylamine in dichloromethane as described above. The ion pair residue was dissolved in 60 μl acetonitrile-water (1 : 1) and passed through the micro column which was rinsed with two 10 μl portions of fresh solvent. The combined eluates were pyrolysed and the recovery calculated by comparing the area under the gas chromatographic peak to that obtained by pyrolysing ACh directly. In this experiment the losses on the micro column are included in the calculation.

b) ACh and PCh (20 nmole each) were analysed as above. In another experiment PCh was omitted in the extraction procedure. An aliquot (6.0 ml) of the organic phase was evaporated and PCh (12 nmole) in MeOH (1.2 ml) was added and evaporated. Dichloromethane (1 ml) was added to the residue and the organic phase was washed with carbonate buffer pH 9.0 and proceeded as described above. The recovery of ACh was calculated from the peak area ratios obtained in the two experiments.

Preparation of 2-acetoxy-1,1-$^2H_2$-1-trimethylammonium iodide (^2H-ACh)

N,N-Dimethylglycolamide was first prepared according to Ratchford and Fisher (8) from ethyl glycolate (Sigma Chemical Co., Missouri) and dimethylamine.

1,1-$^2H_2$-dimethylaminoethanol. LiAl$^2H_4$ (Fluka AG. Switzerland, 99% ^2H) (1.0 g, 0.024 mole) was added to a solution of N,N-dimethylglycolamide (2.6 g, 0.025 mole) in dry ether (40 ml). The mixture was stirred under reflux for 15 h followed by the addition of H_2O (1 ml), 15% NaOH (1 ml) and finally H_2O (3 ml). The filtered ether solution was dried (Na_2SO_4) and used directly in the next step.

1,1-$^2H_2$-dimethylaminoethyl acetate. The ether solution from the previous step was diluted with dry ether (200 ml) and Ac_2O (2.55 g, 0.025 mole) added. The mixture was refluxed for 8 h. After standing over night the ether was evaporated to about 6 ml and the product extracted into 0.5 M citric acid (10 ml). After addition of ammonium citrate buffer (ammonium citrate 2 M, NH_4OH 7.5 M) to pH 9.3 the product was extracted into $CHCl_3$ (10 ml). The $CHCl_3$-extract was dried (Na_2SO_4) and evaporated to dryness.

^2H- ACh. The oily residue from the previous step was dissolved in ethanol (5 ml) and CH_3I (7.1 g, 0.05 mole) was added. After 3 days the crystals obtained weighed 0.72 g, m.p. 157—161°C. After 3 recrystallisations from ethanol the product melted at 159—161°C. The infrared spectrum (KBr) showed characteristic absorption bands at 2240 (C-^2H) and 1767 (C = 0) cm^{-1}. The isotopic purity determined mass fragmentographically on 1,1-$^2H_2$-dimethylaminoethyl acetate formed by demethylation of the product with benzenethiolate was 99 per cent.

RESULTS

Figure 1 shows typical gas chromatograms obtained by pyrolysis and chemical demethylation. ACh was isolated as ion pair with hexanitrodiphenylamine from standard solutions and rat brain, respectively.

The chemical identity of the pyrolysis products of ACh and PCh, dimethylaminoethyl acetate and propionate, respectively was established with an LKB 9000 gas chromatograph — mass spectrometer. The mass spectra obtained at the summit of the gas chromatographic peaks which emerged after pyrolysing extracts from rat brain to which internal standard PCh had been added were identical with those obtained from reference ACh and PCh. Ions at m/e values of 58, 71 and 72, characteristic of these structures (3) were present in ratios identical in both standards and brain extract samples.

Standard curves obtained by analysing standard solutions of ACh and PCh showed good linearity with both techniques (Fig. 2).

The recovery of ACh in the ion pair extraction step was determined by the pyrolysis technique and agreed with the theoretically calculated value of 96 per cent. The mean total recoveries in this procedure for ACh and PCh were 81 and 82 per cent, respectively (n = 6). The main losses occurred in the ion exchange step, which was demonstrated by analysing standard solutions of ACh and PCh which were passed only through this step. The total recovery in the chemical demethylation procedure was 85 per cent (n = 5).

Figure 3 shows a typical mass fragmentogram obtained by focussing on m/e 58 (methylendimethylammonium ion) and m/e 60 (1,1-$^2H_2$-methylendimethylammonium ion) obtained from electron impact on the emerging gas chromatographic peaks of nor-ACh (DMAEA) and nor-^{2}H-ACh (^{2}H-DMAEA), respectively. The mass fragmentographic peak for DMAEA corresponds to 10 pmole of ACh extracted as ion pair from a buffer solution together with 100 pmole of ^{2}H-ACh. The small peak with shorter retention time on channel m/e 60 is unidentified. A good linearity of the standard curve (Fig. 4) was obtained also in this concentration range, which permits quantitation of amounts down to about 10 picomole with good precision.

A comparison of the ACh level in rat brain was made with the methods currently in use in our laboratory (Fig. 5). The different chemical techniques showed good agreement between themselves and with the biological frog rectus method.

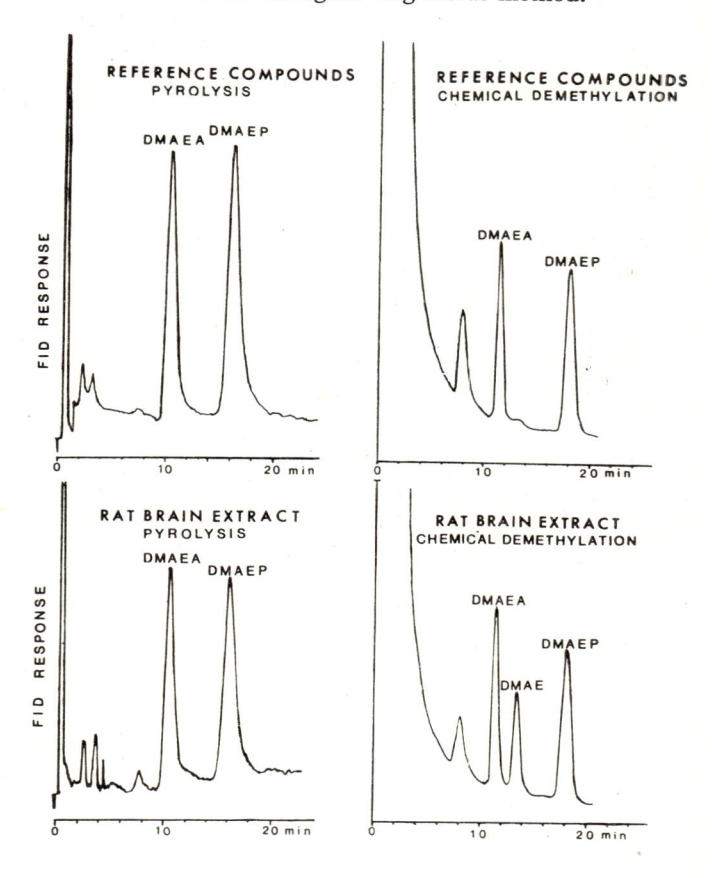

Fig. 1. Gas chromatograms obtained by pyrolysis and chemical demethylation after ion pair extraction of ACh and internal standard PCh, processed as described under "Methods". Upper left quadrant: Pyrolysis products of ACh and PCh (20 nmole each) dimethylaminethyl acetate (DMAEA) and propionate (DMAEP), respectively isolated from buffer solution. Lower left quadrant: Pyrolysis products from rat brain extract to which PCh (20 nmole) had been added. Upper right quadrant: Chemical demethylation products of ACh and PCh (15 nmole each) isolated from buffer solution. Lower right quadrant: Chemical demethylation products from rat brain extract to which PCh (15 nmole) had been added. The third peak (DMAE) has been identifield as the demethylation product, dimethylaminoethanol of choline. Gas chromatographic conditions are described under "Methods".

Discussion

The results demonstrate that ion pair extraction with hexanitrodiphenylamine can be used for isolation of ACh in almost quantitative yield, not only in the nanomole range but also in picomole amounts. The isolated ion pairs can then be demethylated either chemically or by controlled pyrolysis before separation and quantitation in the gas chromatograph.

By a single extraction into dichloromethane about 96 per cent of ACh is recovered. The total recovery of ACh in the whole procedure is about 85 per cent. Other advantages of

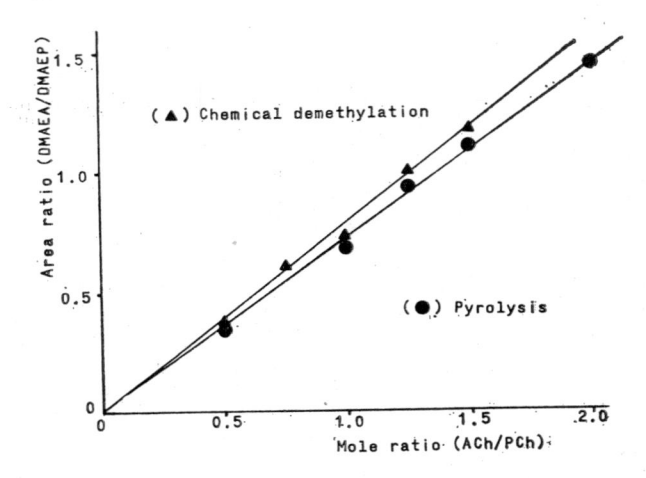

Fig. 2. Linearity of concentration — FID-response ratios for ACh analysed by pyrolysis (●) and chemical demethylation (▲). A constant quantity (20 nmole) of propionylcholine iodide was used in both experiments as internal standard. The gas chromatographic conditions are described under "Methods".

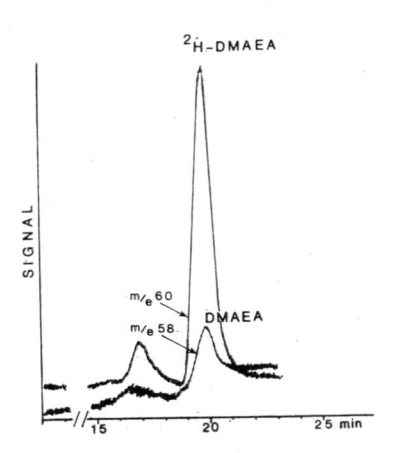

Fig. 3. Mass fragmentogram of ions at $m/e = 58, 60$. ACh (10 pmole) and ^{2}H-ACh (100 pmole) extracted as ion pairs, chemically demethylated and analysed as described under "Methods". One fourth of the CHCl$_3$-extract was analysed. DMAEA (dimethylaminoethyl acetate); ^{2}H-DMAEA (1,1-^{2}H$_2$-1-dimethylaminoethyl acetate). Conditions are described under "Methods".

the ion pair extraction technique are its simplicity, the possibility to work with diluted tissue homogenates, and the selectivity in the extraction of the desired components, which gives clean chromatograms. Furthermore, the isolated ACh is contained in an organic phase easy to evaporate.

The sensitivity of the two gas chromatographic methods is about the same as that for bioassay. The limit of quantitation of ACh with these methods in our laboratory is about one nanomole. The chemical demethylation method has, however, later been modified to about tenfold greater sensitivity (50 picomole) (6). Our difficulties to reproduce the high sensitivity claimed for the pyrolysis method (9) seem to be of a technical nature, probably due to the gas chromatographic equipment and losses in the ion exchange step.

Gas chromatography requires a good internal standard on which the quantitation can be based. We suspect that the variation in the levels of ACh in rat brain obtained with different methods may partly be due to the use of different internal standards. Hexyltri-

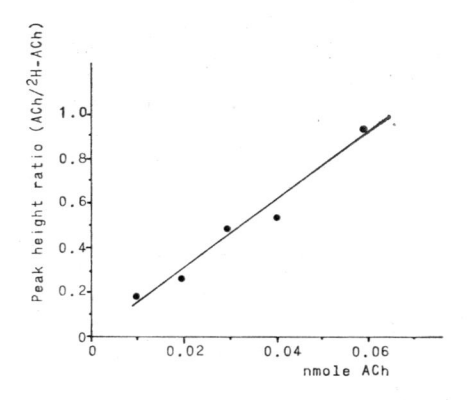

Fig. 4. Linearity of concentration — mass spectrometric response ratios for ACh analysed as described in Fig. 3. A constant quantity (100 pmole) of ^{2}H-ACh was used as internal standard.

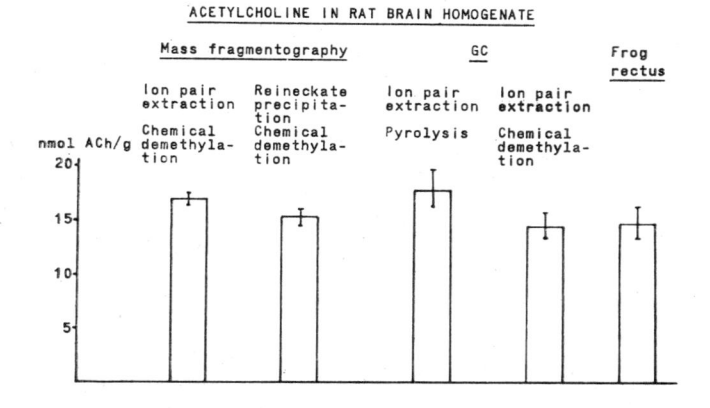

Fig. 5. A comparison of ACh concentrations in rat brain homogenates analysed directly after killing as described under "Methods". The left two bars indicate means of triplicates of four pooled brains. The other bars are means of each ten animals. Extreme values are indicated. The data in the second bar were obtained according to HANIN and JENDEN (1969).

methylammonium bromide and propionylcholine iodide under our conditions gave somewhat different results.

When analysing ACh in the low amounts mentioned above the sensitivity of the hydrogen flame ionisation detection is too low. To obtain sufficient sensitivity we have utilized a mass spectrometer as detector (mass fragmentography). With this method several mass numbers can be monitored continuously, and the ideal internal standard, deuterated ACh, only differing in mass number from endogenous ACh can be used. In this way the sensitivity has been increased, making it possible to estimate samples of biological tissues containing about 10 picomoles of ACh. It is to be expected that this technique will find increasing use in the future.

Acknowledgement

We wish to thank Miss Vivi-Anne Nilsson for expert technical assistance and Professor Donald J. Jenden for a gift of dodecyldiethylenetriamine succinamide polymer. One of us (G.L.) had the pleasure to visit Professor Jack P. Green in his laboratory and learn the pyrolysis technique, which is gratefully acknowledged.

References

1. Eksborg, S. and Persson, B. A. (1971) Photometric determination of acetylcholine in rat brain after selective isolation by ion pair extraction and micro column separation. Acta pharm. Suecica, **8**, 205.
2. Feigenson, M. E. and Saelens, J. K. (1969) An enzyme assay for acetylcholine. Biochem. Pharmacol. **18**, 1479.
3. Hammar, C.-G., Hanin, I., Holmstedt, B., Kitz, R. J., Jenden, D. J. and Karlén, B. (1968) Identification of acetylcholine in fresh rat brain by combined gas chromatography-mass spectrometry. Nature, **220**, 915.
4. Hammar, C.-G. and Hessling, R. (1971) Novel peak matching technique by means of a new combined multiple ion detector-peak matcher device. Anal. Chem. **43**, 298.
5. Hanin, I. and Jenden, D. J. (1969) Estimation of choline esters in brain by a new gas chromatographic procedure. Biochem. Pharmacol. **18**, 837.
6. Jenden, D. J., Campbell, B. and Roch, M. (1970) Gas chromatographic estimation of choline esters in tissues: A modified procedure for microgram quantities. Anal. Biochem. **35**, 209.
7. Jenden, D. J., Roch, M. and Booth, R. (1972) A new liquid phase for the gas chromatographic separation of amines and alkaloids. J. chromatograph. Science **10**, 151.
8. Ratchford, W. P. and Fisher, C. H. (1950) Preparation of N-Substituted lactamides by aminolysis of methyl lactate. J. org. Chem. **15**, 317.
9. Schmidt, D. E., Szilagyi, P. I. A., Alkon, D. L. and Green, J. P. (1970) A method for measuring nanogram quantities of acetylcholine by pyrolysis gas chromatography: the demonstration of acetylcholine in effluents from the rat phrenic nerve — diaphragm preparation. J. Pharmacol. exp. Ther. **174**, 337.
10. Szilagyi, P. I. A., Green, J. P., Monroe Brown, O. and Margolis, S. (1972) The measurement of nanogram amounts of acetylcholine in tissues by pyrolysis-gas chromatography. J. Neurochem. **19**, 2555.
11. Szilagyi, P. I. A., Schmidt, D. E. and Green, J. P. (1968) Microanalytical determination of acetylcholine, other choline esters, and choline by pyrolysis — gas chromatography. Anal. Chem. **40**, 2009.

B.K., Department of Toxicology, Swedish Medical Research Council, Karolinska Institutet, 10401 Stockholm 60, Sweden

BIOSYNTHESIS AND COMPARTMENTATION OF ACETYLCHOLINE IN THE BRAIN

J. SCHUBERTH and A. SUNDWALL

*Psychiatric Research Center, Ulleråker Hospital, Uppsala
and Department of Pharmacology and Toxicology, Biomedical Center, University of Uppsala*

Since the pioneer work of MANN, TENNENBAUM and QUASTEL (39, 40) much effort has been devoted to the study of the biosynthesis and compartmentation of acetylcholine (ACh) in the brain. The purpose of this review is to survey briefly our knowledge of these particular steps in the ACh turnover. We shall discuss the compartmentation of endogenous ACh and related endogenous substances, and evaluate possible routes for the *in vivo* formation of ACh. A comparison of the compartmentation of preformed and newly synthesized ACh will be made so as to enable a discussion of possible mechanisms for biosynthesis, storage and release of brain ACh *in vivo*.

COMPARTMENTATION OF ENDOGENOUS ACh

In vitro experiments with brain mince and slices indicate that the ACh biosynthesis is dependent on the integrity of the cellular organization. MANN, TENNENBAUM and QUASTEL (40) demonstrated the existence in the brain of a "substance" that breaks down to form ACh under a variety of conditions, e.g. treatment of brain homogenates with ether, chloroform and acid. This substance, which was called "combined" or "bound" ACh, is synthesized in brain mince and slices, and reaches very rapidly a limiting value (which is much higher than the normal ACh content of the slices). When the cellular organization is disrupted by treating the brain mince with ether, ACh formation is markedly increased in the presence of a cholinesterase inhibitor (ChEI). The total amount of ACh formed under these conditions is almost exclusively made up of "free" ACh, and greatly exceeds the total amount of ACh (mainly "bound") synthesized in brain mince not treated with organic solvents. Incubation of slices with media containing high concentrations of potassium also accelerated the biosynthesis of mainly free ACh (40).

On high-speed centrifugation of the brain homogenates in the presence of physostigmine to prevent the hydrolysis of ACh, part of the transmitter is found in the supernatant ("free" ACh) and part in the pellet ("bound" ACh). When physostigmine is not present, only "bound" ACh can be detected since only bound ACh is resistant to destruction by cholinesterase. FELDBERG (27) produced some of the earliest evidence that the "bound" ACh was attached to a particle generally identified together with mitochondria. However, by centrifugation in a sucrose gradient, HEBB and WHITTAKER (32) showed that the bound ACh was present in a subcellular fraction distinct from mitochondria, nuclei and microsomes. Morphological examination of the fraction showed that it contained isolated nerve terminals with characteristic elements of the presynaptic region, such as synaptic vesicles, intraterminal mitochondria and postsynaptic membranes (21, 30). The term synaptosome has been introduced by WHITTAKER to denote sealed, pinched off nerve terminals with the postsynaptic membrane attached. When suspended in a hypoosmotic solution, the synaptosomes burst, and the ACh in the cytosol could be separated into at least two fractions by futher centrifugation (22, 70). By this type of separation the ACh of the synaptosome appears to be partly dissolved in the cytosol (labile bound) and partly occluded in the synaptic vesicles (stable bound) (Table 1).

TABLE 1

Subcellular distribution of acetylcholine

Type of acetylcholine	Fraction	Presumed *in vivo* location
Free acetylcholine	High speed supernatant from eserinized sucrose homogenate	Cytoplasm from cell bodies axones and disrupted nerve terminals
Bound acetylcholine	"Crude mitochondrial" or synaptosomal fraction from uneserinized sucrose homogenate	Nerve terminals
Labile ACh	High speed supernatant from eserinized water solution of "crude mitochondrial" or synaptosomal fraction	Cytoplasm from nerve terminals
Stable ACh	High speed pellet from uneserinized water solution of "crude mitochondrial" or synaptosomal fraction	Vesicles from nerve

Essentially according to MARCHBANKS (42)

EFFECT OF DRUGS ON ENDOGENOUS ACh

Certain drugs which influence the central nervous system affect the ACh content of the brain. For example cholinesterase inhibitors, oxotremorine, narcotic analgesics and barbiturates increase the ACh level, while anticholinergic drugs, pentazol, and electroshock decrease the amount of ACh in the brain (29, 34, 51). RICHTER and CROSSLAND (51) also showed that the level of ACh varies with the functional activity of the brain and that following depletion of the brain-ACh store by electroshock, the initial level of ACh was restored within 30 seconds.

To evaluate the possible functional significance of the ACh in the different subcellular fractions, the changes in "free" and "bound" ACh, caused by these drugs, have been measured. The principle results obtained by BEANI et al. (10) and by CROSSLAND and SLATER (18) are summarized in Table 2. As is evident barbiturates do not affect the stable-bound ACh, while physostigmine gives rise to an increase in both stable-bound and labile-bound and in free ACh. Pentazol and scopolamine decrease both types of "bound" ACh but appear to leave "free" ACh unchanged or slightly increased.

TABLE 2

Effects of some drugs on free and bound acetylcholine *in vivo*

	Free	Bound Labile	Bound Stable	L + S	Total (whole brain)
Barbiturates (20—80 mg/kg)	+	+	0	+	+
Physostigmine (1 mg/kg)	+	+	+	+	+
Tremorine (75 mg/kg)	+	?	?	+	+
Atropine (25 mg/kg)	0	?	?	—	—
Scopolamine (5 mg/kg)	(+)	—	—	—	—
Pentazol (80 mg/kg)	0	—	—	—	—

From BEANI et al. (10), CROSSLAND and SLATER (18)

+ increase
— decrease
0 unchanged

SUBCELLULAR DISTRIBUTION OF CHOLINE ACETYLTRANSFERASE

ACh is synthesized from choline (Ch) and acetyl-CoA. This transacetylation reaction is catalyzed by the enzyme choline acetyltransferase (ChAc). HEBB and SMALLMAN (31) found that ChAc sedimented with mitochondria and by further fractionation HEBB and WHITTAKER (32) demonstrated that the enzyme was localized in the synaptosomes. The distribution within the nerve terminals has been the subject of some disagreement. DE ROBERTIS et al. (22) localized the enzyme in the vesicles, following fractionation of osmotically shocked synaptosomes, while WHITTAKER et al. (70) located ChAc in the soluble fraction, which suggested that it was mainly a cytoplasmic enzyme. However, TUČEK (66) observed species differences in the degree of binding of ChAc to particles. He also suggested that ChAc could be bound to some membrane fragments, which contaminate the vesicle fraction to an extent depending on the species used. Experimental proof of this was obtained by FONNUM (28), who found that ChAc is bound nonspecifically to membrane fragments after lysis of the synaptosomes. Furthermore, it was found that the degree of binding was inversely related to the ionic strength. Although the ionic strength within the nerve terminals is not known, it is considered to be sufficient to prevent the binding of ChAc *in vivo*. It must be pointed out, however, that species differences regarding surface charge and isoelectric points have been demonstrated. It is also of considerable interest that multiple forms of ChAc have been found in rat brain (38).

Regarding drug effects on the enzyme there is still rather little information available. Specific inhibitors have recently been discovered (45, 62) but very little is yet known about their pharmacological effects. Product inhibition has been suggested as a regulatory mechanism (35). There are some recent results indicating that a single injection of morphine (30 mg/kg) produces a marked increase in the apparent Michaelis constant of the enzyme (20).

Precursors of ACh in the brain

Acetyl-CoA — The acetyl donor for ChAc is an intermediate in the oxidation of glucose, which is further metabolized mainly through the tricarboxylic acid cycle. This suggests that the formation of acetyl-CoA and of ACh occurs in different compartments of the nerve terminals, since the enzymes for the tricarboxylic acid cycle are localized within the mitochondria (53), whereas ChAc is found outside the mitochondria, as discussed above. The mechanism is unknown by which the intramitochondrial acetyl-CoA becomes available for the ACh biosynthesis. On the basis of experiments with isolated synaptosomes forming ^{3}H, ^{14}C-ACh from double labelled glucose, Sollenberg and Sörbo (63) suggested citrate as the precursor of the acetyl-CoA and ACh. It has also been indicated that intramitochondrial acetyl-CoA *per se* might be transported to the cytoplasm (67).

To elucidate whether drug-induced changes of ACh were reflected by changes in the acetyl-CoA concentration, this ACh precursor was measured in the whole brain of animals treated with some of the drugs which are known to increase or decrease the ACh-level (56). The results are summarized in Table 3. As is evident, only oxotremorine produced a

Table 3

Effects of some drugs on the amount of acetyl-CoA and free choline in the brain

Treatment	Acetyl-CoA*) % of control Schuberth et al. 1966	Choline**) % of control Schuberth et al. 1969	Consolo et al. 1972
Saline	100	100	100
Sarin	91 (0.2 mg/kg)	—	—
Oxotremorine oxalate	74 (1 mg/kg)	130 (1 mg/kg)	146 (3 mg/kg)
Atropine	107 (1 mg/kg)	—	106 (50 mg/kg)
Pentobarbital	89 (30 mg/kg)	109 (60 mg/kg)	97 (55 mg/kg)
Physostigmine sulfate	—	—	127 (0.5 mg/kg)

*) Rat; 5.4 ± 0.17 (11) nanomoles/g.
**) Mouse; 115 ± 2.4 (5) nanomoles/g, Schuberth et al; 62.7 ± 6.52 nanomoles/g, Consolo et al.

a change in the acetyl-CoA concentration. Since oxotremorine increases the brain ACh the decrease in acetyl-CoA may be explained, if it is linked to an increased ACh biosynthesis. However, as discussed later, there are experimental data indicating a decreased formation and release of ACh in oxotremorine-treated animals. It should be mentioned that changes in the rate of ACh synthesis may not result in correspondingly large changes in the acetyl-CoA concentration, due to the fact that the rate of maximal ACh biosynthesis is only about 6% of the rate of the acetyl-CoA formation in the whole brain. Unfortunately, acetyl-CoA undergoes very rapid postmortal changes (54) and therefore it has not yet been possible to measure synaptosomal acetyl-CoA.

TABLE 4

Free choline in the brain according to different investigators

Authors	Date	Material	Method	Content nanomoles/g
ANSELL, SPANNER	1968	Rat brain	Periodide	170 ± 10 (5)
HEBB	1968	Rat brain	Biological	200
MARCHBANKS	1968	Guinea pig cortex	Biological	220
SCHUBERTH, SPARF, SUNDWALL	1969	Mouse brain	ChAc	115 ± 2.4 (5)
SAELENS*)	1969	Mouse brain	ChAc	105
EWETZ, SPARF, SÖRBO	1969	Mouse brain	Phosphokinase	39.3 ± 0.85 (10)
HANIN, MARSELLI, COSTA	1970	Rat brain	Gas chromatography	274 ± 16 (11)
COLLIER	1970	Mouse brain	Biological	67
SCHUBERTH, SUNDWALL	1971	Mouse brain	ChAc	68.1 ± 6.11 (10)
CONSOLO et al.	1972	Mouse brain	ChAc	62.7

*) Personal communication

TABLE 5

Choline compounds in rat brain

	Content nanomoles/g	Author
Free choline	ca 70	cf Table 4
Phosphorylcholine	380—390	PORCELLATI (48); ANSELL and SPANNER (2)
CDP-choline	50	ANSELL and SPANNER (2)
Glycerophosphorylcholine	400	ANSELL and SPANNER (3)
Acetylcholine	15	
Phosphatidylcholine	14700	ANSELL and SPANNER (2)
Choline plasmalogen	620	ANSELL and SPANNER (2)
Sphingomyelin	3650—3670	WELLS and DITTMER (68); ANSELL and SPANNER (2)
	19900	

Choline — The brain appears to contain free choline (Ch). Opinions differ, however, regarding the exact amount. As Table 4 shows, somewhat different values have been obtained by various authors. This may be owing to the presence of the large amount of compounds in the brain which contain choline. Several of these compounds may liberate Ch both prior to and during the extraction of brain tissue (Table 5). A very rapid postmortal Ch increase was in fact demonstrated by SCHUBERTH, SPARF and SUNDWALL (61). Despite this difficulty there are some indications that the Ch-level in the brain is affected by drugs (Table 3). Oxotremorine, physostigmine and haloperidol appear to increase the amount of free Ch whereas atropine and pentobarbital are without effect (17, 59).

A series of experiments by ANSELL and SPANNER (2) indicated that it was improbable that Ch could be synthesized in the brain, from any known Ch precursors. This conclusion was based on the finding, that on intracerebral injection of the labelled Ch precursors, mono- and dimethylaminoethanol, they were not incorporated into Ch metabolites, whereas intracerebral injection of labelled Ch resulted in a pronounced labelling of the phosphorylcholine and choline lipids. Since Ch is not formed in the brain, it must be supplied with Ch from an external source. Thus, it is probable that plasma Ch is incorporated into brain tissue and subsequently metabolized to different Ch metabolites, e.g. ACh.

CHOLINE UPTAKE IN BRAIN TISSUE

That cortex slices (55) and synaptosomes (23, 41, 58) accumulate exogenous Ch has in fact been demonstrated. The Ch incorporation satisfies the kinetics of carrier-mediated transport processes and is, when cortex slices are used, clearly energy dependent. The

TABLE 6

Uptake of choline and acetylcholine by brain cortex slices and by synaptosomes

	Choline		Acetylcholine	
	Slices	Synapt.	Slices	Synapt.
Energy Dependency	+ (55)	0 (23) (+) (41)	+ (36, 49, 57)	
K_T (μmoles/l)	230 (55)	280 (41) 40—80 (49)	83 (57) 108 (36)	80 (49)
Inhibited by (k_I μmoles/l)				
HC-3	60 (57)	19 (49) 40 (23)	5 (57)	
Eserine	No inhib. (55)	137 (23) No inhib. (41)	7 (57) 9 (36)	
Atropine	No inhib. (55)	No inhib. (41)	16 (57) 18 (36)	
Oxotremorine	No inhib. (55)	No inhib. (41) Weak inhib. (36)	23 (57) 6 (36)	

Numbers in parentheses refer to the references.

specificity of the Ch uptake may be doubted, since also ACh is accumulated in slices (46) and in synaptosomes (49) by a similar carrier-mediated process (57). Furthermore, microsomal, mitochondrial and synaptic vesicle fractions take up Ch by a similar carrier-mediated system (24) as well as do kidney slices (64), erythrocytes (8, 43) and diaphragm (1, 15, 50). Recently a high affinity transport system of Ch has been demonstrated in isolated nerve terminals (YAMAMURA and SNYDER, 1972, Science, 78, 626). In brain slices, there is a marked difference in the uptake of ACh and of Ch with regard to the inhibitory effects of drugs (57). As shown in Table 6 physostigmine, atropine, oxotremorine and HC-3 are rather potent inhibitors of the ACh uptake, whereas HC-3 has some and the other drugs no inhibitory effect on the Ch uptake.

In view of the inability of the brain to form Ch, the Ch uptake may be of physiological importance for the ACh biosynthesis. The ACh uptake, on the other hand, is probably only of minor physiological importance as an additional inactivation mechanism of released ACh, since released ACh is very effectively inactivated by cholinesterase.

Newly synthesized ACh

Evidence for the *in vivo* synthesis of labelled ACh after the injection of ^{14}C-Ch into the caudate nucleus of adult rats was obtained by HEBB et al. (33). One hour after the injection between 0.05 and 0.1% of the injected material had been converted to labelled ACh. Pretreatment of the animals with HC-3 injected into the caudate nucleus reduced the formation of ^{14}C-ACh. Similar findings were obtained by CHAKRIN and SHIDEMAN (13) by injection of ^{3}H-Ch into the cortex of rats.

SCHUBERTH, SPARF and SUNDWALL (59) showed that radioactive Ch, injected intravenously into mice, is very rapidly taken up by the brain and metabolized to ACh (Figs. 1 and 2). In conscious mice about 15% of the ^{3}H-Ch, incorporated in the brain, were metabolized to ^{3}H-ACh within 15 seconds after the injection. Similar results have also been published by DIAMOND (24). In barbiturate-anesthetized animals and also in

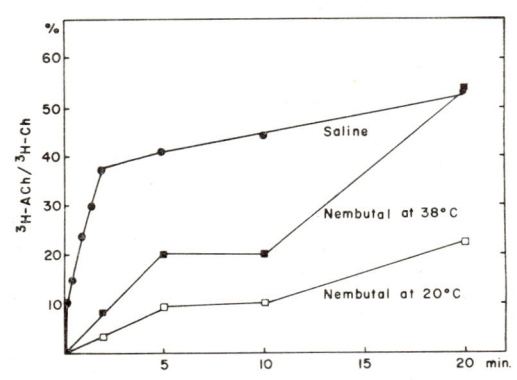

Fig. 1. Synthesis of radioactive acetylcholine in mouse brain *in vitro*. Tritium labelled choline (100 μCi) was given intravenously at zero time. The ratio radioactive ACh/radioactive Ch in whole brain was analyzed at different times. The mice were killed by immersion in liquid nitrogen. Sodiumpentobarbital (60 mg/kg) was given intraperitoneally 30 min before the injection of Ch.

oxotremorine-treated animals a marked retardation in the formation of ^{3}H-ACh was observed. Under these experimental conditions 15% of the ^{3}H-Ch were converted to ^{3}H-ACh not until 4—5 minutes after the ^{3}H-Ch injection (59).

The extremely rapid synthesis of brain ACh from plasma Ch suggests that Ch in plasma is an immediate precursor of ACh in the brain. The presence of 10^{-5} moles/l of very

Fig. 2. Effects of sodium pentobarbital and oxotremorine on the uptake and metabolism of radioactive choline in mouse brain *in vivo*. ^{3}H-tot—total radioactivity; PhCh—phosphorylcholine; Ch—Choline; ACh—acetylcholine. Radioactive choline was given intravenously 30 min after intraperitoneal injection of pentobarbital or oxotremorine. The animals were killed in liquid nitrogen 5 min after the injection of choline.

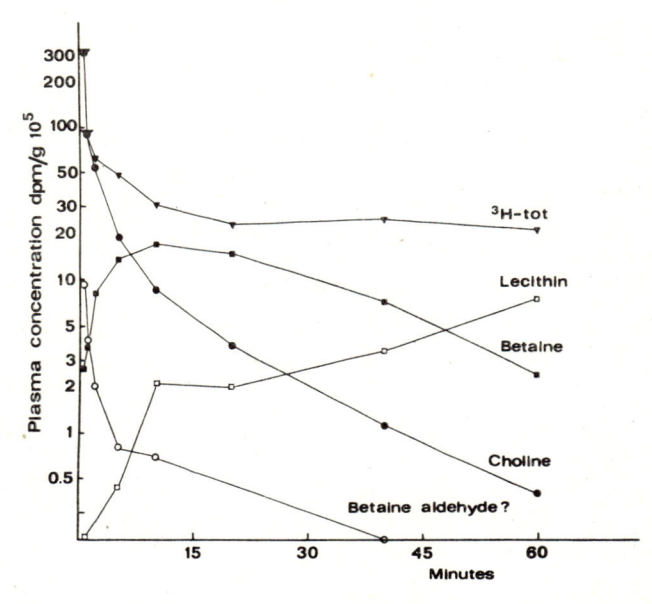

Fig. 3. The concentration of radioactive Ch and its metabolites in plasma of mice as a function of time after intravenous injection of 160 μCi (10 nmoles) [^{3}H]Ch per mouse. 100 μ^3 plasma were taken from the intraorbital plexus at different times after injection.

effectively regulated, endogenous plasma Ch is also consistent with this suggestion (5, 11). In a recent paper by ANSELL and SPANNER (4) the authors claim, however, that Ch is not transported to the brain in a free form, but is supplied by the blood as a Ch lipid, which is split to form free Ch in the brain, prior to utilization. This mechanism was postulated as a result of the finding, that between 1 and 6 hours after intraperitoneal injection of labelled Ch, ethanolamine, dimethylaminoethanol or methionin into rats, lipids in the liver and brain become radioactive although no labelled Ch could be detected in the blood. However, ANSELL and SPANNER did not take into consideration the extremely short half-life of Ch in plasma, as shown in Fig. 3.

COMPARTMENTATION OF NEWLY SYNTHESIZED ACh

Since the brain ACh, which can be labelled from ACh precursors *in vivo*, presumably represents the newly synthesized ACh, it should be possible to study the compartmentation of this particular ACh pool. Experiments to elucidate this have been performed by CHAKRIN and WHITTAKER (14). In following the labelling of brain ACh by intracortical injection of radioactive Ch into anesthetized cats and guinea pigs, synaptosomes and vesicles were prepared from homogenates of the infiltrated cortical area. The specific radioactivity (S.A.) of vesicular ACh was found to be only two-thirds of that of the total synaptosomal ACh. On the assumption that the endogenous ACh in the synaptosomes is distributed 1 : 1 between vesicles and cytoplasm (69) the S.A. of ACh in the cytoplasm should be twice that of the vesicular ACh. On the basis of these experiments the authors postulated that ACh is synthesized from Ch in the cytoplasm, and is then taken up by the vesicles, or that synthesis occurs simultaneously in both cytoplasm and vesicles. The former view is somewhat invalidated by the fact that it has not been possible to demonstrate an uptake of preformed ACh by isolated vesicles (41). Adrenergic vesicles are able to accumulate catecholamines through a mechanism which is dependent on ATP and Mg^{2+} (25).

In a later study by BARKER et al. (9) labelled Ch was administered intraventricularly into conscious guinea pigs under local anesthesia. Synaptosomes were prepared from brain homogenates, and the synaptosomal fraction was further separated into cytoplasm, vesicles and incompletely disrupted synaptosomes, containing vesicles, mitochondria, and external membrane fragments. They obtained some indirect evidence for a small ACh pool with a high S.A., which was lost during the fractionation of the synaptosomes, and which could possibly be recovered in the fraction containing the partially disrupted synaptosomes. The authors postulated that this ACh pool with its rapid turnover was connected in some way with the membrane fragments obtained in the fraction.

SCHUBERTH, SPARF and SUNDWALL (60) who used the probably more physiological method for labelling brain ACh from radioactive Ch in plasma found radioactive ACh in the synaptosomes 90 seconds after intravenous injection of Ch. These studies have been extended in more recent experiments by AQUILONIUS et al. (6). Following intravenous injection of labelled Ch into mice, a rapid incorporation of ACh occurred into both a high molecular weight fraction (HMWF) and a low molecular weight fraction (LMWF) prepared from lysed synaptosomes by gel filtration technique. It was established that the incorporation in the HMWF was exclusively an *in vivo* event and was not due to *in vitro* artefacts. Table 7 gives a summary of our results. As is evident there is a very rapid incorporation of ACh and Ch into both fractions. However, the ratio ^{3}H-ACh/^{3}H-Ch was markedly different in the two fractions, being about 10 times higher in the HMWF than in the LMWF. This strongly indicates that some constituents in the HMWF bind

TABLE 7

Incorporation of labelled choline and acetylcholine in a high and a low molecular weight fraction of brain homogenates following intravenous injection of labelled choline to mice

		Acetylcholine				$\dfrac{\text{Acetylcholine}}{\text{Choline}}$			
		HMWF		LMWF		HMWF		LMWF	
Time min		Control	Barb.	Control	Barb.	Control	Barb.	Control	Barb.
	Radioactive 10^4 DPM/g								
0.25		33	—	65	—	4.7	—	0.38	—
3		28	6	47	31	4.7	2	0.53	0.32
15		8	—	19	—	2.7	—	0.49	—
	Endogenous nanomoles/g	2.2	3.2	5.1	7.4	1.6	2.3	—	—

From AQUILONIUS et al. (6, 7)

newly synthesized ACh. The S.A. of ACh was greater in the high than in the low molecular-weight fraction between 15 seconds and 9 minutes after the injection. In anesthetized animals the incorporation of ^{3}H-ACh 3 minutes after the Ch injection was decreased rather specifically in the HMWF. In the time-interval, from 15 seconds to 9 minutes, a higher S.A. of ACh was obtained in the HMWF than in the LMWF, indicating that the ACh biosynthesis would occur in the HMWF. If this holds good, it must also be assumed that the ACh S.A. is likewise higher in the HMWF than in the LMWF during the time-interval 0—15 seconds which, however, cannot be checked by current techniques. On the other hand, we found that the S.A. of Ch is lower than that of ACh in the HMWF at all the time-intervals studied, a fact which is inconsistent with the hypothesis that the biosynthesis of ACh from Ch occurs in the HMWF. These rather contradictory findings could, however, be explained by ACh being formed in the LMWF, but in close association with the HMWF, which would mean that there is a direct coupling between biosynthesis and the binding of ACh. RITCHIE and GOLDBERG (52), using an *in vitro* system, were able to demonstrate that incorporation of ACh into a vesicle fraction occurred in the presence of concomitant ACh synthesis. The preferentially decreased incorporation of newly synthesized ACh into the HMWF under anesthesia suggests that this pool is of functional importance.

In agreement with BARKER et al. (9) our experiments (6) showed a preferential loss of radioactive ACh from the synaptosomes as compared with the loss of the preformed ACh. In line with several observations that the most recently synthesized ACh is preferentially released (16), our results indicate that newly synthesized ACh is the least stably bound. The morphological distribution of the preformed and the newly synthesized ACh is only a matter of speculation. Although this is not generally accepted, there is much evidence in favor of the hypothesis that vesicles are formed in the cell bodies and then move down the axons to release-sites, where the transmitter is released upon depolarization of the cell membrane. By reloading with newly synthesized transmitter the release cycle may be repeated many times. The life span of catecholamine-containing vesicles has been calculated to be between 35 and 70 days, depending on the species used

(19). This means that there may be a rather heterogeneous population of vesicles in the neurons. After labelling the ACh store under physiological conditions, the functionally most active vesicles, which are located close to the presynaptic membrane, may incorporate ACh of higher S.A. than these vesicles that are more centrally located, which have much lower turnover. The discrepancy in the recovery of endogenous and of labelled ACh may be due to differences in fragility between the two types of vesicles.

REFERENCES

1. ADAMIČ, Š. (1970) Accumulation of acetylcholine by the rat diaphragm. Biochem. Pharmacol. **19**, 2445.
2. ANSELL, G. B. and SPANNER, S. (1968) The metabolism of (Me-^{14}C) choline in the brain of the rat *in vivo*. Biochem. J. **110**, 201.
3. ANSELL, G. B. and SPANNER, S. (1970) The origin and turnover of choline in the brain. In: Drugs and cholinergic mechanisms in the CNS. Proceedings of the conference held at Skokloster, Sweden, February 23—25, 1970. Ed. by E. HEILBRONN & A. WINTER. Försvarets Forskningsanstalt, Stockholm, p. 143.
4. ANSELL, G. B. and SPANNER, S. (1971) Studies on the origin of choline in the brain of the rat. Biochem. J. **122**, 741.
5. APPLETON, H. D., LA DU, B. N., LEVY, B. B., STEELE, J. M. and BRODIE, B. B. (1953) A chemical method for the determination of free choline in plasma. J. biol. Chem. **205**, 803.
6. AQUILONIUS, S. M., FLENTGE, F., SCHUBERTH, J., SPARF, B. and SUNDWALL, A. (1972) Synthesis of acetylcholine in different compartments of brain nerve terminals *in vivo* as studied by the incorporation of choline from plasma. (Submitted for publication.)
7. AQUILONIUS, S. M., FLENTGE, F., SCHUBERTH, J., SPARF, B. and SUNDWALL, A. (1972) The effect of barbiturate anaesthesia on the *in vivo* synthesis of acetylcholine in brain and nerve terminals. (Submitted for publication.)
8. ASKARI, A. (1966) Uptake of some quaternary ammonium ions by human erythrocytes. J. gen. Physiol. **49**, 1147.
9. BARKER, L. A., DOWDALL, M. J., ESSMAN, W. B. and WHITTAKER, V. P. (1970) The compartmentation of acetylcholine in cholinergic nerve terminals. In: Drugs and cholinergic mechanisms in the CNS. Proceedings of the conference held at Skokloster, Sweden, February 23—25, 1970. Ed. by E. HEILBRONN & A. WINTER. Försvarets Forskningsanstalt, Stockholm, p. 193.
10. BEANI, L., BIANCHI, C., MEGAZZINI, P., BALLOTTI, L. and BERNARDI, G. (1969) Drug induced changes in free, labile and stable acetylcholine of guinea-pig brain. Biochem. Pharmacol. **18**, 1315.
11. BLIGH, J. (1952) The level of free choline in plasma. J. Physiol. (London) **117**, 234.
12. BRODIE, B. B. (1964) Physico-chemical factors in drug absorption. In: Absorption and distribution of drugs. Ed. by T. B. BINNS. Livingstone, Edinburgh, p. 16.
13. CHAKRIN, L. W. and SHIDEMAN, F. E. (1968) Synthesis of acetylcholine from labeled choline by brain. Int. J. Neuropharmacol. **7**, 337.
14. CHAKRIN, L. W. and WHITTAKER, V. P. (1969) The subcellular distribution of (N-Me-^{3}H) acetylcholine synthesized by brain *in vivo*. Biochem. J. **113**, 97.
15. CHANG, C. C. and LEE, C. (1970) Studies on the [^{3}H]choline uptake in rat phrenic nerve-diaphragm preparations. Neuropharmacology, **9**, 223.
16. COLLIER, B. and MACINTOSH, F. C. (1969) The source of choline for acetylcholine synthesis in a sympathetic ganglion. Canad. J. Physiol. Pharmacol. **47**, 127.
17. CONSOLO, S., LADINSKY, H., PERI, G. and GARATTINI, S. (1972) Effect of central stimulants and depressants on mouse brain acetylcholine and choline levels. Europ. J. Pharmacol. **18**, 251.
18. CROSSLAND, J. and SLATER, P. (1968) The effect of some drugs on the "free" and "bound" acetylcholine content of rat brain. Brit. J. Pharmacol. **33**, 42.
19. DAHLSTRÖM, A. and HÄGGENDAL, J. (1966) Studies on the transport and life-span of amine storage granules in a peripheral adrenergic neuron system. Acta physiol. scand. **67**, 278.
20. DATTA, K. and WAJDA, I. J. (1972) Morphine-induced kinetic alterations of choline acetyltransferase on the rat caudate nucleus. Brit. J. Pharmacol. **44**, 732.
21. DE ROBERTIS, E., PELLEGRINO DE IRALDI, A., RODRIGUEZ DE LORES ARNAIZ, G. and SALGANICOFF, L. (1962) Cholinergic and non-cholinergic nerve endings in rat brain. I. Isolation and subcellular distribution of acetylcholine and acetylcholinesterase. J. Neurochem. **9**, 23

22. DE ROBERTIS, E., RODRIGUEZ DE LORES ARNAIZ, G., SALGANICOFF, L., PELLEGRINO DE IRALDI, A. and ZIEHER, L. M. (1963) Isolation of synaptic vesicles and structural organization of the acetylcholine system within brain nerve endings. J. Neurochem. **10**, 225.
23. DIAMOND, I. and KENNEDY, E. P. (1969) Carrier-mediated transport of choline into synaptic nerve endings. J. biol. Chem. **244**, 3258.
24. DIAMOND, I. and MILFAY, D. (1972) Uptake of [^{3}H-methyl] choline by microsomal, synaptosomal, mitochondrial and synaptic vesicle fractions of rat brain. The effects of hemicholinium. J. Neurochem. **19**, 1899.
25. EULER, U. S. VON and LISHAJKO, F. (1963) Catecholamine release and uptake in isolated adrenergic nerve granules. Acta physiol. scand. **57**, 468.
26. EWETZ, L., SPARF, B. and SÖRBO, B. (1970) Enzymatic determination of choline in brain with choline phosphokinase and ^{32}P-labelled ATP. In: *In vitro* procedures with radioisotopes in medicine. International Atomic Energy Agency (IAEA). Symposium. Vienna, p. 175.
27. FELDBERG, W. (1945) Present views on the mode of action of acetylcholine in the central nervous system. Physiol. Rev. **25**, 596.
28. FONNUM, F. (1967) The "compartmentation" of choline acetyltransferase within the synaptosome. Biochem. J. **103**, 262.
29. GIARMAN, N. J. and PEPEU, G. (1962) Drug-induced changes in brain acetylcholine. Brit. J. Pharmacol. **19**, 226.
30. GRAY, E. G. and WHITTAKER, V. P. (1962) The isolation of nerve endings from brain: an electron-microscopic study of cell fragments derived by homogenization and centrifugation. J. Anat. (London) **96**, 79.
31. HEBB, C. O. and SMALLMAN, B. N. (1956) Intracellular distribution of choline acetylase. J. Physiol. (London) **134**, 385.
32. HEBB, C. O. and WHITTAKER, V. P. (1958) Intracellular distribution of acetylcholine and choline acetylase. J. Physiol. (London) **142**, 187.
33. HEBB, C. O., LING, G. M., MCGEER, E. G., MCGEER, P. L. and PERKINS, D. (1964) Effect of locally applied hemicholinium on the acetylcholine content of the caudate nucleus. Nature, **204**, 1309.
34. HOLMSTEDT, B., LUNDGREN, G. and SUNDWALL, A. (1963) Tremorine and atropine effects on brain acetylcholine. Life Sci. **2**, 731.
35. KAITA, A. A. and GOLDBERG, A. M. (1969) Control of acetylcholine synthesis — the inhibition of choline acetyltransferase by acetylcholine. J. Neurochem. **16**, 1185.
36. LIANG, C. C. and QUASTEL, J. H. (1969) Uptake of acetylcholine in rat brain cortex slices. Biochem. Pharmacol. **18**, 1169.
37. LIANG, C. C. and QUASTEL, J. H. (1969) Effects of drugs on the uptake of acetylcholine in rat brain cortex slices. Biochem. Pharmacol. **18**, 1187.
38. MALTHE-SØRENSEN, D. and FONNUM, F. (1971) Multiple forms of choline acetyltransferase from rat brain. Nature, New Biol. **229**, 127.
39. MANN, P. J. G., TENNENBAUM, M. and QUASTEL, J. H. (1938) On the mechanism of acetylcholine formation in brain *in vitro*. Biochem. J. **32**, 243.
40. MANN, P. J. G., TENNENBAUM, M. and QUASTEL, J. H. (1939) Acetylcholine metabolism in the central nervous system. The effects of potassium and other cations on acetylcholine liberation. Biochem. J. **33**, 822.
41. MARCHBANKS, R. M. (1968) The uptake of [^{14}C]choline into synaptosomes *in vitro*. Biochem. J. **110**, 533.
42. MARCHBANKS, R. M. (1969) Biochemical organization of cholinergic nerve terminals in the cerebral cortex. In: Cellular dynamics of the neuron. Ed. by S. H. BARONDES. Academic Press, New York, p. 115.
43. MARTIN, K. (1968) Concentrative accumulation of choline by human erythrocytes. J. gen. Physiol. **51**, 497.
44. MARTIN, K. (1969) Effects of quaternary ammonium compounds on choline transport in red cells. Brit. J. Pharmacol. **36**, 458.
45. PERSSON, B. O., LARSSON, L., SCHUBERTH, J. and SÖRBO, B. (1967) 3-Bromoacetonyltrimethylammonium bromide, a choline acetylase inhibitor. Acta chem. scand. **21**, 2283.
46. POLAK, R. L. and MEEUWS (1966) The influence of atropine on the release and uptake of acetylcholine by the isolated cerebral cortex of the rat. Biochem. Pharmacol. **15**, 989.
47. POLAK, R. L. (1969) The influence of drugs on the uptake of acetylcholine by slices of rat cerebral cortex. Brit. J. Pharmacol. **36**, 144.
48. PORCELLATI, G. (1958) The levels of some free nitrogencontaining phosphate esters in nervous tissue. J. Neurochem. **2**, 128.
49. POTTER, L. T. (1968) Uptake of choline by nerve endings isolated from the rat cerebral cortex.

In: A symposium on the interaction of drugs and subcellular components in animal cells. Ed. by P. N. Campbell. Churchill, London, p. 293.
50. Potter, L. T. (1970) Synthesis, storage and release of [^{14}C]acetylcholine in isolated rat diaphragm muscles. J. Physiol. (London) **206**, 145.
51. Richter, D. and Crossland, J. (1949) Variation in acetylcholine content of the brain with physiological state. Amer. J. Physiol. **159**, 247.
52. Ritchie, A. K. and Goldberg, A. M. (1970) Vesicular and synaptoplasmic synthesis of acetylcholine. Science, **169**, 489.
53. Schneider, W. C. (1959) Mitochondrial metabolism. Adv. Enzymol. **21**, 1.
54. Schuberth, J., Sollenberg, J., Sundwall, A. and Sörbo, B. (1965) Determination of acetyl-coenzyme A in brain. J. Neurochem. **12**, 451.
55. Schuberth, J., Sundwall, A., Sörbo, B. and Lindell, J-O. (1966) Uptake of choline by mouse brain slices. J. Neurochem. **13**, 347.
56. Schuberth, J., Sollenberg, J., Sundwall, A. and Sörbo, B. (1966) Acetylcoenzyme A in brain. The effect of centrally active drugs, insulin coma and hypoxia. J. Neurochem. **13**, 819.
57. Schuberth, J. and Sundwall, A. (1967) Effects of some drugs on the uptake of acetylcholine in cortex slices of mouse brain. J. Neurochem. **14**, 807.
58. Schuberth, J. and Sundwall, A. (1968) Differences in the subcellular localization of choline, acetylcholine and atropine taken up by mouse brain slices in vitro. Acta physiol. scand. **72**, 65.
59. Schuberth, J., Sparf, B. and Sundwall, A. (1969) A technique for the study of acetylcholine turnover in mouse brain in vivo. J. Neurochem. **16**, 695.
60. Schuberth, J., Sparf, B. and Sundwall, A. (1970) On the turnover of acetylcholine in the brain. In: Drugs and cholinergic mechanisms in the CNS. Proceedings of the conference held at Skokloster, Sweden, February 23—25, 1970. Ed. by E. Heilbronn & A. Winter. Försvarets Forskningsanstalt, Stockholm, p. 177.
61. Schuberth, J., Sparf, B. and Sundwall A. (1970) On the turnover of acetylcholine in nerve endings of mouse brain in vivo. J. Neurochem. **17**, 461.
62. Smith, J. C., Cavallito, C. J. and Foldes, F. F. (1967) Choline acetyltransferase inhibitors: a group of styryl-pyridine analogs. Biochem. Pharmacol. **16**, 2438.
63. Sollenberg, J. and Sörbo, B. (1970) On the origin of the acetyl moiety of acetylcholine in brain studied with a differential labelling technique using ^{3}H-^{14}C-mixed labelled glucose and acetate. J. Neurochem. **17**, 201.
64. Sung, C. P. and Johnstone, R. M. (1969) Evidence for the existence of separate transport mechanisms for choline and betaine in rat kidney. Biochim. biophys. Acta **173**, 548.
65. Tuček, S. (1966) On subcellular localization and binding of choline acetyltransferase in the cholinergic nerve endings of the brain. J. Neurochem. **13**, 1317.
66. Tuček, S. (1966) On the question of the localization of choline acetyltransferase in synaptic vesicles. J. Neurochem. **13**, 1329.
67. Tuček, S. (1970) Subcellular localization of enzymes generating acetyl-CoA and their possible relation to the biosynthesis of acetylcholine. In: Drugs and cholinergic mechanisms in the CNS. Proceedings of the conference held at Skokloster, Sweden, February 23—25, 1970. Ed. by E. Heilbronn & A. Winter. Försvarets Forskningsanstalt, Stockholm, p. 117.
68. Wells, M. A. and Dittmer, J. C. (1967) A comprehensive study of the postnatal changes in the concentration of the lipids of developing rat brain. Biochemistry, **6**, 3169.
69. Whittaker, V. P. (1959) The isolation and characterization of acetylcholine containing particles from brain. Biochem. J. **72**, 694.
70. Whittaker, V. P., Michaelson, I. A. and Kirkland, R. J. A. (1964) The separation of synaptic vesicles from nerve-ending particles ("synaptosomes"). Biochem. J. **90**, 293.
71. Whittaker, V. P. and Sheridan, M. (1965) The morphology and acetylcholine content of isolated cerebral cortical synaptic vesicles. J. Neurochem. **12**, 363.

A.S., Department of Pharmacology and Toxicology Biomedical Center, University of Uppsala, S-751 23 Uppsala, Sweden

SYNTHESIS AND RELEASE OF ACETYLCHOLINE IN NERVE ELECTROPLAQUE JUNCTIONS FROM *TORPEDO MARMORATA*

M. ISRAEL

Division Risler, Salpêtrière Hospital, Paris

Introduction

Fractionation experiments have shown that in the electric organ of *Torpedo* most of the nerve endings are opened during the homogenization procedure. The enzyme choline acetyltransferase being recovered in a soluble non ocluded form, no synaptosomes are formed. Bound acetylcholine (ACh) present in such homogenates is associated to monodispersed synaptic vesicles, these were purified, and trapped to vesicles in the damaged nerve ending (3, 4, 5). Little or no "free ACh" survives in the homogenate unless a cholinesterase inhibitor is present. "Free ACh" can be estimated as the difference between total ACh determined by extracting the tissue with trichloracetic acid and bound ACh left in the homogenate.

The equivalence of bound ACh to vesicular ACh in such homogenates is verified by the fact that the specific radioactivity of ACh in the vesicular fraction prepared from slices incubated with ^{14}C choline is similar to that of the homogenate (6).

Stimulation of the tissue until the electrical response had fallen was accompanied by a drop in the level of "free ACh". A fall of bound ACh could be elicited after the free had fallen by continuing the stimulation. A rise in the specific radioactivity of ACh (SRA) was demonstrated in the free compartment on stimulation. These results have recently been described (1, 2). Free and bound ACh can now be extracted 10 to 30 seconds after the stimulation period. Attempts to analyse the effects of stimulations during the decay of the electrical response of the tissue are in progress.

Results

1. *Incorporation of radioactive ACh in the free and the vesicular compartments under resting conditions*

If fragments of 0.5 to 0.8 g of electric tissue are incubated in a physiological solution, "free" and bound ACh remain relatively stable during the incubation period. Values of 100 to 300 nM/g are found as "free ACh"; this represents 25 to 50% of the total. In presence of ^{14}C choline (1 μCi/ml) ^{14}C ACh appears in both compartments at similar rates until a plateau reached in the vesicular compartment after 120 minutes. When the plateau is reached, the SRA still rises in the free compartment. The results suggest that diffusion takes place between the two compartments and that the bound pool is saturable.

2. *Effects of stimulation*

About 70% of the discharge (equivalent to the end-plate potential) falls off during the 30 first seconds of a stimulation at 10/s. The amplitude is then stable for 90 seconds, and falls to a negligible level one minute later.

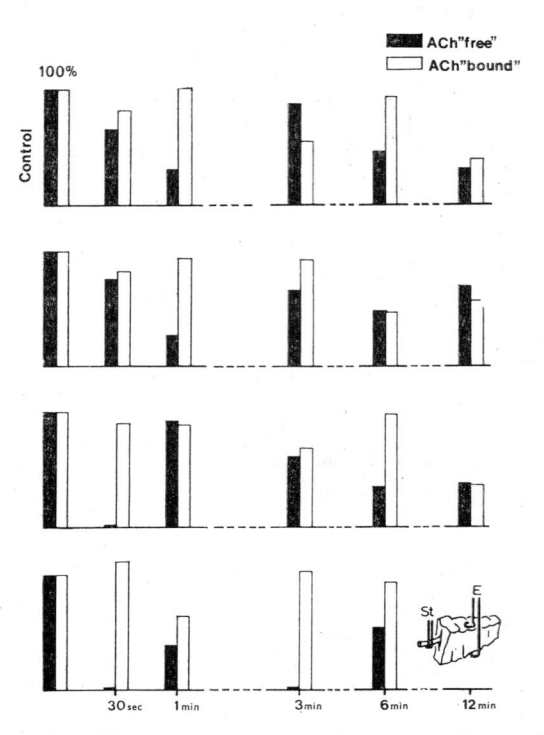

Fig. 1. Stimulation of a slice of electric organ through the nerve. St — stimulating electrodes; E — recording electrodes. A minimum level of "free ACh" is found at 30 sec or 60 sec. "Bound ACh" drops after much longer periods of stimulation. The frequency of stimulation used was 10/s.

When the incubated slice is stimulated through its nerve, low-levels of "free ACh" were found at 30 or 60 seconds, a rise was found after the first minute of stimulation, and at 3 minutes or for longer periods of stimulation falls of about 50% are found in the free compartment (Fig. 1). Bound ACh usually dropped after 6 minutes of stimulation, longer periods of stimulation (up to 12 minutes) were even necessary (Fig. 1).

About 70% of the amplitude of the discharge is abolished during the first 30 seconds of stimulation (10/s). An important drop in "free ACh" with no change in bound ACh or in the number of vesicles was shown after 30 or 60 seconds of stimulation at 10/s.

3. Synthesis of ACh during stimulation

The drop of "free ACh" is accompanied by synthesis occurring from the very radioactive choline pool. The specific radioactivity rises in the free compartment above the controls. The rise was observed as early as 90 seconds after stimulation and was found higher at 6 minutes. The specific radioactivity of bound ACh in the stimulated tissues was found between the values of controls taken before and at the end of the experiment.

Discussion

The results described suggest that "free ACh" represents a readily releasable compartment. Synthesis of transmitter occurred on stimulation in the free compartment. Bound ACh is not immediately available for release, a drop was demonstrated after the free had fallen.

The answer as to what "free ACh" actually represents is still not available: fragile vesicles that would not be demonstrated by our techniques? or acetylcholine in the free form released by a process still unknown?

References

1. Dunant, Y., Gautron, J., Israël, M., Lesbats, B. and Manaranche, R. (1971) Effect de la stimulation de l'organe électrique de la Torpille sur les compartiments "libre et lié" d'acétylcholine. C. R. Acad. Sci. (Paris) **273**, 233.
2. Dunant, Y., Gautron, J., Israël, M., Lesbats, B. and Manaranche, R. (1972) Les compartiments d'acétylcholine de l'organe électrique de la Torpille et leurs modifications par la stimulation. J. Neurochem. **19**, 1987.
3. Israël, M., Gautron, J. and Lesbats, B. (1968) Isolement des vésicules synaptiques de l'organe électrique de la Torpille et localisation de l'acétylcholine à leur niveau. C. R. Acad. Sci. (Paris) **266**, 273.
4. Israël, M., Gautron, J. and Lesbats, B. (1970) Fractionnement de l'organe électrique de la Torpille: localisation subcellulaire de l'acétylcholine. J. Neurochem. **17**, 1441.
5. Israël, M. (1970) Localisation de l'acétylcholine des synapses myoneurales et nerf-électroplaque. Arch. Anat. Microscop. Morphol. exp. **59**, 67.
6. Marchbanks, R. M. and Israël, M. (1971) Aspects of acetylcholine metabolism in the electric organ of Torpedo marmorata. J. Neurochem. **18**, 439.

M.I., Division Risler, Hôpital de la Salpétrière, 47 Bd. de l'Hôpital, Paris 13ᵉ, France

RELEASE OF LOW MOLECULAR SUBSTANCES FROM CHOLINERGIC VESICLES AS A CONSEQUENCE OF PHOSPHOLIPASE A$_2$ ATTACK

E. HEILBRONN

Section of Biochemistry, Research Institute of National Defence, Sundbyberg

Some years ago we introduced phospholipase A$_2$ as a tool in investigations on the chemistry and structure of the cholinergic synaps (7). The enzyme, in our case purified from snake venom (*Naja nigricollis*), attacks phospholipids, preferentially phosphatidyl-ethanolamine, -choline and -serine, and splits off the fatty acid in β-position, thus creating lysophosphatides. The phosphatides themselves are present in neuronal as well as in other membranes.

It was shown on rat brain cortex slices that the acetylcholine uptake and/or storage in this fissue was impaired in the presence of phospholipase A$_2$ (3, 4). Using selected pieces to the motor cortex of the rat for the identification of expected morphological changes, a progressive breakdown of pre- and postsynaptic membranes was observed (2). The synaptic contact area was found to be remarkably stable. Synaptic vesicles were seen to form clusters and a decrease in their total number was observed. Simultaneously a substantial part of the ACh content of the tissue was released.

The loss of ACh from the cortex material was thus largely due to loss of cytoplasmic ACh as a consequence of ruptures in outer synaptosomal membranes. In early stages of enzyme treatment an uptake system for ACh, described by several authors (4, 8, 10) but nevertheless still doubtful, may have been destroyed. The observed clustering of synaptic vesicles, indicating changes in the charge and structure of their membranes, led to further work aiming at an analysis of the sensitivity of the cholinergic vesicle to an enzymic attack as represented by phospholipase A$_2$. A model of a possible enzymic transmitter release was drawn (Fig. 1).

Vesicles, either prepared from rat cerebral cortex synaptosomes which constitute a mixed population derived from both cholinergic membranes, or pure cholinergic vesicles isolated from the electric organ of *Torpedo marmorata* or *nobiliana*, were used. The methods of preparation as well as those used for electron microscopy will be published elsewhere (6). ACh was determined with the leech muscle assay, using a low friction device recently constructed in this laboratory. Contamination with other organelles was less than 1 in a 100.

Cortical synaptic vesicles as well as those from Torpedo were found to be sensitive to phospholipase A$_2$, loosing most of their ACh-content (Table 1). About 10% of the original ACh-content of cortical vesicles remained particle-bound, adsorbed or possibly ionically bound to membrane fractions. Morphologically the vesicles were found to swell and became diffuse, granularity increased and the membranes lost contrast. At a later stage the membranes broke and gave debris with a fibrous appearance (5, 6). In contrast to outer synaptosomal membranes, which we find to reorganize themselves in larger rings or sacs, the vesicle debris never has been observed to fuse again in these *in vitro*

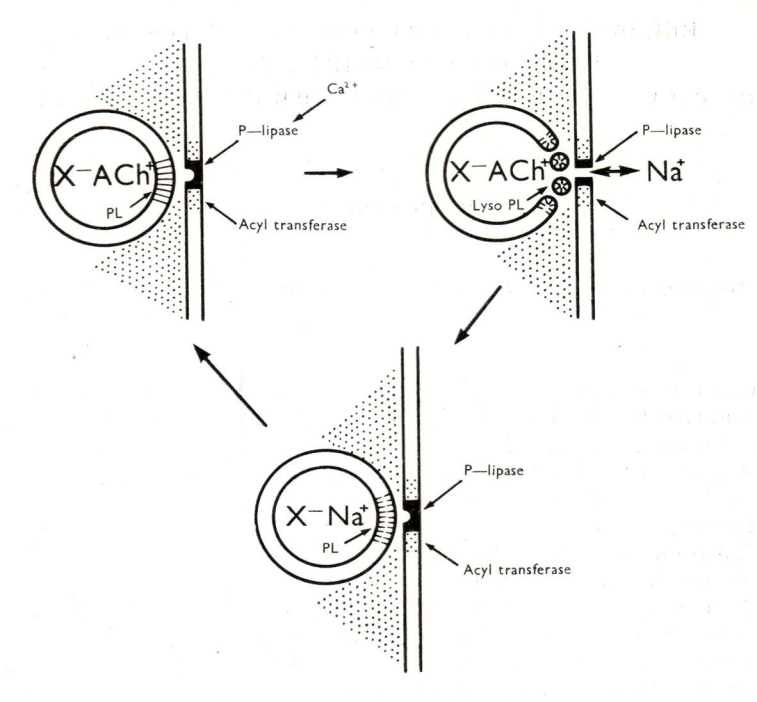

Fig. 1. Model of enzymatically induced ACh release from synaptic vesicles. PL — phosphatidylcholine or other phosphatide.

TABLE 1

Example of ACh release from rat brain cortical synaptic vesicles after 5 min incubation with phospholipase A_2, 1 µg/ml at 25 °C

Sample	"Free" ACh found pmoles/ml
Total after acid boiling	348
Untreated	195
Incubated without P-lipase	192
Incubated with P-lipase	328

experiments. Chemically, immediate and increasing formation of lysolecithine due to enzyme treatment has been observed.

In collaboration with BOYNE and EDWARDS (6) it was found that *Torpedo* vesicles at low temperature (+5°C) in the presence of phospholipase A_2 slowly release ACh. At higher temperature (+26°C) ACh is released more rapidly. ATP, earlier shown by WHITTAKER et al. (11) to be present in *Torpedo* vesicles, is equally released though at a slower rate than ACh (Fig. 2). Morphological investigations show good retention of vesicle structure at low temperature, though perhaps collapse or size reduction of some vesicles is observed. At higher temperature the vesicle structure is lost and the fibrous elements observed with cortex synaptic vesicles are seen.

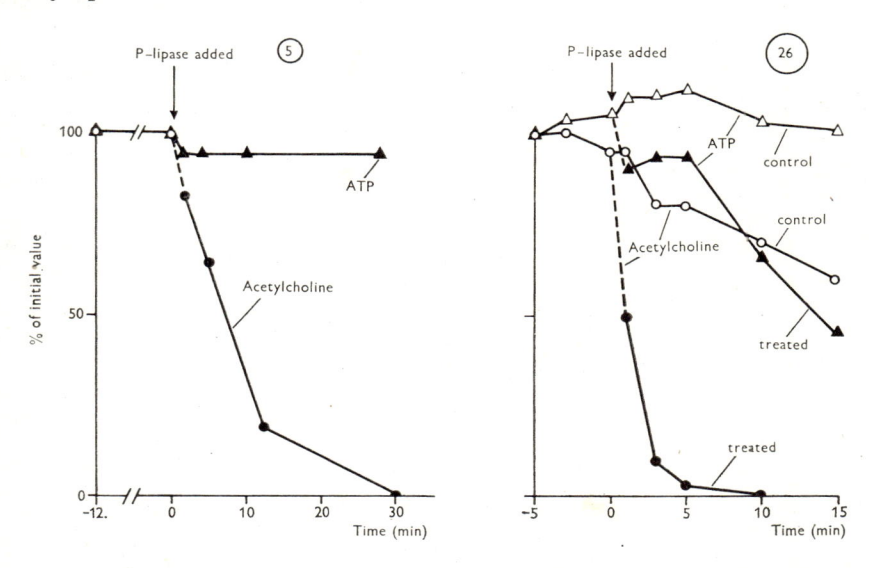

Fig. 2. Phospholipase A_2 induced release of ACh and ATP from cholinergic vesicles isolated from the electric organ of *Torpedo marmorata*. Measurements at two different temperatures. For details see ref. 6.

From the experiments it can be concluded that phospholipids susceptable to phospholipase A_2 are essential for the structure of synaptosomal membranes and cholinergic vesicles. The sensitivity to phospholipase A_2 underlines the importance of hydrophobic protein- phospholipid interaction in the maintenance of a membrane structure. ACh release from isolated synaptic vesicles is facilitated by phospholipase A_2 and occurs in early stages of enzymic attack, as represented by the low temperature experiments, without much destruction of the vesicle. ATP release on the other hand is more dependent on structural breakdown suggesting binding of ATP to vesicle macromolecular compounds, e.g. membrane constituents. The role of lysophosphatides, in the experiments formed due to phospholipase action, has not yet been studied. Theories involving lysolecithin in transmitter release have been forwarded ever since this compound was found in rather high amounts in chromaffin granules (1). Its involvement in membrane fusion has also been discussed (9). In preliminary thin-layer chromatographic analysis of the phospholipid content of cholinergic vesicles we have found very little (0—5% of total phospholipids) lysolecithin. The results presented here keep open the possibility of an enzymic release of ACh at the synaptic junction, either by the formation of pores in the vesicle membrane or by (temporary) fusion of the vesicle with the presynaptic membrane. This may lead to a transfer of ACh from the vesicle to either the presynaptic membrane or the synaptic cleft.

References

1. BLASCHKO, H., FIREMARK, H., SMITH, A. D. and WINKLER, H. (1967) Lipids of the adrenal medulla, lysolecithin a characteristic constituent of chromaffin granules. Biochem. J. **104**, 545.
2. CEDERGREN, E., HEILBRONN, E., JOHANSSON, B. and WIDLUND, L. (1970) Ultrastructural stability of contact regions of phospholipase treated synapses from rat motor cortex. Brain Res. **24**, 139.
3. HEILBRONN, E. (1969) The effect of phospholipases on the uptake of atropine and acetylcholine by slices of mouse brain cortex. J. Neurochem. **16**, 627.
4. HEILBRONN, E. (1970) Further experiments on the uptake of acetylcholine and atropine and the release of acetylcholine from mouse brain cortex slices after treatment with phospholipases. J. Neurochem. **17**, 381.
5. HEILBRONN, E. (1972) Action of phospholipase A on synaptic vesicles. A model for transmitter release? In: Biochemical and Pharmacological Mechanisms Underlying Behaviour. Eds. BRADLEY P. B. and BRIMBLECOMBE R. W., Progress in Brain Research **36**, 29.
6. HEILBRONN, E., BOYNE, A. F. and EDWARDS, W. (1972) The effect of phospholipase A_2 on isolated cholinergic synaptic vesicles. In preparation.
7. HEILBRONN, E. and CEDERGREN, E. (1970) Chemically induced changes in the acetylcholine uptake and storage capacity of brain tissue. In: Drugs and Cholinergic Mechanisms in the CNS. Eds. E. HEILBRONN and A. WINTER, 1970, Distrib. Almqvist and Wiksell, Stockholm, p. 245.
8. POLAK, R. L. and MEEUWS, M. M. (1966) The influence of atropine on the release and uptake of acetylcholine by the isolated cerebral cortex of the rat. Biochem. Pharmacol. **15**, 989.
9. POOLE, A. R., HOWELL, J. I. and LUCY, J. A. (1970) Lysolecithin and cell fusion. Nature (Lond.) **227**, 810.
10. SCHUBERTH, J. and SUNDWALL, A. (1967) Incorporation of exogenous acetylcholine, choline and atropine in mouse brain cortex slices. Abstr. 1st Int. Meeting of the Int. Soc. for Neurochemistry, Strasbourg, p. 187.
11. WHITTAKER, V. P., DOWDALL, M. J. and BOYNE, A. L. (1972) Biochem. Soc. Symp. **36**, in press.

E.H., Section of Biochemistry, Research Institute of National Defence, Dept. 1, 17204 Sundbyberg 4, Sweden

APPLICATION OF MICROCHEMICAL ANALYSIS TO THE CHARACTERIZATION OF NEURONS FROM THE BRAIN OF *HELIX ASPERSA*

P. C. EMSON and F. FONNUM

Division of Toxicology, Norwegian Defence Research Establishement, Kjeller

The neurons of invertebrates are particularly suitable for enzymatic analysis. The large size of some of these neurons means that individual identified neurons can be readily and repeatably dissected out and assayed. Further, the lack of synapses on the cell bodies means the enzyme activity found is due to the neuron itself and not to any adhering terminals. We have attempted to characterize some of the large identifiable neurons in the snail brain by determining whether the presence of enzymes such as choline acetyltransferase (ChAc) and acetylcholinesterase (AChE) is a distinguishing property of cholinergic neurons. This type of approach is necessary because it is not yet feasible to measure directly the content of putative transmitters in single nerve cells.

In the present work we have studied ChAc, the enzyme responsible for the synthesis of acetylcholine (ACh). Previous work (3, 8) has shown that, in *Aplysia* this enzyme is found only in a small fraction of neurons (0.1—0.3 per cent). We have extended this approach to a different mollusc and also to cells which are on average considerably smaller (*Helix* maximum cell diameter 200 µm, *Aplysia* maximum cell diameter 1 mm).

The brain of the snail (*Helix aspersa*) and especially the suboesophageal ganglion has been the subject of a number of pharmacological and electrophysiological investigations (4—6, 14). In particular WALKER, LAMBERT, WOODRUFF and KERKUT (13) have provided a map of approximately 30 large neurons in the suboesophageal ganglion based on action potential shape and firing rate, position and pharmacology. We have measured the activities of AChE and ChAc in most of these identified neurons.

Methods

Sensitive radiochemical methods for the assay of ChAc and AChE have been developed in our laboratory. Choline acetyltransferase was determined by measuring the formation of [1—^{14}C] ACh from [1—^{14}C] acetyl CoA, the labelled acetylcholine was extracted with sodium tetraphenylboron (Kalignost) (2). Acetylcholinesterase was measured by hydrolysis of [1—^{14}C] acetylcholine to [1—^{14}C] acetate (2), the unhydrolysed acetylcholine was removed by Kalignost extraction and the [^{14}C] acetate was counted in a toluene/Triton scintillation mixture. Individual nerve cells (Fig. 1) were dissected from the suboesophageal ganglion, washed in isotonic sucrose and then ruptured by freezing and thawing.

Microdissection was carried out on freeze-dried section of tissue as described by LOWRY (7). All substrate solution contained 0.2% Triton X-100 in order to release all enzyme activity.

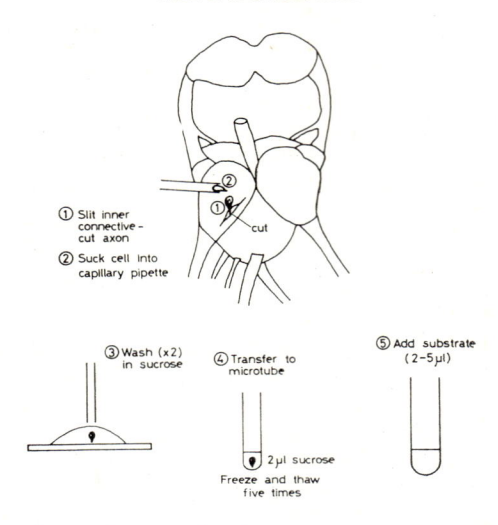

Fig. 1. Summary of procedures used to isolate and assay identified single neurons.

RESULTS

Enzymic properties

The properties of the ChAc from snail brain are summarized in Table 1. The enzyme was strikingly different, in a number of properties, from ChAc's from other vertebrates and invertebrates (10—12). The enzyme was precipitated below 35% ammonium sulphate saturation whereas all previously studied ChAc's, including those from *Aplysia* and the squid precipitate between 40—60% saturation. Attempts to separate the enzyme by

TABLE 1

Properties of the choline acetyltransferase from the snail (*Helix aspersa*)

Apparent Km for acetyl CoA	2.2×10^{-4} M
Apparent Km for choline	1.0 mM
Temperature coefficient	1.2/10 °C
Ammonium sulphate precipitation	Enzyme ppte below 35 % ammonium sulphate saturation
Inhibition by styrylpyridines	Weak inhibition (30 %) at high concentrations (1 mM)

isoeletric focusing failed because of its tendency to precipitate during focusing. The temperature coefficient is unusual in being 1.2/10°C, and this is another difference from other molluscan ChAc's which have more normal coefficients, for example *Aplysia*: 2.4/10°C (3). Inhibition studies using styrylpyridine analogs also showed that snail ChAc is substantially different from vertebrate ChAc in sensitivity to these inhibitors. These compounds were weak inhibitors of the snail enzyme, the best inhibitor producing only 30% inhibition at a concentration of 1 mM. In contrast the rat enzyme was inhibited 50% at 4.7×10^{-5} M. In other properties such as the Michaelis constants, pH optimum and activation by salts, the snail enzyme was similar to other previously studied molluscan ChAc's (3, 12).

The properties of the cholinesterase (ChE) from the snail brain have been studied (1). These results show that at least 90% of the ChE activity is due to a true AChE. The ChE shows substrate inhibition, is inhibited by eserine at a concentration of 10^{-6} M, is not inhibited by iso-OMPA (10^{-4} M) and has a low affinity for butyrylcholine; all properties which indicate the ChE is a true AChE (see Table 2). The ChE has been partially purified

TABLE 2

Properties of the cholinesterase from *Helix aspersa* brain

Substrate specificity	% activity at 1 mM substrate concentration
Acetylcholine	100
Acetylthiocholine	120
Butyrylcholine	5
Apparent Km for acetylthiocholine	5.8×10^{-4} M
I_{50} eserine	9.4×10^{-6} M
Iso-OMPA (1×10^{-4} M)	No inhibition
Substrate inhibition	Above 4 mM
Average activity in whole brain	10.1 mmoles/g of protein/hour

Data from EMSON and KERKUT (1).

and separated into a broad band by gel electrophoresis. The enzyme after purification had a specific activity of 180 m mol/g of protein/hour. Histochemical evidence shows AChE to be present at synaptic junction in *Helix* brain. The enzyme is also found in nerves, muscles and axons.

Regional distribution

We have studied the distribution of ChAc in various snail ganglia (Table 3). When the activities were expressed, per ganglion, there was a two-fold difference between the least active parietal visceral ganglion and the most active cerebral ganglion. However, there is no difference when the results are expressed in terms of wet weight or protein content.

A more detailed investigation of the regional distribution of ChAc was carried out by micro-dissection of freeze-dried sections. Invertebrate brains are particularly suitable for this technique as the neuropile layer is central and surrounded by the cellular lyaer.

TABLE 3

Distribution of choline acetyltransferase in various *Helix aspersa* ganglia

Ganglion	Enzyme activity	
	(nmol/ganglion/h)	(nmole/mg wet weight/h)
Parietal — visceral	45.66	17.91
Cerebral	111.00	20.79
Optic	65.2	21.0
Pedal	54.2	18.42

Each value represents triplicate determination on homogenates of ganglia from five different animals.

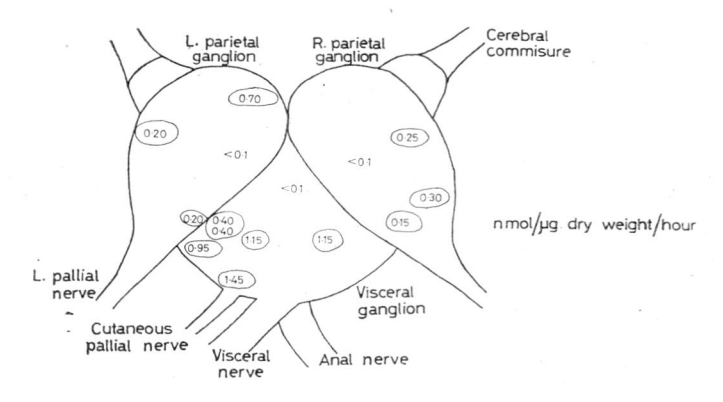

Fig. 2. The distribution of areas of particularly high choline acetyltransferase activity on the surface of the suboesophageal ganglion. The majority of the surface area has low activity (< 0.1 nmole/μg/hour).

This type of approach allowed us to attempt to "map out" areas with higher than average ChAc activity "cholinergic hot spots". Each individual section 40 μm thick, was divided into neuropile and cellular layers, the cellular layer was then further sub-divided. Each tissue sample was assayed for ChAc activity. By analyzing serial sections it was possible to reconstruct the ganglion and indicate regions with high ChAc activity. Figure 2 shows a reconstruction of the upper surface of the suboesophageal ganglion. The numbers on the figure indicate the average ChAc found in regions with particularly high enzyme activities. The neuropile has a uniformly high activity > 0.2 nmol/μg dry weight/hour.

Single cell studies

The information from freeze-dried sections gives an indication of the regions where we would expect to find cholinergic cells. These areas were investigated for large ChAc containing cells. Figure 3 shows two identical identified cells from different preparations, the single axon has been cut just below the axon hillock. Figure 4 shows a map of the large identifiable ChAc containing cells. One should notice that these cells tend to be grouped together and several of them are found in regions where we had found high ChAc activity

(Fig. 2). Of the approximately thirty large neurons described by WALKER et al. (13), five contain ChAc (No. 13, 17, 21, 23, 26). There are five other cells containing ChAc shown on our map. These were not described and numbered by WALKER et al. but can be repeatably found in position shown. Table 4 compares the activities of AChE and ChAc in some of the large neurons described by WALKER et al. Notice that ChAc is found only in certain cells and that the levels of enzyme activity in these cells are fairly constant from preparation to preparation. The majority of cells from the snail brain have no ChAc activity

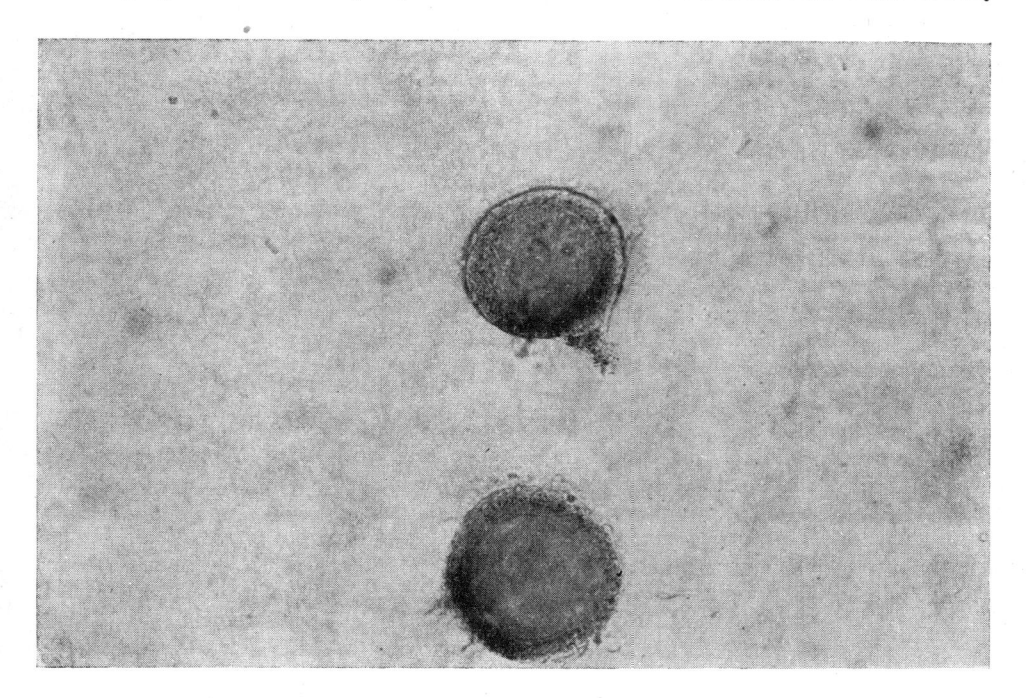

Fig. 3. Two identical neurons from the brain of the snail. The cells are both 100 μm in diameter.

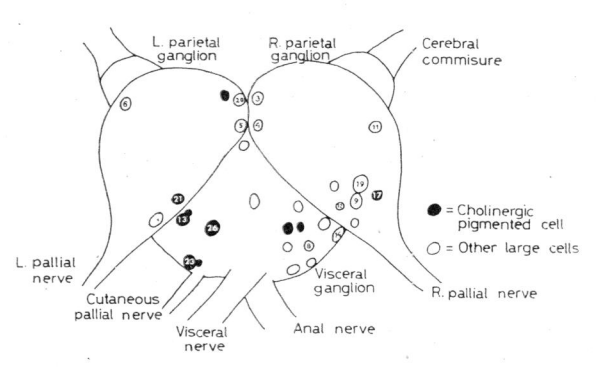

Fig. 4. A map showing the position of pigmented cholinergic cells (shaded black) and some other large cells (unshaded) on the surface of the suboesophageal ganglion.

TABLE 4

Choline acetyltransferase and acetylcholinesterase activity in single identified neurons from *Helix aspersa*

Cell No.	Diameter (μm)	Choline esterase activity	Choline acetyltransferase activity
3	160	150—180 (3)	0 < 2 (5)
4	180	290—320 (3)	0 < 2 (5)
9	150	100—115 (3)	0 < 2 (5)
12	100	100—130 (3)	0 < 2 (5)
13	150	150—170 (3)	99 ± 15 (5)
14	150	120—160 (3)	0 < 2 (5)
17	100	115—135 (3)	94 ± 17 (5)
19	170	260—270 (3)	0 < 2 (5)
23	180	320—380 (3)	45 ± 10 (5)
26	130	80—100 (3)	34 ± 6 (5)

Activities are pmoles/cell/hour. ChE values indicate the range of activities found. ChAc values are means ± standard deviations.

(under 2 pmol/cell/hour). A survey of cells by size was undertaken to see if there might be a greater proportion of cells containing ChAc among the smaller cells in the ganglion. Cells were divided into three groups on the basis of diameter 20—40 μm, 40—60 μm, 60—100 μm. In all these groups approximately 1 cell in 10 contained ChAc. The ChAc activity within each group varied markedly. There was a five-fold difference in enzyme activity between the cells with the highest and lowest ChAc activity within each group.

All the large identifiable cells in the ganglion have been surveyed for AChE activity. In no cases were cells found to lack AChE activity. The cells containing ChAc did not have a higher content of AChE activity. Further work is in progress on the assay of transmitter enzymes such as glutamate decarboxylase and aromatic amino acid decarboxylase in single neurons from the snail and other invertebrate brains.

DISCUSSION

These chemical studies on single neurons from the snail brain show that ChAc is found in only 10% of neurons. This is what we would expect if the enzymes concerned with the synthesis of putative transmitters are specifically localized in the neurons that release them. Our results suggest that the presence of ChAc can be taken as indicating the neuron concerned is cholinergic (i.e. it releases ACh from its nerve terminals). These conclusions agree with previously published work on large cells from *Aplysia* (3, 8). However, the role of AChE is less clear. The presence of AChE in all neurons studied by McCAMAN and DEWHURST (8) led them to suggest that the enzyme might be either present in all neurons as a "safety factor" inactivating any extraneous ACh, or alternatively that AChE is a glial enzyme found in the glial envelope investing and invaginating all invertebrate neurons. In this vein we have always found AChE in all invertebrate neurons we have studied. We cannot conclude definitely that AChE is a glial enzyme in invertebrates until we can separate glia from neurons and this is probably technically impossible.

In conclusion, the presence of ChAc is a distinguishing property of a small number of cells which are probably cholinergic cells, whereas AChE is found in all cells and cannot be used as a marker for cholinergic cells.

ACKNOWLEDGEMENTS

We thank the Royal Society for the award of a European Post-Doctoral Fellowship to one of us (P.C.E.). We are grateful to Drs J. Storm-Mathisen, A. Hamberger, and Professor G. A. Kerkut for advice and encouragement.

REFERENCES

1. EMSON, P. C. and KERKUT, G. A. (1971) Acetylcholinesterase in snail brain. Comp. Biochem. Physiol. **39B**, 879.
2. FONNUM, F. (1969) Radiochemical micro assays for the determination of choline acetyltransferase and acetylcholinesterase activities. Biochem. J. **115**, 465.
3. GILLER, E. JR. and SCHWARTZ, J. H. (1971) Choline acetyltransferase in identified neurons of abdominal ganglion of *Aplysia californica*. J. Neurophysiol. **34**, 93.
4. GLAIZNER, B. (1968) Pharmacological mapping of cells in the suboesophageal ganglia of *Helix aspersa*. In: Neurobiology of Invertebrates (Ed. J. SALANKI), p. 267. New York. Plenum Press.
5. KERKUT, G. A., FRENCH, M. C. and WALKER, R. J. (1970) The location of axonal pathways of identifiable neurons of *Helix aspersa* using the dye Procion Yellow M-4R. Comp. Biochem. Physiol. **32**, 681.
6. KERKUT, G. A. and WALKER, R. J. (1962) The specific chemical sensitivity of *Helix* nerve cells. Comp. Biochem. Physiol. **7**, 277.
7. LOWRY, O. H. (1953) The quantitative histochemistry of the brain. J. Histochem. Cytochem. **1**, 420.
8. MCCAMAN, R. E. and DEWHURST, S. A. (1970) Metabolism of putative transmitters in individual neurons of *Aplysia californica*. J. Neurochem. **17**, 1421.
9. MCCAMAN, R. E. and DEWHURST, S. A. (1971) Metabolism of putative transmitters in individul neurons of *Aplysia californica*. Acetylcholinesterase and catechol-O-methyltransferase, J. Neurochem. **18**, 1329.
10. MEHROTRA, K. N. (1961). Properties of choline acetylase from the house fly *Musca domestica* L. J. Insect. Physiol. **6**, 215.
11. POTTER, L., GLOVER, V. A. S. and SAELENS, J. K. (1968) Choline acetyltransferase from rat brain. J. biol. Chem. **243**, 3864.
12. PRINCE, A. K. (1967). Properties of choline acetyltransferase isolated from squid ganglia. Proc. nat. Acad. Sci. (U.S.) **57**, 1117.
13. WALKER, R. J., LAMBERT, J. D. C., WOODRUFF, G. N. and KERKUT, G. A. (1970) Action potential shape and frequency as criteria for neuron identification in the snail *Helix aspersa*. Comp. gen. Pharmac. **1**, 409.
14. WILGENBURG, H. VAN and LEUWEN, A. A. VAN (1971) Pharmacological characterization of neurons in the visceral and parietal ganglia of *Helix pomatia*. Currents in Modern Biology, **3**, 335.

P.C.E., Division of Toxicology, Norwegian Defence Research Establishment, P. O. Box 25, Kjeller N 2007, Norway

EFFECTS OF DRUGS ON THE REGIONAL DISTRIBUTION AND RELEASE OF ACETYLCHOLINE: FUNCTIONAL SIGNIFICANCE OF CHOLINERGIC NEURONS

G. PEPEU and A. NISTRI

Department of Pharmacology, University of Cagliari School of Pharmacy and Department of Pharmacology, University of Florence Medical School

INTRODUCTION

Acetylcholine (ACh) is present in the C.N.S. of all vertebrates investigated up to the present time, as summarized in Table 1, and it has been found in all brain region. Its distribution is not uniform although regional differences are more evident in the cat than in the rat. In all mammalians species in which regional investigations have been carried out the largest concentration has been found in the striatum and the lowest in the cerebellum (7, 18, 58, 79, 104). Electronmicroscopy and subcellular fractionation studies, have

TABLE 1

ACh content in the brain of different vertebrates

Species	ACh $\mu g/g$	References
Man (cerebral cortex)	0.55	TOWER and ELLIOTT (107)
Monkey (cerebral cortex)	1.5	TOWER and ELLIOTT (107)
Dog (cerebral cortex)	1.6	MALHOTRA and PUNDLIK (60)
Cat (cerebral cortex)	1.12	PEPEU (79)
Rat	2.80	GIARMAN and PEPEU (38)
Guinea pig	2.97	Unpublished
Mouse	1.82	Unpublished
Pigeon	1.59	IGIC (54)
Chicken	1.05	Unpublished
Frog	8.9	GIAMBALVO, MAINARDI and PEPEU (37)
Dogfish	9.0	HEBB (personal communication)

demonstrated the intraneuronal localisation of brain ACh (27, 42, 44). Tobias et al. (105) were the first to report a change in the level of brain ACh following the administration of anaesthetic and convulsant drugs. Their observation was confirmed and extended in the years following (25, 33, 38, 44, 46). Two motives prompted these studies, first the realization that an ever growing number of drugs could affect the brain ACh level, second the hope that studies on the relationship between drug induced variations in behaviour and in the level of brain ACh might offer a clue to the elusive role of this neurotransmitter in the C.N.S. Examples of drug effects on brain ACh, taken from the literature are reported in Table 2. It may be noted that in general C.N.S. depressants tend to increase and C.N.S.

TABLE 2

Effect of some drugs on ACh content in the whole brain of the rat

Drug	Dose mg/kg	% Change	Remarks	References
Pentobarbital	30	+ 16	Sleep	Giarman and Pepeu (38)
Methylpentinol	500	+ 70	Anaesthesia	Pepeu and Giarman (83)
Ether	—	+ 19	Anaesthesia	Crossland and Merrick (25)
Oxotremorine	1	+ 33	Tremors	Unpublished
Metrazol	75	− 22	Convulsions	Giarman and Pepeu (38)
Nicotine	1	− 46	Convulsions	Pepeu (78)
Scopolamine	0.5	− 48	Amnesia	Pazzagli and Pepeu (74)
Atropine	5	− 33	—	Giarman and Pepeu (39)
TEPP	1	+ 117	Toxic symptoms	Giarman and Pepeu (38)
Hemicholinium	50*	− 25	Ataxia, convulsions	Slater (100)
Morphine	50	+ 47	Marked sedation	Giarman and Pepeu (38)

* By intraventricular administration.

stimulants to decrease brain ACh. These changes in ACh levels could basically depend on two different mechanisms: a) an action upon the synthesis of ACh, as in the case of hemicholinium (30, 100), or upon the inactivation as with the cholinesterase inhibitors (38, 64); b) an action upon the output from the cholinergic nerve as shown by studies on the release of ACh either from the cerebral cortex or from subcortical structures (7, 65, 81, 90).

In some instances both actions may take place. The purpose of this review is to present and discuss the existing data on the regional distribution and release of brain ACh, to describe the cholinergic pathways involved in the central action of many drugs and the different sensitivity of cholinergic neurons to different drugs.

Drug effects on regional ACh levels

A survey of the available literature reveals that few papers are devoted to studies on discrete brain areas in comparison to the large number of investigations carried out on the whole brain. Undoubtedly the dissection of the brain in several areas causes relevant losses in ACh, unless special precautions are taken. However, in spite of the diversity of the techniques used, the concentration of ACh reported for various brain regions is remarkably consistent.

CROSSLAND and MERRICK (25) investigated the increase in brain ACh caused by ether and by pentobarbital anaesthesia on the cerebral hemispheres, upper brain stem, cerebellum and pons medulla respectively. They concluded that all parts of the brain undergo an increase in ACh content during both light and deep anaesthesia. During light anaesthesia the increase mostly took place in the cerebrum and in the pons medulla, during deep anaesthesia it extended to the upper brain stem. SCHMIDT (1966) investigating the effect of halothane on brain ACh in rats found that the ACh level during light anesthesia increased in all regions but particularly in the middle brain stem, including the corpora quadrigemina.

GIARMAN and SCHMIDT (95) showed that during the depression induced by the administration of γ-butyro lactone in the rat there is a 96% increase in the ACh content of the cortex and a 42% in the corpora quadrigemina with no change in the other regions.

WESTERMANN et al. (109) found that in the mouse barbital caused an increase in ACh content in the telencephalon and in the brain stem, but the latter increase is less pronounced. The ACh content of all brain regions so far investigated is increased by general anaesthetics, and we are aware of the difficulty of drawing any conclusions on the meaning of these variations. It is tempting to correlate the marked increase in the ACh content of the cerebral cortex observed during anaesthesia with the early impairment of cortical functions. We cannot say to what extent the diminished activity of subcortical structures such as the reticular formation is responsible for such an increase, although a striking rise in cortical ACh levels is observed shortly after midbrain transections (84). Moreover, it is generally assumed that anaesthetics selectively depress the reticular formation (69). Therefore the increased ACh content of the cortex could depend on the reduced activity of the ascending activating system.

The enhanced ACh content produced by some C.N.S. depressants seems to be limited to a few brain regions, not necessarily coincident with those principally affected by general anaesthetics. In fact, tetrabenazine appears to modify ACh levels only in the diencephalon and mesencephalon (106). Similarly, if comparison is made with other regions the highest increase in ACh concentration after treatment with reserpine is described in the hypothalamus (60).

Data on the influence of convulsant drugs on regional brain ACh seem to be lacking. NISTRI and PEPEU (70) studied the effect of strychnine and bicuculline on the ACh level in the spinal cord of the frog. During the convulsions induced by bicuculline there was a short-lasting initial decrease in spinal cord ACh, followed by a recovery to normal levels. On the other hand, there was no immediate decrease in the ACh level during strychnine convulsions, but a delayed increase. A connection between the changes in the ACh level in the spinal cord and the mechanism through which the convulsants are claimed to act could be envisaged. On the contrary in the mammalian brain it is known that convulsions reduce ACh content (9, 94) and that an increased ACh release is produced by strychnine and leptazol (8, 11, 19, 45).

APRISON et al. (1) investigated the changes in ACh concentration in several discrete brain areas of the rat during behavioural excitation induced by the administration of iproniazid and tetrabenazine. A decrease in ACh concentration was found in the telencephalon, in the midbrain and in the pons-medulla. However, the time course of the excitation best correlates with the ACh levels in the telencephalon. During post-excitation depression ACh concentration in the midbrain was higher than prior to the excitation.

It is difficult to attribute these changes to some specific cholinergic pathways. They demonstrate, however, that cholinergic mechanisms are involved in behavioural excitation.

Atropine, scopolamine and other anticholinergic drugs induce a decrease in brain ACh level in the rat (18, 39) and in the cat (26). The decrease is restricted to the cortex and to the caudate nucleus, as shown in the rat by GIARMAN and PEPEU (39) and in the guinea pig by BEANI et al. (7). ACh levels in the thalamus, the midbrain and the medulla-pons are not affected. Electrophysiological studies on the site of action of atropine (56) suggest that this cholinolytic does not act on the midbrain reticular formation, but on higher structures. Furthermore, it should be pointed out that at the relatively low dosage used in most of these experiments, the anticholinergic drugs exert only subtle behavioural effects such as the impairment of learned performances (57) in which neocortical structures play a role. As shown in Table 3, scopolamine decreases brain ACh only in mammals,

TABLE 3

Effect of scopolamine on the ACh content in the whole brain of different animal species

	Dose mg/kg	% Variation
Rat**	0.5	— 48
Mouse*	40	— 23
Chicken	5	+ 4
Frog+	1	— 9

* Atropine
** From PAZZAGLI and PEPEU (74)
+ From GIAMBALVO, MAINARDI and PEPEU (37).

but not in the chicken and in the frog. It is pertinent to mention that scopolamine exerts an adverse facilitatory effect on different types of acquisition and on recent memory in mammals (15, 57), but in pigeons scopolamine shows no effect on either learning or retention (28).

We have seen that centrally acting cholinolytic drugs bring about a decrease in brain ACh concentrations. Conversely, some muscarinic agonists such as tremorine (77), oxotremorine (24, 48) and arecoline (47), induce a rise in brain ACh associated with marked parasympathetic stimulation and with continuous tremors. The structures mostly involved in the ACh increase following oxotremorine administration are the basal ganglia and in particular the caudate nucleus in the cat (3, 79), the caudate nucleus in the rat (18), and the nucleus basalis in the pigeon (54). The latter nucleus may be considered homologous with the striatum of mammals. Arecoline also increases ACh levels, mostly in the forebrain (108). On the basis of the existing experimental work, a relationship between the rise in the ACh level in the basal ganglia and motor incoordination cannot be excluded.

In concluding this survey of the effects of centrally acting drugs on regional levels of ACh, we may underline that the limited amount of information available does not reveal an unified pattern in the localized changes of ACh levels during treatments which cause either depression or excitation. Whether these discrepancies are due to the different properties of the drugs employed or to the different experimental conditions used is still matter of debate.

Drugs effects on regional ACh output

A more dynamic approach to the study of the activity of cholinergic neurons is offered by studies on the ACh release from nervous tissues. This kind of investigation was first undertaken on the cerebral cortex by Elliott et al. (33) and by MacIntosh and Oborin (59). Mitchell (65) gave detailed information on the technique which is now used by most workers and extensively investigated the origin of ACh output from the cerebral cortex. The ACh output from subcortical structure was examined either by means of modifications of Gaddum's cannula (35) or by perfusing the cerebral ventricles (6). In Table 4 the amount of ACh released at rest from various brain regions is shown. In all

TABLE 4

ACh output from different regions of the central nervous system

Region	Animal species	ACh output ng/10 min	References
Cerebral cortex (frontal)	Cat	14.3 ($\times$ cm^2)	Nistri et al. (71)
Cerebellar cortex (vermal)	Cat	0.2 ($\times$ cm^2)	Phillis and Chong (88)
Caudate nucleus	Cat	2.9	McLennan (63)
Thalamus	Cat	1—6	Phillis et al. (89)
Hypothalamus (monkey)	Monkey	0.06—1	Myers and Beleslin (67)
Superior colliculi (monkey)	Monkey	0.1—0.8	Beleslin and Myers (10)
Anterior horn of the lateral ventricles	Cat	8—50	Beleslin and Polak (11)
Spinal subarachnoid space	Cat	0.8	Edery and Levinger (32)

experimental conditions a cholinesterase inhibitor was always present. It may be noted that the highest release occurs from the cerebral and the smallest from the cerebellar cortex. Beleslin et al. (12) showed that greater amount of the ACh which appears in the effluent of the perfused cerebral ventricles comes from the caudate nucleus, the olfactory grey matter and perhaps the septum. The smaller amount of ACh comes from the structures lining the ventral half of the third ventricle including the nuclei of the hypothalamus. However, the direct determination of ACh release from the caudate by means of a push pull cannula gives much lower values (63). According to Mitchell (65) there is no significant difference in ACh output from the somatosensory and parietal cortex in any one animal. Stimulation of the peripheral nerve induces an increase in output only from the controlateral somatosensory cortex. In 3 subsequent papers the existence of two ascending cholinergic systems, one reticulo-cortical and the other thalamo-cortical, was suggested on the basis of experiments on the rabbit cortex (21, 22, 68). A detailed investigation into cortical ACh release after the stimulation of different subcortical regions was offered by Szerb (102) who showed the importance of the septum in the central cholinergic pathways.

The existence of separate reticulo-cortical and thalamo-cortical cholinergic pathways may be questioned in the light of later investigations. In fact PHILLIS (87) found that the basal ACh release is not similar in the different areas of the cortex, the highest being in the somatosensory area. Moreover, stimulation of the reticular formation and of a peripheral sensory nerve causes a widespread increase in cortical ACh output without large qualitative differences whatever stimulation is employed. Similar results have also been obtained by BARTOLINI et al. (4).

In a situation of depressed cortical activity such as that induced by general anaesthetics, the ACh release from the cerebral cortex is impaired, although to a different extent, depending on the drug investigated (65, 87). Here again some correlations appear between the degree of the cortical activity and the ACh release. All these data therefore support the existence of a cholinergic component in the fibres of the non specific and maybe of the specific systems ascending to the cortex. Such a proposal was first advanced by KANAI and SZERB (49) and has also been sustained in some recent reviews (51, 80).

The effects of a large number of drugs on the ACh release from the cortex have been tested and the results have been listed in a recent review (79).

On the other hand the small amount of information available on the effects of drugs on ACh output from subcortical structures comes from studies on the perfused cerebral ventricles in the cat. Leptazol and strychnine markedly increase both the output of ACh into the perfused cerebral ventricles and its release from the parietal cortex (13); atropine and hyoscine have the same effect even following intraventricular administration (90). Conversely, chloralose and morphine depress ACh output into the effluent from the perfused cerebral ventricles (11).

One implication which should be kept in mind when considering the drug-induced variations in cortical ACh release is that the effects are not exerted directly on the cortex, but exerted or modulated by subcortical structures. This is the case of two well-known ACh releasing drugs such as amphetamine and scopolamine (2, 81). NISTRI et al. (71) have in fact shown that a lesion in the septum of the cat abolishes the effect of amphetamine on ACh release and reduces that of scopolamine. However, the EEG patterns induced by the drugs are not modified in the septal animals. These results emphasize the role of the septum in the ascending cholinergic fibers as also revealed by histochemical examinations (52) and demonstrate that electroencephalographic recordings do not necessarily run parallel to the degree of the ACh output, a fact already noted in the case of atropine administration (101).

A COMPARISON BETWEEN THE PHARMACOLOGICAL PROPERTIES OF CENTRAL AND PERIPHERAL CHOLINERGIC NERVE ENDINGS

It is a common assumption that it is possible to compare basic cholinergic mechanisms at central and peripheral levels.

This assumption rests on experimental evidence. MITCHELL (65) for instance, demonstrated a strong similarity between the amount of ACh released per impulse at various stimulus frequencies from the somato-sensory area during stimulation of the controlateral forepaw and from the rat hemidiaphragm during stimulation of the phrenic nerve.

In Table 5 an attempt is made to compare the effects of several drugs on ACh output from the cerebral cortex, the incubated cortical slices, the intestine, the sympathetic ganglia and the heart using data available in literature.

It may be seen that drugs like tetrodotoxin (31, 66, 73) and cocaine (14, 17, 61, 73, 82) or the absence of calcium (17, 29, 66, 73, 93), all of which are able to impair the basic

TABLE 5

Drug-induced variations in ACh output from different parts of the central and peripheral nervous system of the rat

Drug	Cerebral cortex	Cortical slices	Intestine	Sympathetic ganglia	Heart
Scopolamine	+226% (1)	+166% (7)		+ 1%+*(14)	0%•(17)
Oxotremorine	+ 5%*(2)	+ 47% (8)	+19%•(12)		
Morphine	− 71% (3)	− 33% (9)	−81%•(13)		
Absence of Ca^{2+}	− 34%*(4)	− 80% (10)	−89%•(13)	−94%+ (15)	−90%×(18)
Tetrodotoxin	− 74%*(5)	− 9% (10)	−55%•(13)		
Cocaine	− 64%*(6)	+ 6% (11)	−66%•(13)	−81%+°(16)	−45%×(18)

+ Data for the cat
• Data for the guinea-pig
× Data for the rabbit
* Data for atropine
° Data for procaine

The underlined values do not significantly differ from controls. (1) Pepeu et al., (86); (2) Pepeu and Bartolini, (82); (3) Pepeu and Nistri, (85); (4) Randic and Padjen, (93); (5) Dudar and Szerb, (31); (6) Bartolini and Pepeu, (2); (7) Bertels-Meeuws and Polak, (14); (8) Polak, (91); (9) Sharkawi and Schulman, (98); (10) Molenaar and Polak, (66); (11) Bertels-Meeuws and Polak, (14); (12) Cox and Heckner, (23); (13) Paton et al., (73); (14) McKinstry and Koelle, (62); (15) Douglas et al., (29); (16) Matthews and Quilliam, (61); (17) Bartolini et al., (5); (18) Briscoe and Burn, (17).

mechanisms of nerve conduction and of neurotransmitter release, strongly reduce ACh output from both central and peripheral cholinergic nerve endings.

Tetrodotoxin and cocaine, which block the axonal conduction of nervous impulses, are inactive in the cortical slices (14, 66) where the ascending fibres from which ACh is released are severed.

CNS depressants which in Table 5 are represented by morphine since we were unable to find any other data for peripheral tissues, decrease ACh output from the cortex (55, 85),

TABLE 6

Drug-induced variations in the ACh content of the brain and other tissues in the rat.

	Scopolamine	Oxotremorine	Morphine
Brain	−34% (1)	+33% (4)	+47% (6)
Cortical slices	+65%° (2)	−36% (5)	+13% (7)
Heart	− 2%*(3)	+15% (4)	
Ileum			+68%*(8)

° Data for atropine
* Data for the guinea-pig

The underlined values do not significantly differ from controls. (1) Giarman and Pepeu, (39); (2) Molenaar and Polak, (66); (3) Bartolini et al., (5); (4) Nistri, unpublished results; (5) Polak, (91); (6) Giarman and Pepeu, (38); (7) Sharkawi and Schulman, (93); (8) Pepeu, (76).

from the cholinergic nerve endings of the ileum (72, 73, 99) and from the cortical slices (98) with regional differences in potency. Evidence has also been given that this drug impairs the ACh release from the sympathetic ganglia (75), and the heart (50).

Table 6 shows that morphine also increases ACh content in the brain (38) and in peripheral tissues (76), a finding consistent with the decrease in the transmitter output.

Oxotremorine, whose capacity to enhance ACh content varies according to the different regions as discussed previously, increases ACh content (48) (Table 6) without apparently decreasing ACh output *in vivo* (82) (Table 5) and has no effect either on heart ACh content (NISTRI, unpublished) or on the ACh release from the mipafox-treated ileum (23).

The mechanism by which oxotremorine increases ACh content is not fully understood. A mobilization of choline from bound stores has been proposed (47); it might be assumed that oxotremorine only acts in those regions where choline can be easily mobilized. We have already mentioned that scopolamine decreases ACh content in specific brain regions. This decrease can be related to a rise in ACh output. The possibility of reducing the rise in output by subcortical lesions (71) suggests the involvement of specific cholinergic pathways in this effect of scopolamine. The differences between the effects of anticholinergic drugs on the cerebral cortex *in situ* and the cortical slices (91) are difficult to reconcile, and possibly reflect a double mechanism of action of scopolamine revealed by differing experimental conditions.

Furthermore, at peripheral level scopolamine affects neither ACh content nor its release. Oxotremorine and scopolamine constitute, therefore, two examples of pharmacological discrepancies between central and peripheral cholinergic neurons as revealed by centrally acting drugs. On the other hand, it is pertinent to mention that in the sympathetic ganglia preganglionic stimulation causes no change in the ACh content (16). A transient decrease can be found only by using extremely high rates of stimulation which are well beyond any physiological situation (34). Stimulation of the preganglionic nerve therefore induces an increase in ACh synthesis and rapid replenishement of the stores (16, 20). Similarly, the ACh content of the cholinergic terminals in the rat diaphragm (92) and guinea-pig ileum (73), is well preserved under different stimulations.

On the contrary, a marked and persistent decrease in ACh content can be found in the cerebral cortex of animals killed during cortical activation (84) when compared with the levels during synchronization.

These findings and the decrease in ACh levels observed after the administration of central stimulant drugs, point out that ACh synthesis in the cerebral cortex is probably unable to follow closely an initial enhanced transmitter output. This hypothesis, however, would sound unlikely when considering the large number of cortical cholinergic cells and their possibly essential role in the complex functions of the cerebral cortex had the effects of ACh on cholinoceptive cortical cells not been found different from those on the peripheral effectors. In fact, the ACh-induced depolarization in the cortex shows neither the fall in membrane resistance nor the typical short duration observed at the neuromuscular junctions (41). Suggestions have been advanced that ACh action in the cortex depends on an electrogenic mechanism operating through a reduced K^+ conductance (53). The long-lasting depolarization may explain why even a reduced concentration of ACh in the cortex would not easily lead to a failure of the synaptic transmission; in the light of these findings, cortical activities such as the memory processes which probably operate through more persistent neuronal changes (36) than those observed at the peripheral synapses, could be better understood.

Bringing this survey on the regional differences in ACh distribution and release to a close, we can make the following remarks. First, there is still surprisingly little information about regional effects of drugs on cholinergic systems, and no attempt to correlate them with regional distribution of drugs.

We may expect that the development of studies on the ACh turnover (43, 92, 97) and on techniques for killing the animals and dissecting their brains with minimal ACh looses (96) will help to bridge the gap in this field over the next few years.

References

1. APRISON, M. H., KARIYA, T., HINGTGEN, J. N. and TORN, M. (1968) Neurochemical correlates of behavior: changes in acetylcholine, norepinephrine and 5-hydroxytryptamine concentrations in several discrete brain areas of the rat during behavioral excitation. J. Neurochem. **15**, 1131.
2. BARTOLINI, A. and PEPEU, G. (1967) Investigations into the acetylcholine output from the cerebral cortex of the cat in the presence of hyoscine. Brit. J. Pharmacol. **31**, 66.
3. BARTOLINI, A., BARTOLINI, R. and PEPEU, G. (1970) The effect of oxotremorine on the acetylcholine content of different parts of cat brain. J. Pharm. Pharmacol. **22**, 59.
4. BARTOLINI, A., WEISENTHAL, L. M. and DOMINO, E. (1972) Effect of photic stimulation on acetylcholine release from cat cerebral cortex. Int. J. Neuropharmacol. **11**, 113.
5. BARTOLINI, R., AIELLO-MALMBERG, P. and BARTOLINI, A. (1972) Different scopolamine effect on acetylcholine release and content in the central and peripheral nervous systems. Abstract 5th Int. Congr. Pharmacol., San Francisco, 15.
6. BATTACHARYA, B. K. and FELDBERG, W. (1958). Perfusion of cerebral ventricles: effects of drugs on outflow from the cisterna and aqueduct. Brit. J. Pharmacol. **13**, 156.
7. BEANI, L., BIANCHI, C. and MEGAZZINI, P. (1964) Regional changes of acetylcholine and choline acetylase activity in the guinea-pig's brain after scopolamine. Experientia, **20**, 677.
8. BEANI, L., BIANCHI, C., SANTINOCETO, L. and MARCHETTI, P. (1968) The cerebral acetylcholine release in conscious rabbits with semi-permanently implanted epidural cups. Int. J. Neuropharmacol. **7**, 469.
9. BEANI, L., BIANCHI, C., MEGAZZINI, P., BALLOTTI, L. and BERNARDI, G. (1969) Drug induced changes in free, labile and stable acetylcholine of guinea-pig brain. Biochem. Pharmacol. **18**, 1315.
10. BELESLIN, D. B. and MYERS, K. D. (1970) The release of acetylcholine and 5-hydroxytryptamine from the mesencephalon of the unanesthetized rhesus monkey. Brain Res. **23**, 437.
11. BELESLIN, D. and POLAK, R. L. (1965) Depression by morphine and chloralose of acetylcholine release from the cat's brain. J. Physiol. (Lond.) **177**, 411.
12. BELESLIN, D., CARMICHAEL, E. A. and FELDBERG, W. (1964) The origin of acetylcholine appearing on the effluent of perfused cerebral ventricles of the cat. J. Physiol. (Lond.) **173**, 368.
13. BELESLIN, D., POLAK, R. L. and SPROULL, D. H. (1965) The effect of leptazol and strychnine on the acetylcholine release from the cat brain. J. Physiol. (Lond.) **181**, 308.
14. BERTELS-MEEWS, M. M. and POLAK, R. L. (1968) Influence of antimuscarinic substances on "*in vitro*" synthesis of acetylcholine by rat cerebral cortex. Brit. J. Pharmacol. **33**, 368.
15. BIGNAMI, G. (1967) Anticholinergic agents as tools in the investigation of behavioral phenomena. In: Neuropsychopharmacology, Ed. BRILL, H., p. 819. Amsterdam: Excerpta Medica Foundation.
16. BIRKS, R. I. and MACINTOSH, F. C. (1961) Acetylcholine metabolism of a sympathetic ganglion. Can. J. Biochem. Physiol. **39**, 787.
17. BRISCOE, S. and BURN, J. H. (1954) The formation of an acetylcholine-like substance by the isolated rabbit heart. J. Physiol. (Lond.) **126**, 181.
18. CAMPBELL, L. B. and JENDEN, D. J. (1970) Gaschromatographic evaluation of the influence of oxotremorine upon the regional distribution of acetylcholine in rat brain. J. Neurochem. **17**, 1697.
19. CELESIA, G. C. and JASPER, H. H. (1966) Acetylcholine released from the cerebral cortex in relation to state of activation. Neurology, **16**, 1053.
20. COLLIER, B. and MACINTOSH, F. C. (1969) The source of choline for acetylcholine synthesis in a sympathetic ganglion. Can. J. Physiol. Pharmacol. **47**, 127.
21. COLLIER, B. and MITCHELL, J. F. (1966) The central release of acetylcholine during stimulation of the visual pathways. J. Physiol. (Lond.) **184**, 239.
22. COLLIER, B. and MITCHELL, J. F. (1967) The central release of acetylcholine during consciousness and after brain lesions. J. Physiol. (Lond.) **188**, 83.

23. Cox, B. and Hecker, S. E. (1971) Investigation of the mechanism of action of oxotremorine on the guinea-pig isolated ileum preparation. Brit. J. Pharmacol. **41**, 19.
24. Cox, B. and Patkonjak, D. (1969) The relationship between tremor and change in brain acetylcholine concentration produced by injection of tremorine or oxotremorine in the rat. Brit. J. Pharmacol. **35**, 295.
25. Crossland, J. and Merrick, A. J. (1954) The effect of anaesthesia on the acetylcholine content of brain. J. Physiol. (Lond.) **125**, 56.
26. Deffenu, G., Mantegazzini, P. and Pepeu, G. (1966) Scopolamine induced changes of brain acetylcholine and EEG pattern in cats with complete pontine transection. Arch. Ital. Biol. **104**, 141.
27. De Robertis, E., Arnaiz, R. L. G., Salganikoff, L., De Iraldi, A. P. and Zieher, L. M. (1963) Isolation of synaptic vesicles and structural organization of the acetylcholine system within brain nerve endings. J. Neurochem. **10**, 225.
28. Dews, P. B. (1957) Studies on behavior. III. Effects of scopolamine on reversal of a discriminatory performance in pigeons. J. Pharmacol. **119**, 343.
29. Douglas, W. W., Lywood, D. W. and Straub, R. W. (1961) The stimulant effect of barium on the release of acetylcholine from the superior cervical ganglion. J. Physiol. (Lond.) **156**, 515.
30. Dren, A. T. and Domino, E. F. (1968) Effects of hemicholinium (HC_3) on EEG activation and brain acetylcholine in the dog. J. Pharmacol. exp. Ther. **161**, 141.
31. Dudar, J. D. and Szerb, J. C. (1969) The effect of topically applied atropine on resting and evoked cortical acetylcholine release. J. Physiol. (Lond.) **203**, 741.
32. Edery, H. and Levinger, I. M. (1971) Acetylcholine release into the perfused intermeningeal spaces of the cat spinal cord. Neuropharmacol. **10**, 239.
33. Elliott, K. A. C., Swank, R. L. and Henderson, N. (1950) Effects of anaesthetic and convulsants on the acetylcholine content of brain. Amer. J. Physiol. **162**, 469.
34. Friesen, A. J. D. and Khatter, J. C. (1971) The effect of preganglionic stimulation on the acetylcholine and choline content of a sympathetic ganglion. Can. J. Physiol. Pharmacol. **49**, 375.
35. Gaddum, J. H. (1961) Push-pull cannulae. J. Physiol. (Lond.) **155**, 1P.
36. Gerald, R. W. (1955). The biological roots of psychiatry. Amer. J. Psychiat. **112**, 81.
37. Giambalvo, A., Mainardi, G. and Pepeu, G. (1972) Studies on acetylcholine in the frog brain. Pharmacol. Res. Commun. (in press).
38. Giarman, N. J. and Pepeu, G. (1962) Drug-induced changes in brain acetylcholine. Brit. J. Pharmacol. **19**, 226.
39. Giarman, N. J. and Pepeu, G. (1964) The influence of centrally acting cholinolytic drugs on brain acetylcholine levels. Brit. J. Pharmacol. **23**, 123.
40. Giarman, N. J. and Schmidt, K. F. (1963) Some neurochemical aspects of the depressant action of γ-butyrolactone on the central nervous system. Brit. J. Pharmacol. **20**, 563.
41. Godfraind, J. M., Kawamura H. Krnjević, K. and Pumain, R. (1971) Actions of dinitrophenol and some other metabolic inhibitors on cortical neurons. J. Physiol. (Lond.) **215**, 199.
42. Gray, E. G. and Whittaker, V. P. (1962) The isolation of nerve endings from brain: an electron-microscopic study of cell fragments derived by homogenization and centrifugation. J. Anat. **96**, 79.
43. Hanin, I., Massarelli, R. and Costa, E. (1972) An approach to the *in vivo* study of acetylcholine turnover in rat salivary glands by radio gas chromatography. J. Pharmacol. exp. Ther. **181**, 10.
44. Hebb, C. O. and Whittaker, V. P. (1958) Intracellular distributions of acetylcholine and choline acetylase. J. Physiol. (Lond.) **142**, 187.
45. Hemsworth, B. A. and Neal, M. J. (1968) The effect of central stimulant drugs on acetylcholine release from rat cerebral cortex. Brit. J. Pharmacol. **32**, 543.
46. Herken, H. and Neubert, D. (1953) Der Acetylcholingehalt des Gehirns bei Verschiedenen Funktionszuständen. Naunyn-Schmiedeberg's Arch. exp. Path. Pharmak. **219**, 223.
47. Holmstedt, B. (1967) Mobilization of Acetylcholine by cholinergic agents. Ann. N.Y. Acad. Sci. **144**, 433.
48. Holmstedt, B. and Lundgren, G. (1966) Tremorgenic agents and brain acetylcholine. In: Mechanisms of release of biogenic amines, p. 439. Oxford: Pergamon Press.
49. Kanai, T. and Szerb, J. C. (1965) Mesencephalic reticular activating system and cortical acetylcholine output. Nature (Lond.) **205**, 80.
50. Kennedy, B. L. and West, T. C. (1967) Effect of morphine on electrically-induced release of autonomic mediators in the rabbit sino-atrial node. J. Pharmacol. exp. Ther. **157**, 149.
51. Krnjević, K. (1969) Central cholinergic pathways. Fed. Proc. **28**, 113.

52. KRNJEVIČ, K. and SILVER, A. (1965) An histochemical study of cholinergic fibres in the cerebral cortex. J. Anat. **99**, 711.
53. KRNJEVIČ, K., PUMAIN, R. and RENAUD, L. (1971) The mechanism of excitation by acetylcholine in the cerebral cortex. J. Physiol. (Lond.) **215**, 247.
54. IGIĆ, R. (1971) Effect of oxotremorine on the acetylcholine content of whole brain and various brain regions in the pigeon. Brit. J. Pharmacol. **42**, 303.
55. JHAMANDAS, K., PHILLIS, J. W. and PINSKY, C. (1971) Effects of narcotic analgesics and antagonists on the *in vivo* release of acetylcholine from the cerebral cortex of the cat. Brit. J. Pharmacol. **43**, 53.
56. LOEB, C., MAGNI, F. and ROSSI, G. F. (1960) Electrophysiological analysis of the action of atropine on the central nervous system. Arch. Ital. Biol. **98**, 293.
57. LONGO, V. G. (1966) Behavioral and electroencephalographic effects of atropine and related compounds. Pharmacol. Revs. **18**, 965.
58. MACINTOSH, F. C. (1941) The distribution of acetylcholine in the peripheral and the central nervous system. J. Physiol. (Lond.) **99**, 436.
59. MACINTOSH, F. C. and OBORIN, P. E. (1953) Release of acetylcholine from intact cerebral cortex. Abstract XIX Int. Physiol. Congr. 580.
60. MALHOTRA, C. L. and PUNDLIK, P. G. (1959) The effect of reserpine on the acetylcholine content of different areas of the central nervous system of the dog. Brit. J. Pharmacol. **14**, 46.
61. MATTHEWS, E. K. and QUILLIAM, J. P. (1964) Effects of central depressant drugs upon acetylcholine release. Brit. J. Pharmacol. **22**, 415.
62. MCKINSTRY, D. N. and KOELLE, G. B. (1967) Effects of drugs on acetylcholine release from the cat superior cervical ganglion by carbachol and by preganglionic stimulation. J. Pharmacol. exp. Ther. **157**, 328.
63. MCLENNAN, H. (1964) The release of acetylcholine and of 3-hydroxytyramine from the caudate nucleus. J. Physiol. (Lond.) **174**, 152.
64. MILOŠEVIČ, M. P. (1970) Acetylcholine content in the brain of rats treated with Paraoxon and Obidoxime. Brit. J. Pharmacol. **39**, 732.
65. MITCHELL, J. F. (1963) The spontaneous and evoked release of acetylcholine from the cerebral cortex. J. Physiol. (Lond.) **165**, 98.
66. MOLENAAR, P. C. and POLAK, R. L. (1970) Stimulation by atropine of acetylcholine release and synthesis in cortical slices from rat brain. Brit. J. Pharmacol. **40**, 406.
67. MYERS, R. D. and BELESLIN, D. B. (1970) The spontaneous release of 5-hydroxytryptamine and acetylcholine within the diencephalon of the unanaesthetized rhesus monkey. Exp. Brain Res. **11**, 539.
68. NEAL, M. J., HEMSWORTH, B. A. and MITCHELL, J. F. (1968) The excitation of central cholinergic mechanisms by stimulation of the auditory pathway. Life Sci. **7**, 757.
69. NGAI, S. H. (1963). General anesthetics. Effects upon physiological systems. In: Physiological Pharmacology Vol. 1, Part. A. Ed. ROOT, W. S. and HOFMANN, F. G. p. 43. New York: Academic Press.
70. NISTRI, A. and PEPEU, G. (1972) Effects of bicuculline and strychnine on the acetylcholine content of the amphibian spinal cord. Brit. J. Pharmacol. **45**, 173P.
71. NISTRI, A., BARTOLINI, A., DEFFENU, G. and PEPEU, G. (1972) Investigations into the release of ACh from the cerebral cortex of the cat: effects of amphetamine, scopolamine and septal lesions. Neuropharmacology, in press.
72. PATON, W. D. N. (1957) The action of morphine and related substances on contraction and on acetylcholine output of coaxially stimulated guinea-pig ileum. Brit. J. Pharmacol. **12**, 119.
73. PATON, W. D. N., VIZI, E. S. and ABO ZAAR, M. (1971) The mechanism of acetylcholine release from parasympathetic nerves. J. Physiol. (Lond.) **215**, 819.
74. PAZZAGLI, A., PEPEU, G. (1964). Amnesic properties of scopolamine and brain acetylcholine in the rat. Int. J. Neuropharmacol. **4**, 291.
75. PELIKAN, E. W. (1960) The mechanism of ganglionic blockade produced by nicotine. Ann. N.Y. Acad. Sci. **90**, 52.
76. PEPEU, G. (1963) Drug induced changes of intestinal acetylcholine. Biochem. Pharmacol., Suppl. **12**, 262.
77. PEPEU, G. (1963) Effects of "Tremorine" and some anti-Parkinson's disease drugs on acetylcholine in the rat brain. Nature (Lond.) **200**, 895.
78. PEPEU, G. (1965). Nicotina e acetilcolina cerebrale. Arch. Ital. Sci. Farmacol. **15**, 146.
79. PEPEU, G. (1971) Drug interfering with central cholinergic mechanisms. In: Chemistry and brain development. Ed. PAOLETTI, R. and DAVISON, A. N., p. 195. New York: Plenum Press.
80. PEPEU, G. (1972) Cholinergic neurotransmission in the central nervous system. Arch. Int. Pharmacodyn., Suppl. **196**, 229.

81. PEPEU, G. and BARTOLINI, A. (1968) Effect of psychoactive drugs on the output of acetylcholine from the cerebral cortex of the cat. Europ. J. Pharmacol. **4**, 254.
82. PEPEU, G. and BARTOLINI, A. (1969) The effect of oxotremorine on acetylcholine content and release from the cerebral cortex of the cat. Abstract 4th Int. Congr. Pharmacol. Basel, 145.
83. PEPEU, G. and GIARMAN, N. J. (1960) Effect of methylpentynol on acetylcholine in the rat's brain. Nature (Lond.) **186**, 638.
84. PEPEU, G. and MANTEGAZZINI, P. (1964) Midbrain hemisection: effect on cortical acetylcholine in the cat. Science, **145**, 1069.
85. PEPEU, G. and NISTRI, A. (1972) Interaction between morphine and neurotransmitters. In: Int. symposium on recent advances on pain pathophysiology and clinics, Ed. BONICA, J. J., PROCACCI, P. and PAGNI, C. A. Charles, C. Thomas Publ. Springfield, in press.
86. PEPEU, G., MULAS, A. and MULAS, M. L. (1972) Effect of subcortical lesions on acetylcholine output from the cerebral cortex in rats. Abstract 5th Int. Congr. Pharmacol., San Francisco, 179.
87. PHILLIS, J. W. (1968) Acetylcholine release from the cerebral cortex. Brain Res. **7**, 378.
88. PHILLIS, J. W. and CHONG, G. C. (1965) Acetylcholine release from the cerebral and cerebellar cortices: its role in cortical arousal. Nature (Lond.) **207**, 1253.
89. PHILLIS, J. W., TEBECIS, A. K. and YORK, D. H. (1968) Acetylcholine release from the feline thalamus. J. Pharm. Pharmacol. **20**, 476.
90. POLAK, R. L. (1965) Effect of hyoscine on the output of acetylcholine into perfused cerebral ventricles of cats. J. Physiol. (Lond.) **181**, 144.
91. POLAK, R. L. (1971) Stimulating action of atropine on the release of acetylcholine by rat cerebral cortex in vitro. Brit. J. Pharmacol. **41**, 600.
92. POTTER, L. T. (1970) Synthesis, storage and release of ^{14}C acetylcholine in isolated rat diaphragm muscles. J. Physiol. (Lond.) **206**, 145.
93. RANDIC, M. and PADJEN, A. (1967) Effect of calcium ions on the release of acetylcholine from the cerebral cortex. Nature (Lond.) **215**, 990.
94. RICHTER, D. and CROSSLAND, J. (1949) Variation in acetylcholine content of the brain with physiological state. Amer. J. Physiol. **159**, 247.
95. SCHMIDT, K. F. (1966) Effect of halothane anesthesia on regional acetylcholine levels in the rat brain. Anesthesiology, **27**, 788.
96. SCHMIDT, D. E., SPETH, R. C., WELSCH, F. and SCHMIDT, M. J. (1972) The use of microwave radiation in the determination of acetylcholine in the rat brain. Brain. Res. **38**, 377.
97. SCHUBERTH, J., SPARF, B. and SUNDWALL, A. (1969) A technique for the study of acetylcholine turnover in mouse brain in vivo. J. Neurochem. **16**, 695.
98. SHARKAWI, M. and SCHULMAN, M. P. (1969) Inhibition by morphine of the release of ^{14}C acetylcholine from rat brain cortex slices. J. Pharm. Pharmacol. **21**, 546.
99. SCHAUMANN, W. (1957) Inhibition by morphine of the release of acetylcholine from the intestine of the guinea-pig. Brit. J. Pharmacol. **12**, 115.
100. SLATER, P. (1968) The effect of triethylcholine and hemicholinium-3 on the acetylcholine content of rat brain. Int. J. Neuropharmacol. **7**, 421.
101. SZERB, J. C. (1964) The effect of tertiary and quaternary atropine on cortical acetylcholine output and on the electroencephalogram in cats. Can. J. Physiol. Pharmacol., **42**, 303.
102. SZERB, J. C. (1967) Cortical acetylcholine release and electroencephalographic arousal. J. Physiol. (Lond.) **192**, 329.
103. SZERB, J. C., MALIK, H. and HUNTER, E. G. (1970) Relationship between acetylcholine content and release in the cat's cerebral cortex. Can. J. Physiol. Pharmacol. **48**, 780.
104. TAKAHASHI, R. and APRISON, M. H. (1964) Acetylcholine content of discrete areas of the brain obtained by a near freezing method. J. Neurochem. **11**, 887.
105. TOBIAS, J. M., LIPTON, M. A. and LEPINAT, A. A. (1946) Effect of anaesthetics and convulsants on brain acetylcholine content. Proc. Soc. exp. Biol. Med. **61**, 51.
106. TORU, M., HINGTGEN, J. N. and APRISON, M. H. (1966) Acetylcholine concentrations in brain areas of rats during three states of avoidance behaviour. Life Sci. **5**, 181.
107. TOWER, D. B. and ELLIOTT, K. A. C. (1952) Activity of acetylcholine system in cerebral cortex of various unanesthetized mammals. Amer. J. Physiol. **168**, 747.
108. WESTERMANN, K. H., OELSSNER, W. and FISHER, H. D. (1970) Tremor und Hirn-Azetylcholingehalt infantiler und seniler Ratten nach Arekolin. Acta biol. med. germ. **25**, 855.
109. WESTERMANN, K. H., OELSSNER, W. and FISHER, H. D. (1971) Cholinergbeeinflusste Narkose und Hirn-Azetylcholingehalt der Maus. Acta biol. med. germ. **26**, 115.

G.P., Department of Pharmacology, University of Cagliari School of Pharmacy, 09100 Cagliari, Viale Diaz, Italy

METABOLISM OF CNS STIMULATING DRUGS

Chairman: F. SULSER

Associate chairman: S. RASMUSSEN

THE METABOLISM OF THE AMPHETAMINES IN MAN AND LABORATORY ANIMALS[*]

L. G. DRING and J. CALDWELL

Department of Biochemistry, St. Mary's Hospital Medical School, London

The amphetamine group of drugs has been the object of intense pharmacological interest over several decades but, surprisingly, until about fifteen years ago when AXELROD studied several members of this group (2) little was known of their metabolism. In the mid sixties studies on the metabolism of amphetamine itself were published by several workers (1, 7, 10).

From these studies it became clear that two main metabolic options were open to the amphetamine molecule, namely hydroxylation in the aromatic ring, best exemplified by the rat and degradation of the side chain to benzoic acid, best exemplified by the guinea pig. Several other minor metabolites were detected including conjugated forms of benzyl-methyl-carbinol, benzyl-methyl-ketone, 4'-hydroxynorephedrine and unconjugated norephedrine (8). Amphetamine was metabolised in man by both major routes, but the degree of ring hydroxylation was relatively low ($<5\%$) as was production of 4'-hydroxynorephedrine and norephedrine ($<1\%$ and 2% respectively) (6).

Abuse of the amphetamines has become an increasing problem and N-methyl-amphetamine (methamphetamine) is regarded as being particularly dangerous from the point of view of drug dependence and its use has now been restricted to hospitals in the U.K. since 1968 (9). However little work has been done on its metabolism. Axelrod (2) showed that in the dog methamphetamine is demethylated to amphetamine which is hydroxylated to 4'-hydroxyamphetamine. In man only the unchanged drug and amphetamine have been identified and quantitated in the urine, thus, BECKETT and ROWLAND (3) found methamphetamine and amphetamine in the first 24 h urine (about 20% and 4% of the dose respectively).

Labelled [^{14}C]-methamphetamine [($\pm$)-2-methylamino-1-phenyl-[1-^{14}C]-propane hydrochloride] was synthesised from barium [^{14}C] carbonate and administered to rats, guinea pigs and two male human volunteers. The excretion of radioactivity (Table 1) was confined largely to the urine in the rat and man, but there was an appreciable excretion of radioactivity in the faeces of the guinea pig. However, in all three species the bulk of the dose had been excreted in 48 h. Urine from the rat was subjected to paper chromatography (Fig. 1A) and scanned with a radiochromatogram scanner. Two large peaks (peaks c and b) of R_F 0.00 and 0.49 were detected, together with two minor peaks (peaks

---

[*] Supported by a grant from the Medical Research Council

TABLE 1

The excretion of ^{14}C in man, rat and guinea pig after administration of $(\pm)$ [^{14}C]-methamphetamine

	Rat p.o. 45 mg/kg		Guinea pig i.p. 45 mg/kg		Man 20 mg/person	
Day	Urine	Faeces	Urine	Faeces	Urine	
1	46.8	0.6	64.7	18.1	68.8	54.9
2	27.0	1.0	3.5	0.3	21.1	23.2
3	7.0	0.3	0.8	0.1	5.5	7.4
	Total 82.7		Total 87.5		Total 94.4, 85.5	

Figures quoted are as a % of the dose and for the rat and guinea pig the averages of three animals. Radioactivity given was 2—3 µCi in each case.

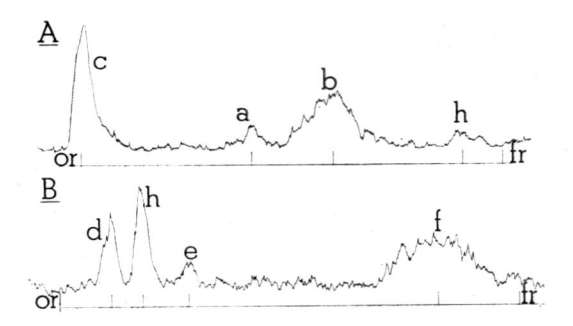

Fig. 1. *A.* Radiochromatogram scan of 0—24 h rat urine after [^{14}C]methamphetamine hydrochloride (45 mg/kg; p.o.; 1.5 µCi). Whatman No 1 paper, using amyl alcohol/tert-amyl alcohol/formic acid/water (5:5:10:2 v/v) as solvent. *B.* Radiochromatogram scan of 0—24 h guinea pig urine after [^{14}C]methamphetamine hydrochloride (45 mg/kg; i.p.; 1.7 µCi). Whatman No 1 paper, using n-butanol saturated with 1.5 M-ammonia-ammonium carbonate buffer (11) as solvent. c — phenolic amine glucuronides, a — phenolic amines, b — amines, h — hippuric acid, d — benzoyl glucuronide, e — benzoic acid, f — 'amines', or — origin, fr — front

a and h) of R_F 0.30 and 0.89. Peak h corresponded to hippuric acid and hydrolysis of peak c gave an equivalent increase in peak a. Peak c was eluted, hydrolysed with β-glucuronidase and subjected to thin layer chromatography. Scanning of the plate revealed three peaks (Fig. 2.1) of R_F 0.04, 0.40 and 0.65 (hne, ha, hma) which corresponded to 4'-hydroxynorephedrine, 4'-hydroxyamphetamine and 4'-hydroxymethamphetamine. Thus peak c probably consisted of the O-glucuronide conjugates of these compounds. Thin layer chromatography of peak a gave a similar pattern to the hydrolysis products of peak c. Therefore peak a contained the same three phenols as hydrolysed peak c. Elution and thin layer chromatography of peak b (Fig. 2.2) yielded two minor and one major peaks of R_F 0.00, 0.43 and 0.80 and these corresponded to an unidentified substance, amphetamine and methylamphetamine respectively.

Guinea pig urine on chromatography (Fig. 1B) using the FEWSTER and HALL (11) solvent system gave four peaks of R_F 0.10, 0.18, 0.28 and 0.82. The first three peaks (d, h and e) corresponded to benzoyl glucuronide, hippuric acid and benzoic acid. The peak R_F 0.82 (f) on elution and rechromatography in thin layer (Fig. 2.2) was resolved into four peaks (u, ne, a and ma) of R_F 0.00, 0.20, 0.47 and 0.79. The origin peak u has not yet been identified but the other three peaks, ne, a and ma corresponded to norephedrine, amphetamine and methamphetamine respectively.

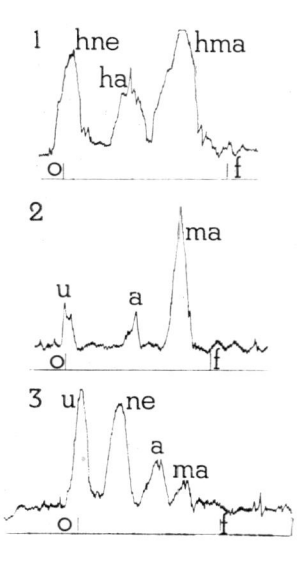

Fig. 2. 1. Radiochromatogram of eluate of peak c from rat urine after ß-glucuronidase treatment. 2. Radiochromatogram of eluate of peak b from rat urine. 3. Radiochromatogram of eluate of peak f from guinea pig urine. In each case the eluate was subjected to thin layer chromatography on Alumina G (Merck A. G., Darmstadt, Germany) 0.25 mm thick using methanol/chloroform (1:1 v/v) (14) as solvent.
hne — 4'-hydroxynorephedrine, ha — 4'-hydroxyamphetamine, hma — 4'-hydroxymethamphetamine, u — unknown, a — amphetamine, ma — methamphetamine, ne — norephedrine, o — origin, f — front.

All the metabolites in both the rat and guinea pig were confirmed by reverse isotope dilution. In man, since only small amounts of radioactivity could be administered, reverse isotope dilution was the primary method of analysis and quantitation.

In order to further confirm the finding of norephedrine as a metabolite of methamphetamine, particularly since some doubt has been cast upon its production by the guinea pig dosed with methamphetamine (4) the amine metabolites were extracted with ether from alkaline (pH 14) guinea pig urine after giving the drug at two dose levels (45 and 10 mg/kg i.p. as hydrochloride). The amines were acetylated at room temperature overnight with acetic anhydride and pyridine in the ethereal solution. After removal of the reagents by evaporation at reduced pressure the acetylated amines were taken up into ethyl acetate and subjected to gas chromatography (Fig. 3). This revealed two peaks with the same retention time as amphetamine and norephedrine. On repeating the separation using combined gas chromatography/mass spectrometry the spectrum of peak 1 (Fig. 4B) was shown to be identical with that of authentic N-acetyl amphetamine (Fig. 4A). Similarly the spectrum of peak 2 (Fig. 5B) was shown to be identical with that of N,O-diacetylnorephedrine (Fig. 5A). Norephedrine could only be found in appreciable quantities in the urine of animals dosed at the higher dose level (45 mg/kg) thus confirming the observations of BECKETT et. al., (4) at the lower dose level. On the other hand at this lower dose level (10 mg/kg) benzyl methyl ketone and benzoic acid (free + conjugated) represented a much greater proportion of the dose than at the higher dose level (10.9 and 63.4% respectively; averages for three animals).

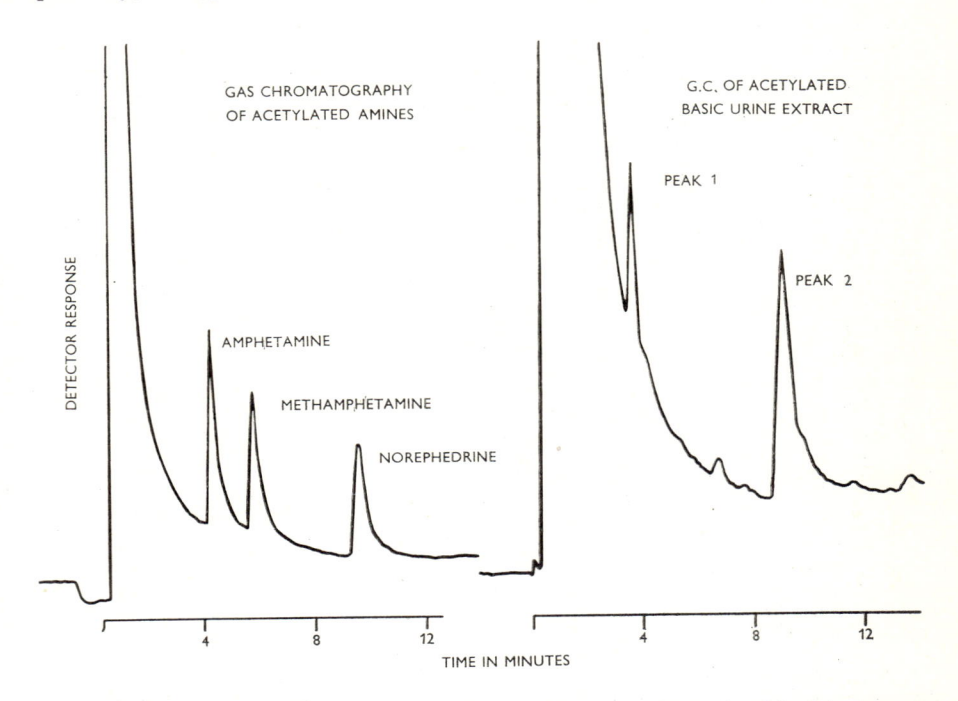

Fig. 3. Gas chromatography of standard acetylated amines and of acetylated basic urine extract. G. C. column: 3% w/w SE-30 on Chromosorb G (100—120 mesh) in a 6 ft glass column. Temperature 150°, then after an initial delay of 8 min the temperature was increased at the rate of 5°/min to an upper limit of 185°.

The quantitative aspects of the metabolism of methamphetamine are given in Table 2. From this table it will be clear that the major metabolites in the rat are 4'hydroxymethamphetamine and 4'-hydroxyamphetamine whereas in the guinea pig benzoic acid and norephedrine are the major excretory products. The presence of a large percentage of the unchanged drug is notable in the human urine and the only other metabolite present in any quantity was 4'-hydroxymethamphetamine.

A summary of the metabolism of methamphetamine is given in Fig. 6. It would seem that the general pattern of metabolism which was found for amphetamine, namely ring hydroxylation in the rat, isopropylamine side chain degradation in the guinea pig and a mixture of both routes in man also holds true for methamphetamine. However there is a greater emphasis on ring hydroxylation in man with methamphetamine.

Hydroxylation at carbon-1 (β-hydroxylation) is of interest since 4'-hydroxynorephedrine and perhaps norephedrine can act as false neurotransmitters (15). Many of the characteristic changes seen on prolonged administration of the amphetamines (13) can be

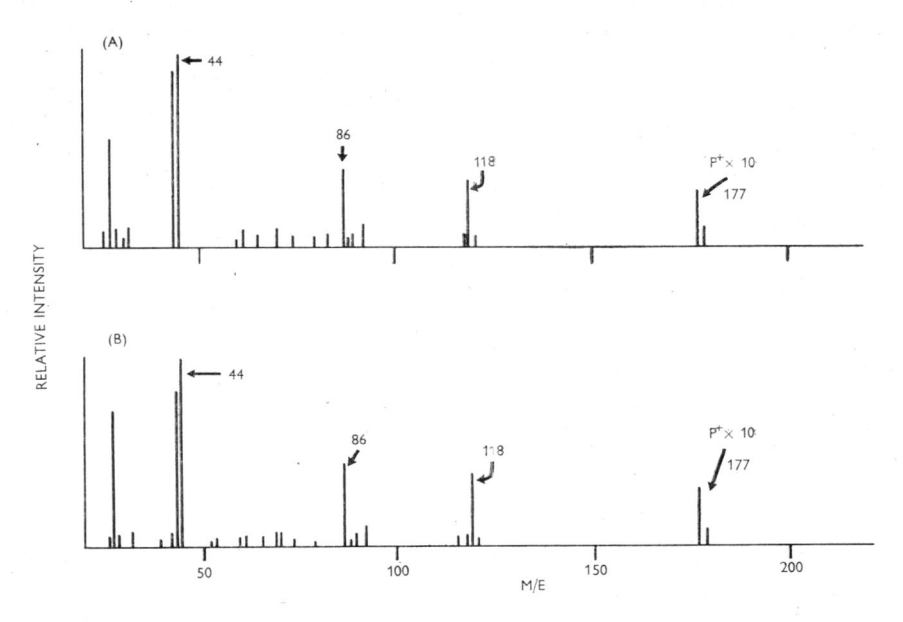

Fig. 4. (A) Mass spectrum of N-acetylamphetamine, retention time 2.0 min. (B) Mass spectrum of peak 1 time 2.0 min (see Fig. 3) from acetylated basic urine extract. In both cases the spectra were recorded with an electron beam energy of 70 eV and the samples were introduced into the mass spectrometer via a Biemann and Watson-type molecular separator from a gas chromatograph using helium carrier gas. The G.C. conditions were essentially the same as quoted for Fig. 3.

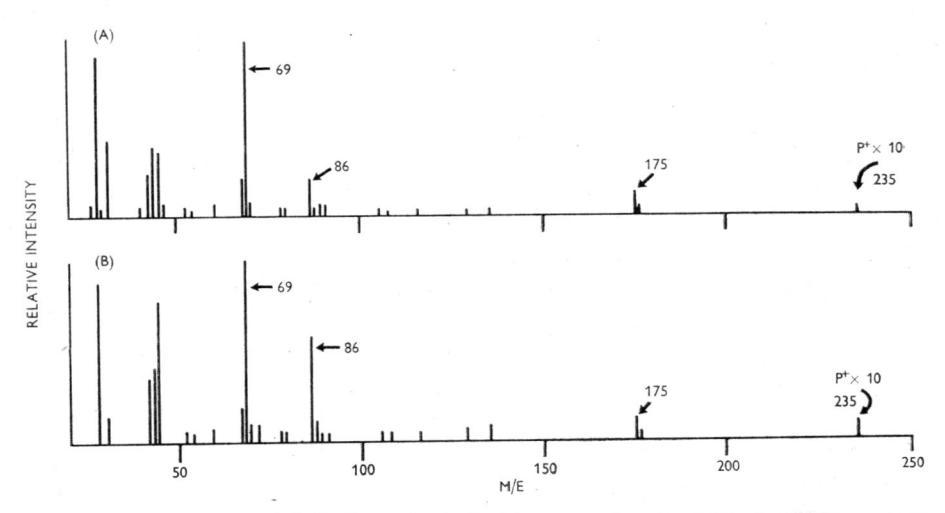

Fig. 5. (A) Mass spectrum of N,O-diacetylnorephedrine, retention time 4.25 min. (B) Mass spectrum of peak 2, retention time 4.25 min (see Fig. 3) from acetylated basic urine extract. The spectra were obtained in the same way as for Fig. 4.

attributed to a loss of adrenergic efficiency and it has been suggested that false transmitter metabolites contribute to this (5, 12). The finding of norephedrines as metabolites of methamphetamine is therefore of interest and it may be that the greater quantities of these compounds formed from methamphetamine as compared with amphetamine may be related to the greater dangers of methamphetamine from the point of view of dependence.

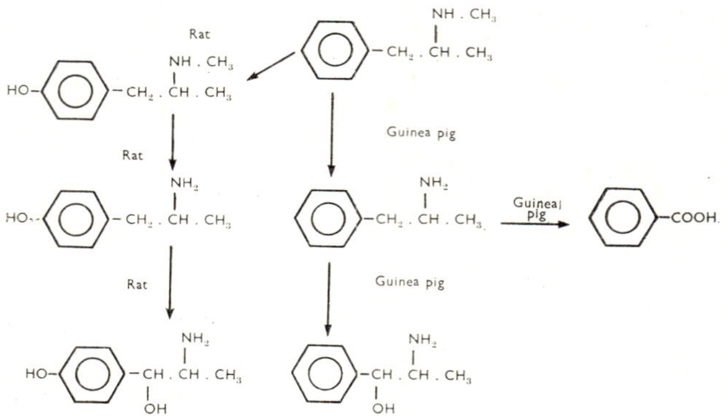

Fig. 6. Possible routes for the metabolism of [^{14}C]-methamphetamine. All the compounds can be detected in human urine.

TABLE 2

The metabolites of (±) [^{14}C]-methamphetamine in rat, guinea pig and man

	Rat p.o. 45 mg/kg	Guinea pig 45 mg/kg		Man 20 mg
	Urine	Urine	Faeces	Urine
Methamphetamine	11.0	2.1	1.3	27.2, 18.1
Amphetamine	3.1	3.1	9.8	2.2, 3.2
4'-Hydroxymethamphetamine	31.4	n.d.	n.d.	14.1, 15.8
4'-Hydroxyamphetamine	5.9	n.d.	n.d.	1.1, 1.0
Norephedrine	n.d.	13.3	5.6	1.7, 2.4
4'-Hydroxynorephedrine	15.8	n.d.	n.d.	1.2, 2.2
Benzoic acid	3.5	30.5	0.0	3.8, 5.6
Total	70.7	86.4*		49.8
Total ^{14}C in excreta	73.7	89.3		61.8

Figures quoted are as a % of the dose and for the rat and guinea pig are the averages of three animals. Radioactivity given was 2—3 µCi in each case. Analyses are for the first two days in the rat and first day in guinea pig and man.

Values are for free + conjugated forms where appropriate.
n.d. — not detected.

* includes an unidentified acidic conjugate present in both urine and faeces to the extent of 12.8 and 7.9 % respectively.

References

1. ALLEVA, J. J. (1963) Metabolism of Tranylcypromine-C^{14} and dl-Amphetamine-C^{14} in the Rat. J. med. Chem. **6**, 21.
2. AXELROD, J. (1954) Studies on sympathomimetic amines. II The biotransformation and physiological disposition of d-amphetamine, d-p-hydroxyamphetamine and d-methamphetamine. J. Pharmacol. exp. Ther. **110**, 315.
3. BECKETT, A. H. and ROWLAND, M. (1965) Urinary excretion kinetics of methylamphetamine in man. J. Pharm. Pharmacol. **17**, 109S.
4. BECKETT, A. H., VAN DYK, J. M., CHISSICK, H. M. and GORROD, J. W. (1971) 'Metabolism' of 'amphetamines' to oximes as a route to deamination. J. Pharm. Pharmacol. **23**, 560.
5. BRODIE, B. B., CHO, A. K. and GESSA, G. L. (1970) Amphetamines and Related Compounds (COSTA, E. and GARATTINI, S. EDS.) p. 217 Raven Press, New York.
6. CALDWELL, J., DRING, L. G. and WILLIAMS, R. T. (1972) Metabolism of [^{14}C]Methamphetamine in Man, the Guinea Pig and the Rat. Biochem. J. **129**, 11.
7. DRING, L. G., SMITH, R. L. and WILLIAMS, R. T. (1966) The fate of amphetamine in man and other mammals. J. Pharm. Pharmacol. **18**, 402.
8. DRING, L. G., SMITH, R. L. and WILLIAMS, R. T. (1970) The Metabolic Fate of Amphetamine in Man and other Species. Biochem. J. **116**, 425.
9. EDITORIAL (1968) Abuse of methylamphetamine Lancet, (ii), 818.
10. ELLISON, T., GUTZAIT, L. and VAN LOON, E. J. (1966) The comparative metabolism of d-amphetamine-C^{14} in the rat, dog and monkey. J. Pharmacol. exp. Ther. **152**, 383.
11. FEWSTER, M. E. and HALL, D. A. (1951) Application of buffered solvent systems to the detection of aromatic acids by paper partition chromatography. Nature (Lond.) **168**, 78.
12. KOPIN, I. J. (1971) Unnatural amino acids as precursors of false transmitters. Fed. Proc. **30**, 904.
13. KOSMAN, M. E. and UNNA, K. R. (1968) Effects of chronic administration of the amphetamines and other stimulants on behavior. Clin. Pharmacol. Ther. **9**, 240.
14. NOIRFALISE, A. (1966) Contribution à la mise au point d'une méthode de recherche des amphétamines dans l'urine. Ann. Biol. clin. (Paris) **24**, 943.
15. THOENEN, H., HUERLIMANN, A., GEY, K. F. and HAEFELY, W. (1966) Liberation of p-hydroxynorephedrine from cat spleen by sympathetic stimulation after pretreatment with amphetamine. Life Sci. **5**, 1715.

L.G.D., Department of Biochemistry, St. Mary's Hospital Medical School, London W. 2., England

METHAMPHETAMINE, FENFLURAMINE AND THEIR METABOLITES: IDENTIFICATION AND SUBCELLULAR LOCALIZATION IN RAT BRAIN HOMOGENATES

F. CATTABENI, G. RACAGNI and E. COSTA

Institute of Pharmacology and Pharmacognosy, School of Pharmacy, University of Milan and Laboratory of Preclinical Pharmacology, National Institute of Mental Health, Saint Elizabeths Hosp., Washington, D.C.

Introduction

In the last decade the combined technique of gas chromatography-mass spectrometry (GC-MS) has emerged as one of the most versatile, sensitive and specific analytical techniques. Its application to organic, inorganic and natural product chemistry is well documented by several papers, recently reviewed by DE JONGH (11). Since appropriate GC-MS instrumentation for quantitative analysis of biological samples is still being developed, its potential impact for future developments of biochemical pharmacology and neurochemistry cannot be assessed appropriately at this time. Nevertheless, it seems realistic to predict that mass fragmentography (MF), a recent development of GC-MS, will become the method of choice to bridge neurochemistry to neurophysiology in the study of neurotransmitters at the synaptic level.

With the introduction of MF as a neurochemical method, a quantal jump has occurred in the sensitivity of methods to measure neurotransmitter concentrations. This technique was described by SWEELY et al. (21) and allows for the absolute identification of drugs (15) and endogenous compounds (2, 6, 7, 9, 9a, 10a, 17, 20) in concentrations smaller than one picomole in brain tissue samples smaller than one mg.

This report concerns the identification of amphetamine (A), methamphetamine (MA), fenfluramine (F) and their metabolites in rat brain tissue. We are also reporting on the subcellular distribution of norfenfluramine (NF), the main metabolite of F present in brain. The localization of F and the changes with time of the brain concentration of F, A and MA metabolites will be related to the time course of brain monoamine depletion elicited by MA, F and A (10, 14, 18) to reach a better understanding of their action on the brain stores of these putative neurotransmitters.

Mass fragmentographic identification of amphetamine, methamphetamine and fenfluramine metabolites[*])

Previous studies on the presence of MA, A and F metabolites in brain tissue had been conducted with radiochemical methods (10b, 18). They revealed that the brain concentrations of these metabolites were as little as a few picomoles per g/tissue (10b, 14, 18).

Since the metabolites of A and MA can be released by nerve impulses and act as false transmitters (10b) and since NF could affect the dynamic equilibrium of 5-hydroxytryptamine (5-HT) in axon terminals (10c), we decided to investigate further the identity and cellular localization of such metabolites.

Conventional GC-MS cannot be satisfactorily applied, for the identification of picomole amounts of chemicals present in tissues for two main reasons: a) the sensitivity of the total ion current is in the nanomole range; this low sensitivity prevents the recording of mass spectra at a given GC retention time when quantities of compounds smaller than one nanomole are being analyzed; b) the presence of organic material in column packings and that of oil vapors and other contaminants in the region of the ion source do not allow the use of the highest possible sensitivity. These limitations can be avoided by focusing continually the instrument on a characteristic fragment (single ion detection) or alternatively focusing on two or three characteristic fragments (multiple ion detection, MID) of the mass spectrum obtained with the authentic compound. With this focusing, the mass spectrometer records the ion density of the fragment(s) generated during the elution time of the compound from the gas chromatographic column. Of course, the mass number (m/e) of the selected fragments must not be generated by other tissue components or by instrument background activity. In this type of analysis, the maximal sensitivity of the GC-MS can be obtained when the instrument is focused on a given fragment continuously, and the overall sensitivity depends on the number of various fragments generated by the electron impact. In optimal conditions, femtomole quantities of a compound can be measured and identified by single ion detection.

In single ion detection analysis the identification of a compound is based upon the appearance of a given fragment at a characteristic gas chromatographic retention time. Better identification is achieved by recording simultaneously two or three fragments (MID); with this procedure identification is enriched by a third parameter: the ion density ratio between the ions; this ratio gives direct information on the cracking pattern of the compound analyzed and, therefore, a criterion of absolute chemical identification. Unfortunately, due to technical limitations, using a magnetic deflection mass spectrometer, MID is feasible only if the fragments to be recorded have m/e values within 10% of each other. This limitation does not apply to the quadruple mass spectrometers.

1. *Methamphetamine*

The simultaneous recording of more than one fragment can also be used for the detection of two or three different compounds present in the same tissue sample. In this case, each ion density measured corresponds to a fragment characteristic of each of the two or three compounds to be determined simultaneously. Obviously this technique is of great value for analyzing tissue content of various drug metabolites. In our experiments, we have simultaneously detected MA and A in brain of MA-treated rats. Three hours after 45 μmol/kg i.p. of d- or l-MA, rat brains were homogenized and extracted as described previously (18). An aliquot of the extract was dried, dissolved in ethylacetate and reacted with trimethylsylyl imidazole and/or heptafluorobutyryl imidazole. The products of this reaction have physicochemical properties which are suitable for GC analysis (16). Under these conditions, reference spectra of MA and A heptafluorobutyryl derivatives (HFB) showed that the most abundant fragment (base peak) of the mass spectrum of each

---

*) Description of the principles of gas chromatography-mass spectrometry and mass fragmentography is not given in the text. The reader is referred to the following references (9, 9a, 10a, 11, 13, 15, 20, 21).

compound is characterized by a m/e 254 and 240, respectively. Both fragments are originated by the cleavage of the α-β carbon bond in the side chain; the positive charge is retained on the nitrogen containing part of the molecule (Table 1). Focusing the GC-MS

TABLE 1

Mass number (m/e) of fragments originated by α—β carbon bond cleavage in amphetamine and analogues

Compounds*	Substituents			Positive charge on	
	R	R'	R"	fragment I m/e (%)	fragment II m/e (%)
Amphetamine-HFB	H	H	H	91 (50)	240 (100)
Methamphetamine-HFB	CH_3	H	H	91 (35)	254 (100)
p-OH-Amphetamine TMS-HFB	H	OH	H	179 (100)	240 (17)
Fenfluramine-HFB	C_2H_5	H	CF_3	159 (20)	268 (100) 240 (40)**
Norfenfluramine-HFB	H	H	CF_3	159 (37)	240 (100)

Conditions: GC-MS LKB 9000, ion source temp. 270°, electron energy 70 eV, trap current 60 μA, accelerating voltage 3.5 kV.

* Trimethylsylyl (TMS) and/or heptafluorobutyryl (HFB) derivatives (16).
** Fragment at m/e 240 is originated by a loss of 28 mass units ($CH_2=CH_2$) from fragment at m/e 268, as confirmed by the presence of a metastable peak at 215.9 ($240.0^2/268.0$).

(LKB 9000) upon these two fragments, we detected MA and the dealkylated product A in the brain of rats receiving MA. We found that the amount of A present in rat brain seems to depend upon the isomer used. This was expected because previous reports had shown that d-MA is dealkylated enzymatically more efficiently than the l-isomer (3, 5). Our results showed that the brain extracts of rats receiving d-MA contain more A than the brain of rats receiving an equal amount of l-MA. In the same extracts, we identified p-hydroxyamphetamine (p-OHA) by focusing the GC-MS on m/e 179. Table 1 shows the origin and relative abundance of this fragment in the spectrum of the trimethylsylyl and heptafluorobutyryl derivative of authentic p-OH-A. Identification was based upon the appearance of a peak at the characteristic retention time, with the instrument recording only fragments with m/e 179. Differentiation of p-OH-A from p-hydroxymethamphet- amine (p-OH-MA) which also generates m/e 179 fragments is possible because p-OH-MA has a longer GC retention time due to the presence of the N-methyl group. Since, in brain extracts of rats receiving MA, we found a peak at m/e 179 only at the retention time of p-OH-A, we may conclude that dealkylation of MA precedes its p-hydroxylation or that the hydroxylation of the dealkylated compound is the preferential metabolic route of MA in the rat.

This conclusion is further supported by preliminary results demonstrating the presence of the β-hydroxylated product of p-OH-A, p-OH-norephedrine in brain extracts of

MA-treated rats. In brain of rats killed three hours after MA, the concentration of p-OH-norephedrine seems to be rather low, when compared with that of p-OH-A. At present, we are investigating whether at later times (18, 24 hours) p-OH-norephedrine concentrations are greater than those of p-OH-A as suggested by earlier reports on radio-chemical measurements of these metabolites in the brain of rats receiving A (10b, 14).

2. Fenfluramine

We have used MF to identify F metabolites in brain tissue. Brains of F-treated rats were homogenized, extracted and reacted as already described (18). The MS was focused upon m/e 240 (Table 1), which is a common fragment for both F-HFB and norfenfluramine-HFB (NF-HFB). We could detect neither phenolic nor alcoholic metabolites of F. The N-dealkylated metabolite of F (4, 8) was the only amine metabolite detected in brain extracts of rats killed 24 hours after injections of l-F (90 μmoles/kg i.p.). We believe that N-dealkylation of F has a certain degree of stereoisomeric specificity because in contrast to the brain of rats receiving l-F, that of rats receiving 90 μmoles/kg i.p. of d-F 24 hours before their sacrifice, contained both the parent compound and NF. Moreover, the concentrations of NF were smaller in rats injected with d-F than in rats receiving l-F. Since 24 hours after the injection of F, the 5-HT concentrations in telencephalon are still reduced (10, 10c, 19), it seemed appropriate to us to investigate the subcellular localization of NF in order to ascertain whether a specific location of NF is involved in the depletion of brain 5-HT elicited by F.

Subcellular localization of norfenfluramine

In rats receiving NF or F, the *in vivo* conversion of labeled tryptophan into 5-HT is greater than normal (10); moreover, neither tryptophan hydroxylase nor aromatic amino acid decarboxylase are inhibited by F or NF (12, 19). Finally, Morgan et al. (19) reported that NF does not inhibit the 5-HT uptake by brain slices. These considerations prompted us to investigate the subcellular localization of NF in brain of rats receiving F, in order to ascertain whether the presence of NF in synaptosomes could explain the long lasting depletion of brain 5-HT elicited by F.

a) *Quantitative analysis with mass fragmentography*: The application of MF to quantitative measurements of compounds in tissue samples has allowed for the measurement of femtomole concentrations of a variety of endogenous compounds such as biogenic amines (9, 9a, 10a, 17), their metabolites (6), steroids (7), and prostaglandins (2, 20).

The pentafluoropropionyl derivative (PFP) of F and NF was formed (1) and the MS focused on m/e 190, corresponding to the base peak (taken as 100% fragment) of NF spectrum and on the same fragment of the spectrum of F (Fig. 1). A typical mass fragmentogram obtained with authentic NF and F is shown in Figure 2, 1.

Mass fragmentography like other quantitative analytical techniques requires the use of an internal standard. Moreover, this technique requires that the chemical structure of the internal standard is as close as possible to that of the compound to be analyzed. Ideally (2, 6, 13, 20) the standard should be the same compound labeled with stable isotopes (^{15}N, ^{13}C, ^{18}O or ^{2}H). Since deuterated NF was not available, we used F as the internal standard of NF.

To calculate the amount of NF present in a given sample, we have reacted with pentafluoropropionic anhydride (PFPA) various mixtures of F and NF; these were prepared by keeping the amount of F constant (0.1 nmole) and changing the quantity of NF from

0.08 to 1.5 nmole. Plotting the ratio of the ion densities (expressed as peak heights of NF versus F) on the ordinates and the moles of NF on the abscissa, the standard reference curve for quantitative measurements of NF in unknown samples was obtained (Fig. 3). We added to each brain sample 0.1 nmoles of F before reacting the sample with PFPA. The ratio of the ion densities obtained was then used to calculate the amount of unknown found in the sample (Fig. 2, 11) by referring to the standard curve (Fig. 3).

b) *Subcellular fractionation*: Rats received NF (90 μmol/kg i.p.) five hours before decapitation. The brain was removed and the telencephalon dissected out. We measured the subcellular localization of NF in this brain tissue because MORGAN et al. (19) have demonstrated that the 5-HT depletion elicited by F is greater in this brain area than in other brain areas. The homogenates of this brain part were fractioned using high speed centrifugation and a discontinuous sucrose gradient as suggested by WHITTAKER (23). Each fraction obtained was extracted with ethyl ether, after addition of 1 ml of N-NaOH. An aliquot of the organic phase was transferred in a vial containing 0.1 nmole of F.

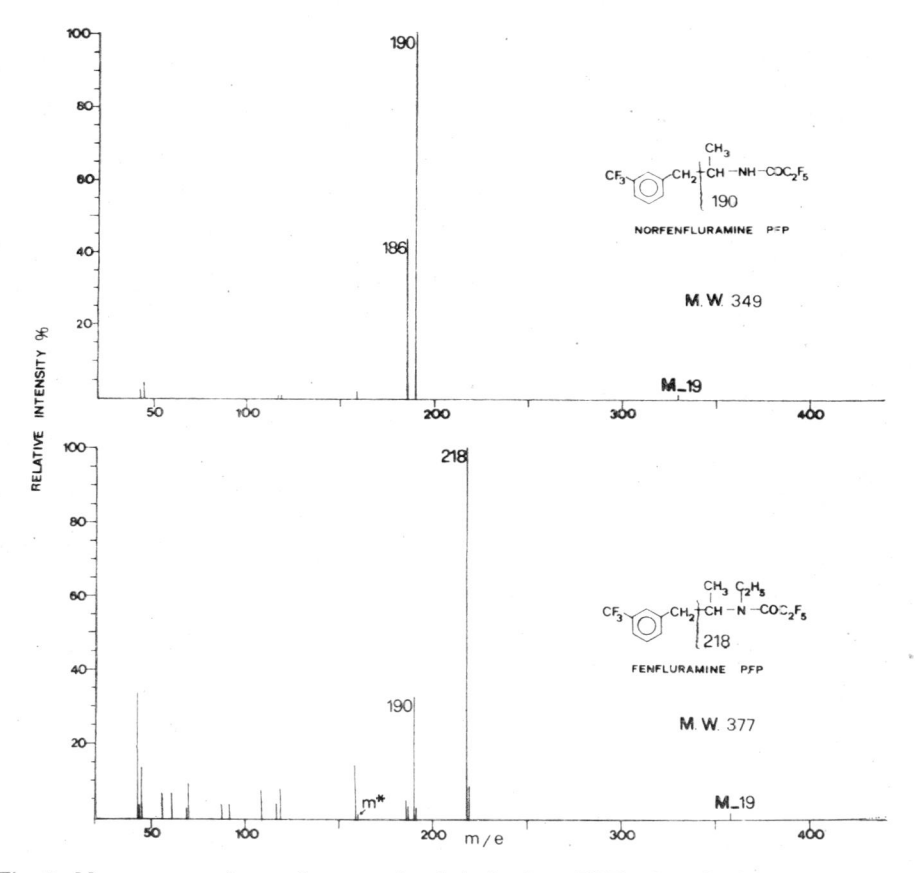

Fig. 1. Mass spectra of pentafluoropropionyl derivatives (PFP) of norfenfluramine and fenfluramine. Fragments at m/e 190 and 218 for NF and F respectively are originated by α—β carbon cleavage, with the positive charge retained on the nitrogen containing part. The peak at m/e 190 in the spectrum of F derives by loss of 28 mass units ($CH_2=CH_2$) from the fragment at m/e 218, as confirmed by the presence of a metastable peak (m*) at m/e 160.5 ($190^2/218$).

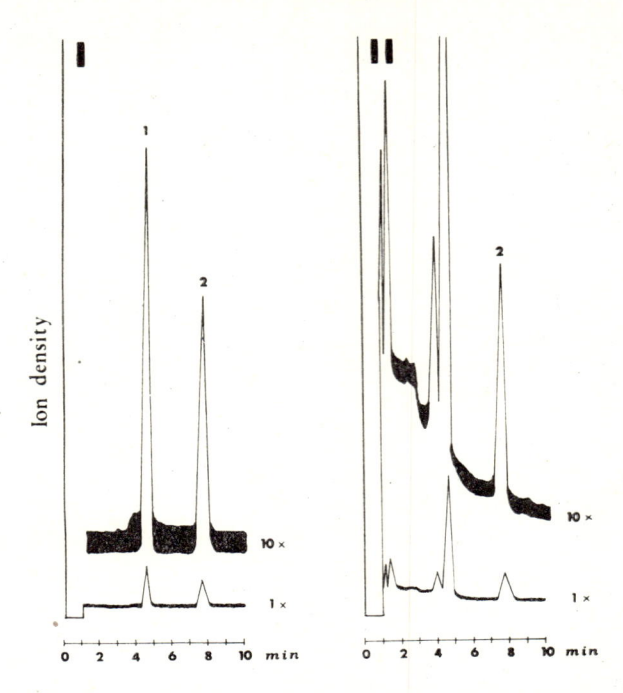

Fig. 2. Mass fragmentogram of: I. Standard norfenfluramine-PFP (0.08 nmol, peak 1) and fenfluramine-PFP (0.1 nmol, peak 2). II. Ether extract of the 0.32M sucrose band subcellular fraction. Peak 2: Fenfluramine standard (0.1 nmol) added prior to the derivatives formation.

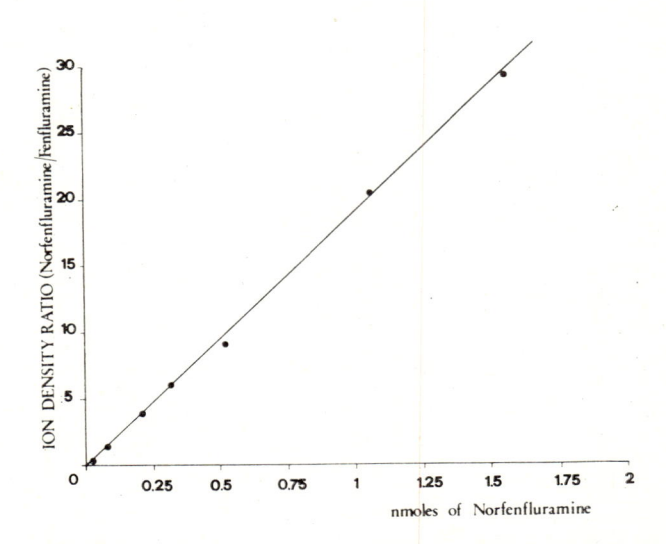

Fig. 3. Using the procedure described in the text, a linear relationship is obtained for norfenfluramine and fenfluramine standards. This calibration curve was used for the quantitative measurements of norfenfluramine in various subcellular fractions.

The ether was evaporated under a stream of nitrogen and the residue reacted with PFPA. After 30 minutes at 60°C, the excess of PFPA was evaporated, the residue redissolved in ethyl acetate and an aliquot injected into the GC-MS to obtain the mass fragmentogram of the unknown.

A mass fragmentogram obtained from one of the subcellular fractions, after the addition of standard F, is shown in Fig. 2, II. The subcellular distribution of NF in the various

TABLE 2

Subcellular distribution of norfenfluramine (NF) in telencephalon of rat

Fractions	nmol. NF	% of total homogenate	nmol/mg protein
Total homogenate	83.81	—	1.58
126,000 g supernatant	15.35	18.37	1.97
126,000 g pellet (microsomal fraction)	1.21	1.44	0.98
12,000 g pellet (crude mitochondrial fraction)	25.12	29.97	1.41
0.32 M sucrose band	0.53	0.63	2.41
Synaptosomal fraction	14.48	17.27	2.44
Mitochondria (pellet)	1.31	1.56	0.29

Each value represents the mean of three experiments.
90 μmol/kg of NF were administered 5 hrs before sacrifice intraperitoneally.

fractions is listed in Table 2 as total NF, as percent of the amount of NF present in the total homogenate (83.81 nmol) and as specific activity in terms of protein content. The crude mitochondrial fraction (12,000 g pellet) contained about 25% of the drug found in total homogenate; after fractionation of this mitochondrial fraction, on a discontinuous sucrose gradient (0.32—0.6—0.8—1—1.2 M), three fractions were collected: in the first, (0.32 M sucrose band), which contains synaptic vesicles and some synaptosomes, we found very little NF (0.53%), but if the content of proteins is considered, this fraction shows an enrichment of the specific activity: 2.41 versus 1.58 of the total homogenate. A similar ratio (2.44) is obtained in the pooled synaptosomal fractions (0.6—0.8—1 M) where 17.3% of the drug is present.

The quantity of NF located in the mitochondria pellet was very low considering either the amount of drug (1.56%) or its specific activity (0.29). The supernatant of the 12,000 g centrifugation was centrifuged at 126,000 g for 60 minutes and the two fractions obtained (supernatant and microsomal fraction) contained together 16.5% of the drug present in the total homogenate. The specific activity of these fractions was lower (microsomal fraction) or equal (supernatant) to that of the total homogenate.

These data suggest that NF is localized in synaptosomes. Because of this location, NF could reduce brain 5-HT concentrations for a long time period by interacting with one of the various mechanisms that maintain the physiological steady-state concentrations of 5-HT in axon terminals. Since either F or NF accelerate 5-HT synthesis (10c), we may suggest that NF may impair storage. To confirm this hypothesis, we are now investigating whether combining F and 6-OH-dopamine treatments (22), we can exclude that NF is bound to noradrenergic nerve terminals.

Summary

The use of mass fragmentography (MF) has been proved to help in identifying picomole amounts or less of methamphetamine (MA) and fenfluramine (F) metabolites in brain tissue. The identification and quantification of these metabolites is of importance since their presence in nerve endings could be involved in the long lasting depletion of brain monoamine stores elicited by MA (18) and F (10, 10c, 19).

Mass fragmentography has been also applied to the quantitative measurement of the subcellular localization in brain homogenates of norfenfluramine (NF), the N-dealkylated metabolite of F. We have shown that NF is localized in synaptosomes and, therefore, because of this location, NF might interfere with specific storage mechanism for 5-HT in nerve terminals. This impairment of 5-HT binding agrees with the independent finding that large doses of F or NF increase the synthesis of brain 5-HT (10c, 14) while they reduce the 5-HT storage (14).

References

1. ANGGÄRD, E. and SEDVALL, G. (1969) Gas chromatography of catecholamine metabolites using electron capture detection and mass spectrometry. Anal. Chem. **41**, 1250.
2. AXEN, U., GREEN, K., HÖRLIN, D. and SAMUELSSON, B. (1971) Mass spectrometric determination of picomole amounts of prostaglandin E_2 and $F_{2\alpha}$ using deuterium labeled carriers. Biochem. biophys. Res. Comm. **45**, 519.
3. AXELROD, J. (1954) Studies on sympathomimetic amines 11. The biotransformation and physiological disposition of D-amphetamine, D-p-hydroxyamphetamine and D-methamphetamine. J. Pharmacol. exp. Ther. **110**, 315.
4. BECKETT, A. H. and BROOKS, L. G. (1967) The absorption and urinary excretion in man of fenfluramine and its main metabolites. J. Pharm. Pharmacol. **19**, 41S.
5. BECKETT, A. H. and ROWLAND, M. (1965) Urinary excretion kinetics of methylamphetamine in man. J. Pharm. Pharmacol. **17**, 109S.
6. BERTILSSON, L., ATKINSON, A. J., JR., ALTHAUS, J. R., HARFAST, A., LINDGREN, J. E. and HOLMSTEDT, B. (1972) Quantitative determination of 5-hydroxyindole-acetic acid in cerebrospinal fluid by gas chromatography-mass spectrometry. Anal. Chem. **44**, 1434.
7. BROOKS, C. J. W. and MIDDLEDITCH, B. S. (1971) The mass spectrometer as a gas chromatographic detector. Clin. chim. Acta. **34**, 145.
8. BRUCE, B. B. and MAYNARD, W. R. (1968) Fenfluramine metabolism. J. pharm. Sci. **57**, 1173.
9. CATTABENI, F., KOSLOW, S. H. and COSTA, E. (1972) Gas chromatographymass spectrometry assay of four indole alkylamines of the rat pineal. Science, **178**, 166.
9a. CATTABENI, F., KOSLOW, S. H. and COSTA, E. (1972) Gas chromatography-Mass fragmentography: a new approach to the estimation of amines and amine turnover. In: Advances in Biochemical Psychopharmacology, Vol. 6, edited by COSTA, E., IVERSEN, L. L. and PAOLETTI, R., Raven Press, New York, p. 37.
10. COSTA, E., GROPPETTI, A. and REVUELTA, A. (1971) Action of fenfluramine on monoamine stores in rat tissues. Brit. J. Pharmacol. **41**, 57.
10a. COSTA, E., KOSLOW, S. H., GREEN, A. R., LEFEVRE, H. F., REVUELTA, A. V. and WANG, C. (1972) Dopamine and norepinephrine in noradrenergic axons: a study *in vivo* of their precursor product relationship by mass fragmentography and radio chemistry. Pharmacol. Rev. **24**, 167.
10b. COSTA, E. and GROPPETTI, A. (1970) Biosynthesis and storage of catecholamines in tissue of rats injected with various doses of d-amphetamine. In: Proceedings of International Symposium on Amphetamines and Related Compounds; Proceedings of the Mario Negri Institute for Pharmacological Research, Raven Press, N.Y., p. 231.
10c. COSTA, E. and REVUELTA, A. (1972) Norfenfluramine and serotonin turnover rate in the rat brain. Biochem. Pharmacol. **21**, 2385.
11. DEJONGH, D. C. (1970) Mass spectrometry, Anal. Chem. Ann. Rev. **42**, 169R.
12. DUHAULT, J. and VERDAVAINNE, C. (1969) Modification du taux de serotonine cerebrale chez le rat par le trifluoromethyl-phenyl-2-ethylamino propane (Fenfluramine 768S). Arch. int. Pharmacodyn. **170**, 276.
13. GAFFNEY, T. E., HAMMAR, C.-S., HOLMSTEDT, B. and McMAHON, R. E. (1971) Ion specific detection of internal standards labeled with stable isotopes. Anal. Chem. **43**, 307.

14. GROPPETTI, A. and COSTA, E. (1969) Tissue concentration of *p*-hydroxynorephedrine in rats injected with d-amphetamine: effect of pretreatment with desimipramine (DMI). Life Sci. **8**, 653.
15. HAMMAR, C.-G., HOLMSTEDT, B. and RHYAGE, R. (1968) Mass fragmentography: identification of chlorpromazine and its metabolites in human blood by a new method. Anal. Biochem. **25**, 532.
16. HORNING, M. G., MOSS, A. M., BOUCHER, E. A. and HORNING, E. C. (1968) The gas liquid chromatographic separation of hydroxy substituted amines of biological importance including catecholamines. Preparation of derivatives for electron capture detection. Anal. Lett. **1**, 311.
17. KOSLOW, S. H., CATTABENI, F. and COSTA, E. (1972) Norepinephrine and dopamine: assay by mass fragmentography in the picomole range Science, **176**, 177.
18. MORGAN, C. D., CATTABENI, F. and COSTA, E. (1972) Methamphetamine, fenfluramine and their N-dealkylated metabolites: effect on monoamine concentrations in rat tissues. J. Pharmacol. exp. Ther. **180**, 117.
19. MORGAN, C. D., LÖFSTRANDH, S. and COSTA, E. (1972) Amphetamine analogues and brain amines. Life Sci. **11**, Part 1, 83.
20. SAMUELSSON, B., HAMBERG, M. and SWEELY, C. C. (1970) Quantitative gas chromatography of prostaglandine E_1 at the nanogram level: use of deuterated carrier and multiple ion analyzer. Anal. Biochem. **38**, 301.
21. SWEELY, C. C., ELLIOT, W. H., FRIES, I. and RHYAGE, R. (1966) Mass spectrometric determination of unresolved components in gas chromatographic effluents. Anal. Chem. **38**, 1549.
22. THOENEN, H. and TRANZER, J. P. (1968) Chemical sympathectomy by selective destruction of adrenergic nerve endings with 6-hydroxydopamine. Naunyn-Schmiedebergs Arch. Pharmakol. **261**, 271.
23. WHITTAKER, V. P. (1969) The subcellular fractionation of nervous tissue. In: Structure and function of the nervous system. G. BOURNE, ED. Vol. 3. Academic Press, New York.
24. ZIANCE, R. J., SIPES, I. G., KINNARD JR, W. J. and BUCKLEY, J. P. (1972) Central nervous system effects of fenfluramine hydrochloride. J. Pharmacol. exp. Ther. **180**, 110.

F.C., Institute of Pharmacology and Pharmacognosy,
School of Pharmacy, University of Milan, 20129
Milan, Italy

METABOLISM OF CYCLOHEXYL-ISOPROPYLAMINES IN MAN IN COMPARISON WITH AMPHETAMINES[*]

T. B. VREE, J. TH. M. VAN DER LOGT, P. TH. HENDERSON
and J. M. VAN ROSSUM

Department of Pharmacology, University of Nijmegen

Introduction

The metabolism of amphetamines and their derivatives with substituents in the propyl side chain have been studied extensively over the past 10 years. (1, 3, 4, 6, 7, 8, 9, 10, 14, 15, 20). The possible routes for metabolism are parahydroxylation, α-C-oxidation (deamination and dealkylation) and N-oxidation. The lipid-solubility plays an important role in directing routes of the total elimination, because a high lipid-solubility results in a less renal clearance, a great volume of distribution, a longer life time in the body and consequently more extensive metabolism. Weak lipophilic properties cause a high renal excretion of the unchanged compound and subsequently low degree of metabolism, such as can be observed with the ephedrines (15, 20).

In general, ring substitution results in an increase of lipid-solubility, accompanied by a greater metabolic clearance. This has been observed for fenfluramine (4), chloroamphetamine (7) and methoxyphenamine (19). Relatively little is known about hydrogen substituted amphetamine, the cyclohexylisopropylamine, and its N-alkyl substituted derivatives, ('saturated amphetamines'), while N-methylcyclohexylisopropylamine, propylhexedrine, is in use as an anti-obesity drug.

The aim of the investigation was to study the influence of the hydrogen substitution on the metabolic pattern. The metabolic fate of the saturated amphetamines in man was compared with the known metabolic pathways of amphetamines and ephedrines.

Experimental

Synthesis: Amphetamine and derivatives (+), (−) were hydrogenated in glacial acetic acid with PtO_2/H_2 (3 atm) in a Parr apparatus. The S (+) amphetamine was converted into S (−) cyclohexylisopropylamine. Ephedrines were treated in the same way to corresponding cyclohexylisopropanolamines. N-cycloalkylamphetamines were prepared by boiling (+) amphetamine in excess of cyclopentanon, cyclohexanon and cycloheptanon,

---

[*] This work was supported in part by grants from the Netherlands Organisation for the Advancement of Pure Research (Z.W.O.) and from the Prevention Fund, Ministry of Health.

resp. with Mg_2SO_4, followed by reduction with sodiumborohydride. All reactions were followed by means of combined GC-MS (LKB 9000).

Gas chromatography: H P 402 gas chromatograph with flame ionisation detector. Columns: 20% Apiezon M, 5% KOH on Gaschrom Q 60—80 mesh and 3% OV 17 on gaschrom Q 60—80-mesh. Amphetamines, ephedrines and its saturated analogues cannot be separated at these columns from each other. The hydroxy metabolites have a retention time of 2.20 times the retention time of the parent compound. After hydrolysis of the urine with 6N HCl, no conjugated amphetamines could be detected.

Mass spectrometry: L.K.B. 9000 combined gas chromatograph- mass spectrometer, equipped with a column of 20% Apiezon-5% KOH on gaschrom Q 60—80 m. Column temperature 160°, separator 200°, ion source 290°, trapcurrent 60 µA, accelerating voltage 3,5 kV, ionisation voltage 20—70 eV. The hydroxy metabolites of the N-cyclohexyl-amphetamine could be separated at the column and the position of the OH group could be identified. With cyclohexylisopropylamines, the separation of the hydroxy metabolites was too poor. Full details will be described elsewhere (19).

Metabolism: 30—60 mg of the HCl salts of the compounds were taken orally by healthy human subjects (25—30 years, 70—85 kg). The urine was kept acidic (pH 5 ±0.3) by the daily intake 4 × 2 grams of ammonium chloride (4 tablets of 0.5 g 4 dd). Each urine sample was collected, made alkaline, extracted with ether and analysed with the GLC as described before (14, 15). Renal excretion rate and cumulative renal excretion was plotted for each urine sample versus the time after administration (see Fig. 1—3) Dissociation constants (Ks) characterizing binding to microsomal enzymes were measured as described by Vree and Henderson (17, 18).

Results and discussion

A. *Excretion of the unchanged compound*

After ingestion of cyclohexylisopropylamine or an N-alkyl substituted derivative by man, a very small amount of the parent compound was excreted unchanged in the urine.

Table 1

Excretion of unchanged amphetamines and cyclohexylisopropylamines in the urine of man

Compound	% dose excreted unchanged and half life time of elimination			
	S configuration	$T^1/_2$	R configuration	$T^1/_2$
Cyclohexylisopropylamine	7%	3 hr	6%	3 hr
.. N-methyl	7	3	7	5
.. N-ethyl	4	3.5	4	3
.. N-isopropyl	1	0.5	3	1
Amphetamine	70	7	90	8
.. N-methyl	65	7	80	7
.. N-ethyl	40	5	90	7
.. N-isopropyl	10	3	85	7

In Table 1 the amounts excreted are given as well as the percentages obtained with the corresponding amphetamines (Fig. 1).

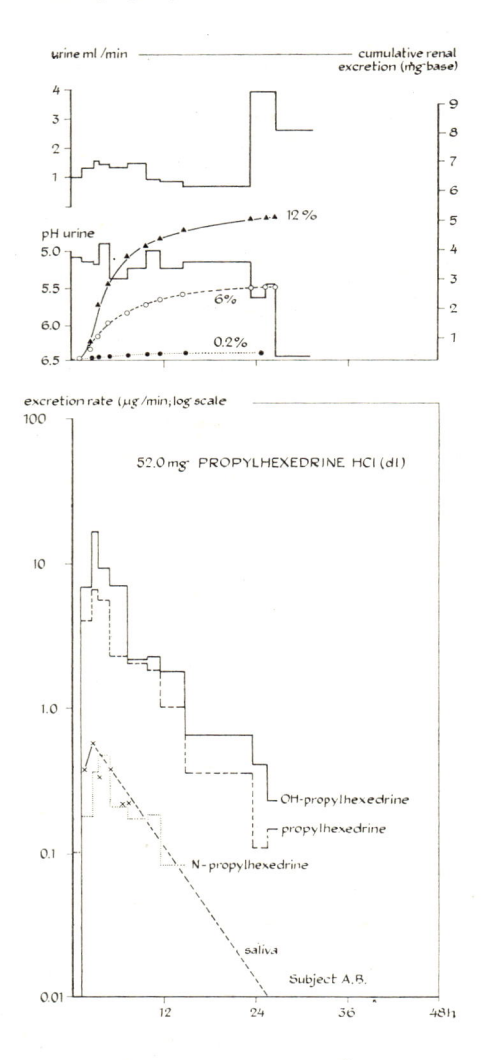

Fig. 1. Renal excretion, urinary pH, average urine production, cumulative renal excretion of N-methylcyclohexylisopropylamine (propylhexedrine) and its metabolites cyclohexylisopropylamine and cyclohexanolisopropylamine. The metabolic processes are very fast, the renal excretion of the metabolites reached a maximum after 2—3 hours.

From the table it can be derived that as the saturated amphetamines are concerned there is no striking difference in metabolic behaviour between the various derivatives and between the different stereochemical configurations of those derivatives. All compounds are very well metabolized and the renal excretion of the unchanged compound is of minor importance. This is in contrast to the amphetamine series, where substantial amounts of unchanged compounds are excreted. For the derivatives with the S configuration the proportional excretion of the unchanged compound decreases with increasing alkyl substituent. However, this excretion is constant for the R configuration (14).

TABLE 2

Percent dose excreted as ring hydroxylated metabolites into the urine of man

Compound	Configuration		
	(—) S	(+) R	S/R
Cyclohexylisopropylamine	0	0	
.. N-methyl	6.0	10	0.60
.. N-ethyl	37	55	0.67
.. N-isopropyl	55	85	0.64

The detection system used, makes it possible to detect the parahydroxylated metabolites of the saturated amphetamine in contrast to parahydroxyamphetamine. In spite of this possibility, no trace of hydroxylated metabolite of cyclohexylisopropylamine was found. It must be concluded that the deamination is an extremely fast metabolic route in the metabolism of this parent compound. Most likely deamination and ring hydroxylation are competitive pathways for elimination. With the amphetamines α-C-oxidation and renal excretion are the two metabolic routes.

B. *Hydroxy metabolites*

In comparison with the amphetamine metabolism, the most striking observation in the metabolism of saturated amphetamines is the hydroxylation of the cyclohexyl ring. The hydroxylation is prevailing when the seize of the substituent increases, concomitantly with increase of the lipid-solubility. The degree of hydroxylation also depends upon the stereochemical configuration, but the ratio of hydroxylation of the R and S configuration is constant (Fig. 2). The results are summarized in Table 2.

TABLE 3

Aromatic hydroxylation of amphetamine antipodes in various species
(after SMITH and DRING, 12)

Species	% dose excreted as p-hydroxyamphetamine		
	S (+)	R (—)	R, S (+, —)
Man	1.1	3.9	2.8
Guinea pig	0	1	
Mouse	14	17	
Rat	48	63	60

The differences in percentage of the hydroxy metabolites in the R and S configuration might be explained with the aid of the competitive metabolic pathways, on the understanding that the S-compound is more susceptible to α-C-oxidation than the R-form.

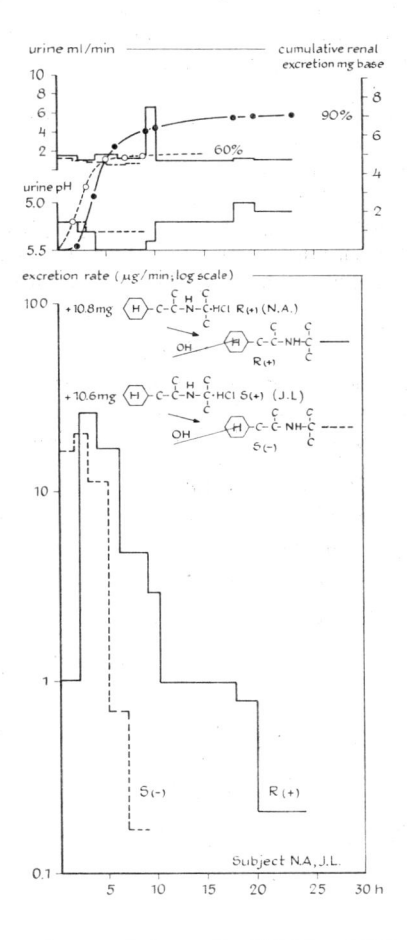

Fig. 2. Difference in renal excretion rate between the R (+) and S (—) configuration of the metabolite N-isopropyl-cyclohexanolisopropylamine. The R (+) configuration ($T^{1}/_{2} = 4$ hr) is much slower metabolized (α-C-oxidation) than the S (—) configuration. The equal maximum renal excretion rate of both metabolites indicates that the rate of hydroxylation is independent of the stereochemical configuration of the side chain.

Deamination is so fast that N-dealkylated metabolites are hardly excreted unchanged in the urine (1—5%). As reported earlier, for amphetamines both reactions were extremely dependent upon the R- and S configuration (14). The same behaviour can be found with saturated amphetamines, the effect in some way is masked by the hydroxylation. DRING (7) showed for some species the amounts of parahydroxylation of S- and R amphetamine, and he found the same differences in hydroxylated products, due to the difference in deamination of the amphetamine (Table 3).

C. The hydroxylating enzyme system

Considering the metabolism of cyclohexylisopropylamines and amphetamines the question arises whether one enzyme performs both α-C-oxidation and ring hydroxylation, or different enzymes, or different active sites of one enzyme system are responsible for the conversion. What is the reason why with increasing size of the N-alkyl substituent with saturated amphetamines the ring hydroxylation increases while with amphetamines the α-C-oxidation increases. An explanation may be that with increasing the seize of the substituent, the lipid-solubility increases too and that 'a certain part' of the enzyme can be reached while with amphetamines the nature of the C—H bond and therefore the rate of the α-C-oxidation is altered. This may be acceptable when one assumes that for all derivatives the rate of aromatic hydroxylation is low. The lipid-solubilities were measured, but it turned out that the corresponding derivatives of saturated and non saturated amphetamines have a fixed ratio of their partition coefficient (Table 4).

TABLE 4

pKa values and partition coefficients of amphetamine, cyclohexylisopropylamine and derivatives

Compound	pKa	TPC_{hept}	TPC_{chlor}	APC_{hept}	APC_{chlor}
Amphetamine	9.90	1.88	146	0.005	0.48
.. N-methyl	10.10	5.14	565	0.015	1.10
.. N-ethyl	10.23	38.6	1790	0.060	2.67
.. N-isopropyl	10.14	117	4460	0.21	8.09
Cyclohexylisopropylamine	10.50	19.0	770	0.015	0.61
.. N-methyl	10.60	92.0	1860	0.058	1.17
.. N-ethyl	10.80	550	8350	0.22	3.34
.. N-isopropyl	10.60	1180	12900	0.74	8.10

TPC – true partion coefficient
APC – apparent partition coefficient
hept – system heptane-water (Teorell buffer, pH 7.4)
chlor – system chloroform-water (Teorell buffer, pH 7.4)

The different saturated amphetamines are about three times more lipid-soluble than the corresponding amphetamines. This difference in solubility does not explain the different enzymatic attack at the molecule. The difference between the two ring systems is the nature of the C-H bond that is attacked, aliphatic and aromatic, and the 'shape' of the molecule.

The phenyl ring is stabilized by its resonance energy of 36 kcal/mol. If one enzyme is postulated for hydroxylation of both phenyl ring and cyclohexyl ring than the resonance energy may act as a threshold. Due to its high activation energy of the hydroxylation of the phenyl the α-C-oxidation get a chance to occur as an alternative metabolic pathway. The cyclohexyl ring behaves like an aliphatic chain, in which the most outstanding C-H bond with the lowest energy is hydroxylated. It may be that different enzyme systems (mechanisms) are metabolizing these amphetamines. The compound ferrocenylisopropyl-amine exerts to be an excellent inhibitor of the metabolism of amphetamines in the rat (17, 18). Ferrocenylisopropylamine binds very strongly to the cytochrome P-450 (Table 5) and in this way inhibits the α-C-oxidation. But, even when the ferrocenylisopropylamine was added in an excess of 50 times the concentration of saturated isopropylamphetamine in rats, the compound failed to inhibit the metabolism of saturated isopropylamphetamine. From this observation it must be concluded that the hydroxylation of the cyclohexyl ring is mediated by an other mechanism than α-C-oxidation. The binding affinities of the amphetamines and its saturated analogues are found to be of the same magnitude in rats. This means that the difference in structure of the phenyl and cyclohexyl ring has no influence at the interaction drug-cytochrome P-450. In Table 5 the binding affinities of the amphetamines and related compounds are given.

TABLE 5

Binding affinities of amphetamines, cyclohexylisopropylamines and related compounds to hepatic cytochrome P-450 of the rat

Compound	Ks value molar	Type
Amphetamine (S)	5.0×10^{-3}	I
Amphetamine (R)	4.5×10^{-3}	I
N-isopropylamphetamine (S)	5.0×10^{-3}	I
N-isopropylamphetamine (R)	4.1×10^{-3}	I
Cyclohexylisopropylamine (S)	4.0×10^{-3}	I
.. N-isopropyl (S)	5.0×10^{-3}	I
Benzphetamine (S)	5.5×10^{-4}	I
Ferrocenylisopropylamine	1.4×10^{-6}	II
.. N-isopropyl	5.0×10^{-6}	II
DPEA	1.4×10^{-6}	I
Imipramine	2.2×10^{-7}	I (2)
Desmethylimipramine	2.7×10^{-6}	I (2)
Amitriptyline	2.5×10^{-7}	I (2)

LEWANDER (11) reported the inhibition of both parahydroxylation (95%) and deamination (50%) of amphetamine by desmethylimipramine. The Ks value of imipramine and desmethylimipramine is of the same magnitude as that of ferrocenylisopropylamine (2) Table 5). This finding supports the idea that if the enzyme is blocked by these strong bounded compounds, all possible metabolic pathways that can be performed by the occupied enzyme entity, are blocked. The same results were obtained by inhibition of the amphetamine metabolism by the compound DPEA (10).

It is postulated by BRODIE (5) and UDENFRIEND (13) that the cytochrome P-450 hydroxylates the aromatic nucleus by the epoxide mechanism. Such a mechanism cannot be involved for the hydroxylation of the cycloalkyl ring.

What are the requirements for an enzymatic hydroxylation of cycloalkyl rings? Is the activation energy of the rupture of the C-H bond the dominating factor or are there also any steric requirements? Is it possible to replace the cyclohexyl ring by a cyclopentyl ring without alteration of metabolic pathways. This should be possible if only the activation energy mentioned is determinant for the hydroxylation.

The compound N-methylcyclopentylisopropylamine, cyclopentamine, is demethylated and excreted into the urine like methylamphetamine (Fig. 3). In man no ring hydroxylation could be observed. The cyclopentyl ring behaves like a phenyl ring, both ring systems appeared to have strong influence at the metabolic routes. The cyclopentyl ring is a planar ring system, chemically stable and without ring tension. It must be concluded that the hydroxylating enzyme can easily attack molecules with a certain flexibility in the C-H bond that can be attacked. This is the case with aliphatic carbon chains and alicyclic ring systems. A cyclopentyl ring is planar and rigid and the same holds for the phenyl ring.

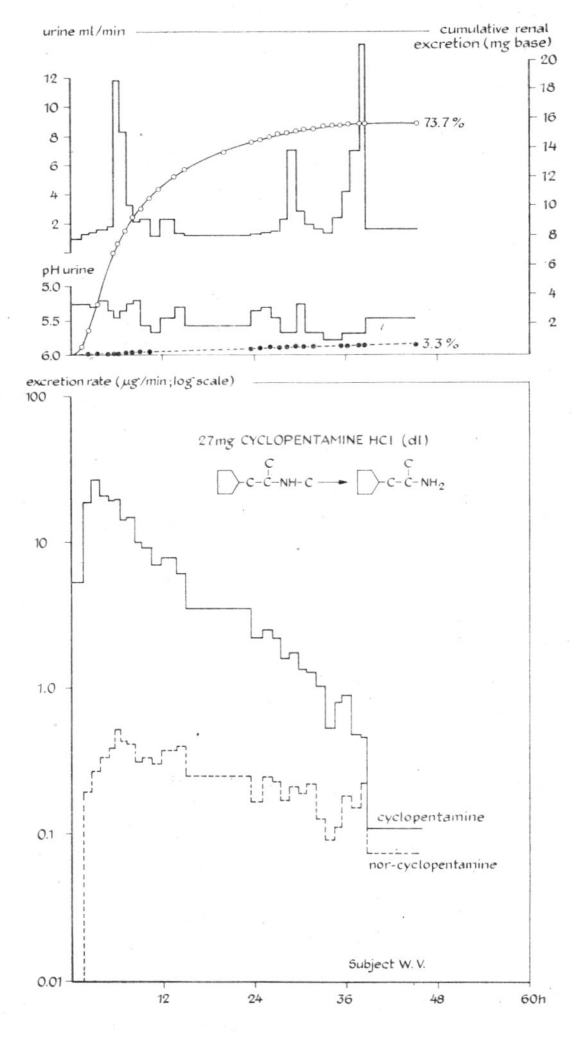

Fig. 3. Renal excretion rate, cumulative renal excretion, urinary pH and average urine production of cyclopentamine. The compound is excreted like methylamphetamine. Cyclopentamine: $T^1/_2 = 7$ hr, 70 % totally excreted unchanged, 5 % α-C-oxidation. Methylamphetamine: $T^1/_2 = 7$ hr, 70 % excreted and 10 % α-C-oxidation. Even the relationship dose mg HCl = μg/min max. excretion rate exists.

D. N-cycloalkyl substituted amphetamines

With amphetamines the main metabolic pathways in man is the α-C-oxidation and with the saturated amphetamines α-C-oxidation competes with ring hydroxylation. Also the 'flexibility' of the ring is demonstrated. In N-cycloalkyl substituted amphetamines, all those competitive pathways are possible. In order to get information about relative rate constants of α-C-oxidation and alicyclic ring hydroxylation, the following compounds were investigated: N-cyclopentyl-, N-cyclohexyl-, and N-cycloheptylamphetamine (S+).

In this series the tertiary C-H bond of the cycloalkyl group has the same outstanding position as the corresponding tertiary C-H in the amphetamine moiety. The rate of formation of the metabolite amphetamine gives an indication about the sterical hindrance of the bulky ring system when the compound is attacked by the cytochrome P-450 for α-C-oxidation. In Table 6 compounds are compared with 2 tertiary C-H bonds available for a α-C-oxidation by the cytochrome.

TABLE 6

Metabolism of N-cycloalkyl substituted amphetamines. Comparison of the availability of the tertiary C-H- bond of the substituent for attack by the cytochrome P-450

Compound	% dose excreted unchanged	% dose excreted as amphetamine	% dose excreted as ring hydroxylated metabolite of N-cycloalkylamph.
(+) isopropylamphetamine	10	40	0
(+) N-cyclopentylamphetamine	3	30	0
(+) N-cyclohexylamphetamine	1	5	18
(+) N-cycloheptylamphetamine	0	5	0

From the table it can be derived that all possible metabolic pathways do occur.

Cyclopentylamphetamine. The amount amphetamine formed and excreted in the urine indicated that the tertiary C-H of the cyclopentyl group can be attacked very easily by the cytochrome P-450. It is almost the same situation as observed with isopropylamphetamine. The ring system exhibits no or very slight sterical hindrance in the interaction with the enzyme. The tertiary C-H binding can be attacked by the cytochrome when this group is adjacent to the nitrogen atom. However, in N-methylcyclopentylisopropylamine, this particular C-H group is not attacked at all (see Fig. 3). This means that the α- C-oxidation only occurs in the aliphatic side chain and that the nitrogen atom must be a 'target' atom for the enzyme. Therefore it is also less probable that α-C-oxidation is responsible for hydroxylation of alicyclic ring systems.

Cyclohexylamphetamine: The low amount of amphetamine formed as metabolite from N-cyclohexylamphetamine indicates that the C-H bond is still accessible for attack by the cytochrome, but also that other metabolic pathways reduce the significance of this contribution to the total elimination. With N-cyclohexylamphetamine, the main metabolite excreted in the urine is N-cyclohexanolamphetamine. The total amount was about 18%, and the OH group was distributed over the ring as follows: 0.8% C2, 2.2% C3 and 15% C4. The situation is the same as observed with the saturated amphetamines. Again, α-C-oxidation and alicyclic ring hydroxylation are the competitive metabolic pathways.

Cycloheptylamphetamine: As compared to the N-cyclohexylamphetamine, the seize of the ring has no influence at the rate of formation of amphetamine. It was not possible to detect alicyclic ring hydroxylated metabolites. The metabolic routes of this compound are not clear.

ACKNOWLEDGEMENTS

The authors are indebted to Miss A. Th. J. M. Muskens, Miss T. Pols, Mr. C. vd Vorstenbosch for their skilful technical assistance, to Mr. P. van Gemert and Dr. B. Ellenbroek for assistance with the synthesis and analysis of the compounds and to Dr. T. D. Yih for assistance with the rat experiments. We also thank the students for their participation in the metabolic studies.

REFERENCES

1. ÄNGGARD, E., GUNNE, L. M., JÖNSSON, L. E. and NIKLASSON, F. (1970) Pharmacokinetic studies on amphetamine dependent subjects. Europ. J. clin. Pharmacol. **3**, 3.
2. BAHR, CH. VON and ORRENIUS, S. (1971) Spectral studies on the interaction of imipramine and some of its oxidized metabolites with rat liver microsomes. Xenobiotica, I, 69.
3. BECKETT, A. H., VAN DYKE, J. M., CHISSICK, H. H. and GORROD, J. W. (1971) Metabolic oxidation on aliphatic basis nitrogens atoms and their α carbon atoms. Some unifying principles. J. Pharm. Pharmacol. **23**, 809.
4. BECKETT, A. H. and BROOKES, L. G. (1967) The absorption and urinary excretion in man of fenfluaramine and its main metabolite. J. Pharm. Pharmacol. **19**, 41 S.
5. BRODIE, B. B., KRISHNA, G., CHO, A. K. and REID, W. D. (1971) Drug metabolism in man: Past, Present and Future. Ann. N.Y. Acad. Sci. **179**, II.
6. DRING, L. G., SMITH, R. L. and WILLIAMS, R. T. (1970) The metabolic fate of amphetamine in man and other species. Biochem. J. **116**, 425.
7. FULLER, R. W. and HINES C. W. (1967) Tissue levels of chloroamphetamines in rats and mice. J. Pharm. Sci. **56**, 302.
8. FULLER, R. W., MOLLOY, B. B. and JOHN PARLI, C. (1972) The effects of ß, ß-difluoro-substitution on the metabolism and pharmacology of amphetamines. Psychopharmacologia, **26** (supp.), 35.
9. HUCKER, H. B., MICHNIEWICZ, B. M. and RHODES, R. F. (1971) Phenylacetone oxime an intermediate in the oxidative deamination of amphetamine. Biochem. Pharmacol. **20**, 2123.
10. GLASSON, B., THOMASSET, M. and BENAKIS, A. (1972) Interaction of DPEA and Iproniazid on the metabolism of d-amphetamine ^{14}C-sulphate in mice. Toxicological problems of Drug combinations. Excerpta Medica Berlin 1971.
11. LEWANDER, T. (1968) Effects of amphetamine on urinary and tissue catecholamines in rats after inhibition of its metabolism with desmethylimipramine. Europ. J. Pharmacol. **5**, 1.
12. SMITH, R. L. and DRING, L. G. (1970) Patterns of metabolism of ß-phenylisopropylamines in man and other species. Amphetamines and related compounds, COSTA, E. and GARRATTINI, S., Eds. p. 121, Raven Press, New York.
13. UDENFRIEND, S. (1971) Arene oxides intermediates in enzymatic hydroxylation and their significance with respect to drug toxicity. Ann. N.Y. Acad. Sci. **179**, 295.
14. VREE, T. B., GORGELS, J.P. M. C. MUSKENS, A. TH. J. M. and VAN ROSSUM, J. M. (1971) Deuterium isotope effects in the metabolism of N-alkyl substituted amphetamines in man. Clin. chim. Acta **34**, 333.
15. VREE, T. B., MUSKENS, A. TH. J. M. and VAN ROSSUM, J. M. (1971) Deuterium isotope effects and stereochemistry in the dealkylation and deamination of amphetamines and ephedrines in man. Xenobiotica, I, 385.
16. VREE, T. B., MUSKENS, A. TH. J. M. and VAN ROSSUM, J. M. (1972) Metabolism of N-alkyl substituted aminopropiophenones in man in comparison to amphetamines and ephedrines. Arch. int. Pharmacodyn. **197**, 392.
17. VREE, T. B., HENDERSON, P. TH. VAN ROSSUM, J. M. and DOUKAS, P. H. (1973) In vivo and in vitro inhibition of the metabolism of amphetamines in rat by ferrocenylisopropylamine. Xenobiotica, **3**, 23.
18. VREE, T. B., HENDERSON, P. TH., DOUKAS, P. H. and VAN ROSSUM, J. M. (1973) Inhibition of

the metabolism of amphetamines in rat by ferrocenylisopropylamine. Psychopharmacologia, **26** (suppl.) 38.
19. VREE, T. B. (1973) Thesis University of Nijmegen.
20. WILKINSON, G. R. and BECKETT, A. H. (1968) Absorption, metabolism and excretion of the ephedrines in man. The influence of urinary pH and urine volume output. J. Pharmacol. exp. Ther. **162**, 139.

T.B.V., Department of Pharmacology, University of Nijmegen, Geert Groote Plein N-21, Nijmegen, The Netherlands

p-CHLOROAMPHETAMINE:
STUDIES ON THE BIOCHEMICAL MECHANISM OF ITS ACTION ON CEREBRAL SEROTONIN[*]

ELAINE SANDERS-BUSH and F. SULSER

Department of Pharmacology, Vanderbilt University School of Medicine and Tennessee Neuropsychiatric Institute, Nashville, Tennessee

Introduction

Since the original observation by Pletscher et al. (19) of the simultaneous decrease in cerebral 5-hydroxytryptamine (5-HT) and 5-hydroxyindole acetic acid (5-HIAA) following the administration of p-chloroamphetamine, the elucidation of the mechanism of these biochemical effects has been the subject of many investigations (3, 6, 8, 10, 13, 14, 20). Previous studies from our laboratory have shown that the administration of p-chloroamphetamine causes a decrease in the rate of turnover of cerebral 5-HT and have suggested that the drug inhibits the synthesis of cerebral 5-HT at the level of the hydroxylation of tryptophan (23). Using isotopic procedures, Costa and Revuelta (4) have confirmed that p-chloroamphetamine reduces the rate of turnover of cerebral 5-HT. Although data on drug-induced changes in the turnover rate of a biogenic amine provide a better indication of the functional state of neurons than do changes in tissue levels, they cannot define the mechanism by which the changes are brought about. In an attempt to elucidate the mechanism by which p-chloroamphetamine decreases the rate of turnover of 5-HT, we have extended our studies to a direct measurement of the activity of cerebral tryptophan hydroxylase and its possible modification by p-chloroamphetamine. The results of these and other recent studies are presented in this paper.

Material and methods

Male Sprague-Dawley rats (180—220 g) were used in all studies. p-Chloroamphetamine hydrochloride was purchased from Regis Chemical Company (Chicago, Illinois) and p-chlorophenylalanine ethylester from Aldrich Chemical Company (Milwaukee, Wisconsin). The drugs were injected intraperitoneally and the doses are expressed in terms of the free base.

In vitro tryptophan hydroxylase activity in brain was assayed by a modification of the method of Lovenberg et al. (12) as described in detail previously (24). Brains were

---

[*] The original investigations reported in this paper have been supported by United States Public Health Service Grant MH-11468.

homogenized in 3 volumes of ice-cold 0.05 M trisacetate buffer (pH 7.4) and the homogenates were centrifuged at 30,000 × g for 20 minutes. Aliquots of the supernatants, equivalent to 100 mg of tissue, were incubated in the presence of L-tryptophan-^{14}C (0.08 mM), pargyline hydrochloride (0.33 mM), 5-HT (0.14 mM) and ferrous ammonium sulfate (0.08 mM) in a final volume of 0.63 ml. The samples were incubated for 1 hour at 37°C and the 5-HT-^{14}C formed was isolated by ion exchange chromatography using Amberlite CG-50 as described by PETERS et al. (17). The activity of tryptophan hydroxylase is expressed as nc 5-HT-^{14}C formed/g/hr.

The conversion of tryptophan-^{3}H to 5-HT-^{3}H in intestine was determined as follows: Rats were injected intravenously with 10 μc of ^{3}H-tryptophan 16 hours after the intraperitoneal injection of p-chloroamphetamine (10 mg/kg) or saline. Animals were sacrificed by decapitation 15 minutes after the administration of ^{3}H-tryptophan, a 10 cm portion of the small intestine was removed, weighed and frozen on dry ice. Endogenous and tritiated 5-HT and tryptophan in the sample of small intestine were isolated by ion exchange chromatography and estimated by spectrophotofluorometry and scintillation radiometry according to a slight modification of the method of SCHUBERT et al. (26).

In the long-term studies, a single dose of p-chloroamphetamine (10 mg/kg) or saline was injected intraperitoneally to rats. At various times after the administration of the drug, the animals were sacrificed and 5-HT, 5-HIAA or the activity of tryptophan hydroxylase were determined. Following removal of the cerebral cortex and cerebellum, the amount of 5-HT in the remaining tissue was analyzed according to BOGDANSKI et al. (2) and 5-HIAA by the method of GIACOLONI and VALZELLI (9).

RESULTS AND DISCUSSION

Effect of p-chloroamphetamine on the activity of tryptophan hydroxylase in brain. When the activity of tryptophan hydroxylase was assayed in brains of rats pretreated with various doses of p-chloroamphetamine, a dose-related reduction in the activity of the enzyme was observed (Table 1). However, the addition of p-chloroamphetamine *in vitro* in concentrations up to 1 mM failed to influence the activity of tryptophan hydroxylase. Under similar conditions, the addition of 0.5 mM p-chlorophenylalanine caused a 65% reduction in the activity of the enzyme (Table 2). The conditions of incubation were

TABLE 1

Effect of the intraperitoneal administration of p-chloroamphetamine on the activity of tryptophan hydroxylase

Dose (mg/kg)	nc[^{14}C] 5-HT formed/g/hr ± S.E.M.	Percent inhibition
0 (5)	31.4 ± 2.9	0
2 (4)	25.2 ± 0.4	20
5 (7)	21.0 ± 1.2	33
7.5 (7)	18.0 ± 2.2	43
10 (7)	12.5 ± 1.2	60

p-Chloroamphetamine was administered i.p. 16 hours prior to sacrifice. The number of animals is shown in parentheses. From SANDERS-BUSH et al. (24).

TABLE 2

Effect of the *in vitro* addition of *p*-chloroamphetamine on the activity of tryptophan hydroxylase

	Tryptophan hydroxylase activity nc[^{14}C]5-HT/g brain/hr
Experiment I	
Control	41.1
p-chloroamphetamine, 1×10^{-5} M	46.9
p-chloroamphetamine, 1×10^{-4} M	48.1
p-chloroamphetamine, 1×10^{-3} M	36.3
p-chlorophenylalanine, 5×10^{-4} M	14.0
Experiment II	
Control	36.4
p-chloroamphetamine, 1×10^{-3} M	31.8
Experiment III	
Control	20.6
p-chloroamphetamine, 1×10^{-4} M	21.4

Values are the mean of duplicate determinations and are representative of several experiments. In Experiment III, the enzyme preparation was preincubated for 30 min. in the presence of *p*-chloroamphetamine. From SANDERS-BUSH et al. (24).

varied in a number of ways (e.g. variation of the concentrations of tryptophan and DMPH$_4$ over a 10-fold range); in no instance was the formation of 5-HT-^{14}C reduced by the addition of *p*-chloroamphetamine. Experiments with *p*-chloromethamphetamine showed that this drug also reduced tryptophan hydroxylase only after its administration *in vivo*. These negative *in vitro* data are in agreement with those of PLETSCHER et al. (21).

The mechanism of the *in vivo* inhibition of cerebral tryptophan hydroxylase by *p*-chloroamphetamine has been investigated (24). The results of these experiments failed to provide evidence that a metabolite of *p*-chloroamphetamine, formed *in vivo*, could be responsible for the decrease in enzyme activity. Experiments involving various combinations of boiled and fresh preparations from treated and control rats did not indicate the presence of a heat-stable inhibitor in the brains of rats pretreated with *p*-chloroamphetamine. In other experiments, it was shown that dialysis of enzyme preparations from control rats and from rats treated with *p*-chloroamphetamine did not reverse the inhibition caused by the drug. Moreover, kinetic studies of tryptophan hydroxylase preparations from control rats and from rats pretreated with *p*-chloroamphetamine showed that the apparent K_m values for tryptophan (3.0×10^{-4}M) and the cofactor, DMPH$_4$, (1.5×10^{-4}M) were the same in both preparations. These results suggest that the drug may have reduced the amount of active enzyme without having altered its properties.

Lack of effect of p-chloroamphetamine on the synthesis of 5-HT in peripheral tissues
The hydroxylation of tryptophan by hepatic preparations has been shown not to be reduced after the *in vivo* administration of *p*-chloroamphetamine or *p*-chloromethamphetamine (5, 19). However, the enzyme in liver which hydroxylates tryptophan is actually phenylalanine hydroxylase and this enzyme has little or no role in the biosynthesis of peripheral

TABLE 3

The effect of p-chloroamphetamine (PCA) on the synthesis of 5-HT in small intestine

Treatment	5-HT			Tryptophan			Conversion index
	nc/g	nmol/g	nc/nmol	nc/g	nmol/g	nc/nmol	nmol/g/min
Saline	2.0 ± 0.1	11 ± 0.3	0.19 ± 0.01	176 ± 7	29 ± 1	6.1 ± 0.4	0.022 ± 0.001
PCA	2.0 ± 0.1	13 ± 0.5	0.16 ± 0.01	166 ± 14	31 ± 3	5.4 ± 0.3	0.025 ± 0.002

Groups of 6 rats were treated with either p-chloroamphetamine (10 mg/kg, i.p.) or saline 16 hours prior to i.v. injection of 150 μc of ^{3}H-tryptophan. Animals were sacrificed 15 minutes later and the specific activity of 5-HT and tryptophan in small intestine was determined.

5-HT (22). In an attempt to more directly assess the effect of p-chloroamphetamine on peripheral tryptophan hydroxylase, we have examined the drug's effect on the synthesis of 5-HT from tryptophan in the intestine. The intraperitoneal administration of p-chloroamphetamine, which maximally reduces the level of 5-HT in brain, did not decrease the steady-state level of 5-HT in the small intestine (Table 3). PLETSCHER et al. (19) have earlier observed that p-chloromethamphetamine exerted no effect on intestinal 5-HT. More importantly, the administration of p-chloroamphetamine did not reduce the conversion of tryptophan-^{3}H to 5-HT-^{3}H in the intestine (Table 3). These results

TABLE 4

Cerebral levels of 5-HT and 5-HIAA and activity of tryptophan hydroxylase at various times after a single dose of p-chloroamphetamine

Time after injection	Percent of control ± S.E.M.		
	5-HT	5-HIAA	Tryptophan hydroxylase
16 hours	39.0 ± 3.6 (4)*	39.6 ± 3.0 (4)*	57.6 ± 1.3 (4)*
4 days	39.6 ± 5.1 (5)*	31.5 ± 2.7 (8)*	52.3 ± 7.9 (5)**
10 days	38.2 ± 3.3 (5)*	—	49.6 ± 1.5 (5)*
2 weeks	47.9 ± 3.2 (9)*	25.8 ± 2.1 (6)*	41.4 ± 7.6 (9)*
4 weeks	62.6 ± 4.5 (11)**	35.3 ± 5.7 (5)*	57.7 ± 6.6 (11)*
6 weeks	73.1 ± 2.3 (4)*	49.2 ± 3.7 (4)*	72.3 ± 7.7 (4)**
2 months	73.2 ± 2.7 (5)**	—	—
4 months	79.5 ± 8.5 (4)***	60.1 ± 3.9 (7)*	60.5 ± 3.0 (4)**

Rats were injected intraperitoneally with a single dose of either saline or 10 mg/kg of p-chloroamphetamine. The animals were sacrificed at various times after the injection. Results are mean values and are expressed as percentage of the respective control values. The number of animals is shown in parentheses. Mean values for all control animals were: 5-HT, 0.69 ± 0.02 μg/gm (n = 43); 5-HIAA, 0.29 ± 0.01 μg/g (n = 33); tryptophan hydroxylase, 78.1 ± 3.9 nc ^{14}C-5HT formed/g/hr (n = 39). From SANDERS-BUSH et al. (25).

*p < 0.001
**p < 0.01
***p < 0.05

demonstrate that *p*-chloroamphetamine does not reduce the turnover rate and the synthesis of 5-HT in peripheral organs, such as the intestine. Moreover, the data suggest that the drug is a selective inhibitor of tryptophan hydroxylase in serotonergic neurons of the CNS.

Long-term effects of p-chloroamphetamine on the metabolism of 5-HT in brain. Results of earlier investigations demonstrated that *p*-chloroamphetamine can cause an irreversible inhibition of cerebral tryptophan hydroxylase (24). Such an inhibition can explain the prolonged, simultaneous decrease of 5-HT and its major metabolite, 5-HIAA, in brain. It was therefore of interest to investigate the long-term changes in enzyme activity and brain 5-HT and 5-HIAA after the administration of *p*-chloroamphetamine.

The effects of a single dose of *p*-chloroamphetamine (10 mg/kg i.p.) on the levels of 5-HT and 5-HIAA and on the activity of tryptophan hydroxylase in brain are shown in Table 4. The maximal decrease in the activity of tryptophan hydroxylase and in the levels of 5-HT and 5-HIAA occurred at about 16 hours. Interestingly, two weeks after the administration of the drug, the activity of tryptophan hydroxylase and the levels of 5-HT and 5-HIAA were still reduced by 50% or more. Four months after the injection of *p*-chloroamphetamine some recovery had occurred, but all three components were still significantly reduced. These results are extremely provocative and require a reevaluation of possible mechanisms by which *p*-chloroamphetamine maintains the prolonged decrease of cerebral 5-HT. Clearly, these biochemical effects persist long after a major portion of the drug has disappeared from the brain (7, 15). Of course, an irreversible inhibition would persist even if the damaging agent is no longer present. However, even though tryptophan hydroxylase is irreversibly inactivated, normal turnover of the enzyme should lead to substantial recovery of activity within 2 weeks, as is the case after the administration of *p*-chlorophenylalanine (Table 5).

TABLE 5

Cerebral levels of 5-HT and activity of tryptophan hydroxylase after a single dose of PCPA

Time after injection	5-HT (μg/g)		Tryptophan hydroxylase (nc 5-HT-^{14}C formed/g/hr)	
	Saline	PCPA	Saline	PCPA
1 day (6)	0.49 ± 0.02	0.14 ± 0.01*	77.9 ± 5.8	6.2 ± 0.6*
2 weeks (7)	0.65 ± 0.01	0.61 ± 0.01	67.6 ± 2.2	53.2 ± 1.9**

Rats were injected intraperitoneally with 300 mg/kg of *p*-chlorophenylalanine ethyl ester (PCPA) or saline either 1 day or 2 weeks prior to sacrifice. The level of 5-HT and the activity of tryptophan hydroxylase in brains were assayed as described in Material and methods. The number of animals is shown in parentheses. From SANDERS-BUSH et al. (25).

*p < 0.001
**p < 0.05

p-Chloroamphetamine is highly localized in the particulate fraction of brain homogenates, where presumably it is bound (7, 18). Interestingly, we have recently found that the ability of synaptosomal preparations to accumulate ^{3}H-5-HT is still markedly reduced 2 weeks after a single dose of *p*-chloroamphetamine, whereas the uptake mechanism for ^{3}H-norepinephrine has, after an initial blockade, fully recovered (unpublished observations from this laboratory). These observations are in agreement with other data that show a temporal relationship between the psychomotor stimulation elicited by *p*-chloroamphetamine and its effect on the metabolism of norepinephrine in brain (27) and a dissociation between the initial excitatory action of the drug and its effect on brain 5-HT (5, 20, 27).

Two other manipulations which have been found to cause a long-lasting reduction in the level of cerebral 5-HT, synaptosomal uptake and in the activity of tryptophan hydroxylase are lesioning of the raphe neurons (11) and the administration of 5,6-dihydroxytryptamine (1), both of which cause a degeneration of serotonergic nerve terminals. Possible mechanisms for the intriguing and extremely long lasting effects elicited by *p*-chloroamphetamine on cerebral 5-HT and tryptophan hydroxylase are presently being investigated. In particular, it has to be seen whether the observed reduction in the level of endogenous cyclic AMP in brain after *p*-chloroamphetamine (16) is in any way causally related to the reduction in the activity of tryptophan hydroxylase.

SUMMARY AND CONCLUSIONS

In many respects, the effects of *p*-chloroamphetamine on cerebral 5-HT and tryptophan hydroxyalse are similar to those elicited by *p*-chlorophenylalanine, a well-known irreversible inhibitor of tryptophan hydroxylase. However, the results presented in this paper clearly demonstrate three important differences between these two drugs:

1. Unlike *p*-chlorophenylalanine, *p*-chloroamphetamine does not inhibit tryptophan hydroxylase *in vitro* in concentrations up to 10^{-3}M.
2. Unlike *p*-chlorophenylalanine, *p*-chloroamphetamine does not reduce the rate of turnover and the biosynthesis of 5-HT in peripheral tissues (e.g. small intestine).
3. The effects of *p*-chloroamphetamine on levels of 5-HT in brain and the activity of cerebral tryptophan hydroxylase last for many months, whereas the effect of *p*-chlorophenylalanine has disappeared within two weeks.

REFERENCES

1. BAUMGARTEN, H. G. and LACHENMAYER, L. (1972) Chemically induced degeneration of indoleamine-containing nerve terminals in rat brain. Brain Res. **38**, 228.
2. BOGDANSKI, D. F., PLETSCHER, A., BRODIE, B. B. and UDENFRIEND, S. (1956) Identification and assay of serotonin in brain. J. Pharmacol. exp. Ther. **117**, 82.
3. CARLSSON, A. (1970) Structural specificity for inhibition of ^{14}C-5-hydroxytryptamine uptake by cerebral slices. J. Pharm. Pharmacol. **22**, 729.
4. COSTA, E. and REVUELTA, A. (1972) (-)-p-Chloroamphetamine and serotonin turnover in rat brain. Neuropharmacology, **11**, 291.
5. FULLER, R. W., HINES, C. W. and MILLS, J. (1965) Lowering of brain serotonin level by chloroamphetamines. Biochem. Pharmacol. **14**, 483.
6. FULLER, R. W. (1966) Serotonin oxidation by rat brain monoamine oxidase: Inhibition by 4-chloroamphetamine. Life Sci. **5**, 2247.
7. FULLER, R. W. and HINES, C. W. (1967) Tissue levels of chloroamphetamine in rats and mice. J. pharm. Sci. **56**, 302.
8. FULLER, R. W. and HINES, C. W. (1970) Inhibition by *p*-chloroamphetamine of the conversion of 5-hydroxytryptamine to 5-hydroxyindoleacetic acid in rat brain. J. Pharm. Pharmacol. **22**, 634.
9. GIACOLONI, E. and VALZELLI, L. (1966) A method for the determination of 5-hydroxyindolyl-3-acetic acid in brain. J. Neurochem. **13**, 1265.
10. KORF, J. and VAN PRAGG, H. M. (1972) Action of *p*-chloroamphetamine on cerebral serotonin metabolism: An hypothesis. Neuropharmacology, **11**, 141.
11. KUHAR, M. J., ROTH, R. H. and AGHAJANIAN, G. K. (1972) Synaptosomes from forebrains of rats with midbrain raphe lesions: Selective reduction of serotonin uptake. J. Pharmacol. exp. Ther. **181**, 36.

12. LOVENBERG, W., JEQUIER, E. and SJOERDSMA, A. (1967) Tryptophan hydroxylation: Measurement in pineal gland, brainstem and carcinoid tumor, Science, 155, 217.
13. MEEK, J. L. and CARLSSON, A. (1971) Blockade of p-chloromethamphetamine induced 5-hydroxytryptamine depletion by chlorimipramine, chlorpheniramine and mepheridine. Biochem. Pharmacol. 20, 707.
14. MEEK, J. L. and FUXE, K. (1971) Serotonin accumulation after monoamine oxidase inhibition. Effect of decreased impulse flow and of some antidepressants and hallucinogens. Biochem. Pharmacol. 20, 693.
15. MILLER, K. W., SANDERS-BUSH, E. and DINGELL, J. V. (1971) p-Chloroamphetamine: Species differences in the rate of disappearance and the lowering of cerebral serotonin. Biochem. Pharmacol. 20, 500.
16. PALMER, G. C., ROBINSON, G. A., MANIAN, A. A. and SULSER, F. (1972) Modification by psychotropic drugs of the cyclic AMP response to norepinephrine in the rat brain *in vitro*. Psychopharmacologia, 23, 201.
17. PETERS, D. A. V., MCGEER, P. L. and MCGEER, E. G. (1968) The distribution of tryptophan hydroxylase in cat brain. J. Neurochem. 15, 1431.
18. PFEIFER, A. K., CSÁKI, L., FODOR, M., GYÖRGY, L. and ÖKRÖS, K. (1969) The subcellular distribution of (+)-amphetamine and (±)-p-chloroamphetamine in the rat brain as influenced by reserpine. J. Pharm. Pharmacol. 21, 687.
19. PLETSCHER, A., BARTHOLINI, G., BRUDERER, H., BURKARD, W. P. and GEY, K. F. (1964) Chlorinated arylalkylamines affecting the cerebral metabolism of 5-hydroxytryptamine. J. Pharmacol. exp. Ther. 145, 344.
20. PLETSCHER, A., DA PRADA, M., BURKARD, W. P., BARTHOLINI, G., STEINER, F. A., BRUDERER, H. and BIGLER, F. (1966) Aralkylamines with different effects on the metabolism of aromatic monoamines. J. Pharmacol. exp. Ther. 154, 64.
21. PLETSCHER, A., DA PRADA, M. and BURKARD, W. P. (1970) The effect of substituted phenylethylamines on the metabolism of biogenic amines, in Amphetamines and Related Compounds, ed. E. COSTA and S. GARATTINI, Raven Press, N.Y., 331.
22. RENSON, J., WEISSBACH, H. and UDENFRIEND, S. (1962) Hydroxylation of tryptophan by phenylalanine hydroxylase, J. biol. Chem. 237, 2261.
23. SANDERS-BUSH, E. and SULSER, F. (1970) p-Chloroamphetamine: *In vivo* investigations on the mechanism of action of the selective depletion of cerebral serotonin, J. Pharmacol. exp. Ther. 175, 419.
24. SANDERS-BUSH, E., BUSHING, J. A. and SULSER, F. (1972) p-Chloroamphetamine — Inhibition of cerebral tryptophan hydroxylase, Biochem. Pharmacol. 21, 1501.
25. SANDERS-BUSH, E., BUSHING, J. A. and SULSER, F. (1972) Long-term effects of p-chloroamphetamine on tryptophan hydroxylase activity and on the levels of 5-hydroxytryptamine and 5-hydroxyindole acetic acid in brain. Europ. J. Pharmacol. in press.
26. SCHUBERT, J., NYBACK, H. and SEDVALL, G. (1970) Accumulation and disappearance of ^{3}H-5-hydroxytryptamine formed from ^{3}H-tryptophan in mouse brain: Effect of LSD-25. Europ. J. Pharmacol. 10, 215.
27. STRADA, S. J., SANDERS-BUSH, E. and SULSER, F. (1970) p-Chloroamphetamine: Temporal relationship between psychomotor stimulation and metabolism of brain norepinephrine. Biochem. Pharmacol. 19, 2621.

E.S.-B., Department of Pharmacology, Vanderbilt University School of Medicine, Nashville, Tennessee, U.S.A.

THE EFFECT OF β,β-DIFLUORO SUBSTITUTION ON THE METABOLISM AND PHARMACOLOGY OF AMPHETAMINES

R. W. FULLER, B. B. MOLLOY and C. J. PARLI

The Lilly Research Laboratories, Eli Lilly and Company, Indianapolis, Indiana

INTRODUCTION

In a recent symposium on amphetamines and related compounds, LE DOUAREC and NEVEU (9) wrote: "It might have been thought that a molecule whose structure has been known as long as amphetamine's has would have been substituted to such a degree that it would be impossible to imagine any further development." Indeed, a wide variety of substituted amphetamines have been prepared and studied. However, few derivatives appear to have been made specifically to investigate the role of ionization in the pharmacologic actions of amphetamine.

The importance of ionization in the effects of many drugs has long been recognized. LEWIS (11) considered the influence of ionization on the activity of sympathomimetic amines, but the amines he studied all had pK_a values well above physiological pH. Among a large group of amphetamine-like compounds that VREE et al. (16) studied, only those with substituents on the nitrogen (like benzylamphetamine or benzphetamine) had pK_a values lower than 9. Recently we have described some fluorinated derivatives of amphetamine that have low pK_a values (6, 7).

Fluorine is a strongly electronegative atom, and when substituted β to the nitrogen of amphetamine it pulls electrons away from the nitrogen and reduces the pK_a. Fluorine is a relatively small atom so that steric influence is slight. The β carbon is not a major site of metabolic attack on amphetamine nor is it known to take part in the attachment of amphetamine to "receptors". Thus, any changes in the pharmacology or metabolism of amphetamine that result from the difluoro substitution are most likely due to differences in ionization. This report deals with those changes.

METHODS

The fluorinated compounds were synthesized in the Lilly Research Laboratories and were used as the soluble hydrochloride salts. The difluoro compounds were racemic mixtures, and the monofluoro compound was one racemic pair of diastereoisomers. dl-Amphetamine sulfate was purchased from the Chemicals Procurement Laboratories, and dl--4-chloroamphetamine hydrochloride was purchased from the Regis Chemical Company.

Male albino rats of the Wistar strain, weighing about 150 g, were obtained from a local breeder. Drugs were injected as aqueous solutions intraperitoneally. The rats were decapitated, and tissues were quickly removed and frozen on dry ice, then stored frozen prior to analysis. Drug levels were measured spectrophotometrically by the methyl orange assay (1, 4). In one experiment, drug levels in the supernatant fraction and in the particulate fraction of brain were determined. In that case, brains were homogenized in 2.5 mM sucrose, and the homogenates were centrifuged at 100,000 $\times$ g for 30 min. The supernatant and the particulate fractions were then assayed for drug in the usual way.

For *in vitro* microsomal studies, liver microsomes were prepared by standard techniques and incubated with drug and a TPNH-generating system. Deaminated products were extracted and determined by gas-liquid chromatography.

Results

Properties of fluorinated amphetamines. Steric influences by substitution of fluorine onto the β carbon of amphetamine appear to be minimal. Figure 1 illustrates that the carbon-

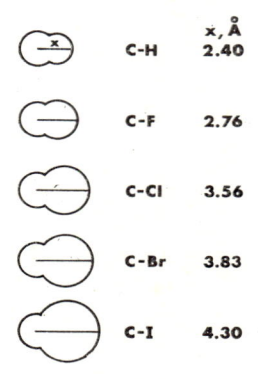

		x, Å
C-H		2.40
C-F		2.76
C-Cl		3.56
C-Br		3.83
C-I		4.30

Fig. 1. Relative sizes of carbon-hydrogen and carbon-halogen groups. The distances ($\times$) were calculated from the tetrahedral covalent radii and the Van der Waals radii given in reference (13).

fluorine group is similar in size to the carbon-hydrogen, with much less steric influence than when other halogen atoms are added. We therefore assume that steric factors contribute little to the altered properties of amphetamine resulting from the introduction of the fluorines.

In contrast to the small change in size of the amphetamine molecule brought about by the fluorines, the basicity of amphetamine is markedly altered (Table 1). A single electron-withdrawing fluorine atom reduces the pK_a by more than one pH unit, and addition of a second fluorine atom further lowers the pK_a by at least as much. Thus the pK_a of β,β-difluoroamphetamine is below physiological pH. At pH 7.4, amphetamine and β-monofluoroamphetamine would exist nearly completely as charged molecules, that is in the cationic form. On the other hand, β,β-difluoroamphetamine would exist mainly (73%) as a neutral molecule. It seemed likely that this altered state of ionization would substantially influence the transport systems and enzymic processes that govern tissue distribution and metabolism, respectively. With that in mind, we examined the distribution and metabolism of these substances in rats.

TABLE 1

Ionization of β-substituted amphetamines

Compound	pK$_a$	At pH 7.4, %	
		RNH$_2$	RNH$_3$
Ph-CH$_2$-CH(CH$_3$)-NH$_2$	9.45	1	99
Ph-CHF-CH(CH$_3$)-NH$_2$	8.35	10	90
Ph-CF$_2$-CH(CH$_3$)-NH$_2$	6.97	73	27

Distribution of fluorinated amphetamines. A comparison of the drug levels in various tissues after the injection of amphetamine, β-monofluoroamphetamine, or β,β-difluoroamphetamine to rats is shown in Fig. 2. The order of tissue distribution for amphetamine was

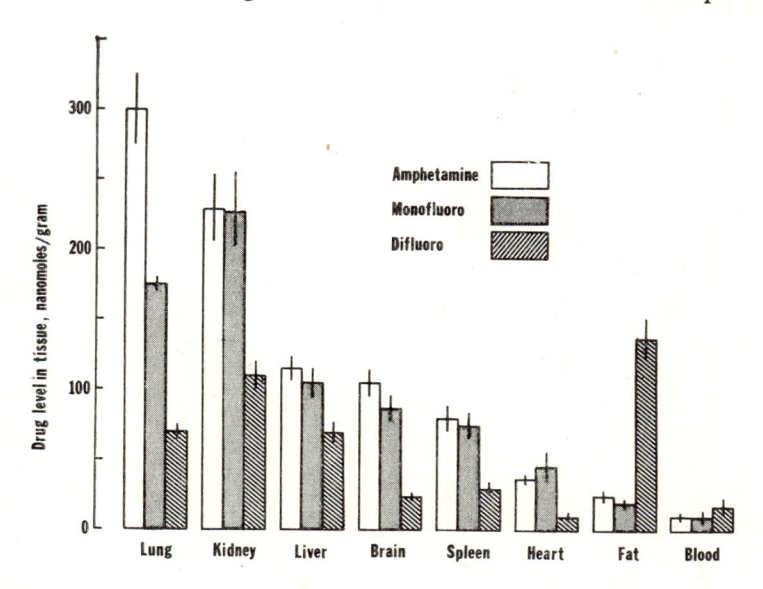

Fig. 2. Tissue distribution of drugs in rats 1 hr after i.p. injection of 0.1 mmole/kg doses of amphetamine, β-monofluoroamphetamine, and β, β-difluoroamphetamine. Mean values and standard errors for 5 rats per group are shown.

lung > kidney > liver > brain > spleen > heart > fat > blood. The distribution of the monofluoro derivative was in general like that of amphetamine; there was less of the monofluoro compound in the lung, but in all other tissues the levels were not significantly different from those of amphetamine. In sharp contrast to this was the distribution of the difluoro compound. β,β-Difluoroamphetamine localized chiefly in epididymal fat, where

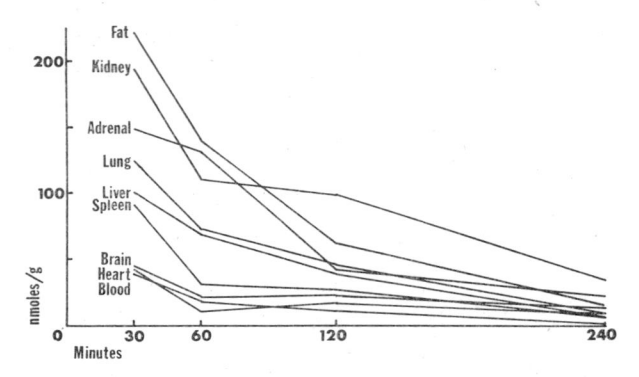

Fig. 3. Disappearance of β,β-difluoroamphetamine from tissues of rats after i.p. injection of 0.1 mmole/kg. Drug levels in all tissues were determined at 30, 60, 120 and 240 minutes. There were 5 rats per group, and the lines connect points representing the mean value for each time. Standard errors are omitted for clarity but were comparable in magnitude to those shown in Fig. 2.

it was present at 5 times the concentration of amphetamine. In all other tissues, the levels of the difluoro compound were much lower than those of amphetamine. In the brain, for example, the difluoro compound was present at only about $\frac{1}{4}$ the concentration of amphetamine. The order of tissue distribution for the difluoro compound, fat > kidney > > liver > lung > spleen > brain > blood > heart, was noticeably different from that of amphetamine or β-monofluoroamphetamine.

To determine if the fat served as a depot for β,β-difluoroamphetamine (referred to hereafter simply as difluoroamphetamine) that would hold the compound for longer times than would other tissues, we measured the tissue levels of that drug at other time intervals (Fig. 3). During the first four hours after drug administration, difluoroamphetamine disappeared from fat as rapidly as from other tissues. The tissue distribution was roughly the same at each of the four time points studied, except that at 2 and 4 hours the kidney had somewhat higher levels of drug.

Previously we had reported that the distribution of amphetamine between the supernatant and particulate fractions of a brain homogenate was markedly altered by 4-chloro substitution (5). Since one effect of the 4-chloro is to increase lipophilicity, we thought the introduction of fluorines might alter this subcellular distribution as well. Fig. 4 shows the distribution of amphetamine and of 4-chloroamphetamine compared to their β,β-difluorinated analogues. The fluorines had no effect on the subcellular distribution of amphetamine; amphetamine was found primarily in the supernatant fraction. The fluorines had only a slight influence on the subcellular distribution of 4-chloroamphetamine, which was found mainly in the particulate fraction. In that case, the addition of the fluorines slightly reduced the degree of association with the particulate material.

Metabolism of fluorinated amphetamines. The disappearance of amphetamine from brain and the influence of molecular substituents on that disappearance rate is shown in Fig. 5.

The addition of the 4-chloro markedly prolonged the half-life, an observation made previously (5) and explained by the fact that the 4-chloro substituent blocks the major route of metabolism of amphetamine in the rat, para-hydroxylation (3). Difluoroamphetamine had a half-life (93 min) similar to that of amphetamine (77 min). In the case of the difluoro compound, however, the introduction of the 4-chloro did not delay the disappearance of the drug at all. Although this observation might be explained in other ways, it first suggested to us that the metabolism as well as the distribution of the difluoro compounds was different from that of amphetamine.

For a number of years, desmethylimipramine (DMI) and similar tricyclic drugs have been known to enhance the levels of amphetamine in rat brain through inhibition of its metabolism by para-hydroxylation (2, 10, 15). Fig. 6 shows data confirming that effect of DMI but revealing that difluoroamphetamine levels were unaffected by DMI. Again,

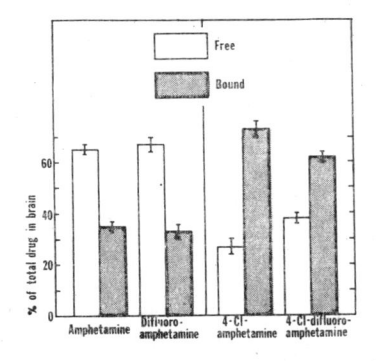

Fig. 4. Subcellular distribution of drugs in rat brain 1 hr after injection of 0.1 mmole/kg doses. Mean values and standard errors for 5 rats per group are shown. "Free" and "bound" drug levels represent the concentrations measured in the supernatant and particulate fractions, respectively, after high speed centrifugation of brain homogenates as described in the text.

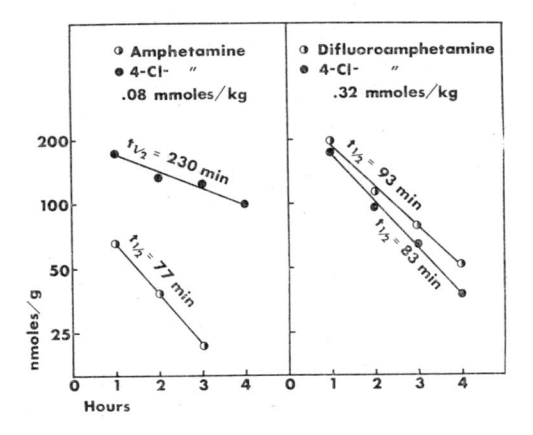

Fig. 5. Rate of disappearance of drugs from rat brain. Mean values for 5 rats per group are shown at each time point. The difluoro compounds were injected at four times the dose of the parent amphetamines to produce comparable drug levels in brain.

these data are most simply explained if the metabolism of difluoroamphetamine occurs by a pathway other than para-hydroxylation.

If different metabolic pathways were involved, we thought it might be possible to find a metabolic inhibitor that would affect difluoroamphetamine but not amphetamine. DPEA (2,4-dichloro-6-phenyl-phenoxyethylamine), a known inhibitor of hepatic microsomal enzymes, was found to be like DMI in that it enhanced brain levels of amphetamine, not difluoroamphetamine. On the other hand, SKF 525A (Fig. 7) had only a slight and not significant effect on amphetamine levels but doubled the levels of difluoro amphetamine. These results suggest that the difluoro compound is metabolized by an SKF 525A-sensitive pathway other than para-hydroxylation.

Fig. 8 illustrates the differences between amphetamine and difluoroamphetamine in terms of the effect of DMI on urinary excretion of drug metabolites. DMI increased by

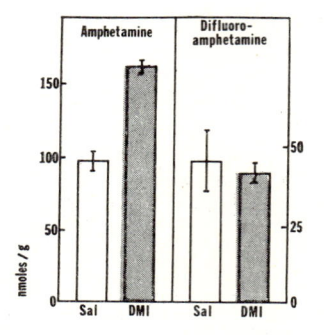

Fig. 6. Enhancement by desmethylimipramine of the levels of amphetamine but not β,β-difluoroamphetamine in rat brain. Amphetamine and β,β-difluoroamphetamine were injected i.p. at 0.1 mmole/kg 1 hr before the rats were killed. DMI was injected i.p. at 5 mg/kg 2 hrs before the rats were killed. Mean values and standard errors for 5 rats per group are shown.

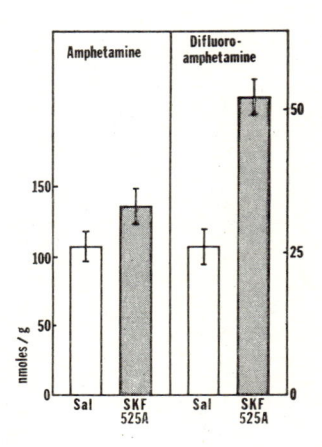

Fig. 7. Enhancement by SKF 525A of the levels of β,β-difluoroamphetamine but not amphetamine in rat brain. Experiments as in Fig. 6 except that SKF 525A (10 mg/kg) was injected in place of DMI. Mean values and standard errors for 5 rats per group are shown.

several-fold the amount of amphetamine excreted unchanged into the urine and reduced the amount of para-hydroxylated metabolite. In contrast, DMI did not influence the amount of difluoroamphetamine excreted unchanged. In control rats, the amount of unchanged difluoroamphetamine excreted was about the same as the amount of unchanged amphetamine indicating both compounds had been metabolized to about the same extent.

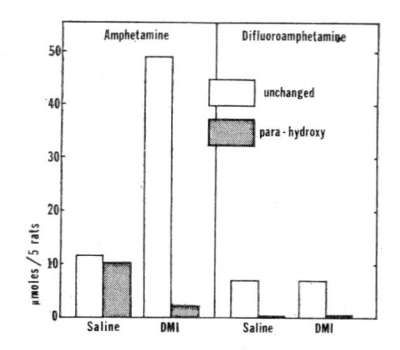

Fig. 8. Effect of desmethylimipramine on the 24-hr urinary excretion of unchanged drug and para-hydroxy metabolites after amphetamine or β,β-difluoroamphetamine injection into rats. Amphetamine or β,β-difluoroamphetamine was injected i.p. at 0.1 mmole/kg, and urine was collected for the next 24 hrs. In one group, DMI had been injected i.p. at 5 mg/kg 1 hr before the other drugs. Urine from 5 rats was combined for analysis.

No para-hydroxylated material could be detected after injection of difluoroamphetamine either with or without DMI; this finding is inconclusive because we had no parahydroxy difluoroamphetamine as a reference standard and suspect that it might be unstable even if it were formed. However, the failure of DMI to influence the excretion of unchanged difluoroamphetamine again indicates that drug is metabolized by a pathway other than para-hydroxylation.

Table 2 compares the rate of deaminated metabolite production from amphetamine and difluoroamphetamine by rat liver microsomes *in vitro*. As can be seen, the rate of metabolism of the difluoro compound was greater than that of amphetamine. These results suggest that the route of metabolism of the difluoro compound in rats is through oxidative deamination, in contrast to the parahydroxylation of amphetamine. In support of that is the finding of the oxime of difluorophenylacetone in free and conjugated form in the urine of rats given difluoroamphetamine (12).

TABLE 2

Comparative rates of oxidative deamination of amphetamine and difluoroamphetamine by rat liver microsomes

Substrate	Nanomoles product formed/g liver/30 min		
	Ketone (alcohol)	Oxime	Total
Amphetamine	7.2	5.6	12.8
Difluoroamphetamine	8.2	63.8	72.0

Pharmacology of fluorinated amphetamines. We have earlier reported (7) that in mice the increased motor activity caused by amphetamine is reduced by β,β-difluoro substitution and the duration of the effect is shortened. These effects of the difluoro substitution seem to be accounted for by (a) the localization of difluoroamphetamine in fat at the expense of tissues like the brain and (b) the very short half-life of difluoroamphetamine in mice. Careful observation of both rats and mice treated with difluoroamphetamine revealed subtle differences in behavioral effects of that compound compared to amphetamine, but further investigation is necessary to define these differences more precisely. Quite possibly the regional distribution of difluoroamphetamine within the anatomical areas of the brain may differ from that of amphetamine.

Difluoroamphetamine shares other pharmacologic properties with amphetamine, i.e., it causes hyperthermia, reduces appetite, and mobilizes free fatty acids into plasma of experimental animals (8). All of the effects that are central in origin (increased motor activity, hyperthermia, anorexia) require higher doses of difluoroamphetamine by a factor of about four to produce effects equal to those of amphetamine. In rats the higher dose appears to be due entirely to the altered tissue distribution of difluoroamphetamine, since its rate of metabolism is about equal to that of amphetamine.

Difluoroamphetamine is essentially equipotent with amphetamine in elevating plasma free fatty acids in rats (8; SHAW, unpublished studies). Since difluoroamphetamine localizes in fat to a much higher degree than amphetamine, one might have expected the difluoro compound to be a more potent lipolytic agent. The exact mechanism by which amphetamine stimulates lipolysis is unknown (14), but the lack of *in vitro* activity would suggest that it does not act directly on the adipocyte. Thus the presence of high concentrations of difluoroamphetamine in fat, if the compound is contained within the adipocytes, could not be expected to lead to greater mobilization of free fatty acids. In any case, it is possible to elevate circulating free fatty acids with doses of difluoroamphetamine that are essentially devoid of CNS stimulant activity; as a lipolytic agent, difluoroamphetamine is freer of side effects than is amphetamine.

Discussion

The substitution of two fluorines on the β carbon of amphetamine markedly alters its distibution in tissues, its metabolism, and its pharmacologic profile. Inasmuch as the steric influence (of the fluorines) is small, the major factor leading to the altered biologic properties probably relate to the reduction of the pK_a caused by the electron withdrawing effect of fluorine. Difluoroamphetamine exists at physiologic pH primarily as a neutral molecule, whereas amphetamine is almost completely cationic. Thus the tendency of difluoroamphetamine to localize in adipose tissue is understood on the basis of its non-charged nature. All other tissues contain less difluoroamphetamine than amphetamine after equimolar doses. This result probably does not indicate any difficulty of the difluoro compound in penetrating other tissues, but simply the rapid equilibration between tissues, with fat accumulating higher levels at the expense of the other organs.

The metabolism of amphetamine in mice is markedly accelerated by the difluoro substitution (7). In rats the rate of metabolism is not changed much by the difluoro substitution but the route of metabolism appears to be shifted. Whereas rats metabolize amphetamine almost entirely by para-hydroxylation, they metabolize difluoroamphetamine by oxidative deamination.

Complete evaluation of the changes in pharmacologic activity brought about by the difluoro substitution remains to be completed, but present results suggest that difluoroamphetamine and amphetamine produce similar effects, the differences in their pharmacologic profiles probably relating mainly to the different tissue distribution of the two compounds. For example, central actions of difluoroamphetamine require higher doses than with amphetamine because a greater proportion of the difluoro compound localizes in tissue other than the brain, i.e., fat. These studies underscore the importance of ionization of basic drugs in influencing their biologic fate and their pharmacologic properties.

SUMMARY

Substitution of a fluorine on the β carbon of amphetamine reduces the pK_a because of the electron-withdrawing nature of fluorine. β,β-Difluoroamphetamine has a pK_a lower than physiologic pH and so exists mainly as a neutral molecule whereas amphetamine is cationic. As a result, both tissue distribution and metabolism are altered. Difluoroamphetamine is localized predominantly in adipose tissue, the tissue in which amphetamine is least abundant. Difluoroamphetamine is metabolized by deamination, whereas amphetamine is metabolized by para-hydroxylation. Difluoroamphetamine has many of the same pharmacologic actions as amphetamine (motor stimulation, anorexia, hyperthermia, lipolysis) but the dose-response curves for the central actions are different.

ACKNOWLEDGMENTS

We are grateful for the assistance of Kenneth L. Hauser, Harold D. Snoddy, and Nancy Wang Lee in the experiments described herein.

REFERENCES

1. AXELROD, J. (1954) Studies on sympathomimetic amines. II. The biotransformation and physiological disposition of d-amphetamine, d-p-hydroxyamphetamine and d-methamphetamine. J. Pharmacol. exp. Ther. **110**, 315.
2. CONSOLO, S., DOLFINI, E., GARATTINI, S. and VALZELLI, L. (1967) Desipramine and amphetamine metabolism. J. Pharm. Pharmacol. **19**, 253.
3. DRING, L. G., SMITH, R. L. and WILLIAMS, R. T. (1970) The metabolic fate of amphetamine in man and other species. Biochem. J. **116**, 425.
4. DUBNICK, B., LEESON, G. A., LEVERETT, R., MORGAN, D. F. and PHILLIPS, G. E. (1963) Sympathomimetic properties of chlorphentermine: metabolism, metabolic effects, interaction with reserpine and biogenic amines. J. Pharmacol. exp. Ther. **140**, 85.
5. FULLER, R. W. and HINES, C. W. (1967) Tissue levels of chloroamphetamines in rats and mice. J. pharm. Sci. **56**, 302.
6. FULLER, R. W. and MOLLOY, B. B. (1971) Tissue distribution and metabolism of amphetamine, ß-fluoroamphetamine, and ß, ß-difluoroamphetamine in the rat. Pharmacologist, **13**, 294.
7. FULLER, R. W., MOLLOY, B. B., ROUSH, B. W. and HAUSER, K. L. (1972) Disposition and behavioral effects of amphetamine and ß, ß-difluoroamphetamine in mice. Biochem. Pharmacol. **21**, 1299.
8. FULLER, R. W., SHAW, W. N. and MOLLOY, B. B. (1972) Dissociation of the lipid mobilizing and hyperthermic effects of amphetamine by ß-fluoro substitution. Arch. int. Pharmacodyn. **199**, 194.
9. LE DOUAREC, J. C. and NEVEU, C. (1970) Pharmacology and biochemistry of fenfluramine. In COSTA, E. and GARATTINI, S. (Eds.). Amphetamines and Related Compounds (Raven Press). New York.
10. LEWANDER, T. (1969) Influence of various psychoactive drugs on the *in vivo* metabolism of d-amphetamine in the rat. Europ. J. Pharmacol. **6**, 38.
11. LEWIS, G. P. (1954) The importance of ionization in the activity of sympathomimetic amines. Brit. J. Pharmacol. **9**, 488.

12. PARLI, C. J. and LEE, N. W. (1972) Oxidative deamination of amphetamine and ß, ß-difluoro-amphetamine by rat liver microsomes. Abstracts of Fifth International Congress on Pharmacology.
13. PAULING, L. (1960) The Nature of the Chemical Bond, 3rd Edition. (Cornell University Press). Ithaca, New York.
14. SHAW, W. N., FULLER, R. W. and MATSUMOTO, C. (1972) Studies on the mechanism of amphetamine-induced lipolysis in the rat. Europ. J. Pharmacol. **19**, 98.
15. SULSER, F., OWENS, M. L. and DINGELL, J. V. (1966) On the mechanism of amphetamine potentiation by desimipramine (DMI). Life Sci. **5**, 2005.
16. VREE, T. B., MUSKENS, A. TH. J. M. and VAN ROSSUM, J. M. (1969) Some physico-chemical properties of amphetamine and related drugs. J. Pharm. Pharmacol. **21**, 774.

R.W.F., The Lilly Research Laboratories, Eli Lilly & Co., Indianapolis, Indiana, U.S.A.

DRUGS AND CERTAIN CONDITIONS INTERFERING WITH THE METABOLISM AND EXCRETION OF AMPHETAMINE IN THE RAT[*]

T. LEWANDER and J. JONSSON

Psychiatric Research Center, University of Uppsala,
Ulleråker Hospital, Uppsala

Introduction

The main pathway of metabolism of amphetamine in the rat is through p-hydroxylation; a minor pathway being the oxidative deamination of the drug to benzoic acid, which is conjugated with glycine to hippuric acid (1, 3, 19, 20, 21). (20) The degree of p-hydroxylation varies widely among the species.

Sulser, Owens and Dingell (42) and Valzelli, Consolo and Morpurgo (47) showed, that pretreatment of rats with desmethylimipramine (DMI) caused an increase in the brain concentration of subsequently administrered amphetamine. This finding was explained by the demonstration, that DMI inhibits the p-hydroxylation of amphetamine (11, 32).

Since then, a large number of chemically and pharmacologically different agents have been shown to interfere with the disposition and metabolism of amphetamine in the rat. Many of these drugs are thought to have rather specific effects on monoaminergic mechanisms and have been used as pharmacological tools for elucidation of the mechanisms of action of amphetamine. In a number of cases erroneous conclusions have been reached, due to negligence of the possibility of a metabolic interaction with amphetamine. Furthermore, one of the generally used screening tests of antidepressive properties of new drugs has been the determination of potentiation of amphetamine excitation in rats. It is the aim of the present communication to help avoid these errors in future research by reviewing the literature on this subject. In addition, a few new drugs are added to the list of inhibitors of amphetamine metabolism in the rat.

Methods

^{14}C- and ^{3}H-labelled amphetamine (CEA, Saclay, Gif-sur-Yvette and New England Nuclear respectively) was administered after which samples of urine or tissues were taken

---

[*] Original data are from studies supported by the Swedish Medical Research Council (project no B 73-04X-1017-09, TL) and The Tricentennial Fund of the Bank of Sweden (project No 150).

for determination of amphetamine and its metabolites. The radiopurity of each batch of labelled drug was checked and when necessary impurities were separated from amphetamine by ion exchange chromatography (34).

Determination of amphetamine in tissues

Single rat brains were homogenized in 0.4 M perchloric acid. Plasma was prepared by centrifugation of blood samples in heparinized tubes. Amphetamine-^{3}H was extracted into toluene at pH $>$ 12 (recovery $>$ 90%). An aliquot of the toluene phase was than directly transferred into a counting vial containing the scintillation mixture for measurement of radioactivity (23, 34). This procedure seems to be selective for amphetamine as no metabolites of the drug or nonspecific radioactivity were present in the final extracts on checking with ion-exchange chromatography (34).

Determination of urinary metabolites of amphetamine

The pattern of distribution of radioactive amphetamine metabolites in urine was determined by paper chromatography. The system described by ELLISON, GUTZAIT and VAN LOON (21) has been found very useful, since an aliquot of urine is applied directly on the paper strip without prior purification. In this system amphetamine, p-hydroxyamphetamine (free and conjugated), hippuric acid and some unidentified metabolites are well separated. Parahydroxynorephedrine and norephedrine, if present, do not interfere with the p-hydroxy-amphetamine or amphetamine peaks in this system.

RESULTS AND DISCUSSION

Approaches of establishing metabolic interactions with amphetamine in rats

1. *Disappearance rate of amphetamine.* The tissue (mostly brain, liver or plasma) concentration of amphetamine has been determined at a few time intervals after the administration of the drug or drug combinations. On the assumption of a monoexponential decline of amphetamine a straight line has generally been adapted to the points obtained in a semilogaritmic plot. Amphetamine disappears, however, in 2 or 3 phases with different $T\frac{1}{2}$, between 15 minutes and 12 hours after its intraperitoneal administration (Fig. 1) as shown by MAICKEL et al. (37) for a series of doses of amphetamine and later confirmed by LEWANDER (34). The genesis of the multiexponential decline of amphetamine is not known although the initial phase might possibly be one of distribution.

Due to the polyphasic disappearance of amphetamine in rats changes in the $T\frac{1}{2}$ of amphetamine should be interpreted with caution, unless significant differences in tissue concentrations of amphetamine at 2 or more time points are present.

The effect of 780 SE, a fenfluramine derivative (see Table 1), on brain and plasma concentrations of amphetamine is shown in Fig. 1. This substance, like e.g. DMI and fenfluramine, causes both increases in the amphetamine levels and slower rates of disappearance of amphetamine in the initial phases. The relation between urinary p-hydroxyamphetamine and amphetamine is reversed by 780 SE, which indicates inhibition of p-hydroxylation (24).

2. *Pattern of urinary metabolites of amphetamine.* Urine is collected for 4—24 hours after administration of radioactively labelled amphetamine. The percentage of the administered dose excreted is calculated and the different metabolites are quantitated and calculated as percentages of administered or excreted dose. Typical radiochromatograms

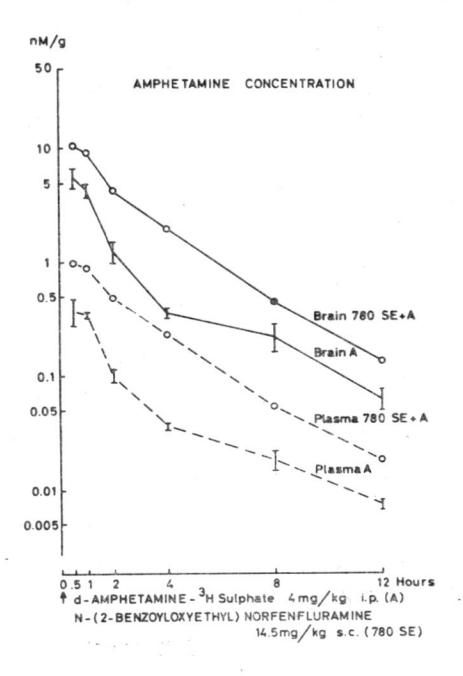

Fig. 1. Effect of 780 SE, a fenfluramine derivative (see Table 1), on the disappearance of amphetamine from brain and plasma in rats. Four mg/kg of d-amphetamine-^{3}H sulphate, 12 μCi/rat, was administered i.p., 780 SE, 14,5 mg/kg s.c., was given 1 hour before the amphetamine injection. Points and vertical bars represent means of 3—4 observations $\pm$ SEM. Open symbols represent statistically significant differences (p $<$ 0.05, Student's t-test) from control rats.

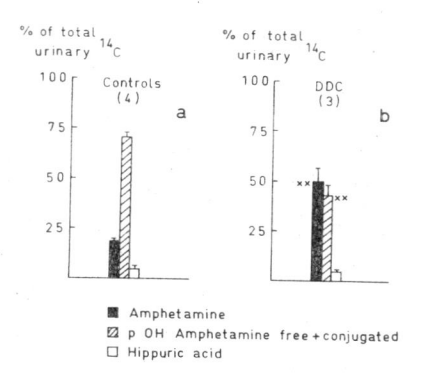

Fig. 2a. Pattern of distribution of urinary metabolites of d-amphetamine-^{14}C in control rats. Unchanged amphetamine p-hydroxyamphetamine (free + conjugated) and hippuric acid are expressed as percentages ($\pm$ SEM) of excreted radioactivity during 24 hours after i.p. injection of 5 μCi of d-amphetamine-^{14}C per rat. Figures within brackets represent number of observations.

Fig. 2b. Changes in the pattern of urinary metabolites of amphetamine caused by diethyldithiocarbamate (DDC), 400 mg/kg, given s.c. 1 hour before d-amphetamine-^{14}C.

of rat urine samples, are to be found in ELLISON et al. (21) and LEWANDER (32). The pattern of metabolites of amphetamine (amphetamine *p*-hydroxyamphetamine free + conjugated, hippuric acid) may be depicted as in Fig. 2a.

Fig. 2b shows the changes in the distribution of metabolites of amphetamine induced by diethyldithiocarbamate (DDC), a metabolite of disulfiram known as a dopamine-β-hydroxylase inhibitor (9). This agent apparently inhibits *p*-hydroxylation of amphetamine and thereby causes increased brain and plasma concentrations of amphetamine when the two drugs are given together (25).

3. *Studies on amphetamine metabolism in vitro*. The isolated perfused rat liver has been reported to be a suitable preparation for studies of amphetamine metabolism *in vitro* (16). Ordinary preparations of rat liver microsomes hydroxylate amphetamine at very slow rates (15, 16, 22) for thus far unknown reasons. Deamination of amphetamine however, proceeds easily with microsomal preparations from rabbit liver (4). Rabbits do not hydroxylate amphetamine (3, 20).

Influence of age, sex and some other factors on the disappearance rate and metabolism of amphetamine

According to GROPPETTI and COSTA (22) the rate of decline of amphetamine in whole young male rats (40—60 g) seem to be slower than in adult (200—250 g) rats. In "young" female rats (150—200 g), the $T\frac{1}{2}$ of amphetamine was slightly more rapid than in "old" females (300 g rats) (49). A difference in $T\frac{1}{2}$ of amphetamine between male (76 minutes) and female (130 minutes) rats has also been reported by GROPPETTI and COSTA (22).

As shown in Fig. 3 there were no significant differences in the pattern of distribution of urinary metabolites of amphetamine between ages and sexes. However small changes in the initial rate of metabolism of amphetamine *in vivo* may be masked when 24 hour urine samples are collected for studies of amphetamine metabolites.

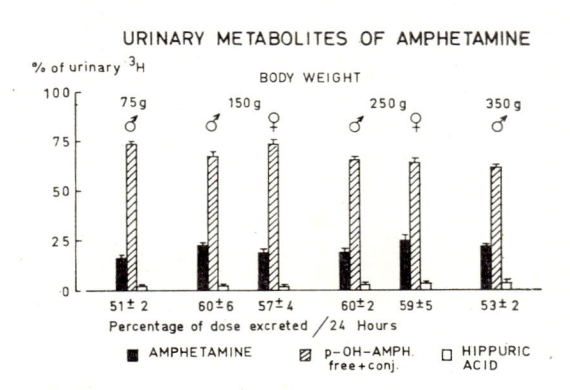

Fig. 3. Pattern of distribution of urinary metabolites of amphetamine in groups of 5 Sprague-Dawley rats of different ages and sexes. Male rats: body weight 75 g appr. 30 days, 150 g appr. 40 days, 250 g appr, 65 days and 350 g appr. 105 days. Female rats: body weight 150 appr. 55 days, 250 g more than 120 days. Tritiated d-amphetamine sulphate 5 mg/kg, 25 μCi/rat, was administered i.p. and urine was collected for 24 hours. The columns represent percentages (mean $\pm$ SEM) of excreted radioactivity as described in the text to Fig. 2a. Below the columns are given the percentages of the total administered dose excreted during 24 hours.

ASATOOR et al. (2) showed that the urinary excretion of metabolically unchanged amphetamine, a weak base, is dependent on the urinary pH in the rat. Due to non-ionic diffusion, an acid urine accelerates the renal excretion of the drug, while an alkaline urine retards it. Recently, BORELLA and HERR (6) confirmed this findings and showed that brain concentrations of amphetamine were lower in rats treated with ammonium chloride, in order to acidify the urine, than in control rats.

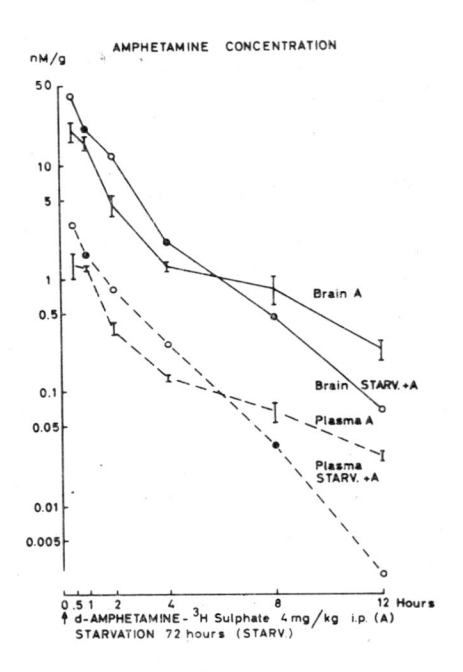

Fig. 4. Effect of 72 hours of starvation on the disappearance of amphetamine in male Sprague-Dawley rats, Four mg/kg of d-amphetamine-^{3}H sulphate, 12 μCi/rat, was administered i.p. and groups of 3—4 rats were killed at the indicated time intervals. Open symbols represent statistically significant differences (p $<$ 0.05 or less, Students t-test) from control rats. Points and vertical bars represent means $\pm$ SEM.

Inoculation of rats with tumour cells has been shown to impair p-hydroxylation of amphetamine and cause increased tissue concentrations of the drug (39).

Electric shock stress but not cold stress or revolving drum stress administered after the injection of amphetamine, causes increased brain concentrations of amphetamine (40). Recently CAMPBELL and FIBIGER (8) reported potentiation of amphetamine induced psychomotor excitation by starvation in rats. We therefore undertook a study on the effect of 72 hours of starvation on the disappearance of amphetamine from brain and plasma. As seen in Fig. 4 the multiexponential decline of amphetamine was altered; the later phase was markedly accelerated. The potentiation of amphetamine effects in starved rats might be due to the increased brain concentrations of the drug at 0.5—2 hours after administration of the drug.

Influence of drugs on the disappearance rate and metabolism of amphetamine

For convenience all drugs or other chemical agents that, to our knowledge, have been investigated with respect to metabolic interaction with amphetamine in rats are listed in Table 1. Either the drug has been shown to cause increased brain concentrations, changes

TABLE 1

Drugs and other chemicals interfering with the metabolic disposition of amphetamine in rats. Capitals B, U and PL in the fifth column indicates changes in brain concentrations of amphetamine, urinary pattern of metabolites and in the fate of amphetamine in perfused liver experiments

Drug	Pharmacological action	Interaction: yes or no	Reference	Brain (B) Urine (U) Perfused liver (PL)
Desipramine[1]	Antidepressant	Yes	(47)	B
			(42)	B
			(11)	U
			(32, 33)	U
			(18)	B
			(16)	PL
			(28), 29)	B
Imipramine	Antidepressant	Yes	(47)	B
			(33)	U
Amitriptyline	Antidepressant	Yes	(48)	B
Nortriptyline	Antidepressant	Yes	(48)	B
			(33)	U
Dibenzepine	Antidepressant	Yes	(48)	B
Protriptyline	Antidepressant	Yes	(33)	U
Lu 3-010[2]	Antidepressant	Yes	(33)	U
Iprindole	Antidepressant	Yes	(38)	B
			(29)	B
B.W. 65-54[3]	Antidepressant	Yes	(29)	B
Chlorpromazine	Neuroleptic	Yes	(43, 44)	B
			(48)	B
			(33)	U
			(7)	B
			(5)	U
			(29)	B
Propericiazine	Neuroleptic	Yes	(48)	B
Promethazine	Neuroleptic	Yes	(33)	U
Chlorprothixene	Neuroleptic	Yes	(33)	U
			(27)	B
Prochlorperazine	Neuroleptic	Yes	(33)	U
Promazine	Neuroleptic	Yes	(27)	B
Trifluorpramzine	Neuroleptic	Yes	(27)	B
Perphenazine	Neuroleptic	No	(27)	B
Haloperidol[4]	Neuroleptic	No	(33)	U
			(29)	B

Table 1 (Cont.)

Drug	Pharmacological action	Interaction: yes or no	Reference	Brain (B) Urine (U) Perfused liver (PL)
Reserpine	Neuroleptic	No	(48)	B
			(41)	B
			(33)	U
α-Methyltyrosine	Tyrosine-OHase inhibitor	No	(17)	B
			(45)	B
			(48)	B
Disulfiram	Dopamine-β-OHase inhibitor + aldehyde dehydrogenase inhibitor	Yes	(14)	U
Diethyldithio-carbamate DDC	Dopamine-β-hydroxylase inhibitor	Yes	This paper	U
		Yes	(25)	B+U
FLA-63[5]	Dopamine-β-hydroxylase inhibitor	Yes	(26)	B
		No	(26)	U
Nialamide	Monoamine-oxidase inhibitor[6]	Yes	(33)	U
Phenelzine	Monoamine-oxidase inhibitor[6]	No	(48)	B
Methysergide	Antiserotoninergic	Yes	(36)	U
Atropine	Anticholinergic	Yes	(33)	U
Cocaine	Central stimulant	Yes	(33)	U
Chlordiazepoxide	Sedative	Yes	(33)	U
Diazepam	Sedative	Yes	(33)	U
Meprobamate	Sedative	No	(33)	U
Secobarbital	Hypnotic	No	(33)	U
Phenobarbital	Hypnotic	No	(33)	U
Diphenylhydantoin	Antiepileptic	Yes	(22)	[13]
Ethanol		Yes	(13)	U
		Yes	(14)	U
			(25)	B
Pyrazole	Alcohol dehydrogenase inhibitor	Yes	(14)	U
SKF-525 A[7]	Inhibitor of liver microsomal enzymes	Yes	(22)	B
			(14)	U
			(10)	B
DPEA[8]	Inhibitor of liver microsomal enzymes	Yes	(14)	U
Lilly 18947[9]	Inhibitor of liver microsomal enzymes	Yes	(14)	U
Benzopyrene[10]	Liver microsomal enzyme inducer	No	(14)	U
Phenobarbital	Liver microsomal enzyme inducer	Yes[11]	(33)	U
		No	(14)[12]	U
		No	(22)[13]	
3-Methylcholan-threne	Liver microsomal enzyme inducer	No	(22)	B

Table 1 (Cont.)

Drug	Pharmacological action	Interaction: yes or no	Reference	Brain (B) Urine (U) Perfused liver (PL)
Amphetamine, chronic treatment		No	(31) (35)	U B
Fenfluramine	Anorexigenic	Yes	(23) (24)	B U
780 SE = S992[14])	Anorexigenic	Yes	(24) This paper	U B
p-Chloro-amphetamine		No	(24)	U
p-Chlorometh-amphetamine		No	(24)	U
Noradrenaline		Yes	(50)	B
Adrenaline		Yes	(50)	B

[1]) Not in mice (18, 30), that do not p-hydroxylate amphetamine to any great extent (20).
[2]) Lu 3-010: 1-phenyl-1-(3'-methylaminopropyl) 3,3-dimethylphtalane HCl (H. Lundbeck & Co., Copenhagen).
[3]) B.W. 65—54: DL-erythro-α-(3,4-dichlorophenyl)-ß-(t-butylamino)propanol HCl (Burroughs Wellcome & Co, USA).
[4]) Except in doses > 10 mg/kg, which increases brain concentrations.
[5]) FLA-63: bis-(1-methyl-4-homopiperazinyl thiocarbonyl)-disulfide (12).
[6]) Nialamide, pargyline, tranylcypromine affects amphetamine metabolism in isolated perfused cat liver (46). Iproniazid, pheniprazine, but not pargyline, increases brain concentrations of amphetamine in mice (30).
[7]) SKF-525 A: 2-diethylaminoethyl-2,2-diphenylvalerate.
[8]) DPEA: 2,3-dichloro-4-phenylphenoxyethylamine.
[9]) Lilly 18947: 2,4-dichloro-6-phenylphenoxy-N,N-diethylethylamine.
[10]) 2 mg/kg daily for 3 days.
[11]) 80 mg/kg daily for 5 days, slight increase in p-hydroxylation.
[12]) 80 mg/kg daily for 3 days.
[13]) 1,5 mg/kg daily for 5 days (phenobarbital), 20 mg/kg (3-methylcholanthrene). Whole rat amphetamine concentrations.
[14]) 780 SE = S992: N(2-benzoyloxyethyl)norfenfluramine.

in the urinary pattern of metabolites of amphetamine or has been tested in the isolated perfused rat liver. Obviously a large number of chemically widely different drugs and other chemicals alter the metabolic disposition of amphetamine in the rat. The mechanisms by which the hydroxylation of amphetamine is inhibited by these drugs are not known, like the p-hydroxylation reaction itself (see above), and deserve further study.

Measurements of the brain and plasma concentrations of amphetamine give the best information of a possible interaction in our experience. Drugs that are short-acting with regard to inhibition of the metabolism of amphetamine might cause an increase in the drug level of short duration without significantly changing the pattern of metabolites of amphetamine in 24 hour urine samples. Altered brain concentrations of amphetamine do not always, of course, indicate inhibition of the metabolism of amphetamine, but may be caused by other mechanisms (see above).

Conclusions

From the available information it is concluded that all drugs or other experimental conditions, which change the intensity and/or duration of action of amphetamine in the rat should be suspected of interaction with the metabolism and/or excretion of the drug. This statement has probably a more general bearing on studies of most other drug combinations.

Acknowledgements

The authors wish to thank Mrs Sonja Ahlén and Mrs Inger Jansson for their expert technical assistance.

References

1. ALLEVA, J. J. (1963) Metabolism of Tranylcypromine-^{14}C and dl-Amphetamine-^{14}C in the rat. J. med. Chem. **6**, 621.
2. ASATOOR, A. M., GALMAN, B. R., JOHNSON, J. R. and MILNE, M. D. (1965) The excretion of dexamphetamine and its derivatives. Brit. J. Pharmacol. **24**, 293.
3. AXELROD, J. (1954) Studies on sympathomimetic amines. II. The biotransformation and physiological disposition of D-amphetamine, D-p-hydroxyamphetamine and D-methamphetamine. J. Pharmacol. exp. Ther. **110**, 315.
4. AXELROD, J. (1955) The enzymatic deamination of amphetamine (Benzedrine). J. biol. Chem. **214**, 753.
5. BORELLA, L. E. (1969) Effect of chlorpromazine on the urinary excretion of amphetamine in rats. Pharmacologist, **11**, 292.
6. BORELLA, L. E. and HERR, F. (1971) Effect of ammonium chloride on the potentiation of amphetamine by psychotropic drugs in the rat. Biochem. Pharmacol. **20**, 589.
7. BORELLA, L. E., HERR, F. and WOJDAN, A. (1969) Prolongation of certain effects of amphetamine by chlorpromazine. Can. J. Physiol. Pharmacol. **47**, 7.
8. CAMPBELL, B. A. and FIBIGER, H. C. (1971) Potentiation of amphetamine induced arousal by starvation. Nature, **233**, 424.
9. CARLSSON, A., FUXE, K., HÖKFELT, T. and LINDQVIST M. (1967) Histochemical and biochemical effects of diethyldithiocarbamate on tissue catecholamine. J. Pharm. Pharmacol. **19**, 481.
10. CLAY, G. A., CHO, A. K. and ROBERFROID, M. (1971) Effect of diethylaminoethyl diphenylpropylacetate hydrochloride (SKF-525A) on the norepinephrinedepleting actions of d-amphetamine. Biochem. Pharmacol. **20**, 1821.
11. CONSOLO, S., DOLFINI, E., GARATTINI, S. and VALZELLI, L. (1967) Desipramine and amphetamine metabolism. J. Pharm. Pharmacol. **19**, 253.
12. CORRODI, H. and FLORVALL, L. (1970) Dopamine-ß-hydroxylase inhibitors. The preparation and the dopamine-ß-hydroxylase inhibitory activity of some compounds related to dithiocarbamic acid and thiuramdisulphide. Acta pharm. Sued. **7**, 7.
13. CREAVEN, P. J. and BARBEE, T. (1969) The effect of ethanol on the metabolism of amphetamine by the rat. J. Pharm. Pharmacol. **21**, 859.
14. CREAVEN, P. J., BARBEE, T. and ROACH, M. K. (1970) The interaction of ethanol and amphetamine metabolism. J. Pharm. Pharmacol. **22**, 828.
15. DALY, J., GUROFF, G., UDENFRIEND, S. and WITKOP, B. (1967) Hydroxylationinduced migrations of tritium in several substrates of liver aryl hydroxylases. Arch. Biochem. Biophys. **122**, 218.
16. DINGELL, J. V. and BASS, A. D. (1969) Inhibition of the hepatic metabolism of amphetamine by desipramine. Biochem. Pharmacol. **18**, 1535.
17. DINGELL, J. V., OWENS, M. L., NORVICH, M. R. and SULSER, F. (1967) On the role of norepinephrine biosynthesis in the central action of amphetamine. Life Sci. **6**, 1155.
18. DOLFINI, E., TANSELLA, M., VALZELLI, L. and GARATTINI, S. (1969) Further studies on the interaction between desipramine and amphetamine. Europ. J. Pharmacol. **5**, 185.
19. DRING, L. G., SMITH, R. L. and WILLIAMS, R. T. (1966) The fate of amphetamine in man and other mammals. J. Pharm. Pharmacol. **18**, 402.

20. DRING, L. G., SMITH, R. L. and WILLIAMS, R. T. (1970) The metabolic fate of amphetamine in man and other species. Biochem. J. **116**, 425.
21. ELLISON, T., GUTZAIT, L. and VAN LOON, E. J. (1966) The comparative metabolism of d-amphetamine-C^{14} in the rat, dog and monkey. J. Pharmacol. exp. Ther. **152**, 383.
22. GROPPETTI, A. and COSTA, E. (1969) Factors affecting the rate of disappearance of amphetamine in rats. Int. J. Neuropharmac. **8**, 209.
23. JONSSON, J. and GUNNE, L.-M. (1972) Interaction of fenfluramine with d-amphetamine induced excitatory behaviour and hyperthermia. Europ. J. Pharmacol. **19**, 52.
24. JONSSON, J. (1972) Interaction of fenfluramine analogues with the *in vivo* metabolism of d-amphetamine in the rat. J. Pharm. Pharmacol. In press.
25. JONSSON, J. and LEWANDER, T. (1972a) The effects of ethanol and diethyldithiocarbamate (DDC) on the brain and plasma concentrations of amphetamine in the rat. J. Pharm. Pharmacol. In press.
26. JONSSON, J. and LEWANDER, T. (1972b) Increased brain concentrations of amphetamine in rats pretreated with FLA-63, a dopamine-ß-hydroxylase inhibitor. To be published.
27. LAL, S., MISSALA, K. and SOURKES, T. L. (1971) Effect of neuroleptics on brain amphetamine concentrations in the rat. J. Pharm. Pharmacol. **23**, 967.
28. LEMBERGER, L., SERNATINGER, E. and KUNTZMAN, R. (1970) Effect of desmethylimipramine, iprindole and DL-erythro-α-(3, 4-dichlorophenyl)-ß-(t-bytyl amino) propanol HCl on the metabolism of amphetamine. Biochem. Pharmacol. **19**, 3021.
29. LEMBERGER, L., WITT, E. D., DAVIS, J. M. and KOPIN, I. J. (1970) The effects of haloperidol and chlorpromazine on amphetamine metabolism and amphetamine stereotype behaviour in the rat. J. Pharmacol. **174**, 428.
30. LEW, C., IVERSEN, D. and IVERSEN, L. L. (1971) Effects of imipramine, desipramine and monoamine oxidase inhibitors on the metabolism and psychomotor stimulant actions of d-amphetamine in mice. Europ. J. Pharmacol. **14**, 351.
31. LEWANDER, T. (1968a) Urinary excretion and tissue levels of catecholamines during chronic amphetamine intoxication. Psychopharmacologia (Berl.) **13**, 394.
32. LEWANDER, T. (1968b) Effects of amphetamine on urinary and tissue catecholamines in rats after inhibition of its metabolism with desmethylimipramine. Europ. J. Pharmacol. **5**, 1.
33. LEWANDER, T. (1969) Influence of various psychoactive drugs on the *in vivo* metabolism of d-amphetamine in the rat. Europ. J. Pharmacol. **6**, 38.
34. LEWANDER, T. (1971a) On the presence of p-hydroxynorephedrine in the rat brain and heart in relation to changes in catecholamine levels after administration of amphetamine. Acta pharmaco. toxicol. **29**, 33.
35. LEWANDER, T. (1971b) Effects of chronic amphetamine intoxication on the accumulation in the rat brain of labelled catecholamines synthesized from circulating tyrosine-^{14}C and dopa-^{3}H. Naunyn Schmiedebergs Arch. Pharmak. **271**, 211.
36. LEWANDER, T. and JONSSON, J. (1972) On the simultaneous interactions with the neurochemical and pharmacological effects of amphetamine by some drugs in rats. Psychopharmacologia (Berl.) **26**, suppl. p 36.
37. MAICKEL, R. P., COX R. H. Jr., MILLER, F. P., SEGAL, D. S. and RUSSEL, R. W. (1969) Correlation of brain levels of drugs with behavioural effects. J. Pharmacol. exp. Ther. **165**, 216.
38. MILLER, K. W., FREEMAN, J. J., DINGELL J. V. and SULSER, F. (1970) On the mechanism of amphetamine potentiation by iprindole. Experientia **26**, 863.
39. ROSSO, R., DOLFINI, L. and FRANCHI, G. (1968) Metabolism of amphetamine in tumour bearing rats. Biochem. Pharmacol. **17**, 633.
40. SALAMA, A. I. and GOLDBERG, M. E. (1969) Effect of several models of stress and amphetamine on brain levels of amphetamine and certain monoamines. Arch. int. Pharmacodyn. **181**, 474.
41. STOLK, J. M. and RECH, R. H. (1969) Effect of reserpine on accumulation and removal of d-amphetamine-^{3}H. Biochem. Pharmacol. **18**, 2786.
42. SULSER, F., OWENS, M. L. and DINGELL, J. V. (1966) On the mechanism of amphetamine potentiation by desipramine (DMI). Life Sci. **5**, 2005.
43. SULSER, F. and DINGELL, J. V. (1968a) Adrenergic mechanisms in the central action of tricyclic antidepressants and substituted phenothiazines. Agressologie, **IX**-2, 1.
44. SULSER, F. and DINGELL, J. V. (1968b) Potentiation and blockade of the central action of amphetamine by chlorpromazine. Biochem. Pharmacol. **17**, 634.
45. SULSER, F., OWENS, M. L., NORVICH, M. R. and DINGELL, J. V. (1968) The relative role of storage and synthesis of brain norepinephrine in the psychomotor stimulation evoked by amphetamine or by desipramine and tetrabenazine. Psychopharmacologia (Berl.) **12**, 322.
46. TRINKER, F. R. and RAND, M. J. (1970) The effect of nialamide, pargyline and tranylcypromine on the removal of amphetamine by the perfused liver. J. Pharm. Pharmacol. **22**, 496.

47. VALZELLI, L., CONSOLO, S. and MORPURGO, C. (1967) Influence of imipramine-like drugs on the metabolism of amphetamine. In: Antidepressant Drugs. Eds. S. Garattini & M. N. G. Dukes, Excerpta Medica Foundation. Amsterdam, New York, London, Milan, Tokyo, Buenos Aires. pp. 61.
48. VALZELLI, L., DOLFINI, E., TANSELLA, M. and GARATTINI, S. (1968) Activity of centrally acting drugs on amphetamine metabolism. J. Pharm. Pharmacol. **20**, 595.
49. ZIEM, M., COPER, H., BROERMANN, I. and STRAUSS, S. (1970) Vergleichende Untersuchungen ueber einige Wirkungen des Amphetamins bei Ratten verschiedenen Alters. Naunyn-Schmiedebergs Arch. Pharmak. **267**, 208.
50. YOUNG, R. L. and GORDON, M. W. (1961) The influence of epinephrine and norepinephrine on the accumulation of amphetamine -1-^{14}C rat brain. Biochem. Pharmacol. **6**, 273.

T.L., Psychiatric Research Center, University of Uppsala
Ulleråker Hospital, Uppsala, Sweden

PHARMACOLOGICAL IMPLICATIONS OF THE CHANGES OF BRAIN MONOAMINE TURNOVER RATES ELICITED BY (+) AMPHETAMINE AND SOME CHEMICALLY RELATED COMPOUNDS

E. COSTA

Laboratory of Preclinical Pharmacology, National Institute of Mental Health, Saint Elizabeth's Hospital, Washington, D.C.

Introduction

Although several publications (4, 5, 13) have reported that (+) amphetamine causes a number of biochemical changes in central and peripheral catecholaminergic nerves, only few reports attempt to establish quantitative correlations between neurochemical and behavioral (23, 21) responses elicited by (+) amphetamine. Many neurochemical studies fail to include dose response relationships thus limiting the possibility to relate these data to behavioral studies (24). Some of the neurochemical effects of (+) amphetamine are elicited only by maximal tolerated doses of the drug but not by the effective doses of (+) amphetamine to elicit anorexia or to increase motor activity (34, 51).

The view that the CNS actions of (+) amphetamine are related to the release of norepinephrine (NE) from central neurons mainly derives from the selective depletion of brain NE caused by 20 to 40 µmoles/kg i.p. of (+) amphetamine (5, 13, 34) given to rodents. In rat, small doses of (+) amphetamine (3 µmoles/kg i.v.) increase the turnover rate of brain dopamine (DM) but not that of NE (21). However, comparatively large doses of (+) amphetamine (10 µmoles/kg i.v.) slightly decrease brain NE concentrations and do not affect the concentrations of brain DM. Since 3 µmoles/kg i.v. of (+) amphetamine cause anorexia and increase motor activity one can hardly use the decrease of brain NE concentrations elicited by (+) amphetamine to implicate NE in mediating the (+) amphetamine effects on motor activity and food intake. Nevertheless, it is usually assumed that these effects of (+) amphetamine are mediated by an action on brain noradrenergic axons. Another action of (+) amphetamine that is seldom taken into account when the action of (+) amphetamine on brain NE turnover rate is assessed is the hyperthermic effect caused by this drug (9). The dynamics of transmitters stored in monoaminergic neurons may be altered by hyperthermia, because the control of thermoregulation involves monoaminergic neuronal function. Changes of monoamine turnover rate elicited by hyperthermic doses of (+) amphetamine may not necessarily indicate a specific neuronal action involved in the increase of motor activity or decrease of food intake elicited by the drug, rather they could be the consequence of enhanced afferent input reaching noradrenergic neurons, which participate in thermoregulation.

When behavioral responses elicited by drugs are related to changes of monoamine turnover rates measured *in vivo*, it is assumed that the changes in turnover rates reflect changes in rates of neuronal activity. However, these studies must be carried out with the understanding that there are many mechanisms whereby drugs reduce or increase the turnover rate of a monoamine stored in a given neuronal population.

The turnover rate of a brain monoamine may be decreased by drugs which: a) inhibit the rate limiting enzyme for the biosynthesis of the monoamine; b) occupy postsynaptic receptors and function as agonists of the transmitters; c) decrease the afferent excitatory input in the neuronal population under consideration; d) increase the afferent inhibitory input in the neuronal population under consideration; e) reduce the release of transmitter by nerve impulses because they activate regulatory receptors in the nerve ending; f) increase the monoamine concentration (this applies to the specific instance that the monoamine concentration controls its own biosynthesis by product inhibition).

The turnover rate of a brain monoamine stored in a given neuronal population can be increased by drugs which: a) block the reuptake of the monoamine by presynaptic endings; b) block the postsynaptic receptors; c) decrease the concentration of the monoamine if the latter can control its own biosynthesis by product inhibition; d) increase the activity of the rate limiting enzyme by transynaptic activation; e) decrease the afferent synaptic input generating inhibitory postsynaptic potentials; f) increase the afferent synaptic input generating excitatory postsynaptic potentials.

These considerations suggest that turnover rate measurements cannot by themselves define the mode of action of (+) amphetamine but they have to be considered in the context of other pertinent information concerning the possible mechanisms whereby (+) amphetamine can interact with monoaminergic nerves.

Depletion of brain NE by (+) amphetamine

It is usually assumed that (+) amphetamine causes its pharmacological effects by enhancing the release of NE from noradrenergic neurons (51). This assumption derives from the finding that brain NE concentration is reduced in rats receiving 5 μmoles/kg i.v. of (+) amphetamine (Table 1). However, the threshold dose for the decrease of brain NE content seems unrelated to that eliciting anorexia, increasing locomotor activity and causing hyperthermia (Table 1).

TABLE 1

Pharmacological responses to various doses of (+) amphetamine*

μmoles/kg i.v.	Brain NE nmoles/g ± SEM	Motor activity events/minute ± SEM	Food intake g/2 hr ± SEM	Body temperature °C ± SEM
0	2.3 ± 0.15	19 ± 10	18 ± 3.0	36.2 ± 0.42
1	2.4 ± 0.20	42 ± 18	14 ± 2.5	36.5 ± 0.32
3	2.2 ± 0.18	84 ± 15**	12 ± 2.0**	37.0 ± 0.53
5	1.7 ± 0.15**	180 ± 20**	9 ± 1.7**	38.0 ± 0.23**

* Brain NE concentrations and various pharmacological responses were measured in groups of 5 animals each at two hours or during two hours after the drug injection. To measure food intake rates were trained to eat their daily food intake in 2 hours.

** $P < 0.05$ when compared to rats receiving only saline.

This lack of relationship was not sufficient to exclude that an interaction of (+) amphetamine with brain noradrenergic neurons is involved in its central action. In fact, this drug may increase or decrease the turnover rate of brain NE without affecting the steady state concentration of this amine. Such a mechanism became a distinct possibility when it was found that (+) amphetamine blocks uptake of catecholamines in noradrenergic neurons (11). Before discussing the (+) amphetamine effects on catecholamine turnover rate let us consider with greater detail the mechanism of the catecholamine depletion elicited by (+) amphetamine. A careful inspection of the time courses of the decrease of brain NE elicited by large doses of (+) amphetamine (Table 2) suggests that a blockade of NE uptake by neurons or any other direct action of (+) amphetamine on noradrenergic neurons cannot explain the long lasting depletion of brain NE elicited by (+) amphetamine. The data reported in Table 2 shows that brain NE is still depleted 28 to 48 hours after (+) amphetamine (37 μmoles/kg i.p.); however at this time, (+) amphetamine has virtually disappeared from brain. The data reported in Table 2 show that a metabolite

TABLE 2

Brain concentrations of norepinephrine, amphetamine and p-OH-norephedrine in rats receiving 37 μmoles/kg i.p. of $(+)^3$H amphetamine

Hours after injection	$(+)^3$H amphetamine nmoles/g $\pm$ SEM	p-OH-norephedrine nmoles/g $\pm$ SEM	Norepinephrine nmoles/g $\pm$ SEM
0	—	—	2.7 $\pm$ 0.18
1	46 $\pm$ 3.2	0.12 $\pm$ 0.013	2.2 $\pm$ 0.12*
3	9.7 $\pm$ 1.2	0.42 $\pm$ 0.037	1.8 $\pm$ 0.15*
5	3.7 $\pm$ 0.27	0.66 $\pm$ 0.043	1.7 + 0.10*
17	0.11 $\pm$ 0.031	0.53 $\pm$ 0.038	1.6 $\pm$ 0.12*
28	< 0.037	0.35 $\pm$ 0.045	1.8 $\pm$ 0.15*
48	< 0.037	0.24 $\pm$ 0.017	2.2 $\pm$ 0.21*

Each value is the mean of four animals.
* $P < 0.05$ when compared to the NE concentrations of rats receiving saline.

of (+) amphetamine (25, 45), p-OH-norephedrine, persists in the brain longer than amphetamine (28). At a first glance, these data appear to indicate that p-OH-norephedrine is not stoichiometrically replacing brain NE. However, one should refrain from hasty conclusions because we cannot estimate the relative proportion of NE and p-OH-norephedrine that is present in cell bodies, in axons and in axon terminals. Presumably, most of the p-OH-norephedrine is localized in nerve terminals whereas NE is distributed in cell bodies, axons and nerve terminals.

We then tried to obtain additional supportive evidence to the proposal that the long lasting decrease of brain NE concentrations elicited by (+) amphetamine in rats was related to the accumulation of p-OH-norephedrine (27, 16). Guinea pig, unlike the rat, fails to p-hydroxylate (+) amphetamine (16); hence if p-OH-norephedrine were involved in the long lasting depletion of NE, in guinea pig, the time course of the decrease of brain NE should not outlast that of the disappearance of (+) amphetamine concentrations from brain.

The data reported in Table 3 show this to be the case; in the guinea pig brain the decrease of NE concentrations is no longer evident when the concentrations of amphet-

TABLE 3

Concentrations of norepinephrine and (+) amphetamine in brain of guinea pig receiving 37 μmoles/kg i.p. of (+) amphetamine-^{3}H

Hours after injection	(+) Amphetamine nmoles/g ± SEM	Norepinephrine nmoles/g ± SEM
0	—	1.9 ± 0.092
1	44 ± 1.8	1.4 ± 0.084*
3	23 ± 5.2	1.3 ± 0.078*
6	17 ± 4.2	1.4 ± 0.094*
17	1.1 ± 0.12	1.8 ± 0.10

*) $P < 0.05$ when compared to NE concentrations of rats receiving saline. Each value is the average of four animals.

amine are smaller than 1.1 nmoles/g. This finding contrasts with the data on the rat brain reported in Table 2. In this species the brain NE concentrations are still depleted when the concentrations of (+) amphetamine are below the limit of detection (0.037 nmoles/g).

Another line of evidence supporting a relationship between the accumulation of p-OH-norephedrine and the long lasting reduction of NE concentrations elicited by (+) amphetamine in the rat brain comes from studies of the interaction between desmethylimipramine (DMI) and (+) amphetamine (27, 28). It was reported (26, 43) that DMI slows down the rate of disappearance of (+) amphetamine from rat tissues including brain, because DMI inhibits p-hydroxylation of (+) amphetamine by liver microsomal enzymes. When rats are pretreated with DMI (38 μmoles/kg i.p.) and one hour later they receive (+) amphetamine (22 μmoles/kg i.p.), the brain NE concentrations are not reduced although the amphetamine concentrations in brain are greater in these rats than in rats receiving only (+) amphetamine (Table 4). Therefore these data indicate that in rats

TABLE 4

Amphetamine, p-OH-norephedrine, and norepinephrine concentrations in brain of rats receiving (+) amphetamine (22 μmoles/kg i.p.) with or without a pretreatment with desmethylimipramine (38 μmoles/kg i.p.)

Treatment	(+) Amphetamine nmoles/kg ± SEM	p-OH-Norephedrine nmoles/g ± SEM	Norepinephrine nmoles/g ± SEM
(+) Amphetamine	0.42 ± 0.021	0.19 ± 0.008	1.8 ± 0.091*
(+) Amphetamine + desmethylimipramine	10 ± 0.18	< 0.029	2.3 ± 0.078

Rats received (+) amphetamine and desmethylimipramine 9 and 10 hours before sacrifice.
*) $P < 0.05$

receiving (+) amphetamine the time course of the concentration of p-OH-norephedrine, an important metabolite of (+) amphetamine in this species, relates to that of the depletion of brain NE. Moreover, these data show that the depletion of brain NE is independent from the concentration of the parent compound. However, we should make it clear that (+) amphetamine *per se*, if given in sufficient doses, can cause a reduction of brain NE which is dependent from the formation of p-OH-norephedrine (18). This possibility is illustrated by the data shown in Table 5. In rats treated with the combination of DMI

TABLE 5

Brain norepinephrine concentration in rats receiving (+) amphetamine alone or after pretreatment with desmethylimipramine

Treatment*)	NE nmoles/g ± SEM		
	0	4 hr	16 hr
Amphetamine (22 μmoles/kg i.p.)	2.3 ± 0.078	2.0 ± 0.081*	1.8 ± 0.091*
Amphetamine (22 μmoles/kg i.p.) and Desmethylimipramine (38 μmoles/kg i.p.)	2.4 ± 0.087	2.1 ± 0.063*	2.4 ± 0.010

(+) Amphetamine was injected intraperitoneally 1 hr after desmethylimipramine. The latter drug when given alone, fails to change steady state concentration of brain NE.

$P < 0.05$ when compared to animals receiving only saline or desmethylimipramine.

and (+) amphetamine, p-OH-norephedrine is not formed but the concentration of brain NE is reduced for a short time following the injection of the drug. These results prompted us to suggest that the long lasting decrease of NE (Table 2 and 5) elicited by (+) amphetamine (22 to 37 μmoles/kg) may depend on the accumulation of its hydroxylated metabolite p-OH-norephedrine. However, (+) amphetamine *per se* can reduce the concentrations of NE (Table 5) as long as it is present in the tissues in concentrations greater than 14 nanomoles/g of tissue. While we could postulate that the long lasting depletion of brain NE elicited by (+) amphetamine is probably mediated by an accumulation of p-OH-norephedrine, we could not suggest any possible mechanism to explain the short lasting reduction of brain NE elicited by (+) amphetamine when its hydroxylation to form p-OH-norephedrine is prevented. The blockade of NE uptake by nerve terminals (11) elicited by (+) amphetamine could not be invoked because this drug has a greater affinity for the uptake mechanism of dopaminergic neurons (44). Therefore, if uptake blockade were operational in the reduction of brain NE concentrations, one might have expected that brain DM concentrations could also be depleted by (+) amphetamine doses that deplete brain NE. Since this is not the case (6), to explain the depletion of NE elicited by (+) amphetamine in guinea pigs, we can only speculate on a possible action of (+) amphetamine on catecholamine biosynthesis (32). In this species the amphetamine hydroxylation is negligible and the parent compound is present in brain in high concentrations.

NEURONAL LOCALIZATION OF p-OH-NOREPHEDRINE, A METABOLITE OF (+) AMPHETAMINE

To establish whether or not p-OH-norephedrine plays a role in the reduction of brain norepinephrine concentrations caused by (+) amphetamine, we had to show that this metabolite localizes in neurons. We performed experiments to show that: a) the rates of neuronal activity are related to the efflux rates of p-OH-norephedrine from tissues; b) the efficiency of NE retrieval by sympathetic neurons is related to the efflux rates of p-OH-norephedrine; c) the injections of (+) amphetamine in doses that release neuronal NE also release p-OH-norephedrine-^{3}H formed from previously injected (+) amphetamine-^{3}H.

A. *Efflux of p-OH-norephedrine from tissues during increased sympathetic neuronal activity*

Since a blood brain barrier hinders the efflux of p-OH-norephedrine from brain, we could not study how the p-OH-norephedrine efflux from brain relates to neuronal activity. Therefore, we studied the efflux of p-OH-norephedrine from peripheral sympathetic neurons where, unlike the brain, the p-OH-norephedrine released from neuronal binding sites during nerve activity in part leaves the tissues when the concentrations of p-OH-norephedrine released exceed the capacity of the specialized uptake mechanisms. Rats were injected with (+)^{3}H amphetamine (37 μmoles/kg i.p.) and kept at 20°C for eight hours. At this time, a group of 5 rats was killed and their hearts and salivary glands were analyzed for p-OH-norephedrine. Similar analyses were performed in the tissues of another group of 5 rats kept at 20°C for an additional 16 hours and in the tissues of a third group of rats kept for an equal length of time at 4°C. The results of these analyses are reported in Table 6. These data show that in rats exposed for 16 hours at 4°C the cardiac

TABLE 6

Concentrations of p-hydroxynorephedrine in tissues of rats receiving (+) ^{3}H amphetamine (37 μmoles/kg i.p.) and kept at various environmental temperatures

Hours after (+)^{3}H amphetamine	Hours at 4 °C	p-Hydroxynorephedrine nmoles/g $\pm$ SEM Heart	Salivary gland
8	None	2.0 $\pm$ 0.25	2.3 $\pm$ 0.29
24	None	1.7 $\pm$ 0.047	1.6 $\pm$ 0.26
24	16	0.72 $\pm$ 0.14★	1.7 $\pm$ 0.31

★) $P < 0.01$ when compared with rats kept at 20 °C for 24 hours after (+)^{3}H amphetamine.

concentrations of p-hydroxynorephedrine decrease at a faster rate than those of the salivary glands. Rats pretreated with tracer doses of ^{3}H NE were kept at 20°C and 4°C for various time periods and the decline of NE specific radioactivity in heart and salivary gland was measured (Table 7). Cold exposure increases significantly the fractional rate constant for the decline of heart NE specific activity but not that for salivary gland. Since steady state concentrations of NE are maintained during cold exposure by applying principles of steady state kinetics, we can calculate the turnover rate of heart NE in rats kept at 20°C and 4°C. These calculations show that the turnover rate of heart NE is increased during cold exposure; however, in the same animals the turnover rate of salivary gland NE is not increased (Table 7). Since cold exposure accelerates the rate of neuronal activity of sympathetic axons innervating the heart but not that of axons innervating the salivary gland, we can relate the increase of heart NE turnover rate to the increase of neuronal activity. If this interference is extended to the data reported in Table 6

TABLE 7

Turnover rate of heart and salivary gland norepinephrine in rats exposed to different environmental temperatures

Environmental temperature	NE concentrations nmoles/g ± SEM		k/hr for ^{3}H-NE disappearance		Turnover rate nmoles/g/hr	
	Heart	Salivary gland	Heart	Salivary gland	Heart	Salivary gland
4°C	3.9 ± 0.30	5.7 ± 0.89	0.12 ± 0.03*	0.11 ± 0.03	0.46	0.63
22°C	4.3 ± 0.89	6.1 ± 0.71	0.064 ± 0.007	0.10 ± 0.02	0.27	0.61

Rats were placed at 4°C or maintained at 20°C for 16 hours before an intravenous injection of DL-^{3}H NE (2.5 nmoles/kg). Groups of four to six rats were killed at 2, 4, 14 and 23 hours after injection. Data are presented as mean ± S.E.M. k/hr was calculated from the exponential decline of NE specific activity.

*) $P < 0.05$

we can suggest that the increase of the efflux rate of p-OH-norephedrine elicited by cold is related to the increased rate of neuronal activity. Since the efflux rate of this amphetamine metabolite mirrors that of the transmitter in two different tissues, we can infer that p-OH-norephedrine might be stored in sympathetic nerves.

B. *Efflux of p-OH-norephedrine from tissues after pharmacological blockade of transmitter is retrieved*

DMI blocks the uptake of NE into sympathetic neurons (11). Retrieval of NE plays an important role in terminating the response of postsynaptic cells to the NE released during sympathetic activity (3). Since synthesis, metabolism and reuptake of NE contribute to maintain the constancy of the amine concentration in neurons in the face of changing rates of nerve activity, if reuptake is pharmacologically blocked the NE concentration can be maintained at steady state only if its rate of synthesis is increased (15). Data in the literature (14) show that if NE of sympathetic nerves is substituted by another amine, the efflux rate of the latter is increased during cold exposure or when its reuptake by nerve terminals is blocked by DMI. The results reported in Table 8 show that DMI

TABLE 8

Efflux of p-OH-norephedrine from heart and salivary gland of rats receiving (+)^{3}H amphetamine with or without DMI

Treatment	p-OH-norephedrine nmoles/kg ± SEM	
	Heart	Salivary gland
Amphetamine (37 μmoles/kg i.p.)	0.93 ± 0.10	0.99 ± 0.16
Amphetamine (37 μmoles/kg i.p.) and DMI (38 μmoles/kg i.p.)	0.57 ± 0.059*	0.59 ± 0.060*

* $P < 0.05$ when compared to rats receiving only (+)^{3}H amphetamine.

DMI was injected 24 hr after (+)-H-amphetamine. All animals were killed 30 hrs after (+)^{3}H-amphetamine.

increases the efflux rate from heart and salivary gland of p-OH-norephedrine formed from previously injected (+) amphetamine. These data contribute another line of evidence to support the view that p-OH-norephedrine is localized in sympathetic nerves. Moreover, they reinforce the significance of the results reported in Table 6 on the difference of the efflux of p-OH-norephedrine from salivary gland and heart during cold exposure by showing that in these two tissues sympathetic nerves behave similarly with regard to the acceleration of p-OH-norephedrine efflux elicited by pharmacological blockade of the transmitter reuptake.

C. *Release of ^{3}H p-OH-norephedrine by injections of (+) amphetamine*

The peripheral sympathomimetic effects elicited by (+) amphetamine are associated with a release of neuronal NE (2). If p-OH-norephedrine formed in heart tissue from (+)^{3}H amphetamine were accumulated in sympathetic nerves, one might expect that successive doses of (+) amphetamine would release the (+)^{3}H amphetamine metabolite. Table 9 lists the concentrations of p-OH-norephedrine found in heart and brain of rats receiving various combinations of (+) amphetamine and (+)^{3}H amphetamine.

TABLE 9

p-OH-norephedrine concentrations in heart and brain of rats injected with two successive injections of (+)^{3}H amphetamine

Experiment No.	(+) Amphetamine (μmoles/kg i.p.) Injection 1	Injection 2	Hours between first injection and sacrifice	p-OH-norephedrine (nmoles/g ± SEM) Heart	Brain
1	37 (^{3}H)	22 (^{3}H)	22	1.9 ± 0.38	0.38 ± 0.030
2	37 (^{3}H)	—	22	2.1 ± 0.053	0.16 ± 0.012
3	22 (^{3}H)	—	1	0.61 ± 0.042	0.23 ± 0.042
4	37	22 (^{3}H)	22	0.66 ± 0.036	0.28 ± 0.066

Concentrations of p-OH-norephedrine shown are the average of at least 4 rats. The rats receiving two injections were sacrificed 1 hour after the second injection.

One hour after receiving 22 μmoles/kg of (+)^{3}H amphetamine, the rats store in their hearts 0.61 nanomoles/g of ^{3}H p-OH-norephedrine, but twenty one hours after 37 μmoles of (+)^{3}H amphetamine their hearts contain 2.1 nanomoles/g of the amphetamine metabolite. The heart of rats receiving doses of ^{3}H amphetamine with an identical time schedule contain 1.9 nanomoles/g of ^{3}H p-OH-norephedrine instead of the expected 2.7 nanomoles/g (Table 9). As expected, the concentrations of ^{3}H p-OH-norephedrine in brain of the rats receiving the two injections of (+)^{3}H amphetamine are equal to the total of the concentrations found in the brain of the rats receiving each of the two doses of (+)^{3}H amphetamine (Table 9). Since an injection of (+) amphetamine (37 μmoles) 22 hours before does not prevent the accumulation in heart or brain of p-OH-norephedrine formed from 22 μmoles/kg i.p. of (+)^{3}H amphetamine given 1 hour before death, we conclude that in the first experiment reported in Table 9, the second dose of (+)^{3}H amphetamine releases the amphetamine metabolite accumulated in heart after the first dose of ^{3}H (+) amphetamine. The differences in the physicochemical properties of

(+) amphetamine and p-OH-norephedrine suggest that their binding sites to nonspecific tissue constituents may not be identical; therefore, the release of the accumulated metabolite by the parent compound corroborates the view that p-OH-norephedrine is stored in neurons. In contrast, two successive doses of (+)^{3}H amphetamine cause the accumulation of p-OH-norephedrine formed from each of the two amphetamine doses in brain (Experiment No. 1, Table 9). Since the p-OH-norephedrine also in brain may accumulate in noradrenergic neurons it can be inferred that the presence of p-OH-norephedrine in brain should be considered in discussing mechanisms whereby chronic (+) amphetamine in high doses can change brain function.

D. *Functional implications of p-OH-norephedrine accumulation in sympathetic neurons*

Tachyphylaxis to the peripheral sympathetic responses elicited by (+) amphetamine has been described (8). This adaptation to the pharmacological effect of (+) amphetamine can be explained if p-OH-norephedrine (formed from (+) amphetamine and stored in sympathetic neurons) were released by the parent compound in lieu of the transmitter, NE. Successive injections of (+) amphetamine result in a progressive reduction of the adrenergic response because increasing amounts of p-OH-norephedrine released by successive doses of (+) amphetamine. Since p-OH-norephedrine is endowed with a limited intrinsic activity on postsynaptic sympathetic receptors, the intrinsic activity of the transmitter released by successive doses of (+) amphetamine will become smaller and smaller after successive injections of (+) amphetamine. It is conceivable that nerve impulses release p-OH-norephedrine from brain neurons, with chronic (+) amphetamine injections the amount of p-OH-norephedrine participating to sympathetic function and bound to postsynaptic noradrenergic receptors may continually increase. The occupancy of noradrenergic receptors by a compound with weak intrinsic activity may be involved in triggering transynaptically by a neuronal loop the increase of tyrosine hydroxylase reported to occur (31) either after high doses of (+) amphetamine, or after its chronic administration. Although, in man, p-OH-norephedrine is a minor metabolite of (+) amphetamine, still it is conceivable that when (+) amphetamine is abused either for long periods of time in moderate oral doses or is injected itravenously in large doses, p-OH-norephedrine may accumulate in the brain of man. Perhaps the accumulation of this metabolite may be a factor in eliciting the psychotic episodes with paranoid overtones that are frequently described in amphetamine abusers. The slow efflux of p-OH-norephedrine from brain is in keeping with the time course of the clinical episodes which generally do not exceed in the duration the time period expected from the half life of the compound. The slow efflux rate of this metabolite from brain may also account for the difficulties encountered in detecting p-OH-norephedrine in the spinal fluid of amphetamine abusers.

EFFECTS OF AMPHETAMINE ON THE TURNOVER RATE OF BRAIN CATECHOLAMINES AND MOTOR ACTIVITY

WEISSMAN, KOE and TENEN (49) first suggested that the increase of locomotor activity caused by (+) amphetamine in rats can be observed only if the biosynthesis of brain catecholamines is unimpaired. This suggestion has focused the attention of several investigators on the possibility that amphetamine disrupts the dynamic equilibrium of catecholamine stores favoring the efflux of catecholamines from presynaptic axon terminals into their respective postsynaptic receptors. However, the data available fail to specify whether brain NE or brain DM or both are involved in the increase of locomotor activity elicited by (+) amphetamine. Locomotor activity is affected differently by various doses of (+) amphetamine. Following small doses of the drug the exploratory and rearing movements become more and more frequent. When the doses of (+) amphetamine are increased the exploratory movements are reduced because the rats exhibit characteristic stereotyped motions (biting the cage wires, licking, circular movements of the head, etc.).

RANDRUP and SCHEEL-KRUGER (39) suggested that an action on dopaminergic neurons may explain the stereotyped behavior elicited by high doses of (+) amphetamine whereas the increase in exploratory activity observed after low doses of (+) amphetamine may be associated with an action on noradrenergic neurons. However, UNGERSTEDT and ARBUTH-NOTT (47) have shown that small doses of (+) amphetamine act on brain dopaminergic axons. CARLSSON (12) has shown that the stimulation of motor activity caused by (+) amphetamine in mice involves the release of brain DM.

The data reported in Table 10 concern experiments designed to measure dose response relationships between the effects of (+) amphetamine on motor activity, turnover rate of striatal DM and tel-diencephalic NE.

TABLE 10

Effects of two doses of (+) amphetamine on locomotor activity and turnover rate of brain catecholamines

(+) Amphetamine μmoles/kg i.v.	Motor activity (events/min $\pm$ SEM)	Striatum NE nmoles/g $\pm$ SEM	Striatum DM nmoles/g/hr $\pm$ SEM	Telencephalon NE nmoles/g $\pm$ SEM	Telencephalon DM nmoles/g/hr $\pm$ SEM
Saline (5)	4.5 $\pm$ 1.7	59 $\pm$ 3	38 $\pm$ 3.2	3.1 $\pm$ 0.2	2.1 $\pm$ 0.3
2.2 (5)	25 $\pm$ 7.4*	59 $\pm$ 8	77 $\pm$ 7.2*	3.3 $\pm$ 0.06	2.3 $\pm$ 0.4
Saline (5)	2.5 $\pm$ 0.71	63 $\pm$ 6	29 $\pm$ 3.5	2.8 $\pm$ 0.08	1.5 $\pm$ 0.3
1.4 (5)	5.8 $\pm$ 1.2	55 $\pm$ 2	24 $\pm$ 2.9	2.7 $\pm$ 0.05	1.7 $\pm$ 0.2

Rats were injected with 26 nmoles/kg i.v. (0.8 mCi) of 3,5-^{3}H L-tyrosine and ten minutes later with either saline (5 ml/kg i.v.) or one of the doses of (+) amphetamine and killed 15 minutes later. Turnover rate (TR) of NE or DM (M) was calculated from

$$M \text{ nmoles/g/hr} = \frac{M \text{ dpm/g/hr}}{SA \text{ tyrosine}}$$

Motor activity was recorded during the 15 minute interval between injection of (+) amphetamine and death.

* $P < 0.05$. Number of animals in parentheses.

From the data listed in Table 10 it appears that 2.2 μmoles/kg i.v. of (+) amphetamine increases motor activity and simultaneously enhances the turnover rate of striatal DM; the smaller dose of (+) amphetamine fails to increase motor activity and does not change the conversion index of striatal tyrosine into DM. Neither dose of (+) amphetamine increases the turnover rate of NE in tel-diencephalon (Table 10). These results differentiate between the pharmacological and neurochemical effects of the two doses of (+) amphetamine we selected. In other experiments, the dose of 2.2 μmoles/kg i.v. of (+) amphetamine stimulated motor activity and caused anorexia but not hyperthermia

(Table 11). In contrast, 1.4 μmoles/kg i.v. of (+) amphetamine does not increase motor activity but causes anorexia (Table 11). Our data suggest that an accelerated rate of striatal DM may be involved in the increase of motor activity elicited by 2.2 μmoles/kg i.v.

TABLE 11

Effect of (+) amphetamine, (—) amphetamine and cocaine on motor activity, body temperature, food intake and turnover rate of striatal DM

Drug injected (μmole/kg i.v.)	DM nmoles/g ± SEM	DM nmoles/g/hr	Body temperature C° ± SEM	Events/min ± SEM	Food intake g ± SEM
Saline	53 ± 9	36 ± 4.8	36.7 ± 0.21	3.4 ± 0.5	14 ± 2
(+) Amphetamine (2.2)	60 ± 3	65 ± 4.8*	36.5 ± 0.42	12 ± 2.3*	7.8 ± 1.3*
Cocaine (8.8)	62 ± 4	58 ± 3.8*	37.6 ± 0.15*	22 ± 4.2*	14 ± 1.7
(—) Amphetamine (7.4)	54 ± 2	40 ± 3.8	37.8 ± 0.15*	4.2 ± 1.3	9.1 ± 1.5*

Rats (5 per group) received 1 mCi/kg i.v. of 3,5 ^{3}H tyrosine and 10 minutes later either saline (5 ml/kg i.v.) or one of the drugs listed in the table. The rats were decapitated 15 minutes after the drug injection.

* $P < 0.05$ when compared to saline treated rats.

of (+) amphetamine. The data reported in Table 11 validate such a correlation by showing that 7.4 μmoles/kg i.v. of (—) amphetamine which causes anorexia and hyperthermia but does not increase motor activity fails to accelerate the turnover rate of striatal DM. In contrast, cocaine (8.8 μmoles/kg i.v.) fails to elicit anorexia but increases motor activity, causes hyperthermia, and increases the turnover rate of striatal DM. Since both doses of (+) amphetamine neither change the steady state concentrations of tel-diencephalic NE nor increase its turnover rate (Table 10) we can conclude that the anorexia and the increase of motor activity elicited by (+) amphetamine are not related to a change in the turnover rate of tel-diencephalic NE.

Data shown in Table 11 suggest a dissociation between anorexia and increase of the turnover rate of striatal DM because cocaine causes anorexia and does not increase turnover rate of striatal DM while (—) amphetamine elicits anorexia and does not increase turnover rate of striatal DM. The data shown in Table 12 show that (—) amphetamine

TABLE 12

Effect of cocaine, (+) and (—) amphetamine on the turnover rate of NE in tel-diencephalon

Drug μmoles/kg i.v.	NE nmoles/g ± SEM	NE nmoles/g/hr ± SEM
Saline	2.2 ± 0.14	0.91 ± 0.12
(+) Amphetamine (2.2)	2.5 ± 0.15	0.98 ± 0.096
(—) Amphetamine (7.4)	2.8 ± 0.16	0.94 ± 0.096
Cocaine (8.8)	2.6 ± 0.09	1.0 ± 0.096

Rats received 1 mCi/kg i.v. of 3,5-^{3}H tyrosine and 10 minutes later either saline or the drug listed in the table; they were killed 15 minutes after drug injections.

(7.4 μmoles/kg i.v.) and cocaine (8.8. μmoles/kg i.v.), like (+) amphetamine (2.2 μmoles/kg i.v.) do not increase the turnover rate of tel-diencephalic NE. By comparing the data reported in Table 12 to those reported in Table 11 we could infer that the increase of turnover rate of tel-diencephalic NE is dissociated from anorexia, hyperthermia, and increase of motor activity elicited by (+) amphetamine.

Effect of Amphetamine Analogues on Anorexia, Motor Activity, and Turnover Rate of Brain Catecholamines

Probably, (+) methamphetamine is the amphetamine analogue most commonly used as a substitute of (+) amphetamine. The availability of this compound in the black market probably exceeds that of (+) amphetamine; therefore, methamphetamine is the drug frequently available to drug abusers. This consideration prompted us to study the biochemical pharmacology of this compound.

Rats were injected intraperitoneally with (±) methamphetamine (90 μmol/kg) and brain DM, NE and 5-HT were measured at various times after the injection. The results of these experiments are reported in Table 13.

Table 13

Percent change of NE, DM and 5-HT in brain of rats receiving 90 μmoles/kg i.p. of (±) methamphetamine

Brain monoamine	Hours after injection						
	0	1	2	6	10	24	48
NE	100	60	50	66	65	82	84
5-HT	100	49	42	82	78	90	89
DM	100	118	110	118	—	108	106

Amine concentrations at 0 time (nmoles/g ± SE): NE (2.0 ± 0.16); 5-HT (1.2 ± 0.070); DM (4.1 ± 0.010).

The reduction of brain NE concentrations elicited by (±) methamphetamine at 1 and 2 hours is statistically significant ($P < 0.01$) but at 6 hours or later this change is no longer statistically significant; the changes in brain DM noted in these experiments were never significant. The decrease of brain 5-HT concentrations were significant at 1 and 2 hours but they were no longer significant at 24 hours after the injection or later. A decrease of brain 5-HT concentrations was never found after equimolar doses of (±) amphetamine. Furthermore equimolar doses of (+) or (−) methamphetamine were as effective as (±) methamphetamine in reducing brain 5-HT concentrations. While a single dose of (±) methamphetamine (90 μmoles/kg i.p.) reduced heart NE concentrations for longer than 48 hours (Table 14) the brain NE concentrations were reduced for less than 24 hours (Table 13).

Data of Table 14 document how methamphetamine deviates from the effects on brain monoamines elicited by (+) amphetamine both qualitatively and with regard to the time course of the response. Since it was known that methamphetamine is rapidly dealkylated

TABLE 14

Heart NE concentrations in rats after (±) methamphetamine injection (90 μmol/kg i.p.)

Hours	nmoles/g ± SEM	P
0	4.5 ± 0.50	—
5	2.0 ± 0.08	< 0.005
25	1.7 ± 0.26	< 0.005
50	2.4 ± 0.14	< 0.005

Each point is the average of four determinations.

(1) we thought it important to study the metabolism of methamphetamine to learn whether the metabolic degradation of this molecule could explain the difference in the effects on tissue monoamines described above for methamphetamine and amphetamine.

In this symposium, Dr. CATTABENI reports in detail the results of these studies (35). Here, it will be sufficient to say that by mass fragmentography we could detect both methamphetamine and amphetamine in brain homogenates of rats killed three hours after treatment with (+) or (−) amphetamine (45 μmol/kg i.p.). The presence of amphetamine in these tissues confirmed that methamphetamine is metabolized by dealkylation and our results suggest that there is a preferential dealkylation of the d-isomer. In these brain homogenates, we could also detect p-hydroxyamphetamine. No tracers of the p-hydroxylated derivative of methamphetamine could be found in these homogenates. Using ^{14}C-methamphetamine, we could detect the persistance of polar metabolites (probably p-OH-norephedrine) for 24 hours in tissues of rats receiving methamphetamine. The maximal concentrations of these metabolites found in heart were approximately 7-fold greater than those found in brain. In heart of rats receiving (+) methamphetamine we found we could identify p-OH-norephedrine by multiple ion detection.

In conclusion, our studies (35) show that rats promptly dealkylate methamphetamine, the rate of dealkylation is probably a limiting process for the successive hydroxylation of amphetamine in p- and β-position. Since these hydroxylations are first order process the concentration of the substrate (amphetamine) determines the amount per time of drug hydroxylated. Therefore, in strains of rats injected with equal amounts of amphetamine and methamphetamine we could not find the same quantity of p-hydroxyamphetamine because the rate of hydroxylation of methamphetamine presumably depends upon the rate of its dealkylation. Since the diffusion of p-OH-norephedrine from blood to brain depends on the concentration of the drug in blood, the amount of p-OH-norephedrine in brain of rats receiving methamphetamine was less than that present in rats receiving equal molar doses of amphetamine. This conclusion does not apply to the heart. Since p-OH-amphetamine is taken up and concentrated by heart neurons the rate of its formation may not influence the quantity of p-OH-norephedrine that will be stored in heart; thus equamolar quantities of amphetamine and methamphetamine produce a depletion of heart NE with a similar time course and by the same extent.

Effect of phenmetrazine, aminorex, and p-chloramphetamine, p-Cl-methamphetamine and chlorphentermine on the steady state concentrations of brain monoamines

The chemical structures of these compounds is shown in Fig. 1.

We detected stereotyped behavior neither in rats receiving intravenously 5, 11, 17 μmoles/kg nor in animals injected intraperitoneally with 44, 62 and 112 μmoles/kg

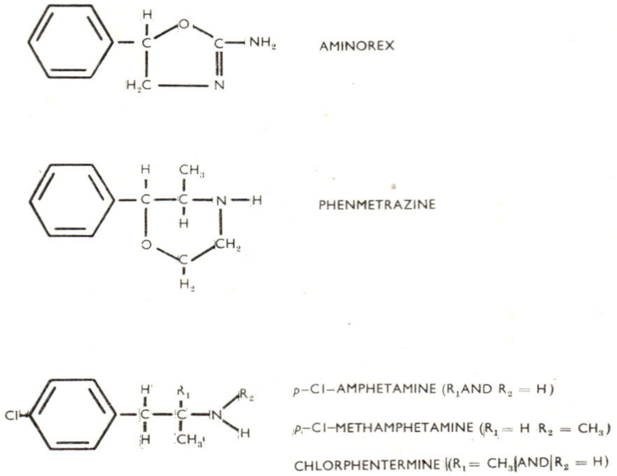

Fig. 1.

TABLE 15

Effect of p-Cl-amphetamine on the concentrations of 5-HT and NE of rat tel-diencephalon

Isomer tested (μmoles/kg i.p.)	NE nanomoles/g ± SEM			
	4 hr.	24 hr.	48 hr.	72 hr.
± (44)	3.0 ± 0.34	3.2 ± 0.28	3.1 ± 0.25	2.9 ± 0.18
+ (25)	2.8 ± 0.13			
− (25)	2.7 ± 0.14			

Isomer tested (μmoles/kg i.p..	5-HT nanomoles/g ± SEM			
	4 hr.	24 hr.	48 hr.	72 hr.
± (44)	0.91 ± 0.081	0.89 ± 0.078	0.95 ± 0.089	0.98 ± 0.083
+ (25)	0.83 ± 0.062			
− (25)	0.53 ± 0.021			

Concentrations (namomoles/g ± SEM) of NE (3.1 ± 0.23) and 5-HT (2.1 ± 0.19) in rats used as controls. Each mean is the average of at least four experiments.

of ($\pm$) p-Cl-amphetamine, aminorex and phenmetrazine, respectively. The large doses of these three amphetamine congeners were tested for their action on tissue monoamine content. Only ($\pm$) p-Cl-amphetamine decreases the concentration of tel-diencephalon 5-HT and this decrease lasted several days (Table 15).

We compared the effects of ($+$) and ($-$) p-Cl-amphetamine (25 μmoles/kg i.p.) on the concentrations of 5-HT in rat telencephalon and found that the ($-$) isomer is more active than the ($+$) isomer in reducing the concentrations of this amine (Table 15). Both compounds were less active in reducing the hypothalamic concentrations of 5-HT 65% ($+$ isomer) and 60% ($-$ isomer) of normal animals; the 5-HT content of brain stem was reduced by a similar extent. The N alkylated derivative of p-Cl-amphetamine (35 μmoles/kg i.p.) only reduced the tel-diencephalic concentrations of 5-HT to about 60% of controls but failed to modify the 5-HT concentrations of brain stem and hypothalamus. Contrary to amphetamine and methamphetamine (Table 13), the ability to reduce brain 5-HT concentrations is greater for p-Cl-amphetamine than for p-Cl-methamphetamine. The presence of two methyl groups linked to the α-carbon of p-Cl-amphetamine (chlorphentermine; 35 μmoles/kg i.p.) reduces the ability of the compound to decrease the 5-HT concentrations of telencephalon. Chlorphentermine, ($+$) and ($-$) p-Cl-amphetamine only slightly reduced the NE concentrations in telencephalon, p-Cl-methamphetamine failed to change the telencephalic concentrations of NE. In conclusion, the two compounds with the side chain rearranged into a ring (aminorex and phenmetrazine) although mimic pharmacologically ($+$) amphetamine, fail to change the steady state concentration of brain monoamines and in the doses mentioned did not elicit stereotype behavior. The presence of a Cl in p-position lowers the concentrations of brain 5-HT, this effect is reduced by either N-alkylation or by the presence of two methyl groups in the α-C. All the p-Cl derivatives tested preferentially lower brain 5-HT but they also slightly reduce brain 5-HT concentrations. The only exception to this rule is p-Cl-methamphetamine.

Effect of phenmetrazine, aminorex, and ($\pm$) p-Cl-amphetamine on the motor activity and turnover rate of brain catecholamines

The data reported in Table 16 support the view that a lowering of brain 5-HT is independent of the increase in motor activity elicited by ($\pm$) p-Cl-amphetamine. Moreover, these experiments reveal that motor activity of rats can be increased by doses of ($\pm$) p-Cl-amphetamine, and aminorex which do not accelerate the turnover rate of brain NE (Table 16). We found that aminorex, injected in doses which increase motor activity can increase the turnover rate of striatal DM; therefore, an action of dopaminergic axons can still be entertained as a possible indirect mechanism involved in the motor stimulation elicited by aminorex. Moreover, our results suggest that an increase of striatal DM turnover rate may be involved in the increase of motor activity elicited by ($\pm$) p-Cl-amphetamine. In this regard our studies modify the suggestion previously made by Strada et al. (42) that the stimulatory effect of p-Cl-amphetamine relates to an accumulation of brain NE metabolites by showing that threshold doses of the drug to increase motor activity increase striatal DM turnover rate. We found that phenmetrazine (Table 17) fails to change the turnover time of hypothalamic NE and striatal DM when injected into rats in doses that increase locomotor activity. Therefore, this drug should be considered capable of stimulating motor activity without acting on brain noradrenergic and dopaminergic axons. Studies of Thoma and Wick (46) had indicated that phenmetrazine is a direct acting sympathomimetic amine since its pressor effect and its

TABLE 16

Effect of aminorex and (±) p-Cl-amphetamine on rat motor activity and turnover rate of catecholamines

Drug (μmoles/kg i.v.)	Motor activity events/min	Turnover time (hr.) Tel-diencephalon NE	Brain stem NE	Striatum DM
Saline	17 ± 3	2.6	2.7	2.9
Aminorex (1.5)	77 ± 12★	2.4	2.4	1.5★
(±) p-Cl-amphetamine (3.5)	57 ± 16★	2.2	2.6	1.7★

These data were compiled from Costa et al. (17). Turnover time measured with an isotopic method (pulse injection ^{3}H tyrosine).

★ $P < 0.05$. The significance of turnover time was calculated on the k value. The steady state concentrations of these amines are unchanged.

TABLE 17

Effects of phenmetrazine on rat motor activity and on turnover time of hypothalamic NE and striatal DM

μmoles/kg i.v.	Motor activity events/min	Turnover time (hr.) Hypothalamic NE	Striatal DM
—	23 ± 6.8	3.2	3.6
5.6	61 ± 6.8★	2.6	3.2
2.8	42 ± 6.2★	2.9	2.8

These data were compiled from Costa et al. (17). Turnover time was measured with isotopic methods (pulse injection ^{3}H tyrosine). Steady state concentration of monoamines was not affected by drugs.

★ $P < 0.05$.

effect on nictitating membrane were enhanced rather than antagonized by cocaine. A recent report on the action of phenmetrazine in man (33) tends to contraindicate that its central action is a consequence of the NE release in brain.

In conclusion, our results support and extend to aminorex and p-Cl-amphetamine the proposal made by Van Rossum et al. (48) that the central action of minimal effective doses of (+) amphetamine involves a presynaptic action on central dopaminergic axons. Moreover, phenmetrazine when given in minimal effective doses to increase locomotor activity and to decrease drive for food may act directly on brain postsynaptic catecholaminergic receptors.

Action of Fenfluramine on Monoamine Stores of Rat Tissues

In rodents, fenfluramine depresses locomotor activity (10) but reduces the drive for food (7) thus establishing that phenylethylamines can cause anorexia without central stimulation (7). Fenfluramine decreases the 5-HT concentrations of brain tissue (37); the depletion of tel-diencephalic 5-HT stores persists for several days after a single injection of fenfluramine (17). Fenfluramine is rapidly N-dealkylated in rat tissues (35) but its dealkylated metabolite (Table 18) also reduces telencephalic 5-HT concentrations

TABLE 18

5-HT and NE content of rat telencephalon at various times after fenfluramine (90 μmoles/kg i.p.) and norfenfluramine (40 μmoles/kg i.p.)

Drug	% of controls after hr										
	1		2		4		16		32		48	
	NE	5-HT	NE	5-HT	NE	5-HT	NE	5-HT	NE	5-HT	NE	5-HT
Fenfluramine	78	68	80	50	70	40	90	52	95	65	98	73
Norfen-fluramine	84	46	92	42	90	38	92	58	96	72	94	67

The 5-HT and NE concentrations in the telencephalon of rats used as control were 1.4 ± 009 and 1.4 ± 0.17 respectively.

selectively. The time course of fenfluramine and norfenfluramine action on monoamine stores of telencephalon is reported in Table 18. The effect of these two drugs on telencephalon DM concentrations is not reported in the table because the concentrations of this amine did not change after the injections of either drug. The concentration of telencephalon NE were decreased only after fenfluramine but this reduction was no longer significant at 16 hrs after the injection. In contrast, both drugs significantly decreased the concentrations of telencephalon 5-HT for longer than 48 hours. From the data reported in Table 18 it appears that norfenfluramine is more active than fenfluramine in decreasing telencephalon 5-HT. This indication was substantiated by a dose response study carried out at three hours after the drug injections. This study revealed that the dose of fenfluramine to lower telencephalon 5-HT by 50% was 75 μmoles/kg i.p. whereas that of norfenfluramine was 24 μmoles/kg i.p. Since the decrease of telencephalic 5-HT elicited by norfenfluramine reaches maximal values one hour after the injection, whereas that of fenfluramine is maximal at three to four hours (Table 18) we can infer that N-dealkylation may be important in mediating the decrease of brain 5-HT elicited by fenfluramine. The ED_{50} of fenfluramine to elicit an anorexic effect in the rat is 6 μmoles/kg i.p. with a fiducial limit of 4.9—8.2 that of amphetamine 3.4 μmoles/kg i.p. (F.L. 2.5—5.2) (29). We have investigated whether 12 μmoles/kg of fenfluramine which given intraperitoneally produces anorexia in 100% of the animals, changed the steady state concentrations or the turnover rate of various telencephalic brain monoamines (Table 19). The data reported in Table 19 show that the anorexic dose of fenfluramine tested increases the turnover rate of NE but it fails to change that of 5-HT or of DM. Moreover, this dose fails to decrease the steady-state concentration of the three brain monoamines studied. The findings reported in Table 19 offer another line of evidence supporting a dissociation

TABLE 19

DM, 5-HT and NE content and turnover rate in telencephalon of rats receiving two hours earlier 12 μmoles/kg i.p. of fenfluramine

Drug	DM		
	nmoles/g/hr	k hr^{-1} ± SEM	nmoles/g ± SEM
Saline	1.2	0.31 ± 0.10	4.8 ± 0.031
Fenfluramine	1.5	0.32 ± 0.08	4.8 ± 0.83

Drug	5-HT		
	nmoles/g/hr	k hr^{-1} ± SEM	nmoles/g ± SEM
Saline	0.95	0.68 ± 0.03	1.4 ± 0.17
Fenfluramine	1.2	0.85 ± 0.07	1.4 ± 0.19

Drug	NE		
	nmoles/g/hr	k hr^{-1} ± SEM	nmoles/g ± SEM
Saline	0.56	0.40 ± 0.01	1.4 ± 0.09
Fenfluramine	0.75	0.53 ± 0.01	1.3 ± 0.18

Turnover rate was calculated from the change with time of the precursor and product specific radioactivity after a tracer dose of labeled tyrosine and tryptophan (29).

of the increase of brain NE turnover rate from the increase of locomotor activity. In fact, the anorexic dose of fenfluramine (12 μmoles/kg) may actually reduce locomotor activity in the rat (29). Consistently with the data reported in this paper for a number of phenylethylamine derivatives, also fenfluramine does not increase locomotor activity and fails to increase the turnover rate of tel-diencephalic DM.

ACTION OF NORFENFLURAMINE AND (−) p-Cl-AMPHETAMINE ON TEL-DIENCEPHALIC 5-HT STORES

(−) p-Cl-amphetamine (38) (Table 15) and norfenfluramine (Table 20) cause a long lasting decrease of telencephalic concentrations of 5-HT. Despite this similarity the pharmacological profile of p-Cl-amphetamine differs from that of norfenfluramine in several respects. Norfenfluramine decreases locomotor activity, increases the duration of slow waves EEG activity and causes hyperthermia and tremors (30) whereas p-Cl-amphetamine increases locomotor activity (38) and reduces the duration of behavioral and slow wave EEG sleep. Currently, it is believed that the duration of slow wave EEG and behavioral sleep are inversely related to brain 5-HT concentrations (30). Since norfenfluramine and p-Cl-amphetamine deplete brain 5-HT by an equal extent and persist-

TABLE 20

Action of (+)(—) norfenfluramine (40 μmoles/kg i.p.) or (—) p-Cl-amphetamine (25 μmoles/kg i.p.) on the turnover rate of telencephalic 5-HT

Drug	5-HT nmoles/g ± SEM	k/hr	5-HT nmoles/g/hr
Saline	1.7 ± 0.07	0.89	1.5
p-Cl-amphetamine	0.5 ± 0.04	1.6	0.86
Saline	1.9 ± 0.025	0.69	1.3
Norfenfluramine	0.75 ± 0.015	3.6	2.7

Turnover rate was calculated from the change with time of the precursor and product specific radioactivity after a tracer dose of labeled tryptophan (19, 20).

ence but affect the sleep pattern in opposite ways, one might conclude that 5-HT stores of brain are not involved in the control of sleep. Before concluding that the action of these two drugs on sleep patterns is unrelated to their action on brain 5-HT stores we measured how these two drugs change the turnover rate of 5-HT stores in telencephalon. The results obtained in these experiments are reported in Table 20. They show that the lowering of telencephalic 5-HT stores elicited by p-Cl-amphetamine must derive from a mechanism different from that of norfenfluramine. In rats receiving p-Cl-amphetamine (Table 20) the rate of 5-HT synthesis is slower than in normal rats, suggesting that less transmitter is made per unit of time as a result of the drug injection. This finding confirms previous reports (20, 41, 40), suggesting that p-Cl-amphetamine inhibits the synthesis of brain 5-HT. In contrast, norfenfluramine administered to rats in doses that reduce selectively brain 5-HT concentrations actually increases brain 5-HT turnover rate (Table 20). This finding may help to explain why two drugs which reduce brain 5-HT concentrations may affect sleep patterns differently; the long lasting absence of slow frequency high voltage EEG activity elicited by p-Cl-amphetamine is in line with a long lasting reduced availability of 5-HT to the active sites due to the long lasting reduced rate of 5-HT biosynthesis (41). In contrast, norfenfluramine which lowers 5-HT concentrations without reducing its formation actually causes a persistence of slow wave sleep (22).

Conclusions

1. The depletion of brain NE elicited by (+)amphetamine in rats stems from 2 types of actions: a direct one related to the tissue concentrations of the drug (more than 10^{-3} M) and an indirect one related to the formation of p-OH-norephedrine, an amphetamine metabolite which accumulates intraneuronally. The duration of the direct action is short lasting because it depends on the rate of the physiological disposition of the drug. For this reason the time course of this action is different in different species. For instance, the direct action lasts longer in the guinea pig (16) than in the rat (26) because the T 1/2 of amphetamine in this species is three times faster than in guinea pigs (16). The mechanism of this direct action is not understood. It does not appear to involve the blockade of the reuptake of the NE released by nerve impulses because (+) amphetamine does not deplete brain DM concentrations although the uptake of DM is preferentially blocked by (+) amphetamine (44). The indirect action is related to the rate of physiological disposition of p-OH-norephedrine, which in the rat has a half life of about 22 hours (16). In man,

p-OH-norephedrine is a minor metabolite of (+) amphetamine (50) but it may play a role in the symptomatology associated with the habituation to this drug. Mass spectrometry gas chromatographic assay of p-OH-norephedrine (CATTABENI, this symposium) in spinal fluid of drug abusers may help to resolve whether the accumulation in brain of this amphetamine metabolite plays a role in the psychoses elicited by (+) amphetamine.

2. p-OH-norephedrine formed from (+) amphetamine not only accumulates in brain neurons of rats receiving this drug but it acts as a false neurochemical transmitter. This finding enhances the interest of ascertaining whether in man this metabolite is also accumulated in brain neurons. Guinea pigs receiving (+) amphetamine fail to form and accumulate p-OH-norephedrine (16).

3. In rats and presumably in man, methamphetamine is rapidly dealkylated to form amphetamine. The latter is then metabolized according to the usual pattern by a first order process. The dealkylation rates determine the amount of p-OH-norephedrine and its concentration in blood. Since this is important for the passage of the drug from blood to brain, dealkylation in turn determines the duration and extent of brain NE depletion. Unlike (+) amphetamine, (+) methamphetamine lowers brain 5-HT but this action is short lasting.

4. The increase in motor activity elicited by maximal effective doses of (+) amphetamine appears unrelated to an increase of brain NE turnover rate but is related to an increase of the turnover rate of striatal DM. This conclusion is supported by studies with the (−) isomer of amphetamine and with cocaine. The (−) isomer is less active than the (+) isomer in increasing motor activity and in accelerating the turnover rate of brain DM.

5. Anorexia elicited by minimal effective doses of (+) amphetamine fails to involve a drug action on presynaptic catecholaminergic neurons. A direct effect of (+) amphetamine on postsynaptic receptors should be considered.

6. The increase of motor activity elicited by aminorex and (±) p-Cl-amphetamine appears to be associated to an increase of the turnover rate of striatal DM. An action on the dopaminergic striatal system does not appear to be involved in the locomotor stimulation elicited by phenmetrazine. Phenmetrazine and aminorex do not decrease brain amines concentrations even if they are injected in high doses suggesting that in the series of compounds discussed in this paper, the depletion of brain NE requires the presence of a straight side chain in the ring.

7. The presence of a Cl atom in the p-position of amphetamine is associated with a preferential depletion of telencephalic 5-HT stores (38). The 5-HT stores of other brain structures appear more resistent to the depleting action of this chlorinated analogue of amphetamine (36). The (+) is less effective than the (−) isomer; the N methyl or α-methyl analogue of p-Cl-amphetamine are less active than the parent compound in depleting telencephalic 5-HT stores (36).

8. Fenfluramine in small doses (12 μmoles/kg i.p.) reduces locomotor activity, causes anorexia and increases brain 5-HT turnover rate, but it does not change brain DM turnover rate. In high doses (40 μmoles/kg i.p.) fenfluramine preferentially depletes telencephalic 5-HT stores. A single dose of fenfluramine reduces 5-HT concentrations of telencephalic stores for several days. Fenfluramine is metabolized into norfenfluramine which persists for a long time in tissues of rats receiving fenfluramine. Norfenfluramine may mediate the action of fenfluramine in telencephalic stores of 5-HT.

9. p-Cl-Amphetamine and norfenfluramine reduce tel-diencephalic 5-HT. Norfenfluramine increases the turnover rate of the 5-HT stores whereas p-Cl-amphetamine decreases it. This difference in the mode of action of the two drugs on brain 5-HT may help to explain their different pharmacological profile.

References

1. Axelrod, J. (1954) Studies on Sympathomimetic Amines 11. The biotransformation and physiological disposition of d-amphetamine, d-p-hydroxyamphetamine, and d-methamphetamine. J. Pharmacol. exp. Ther. **110**, 315.
2. Axelrod, J. (1964) The uptake and release of catecholamines and the effect of drugs. Progr. Brain Res. 8, 81.
3. Axelrod, J. (1971) Noradrenaline fate and control of its biosynthesis. Science, **173**, 598.
4. Axelrod, J. and Tomchick, R. (1960) Increased rate of metabolism of epinephrine and norepinephrine by sympathomimetic amines. J. Pharmacol. exp. Ther. **130**, 367.
5. Baird, J. R. C. (1968) The effects of (+)-amphetamine and (±) phenmetrazine on the NE and DM levels of the hypothalamus and corpus striatum of the rats. J. Pharmacol. **20**, 234.
6. Baird, J. R. C. and Lewis, J. J. (1963) Effects of drugs on noradrenaline and 3-hydroxytryptamine (dopamine) levels and on the noradrenaline to dopamine ratio in the rat brain. Biochem. Pharmacol. **12**, 579.
7. Bernier, A., Sicot, N. and LeDouarec, J. C. (1969) Action comparée de la fenfluramine et de l'amphetamine chez les rats obèses hypothalamiques. Rev. franç. Etud. clin. biol. **14**, 762.
8. Bhagat, B. (1965) Pressor response to amphetamine in the spinal cord and its influence on tachyphylaxis to tyramine. J. Pharmacol. exp. Ther. **149**, 206.
9. Bizzi, A., Bonaccorsi, A., Jespersen, S., Iori, A. and Garratini, S. (1970) Pharmacological studies on amphetamine and fenfluramine. In: Amphetamines and Related Compounds. Edited by Costa, E. and Garattini, S. Raven Press, New York, p. 577.
10. Boissier, J. R., Simon, P., Fichelle, J. and Hervonet, E. (1956) Action psychoanaleptique de quelques anorexigènes derivés de la phenylethylamine. Thérapie, **20**, 297.
11. Burgen, A. S. V. and Iversen, L. L. (1965) The inhibition of noradrenaline uptake by sympathomometic amines in the rat isolated heart. Brit. J. Pharmacol. **25**, 34.
12. Carlsson, A. (1970) Amphetamine and brain catecholamines. In: International Symposium on Amphetamines and Related Compounds. Edited by Costa, E. and Garattini, S. p. 217—230, Raven Press, New York.
13. Carlsson, A., Fuxe, K., Hamberger, B. and Lindqvist, M. (1966) The effect of (+)-amphetamine-containing neurons. J. Pharm. Pharmacol. **18**, 128.
14. Costa, E., Neff, N. H. and Ngai, S. H. Regulation of metaraminol efflux from rat heart and salivary gland. Brit. J. Pharmacol. **36**, 153.
15. Costa, E. and Neff, N. H. (1966) The dynamic process for catecholamine storage as a site for drug action. Prof. V. Int. C.I.N.P. Meeting, Excerpta Medica International Congress Series 129, 959.
16. Costa, E. and Groppetti, A. (1970) Biosynthesis and storage of catecholamines in tissues of rats injected with various doses of d-amphetamine. In: Amphetamines and Related Compounds. Edited by Costa, E. and Garattini, S. Raven Press, New York, p. 231—255.
17. Costa, E., Groppetti, A. and Revuelta, A. (1971) Action of fenfluramine on monoamine stores of rat tissues. Brit. J. Pharmacol. **41**, 57.
18. Costa, E. and Groppetti, A. (1972) Relationship between biochemical and pharmacological responses elicited by d-amphetamine. Proceedings of a Symposium on "Current Concepts of Amphetamine Abuse" held at Duke University, N. Carolina, June 5—6, 1970. In: Keup, W. (Ed.): Drug Abuse — Current Concepts in Research. Springfield, Ill., Charles C. Thomas, 1971.
19. Costa, E. and Revuelta, A. (1972) Norfenfluramine and serotonin turnover rate in the rat brain. Biochem. Pharmacol. In press.
20. Costa, E. and Revuelta, A. (1972) (—) p-Cl-amphetamine and serotonin turnover in rat brain. Neuropharmacology, **11**, 291.
21. Costa, E., Groppetti, A. and Naimzada, M. K. (1972) Effects of amphetamine on the turnover rate of brain catecholamines and motor activity. Brit. J. Pharmacol. **44**, 742.
22. Foxwell, M., Funderbruck, W. H. and Werd, J. W. (1969) Studies on the site of action of a new anorectic agent, fenfluramine. J. Pharmacol. exp. Ther. **165**, 60.
23. Fuxe, K. and Ungerstedt, U. (1970) Histochemical, biochemical, and functional studies on central monoamine neurons after acute and chronic amphetamine administration. In: Amphetamine and Related Compounds. Edited by Costa, E. and Garattini, S., Raven Press, New York p. 257—288.
24. Glowinski, J. and Axelrod, J. (1965) Effects of drugs on the uptake, release, and metabolism of ^{3}H-norepinephrine in the rat brain. J. Pharmacol. exp. Ther. **149**, 43.
25. Goldstein, M. and Anagnoste, B. (1965) The conversion in vivo of d-amphetamine to (+)-p-hydroxynorephedrine. Biochem. Biophys. Acta, **107**, 166.

26. GROPPETTI, A. and COSTA, E. (1969) Factors affecting the rate of disappearance of amphetamine in rats. Int. J. Neuropharmacol. **8**, 209.
27. GROPPETTI, A. and COSTA, E. (1969) Effects of cold exposure and DMI on the p-hydroxynorephedrine-^{3}H concentrations in tissues of rats injected with d-amphetamine-^{3}H. Atti Accad. med. lombarda, **23**, 1105.
28. GROPPETTI, A. and COSTA, E. (1969) Tissue concentrations of p-hydroxynorphedrine in rats injected with d-amphetamine: Effect of pretreatment with desipramine. Life Sci. **8**, 653.
29. GROPPETTI, A., MISHER, A., NAIMZADA, M., REVUELTA, A. and COSTA, E. (1972) Evidence that in rats 1 N-benzyl-β-methoxy-3-trifluoromethylphenethylamine dissociates anorexia from central stimulation and actions on brain monoamine stores. J. Pharmacol. exp. Ther. In press.
30. JOUVET, M. (1968) Insomnia and decrease of cerebral 5-hydroxytryptamine after destruction of the raphe system in the cat. Advances in Pharmacol. **6B**, 265.
31. KUCZENSKI, R. T. and MANDELL. A. J. (1972) Regulatory Properties of Soluble and Particulate Rat Brain Tyrosine Hydroxylase, J. biol. Chem. **247**, 3114.
32. MANDEL, A. J., KNAPP, S., KUCZENSKI, R. T. and SEGAL, D. S. (1972) Methamphetamine induced alteration in the physical state of rat caudate tyrosine hydroxylase. Biochem. Pharmacol. **21**, in press.
33. MARTIN W. R., SLOAN, J. W., SAPIRE, J. D. and JASINSKI, A. R. (1971) Physiologic, subjective, and behavioral effects of amphetamine methamphetamine, ephedrine, phenmetrazine, and methylphenidate in man. Chem. Pharmac. **12**, 245.
34. MOORE, K. E. and LARIVIERE, E. W. (1963) Effects of d-amphetamine and restraint on the content of norepinephrine and dopamine in rat brain. Biochem. Pharmacol. **12**, 1283.
35. MORGAN, C. D., CATTABENI, F. and COSTA, E. (1972) Methamphetamine, fenfluramine, and their N-dealkylated metabolites: Effect on monoamine concentrations in rat tissues. J. Pharmacol. exp. Ther. **180**, 127.
36. MORGAN, C. D., LOFSTRANDH, S. and COSTA, E. (1972) Amphetamine analogues and brain amines. Life Sci. **11**, 83.
37. OPITZ, K. (1967) Anoroxigene Phenylalkylamine und Serotoninstoffwechsel. Naunyn-Schmiedeberg's Arch. Pharmakol. **258**, 56.
38. PLETSCHER, A., DAPRADA, M., BATHOLINI, G., BURKARD, W. P. and BRUDERER, H. (1965) Two types of monoamine liberation by chlorinated aralkylamines. Life Sci. **4**, 2301.
39. RANDRUP, A. and SCHEEL KRUGER, J. (1966) Diethyldithiocarbamate and amphetamine stereotype behavior. J. Pharm. Pharmacol. **18**, 752.
40. SANDERS-BUSH, E. and SULSER, F. (1970) p-Cl-amphetamine *in vivo* investigations on the mechanism of action of the selective depletion of cerebral 5-HT. J. Pharmacol. exp. Ther. **175**, 419.
41. SANDERS-BUSH, E. and BUSHING, J. A. (1971) Inhibition of cerebral tryptophan hydroxylase by p-Cl-amphetamine. Fed. Proc. Fed. Amer. Soc. exp. Biol. **30**, 381.
42. STRADA, S. J., SANDERS-BUSH, E. and SULSER, F. (1970) p-Chloramphetamine: Temporal relationship between psychomotor stimulation and metabolism of brain norepinephrine. Biochem. Pharmacol. **19**, 2621.
43. SULSER, F., OWENS, M. L. and DINGELL, J. V. (1966) On the mechanism of amphetamine potentiation by desipramine (DMI). Life Sci. **5**, 2005.
44. TAYLOR, K. M. and SNYDER, S. H. (1970) Amphetamine: Differentation by d- and l-isomers of behavior involving brain norepinephrine or dopamine. Science, **168**, 1487.
45. THOENEN, H., HÜRLIMANN, A., GEY, K. F. and HAEFELY, W. (1966) Liberation of p-hydroxynorephedrine from cat spleen by sympathetic nerve stimulation after pretreatment with methamphetamine. Life Sci. **5**, 1715.
46. THÖMA, O. and WICK, H. (1954) Über einige tetrahydro-1,4-oxazine mit sympatohicommimetischen Eigenschaften. Naunyn-Schmiedeberg's Arch. Pharmakol. **222**, 540.
47. UNGERSTEDT, U. and ARBUTHNOTT, G. W. (1970) Quantitative recording of rotational behaviour in rats after 6-hydroxydopamine lesions of the gliostriatal dopamine system. Brain Res. **23**, 485
48. VAN ROSSUM, J. M., VAN DER SCHOOT, J. B. and HURKMANS, J. A. T. (1962) Mechanism of action of cocaine and amphetamine in brain. Experientia. **18**, 229.
49. WEISSMAN, A., KOE, B. K. and TENEN, S. (1966) Anti-amphetamine effects following inhibition of tyrosine hydroxylase. J. Pharmacol. exp. Ther. **151**, 339.
50. WILLIAMS, R. T. (1967) Comparative patterns of drug metabolism. Fed. Proc. **26**, 1029.
51. WISE, C. D. and STEIN, L. (1970) Amphetamine: facilitation of behaviour by augmented release of norepinephrine from the medial forebrain bundle. In: Amphetamine and Related Compounds. Edited by COSTA, E. and GARATTINI, S., Raven Press, New York, p. 463.

E.C., Laboratory of Preclinical Pharmacology, National Institute of Mental Health, Saint Elizabeth's Hospital, Washington, D. C., U.S.A.

MECHANISMS BY WHICH AMPHETAMINES PRODUCE STEREOTYPY, AGGRESSION AND OTHER BEHAVIOURAL EFFECTS

A. RANDRUP, I. MUNKVAD and J. SCHEEL-KRÜGER

Psychopharmacological Laboratory, E Sct. Hans Hospital, Roskilde

INTRODUCTION

The excitatory or stimulant effect of amphetamines (incl. apomorphine) is not a general one affecting all kinds of behaviour alike, but it is selective; certain items of behaviour are quantitatively increased while others are concurrently decreased or abolished. This selectivity of effect is seen already after small doses of amphetamine but becomes more pronounced after larger doses (84, 95). Many, probably all kinds of behaviour are affected, resulting in a profound change in the whole behavioural pattern (65, 66, 82, 84, 95). Stereotypy, i.e. lack of variation and apparent aimlessness, is a characteristic feature of the pattern that emerges; in the extreme the behaviour consists in the continuous repetition of one or a few acts.

One mg/kg of d-amphetamine given subcutaneously to rats thus produces selective stimulation of sniffing, locomotion and rearing, while there is little grooming activity (32). Gradual increase of the amphetamine dose in the interval 1—10 mg/kg leads first to further decrease and eventually to disappearance of grooming activity; then locomotion and rearing are also decreased and finally disappear so that only sniffing remains. Before disappearing, locomotion shows stereotyped features consisting in repetitive running forth and back or along a fixed route in a restricted part of the cage (52, 84, 97). At 10 mg/kg the behavioural pattern is extremely stereotyped. Sniffing, often accompanied by licking and biting, is performed continuously and usually covers a small area at or near the bottom of the cage; occasionally backward locomotion is seen. (5, 32, 61, 75, 92).

With the higher doses the stereotyped behaviour does not appear immediately after a subcutaneous injection but develops gradually through a pre-phase with selective stimulation and inhibition comparable to that seen with the smaller doses; after the period of maximal stereotypy there is again a post-phase which is similar to the pre-phase (see Figs. 1 and 3).

Selective stimulation and inhibition, and with higher doses extremely stereotyped behaviour has been produced by amphetamine in many mammalian species including man. Thus dogs make i.a. locomotion stereotypies: continuous circling or running forth and back along a fixed route (17, 68, 79, 118, 119), while cats perform continuous head-movements (as if looking around) sniffing or certain grooming responses. (24, 27, 79, 116, 117). With monkeys we have seen repetitive locomotion along a fixed route, continuous picking or preening of a limb, hand-looking, limb-movements, etc. (25, 49, 79, 81). With humans there are reports of continuous performance of various tasks: washing and rewashing of plates, dismantling and reassembling of clocks, combing of hair, marching around in circles, plucking at fingers etc. (28, 79, 81, 82, 84, 88).

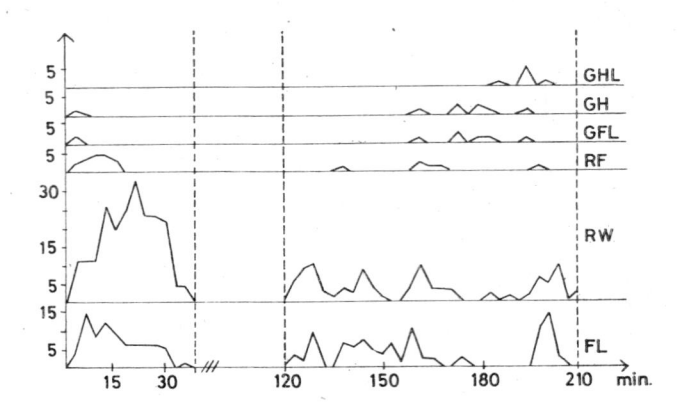

Fig. 1. Selective behavioural stimulation of a rat by amphetamine. Each horizontal section represents an item of behaviour. From top to bottom: grooming with the hind legs, grooming with the head (mouth), grooming with the forelegs, rearing in the free, rearing at the wall, forward locomotion. The number of times the first five elements occurred were counted in each three-minute period, locomotion measured as the numbers of lines (50 cm distance, the cage was 3×3.5 m^2) the rat crossed in three minutes. These numbers are represented on the ordinate. Time is on the abscissa, the whole period being 210 min beginning just after the injection of amphetamine. During the phase of maximal stereotypy (shown between vertical broken lines in the diagram) none of the six behavioural elements recorded were performed but only continuous sniffing, licking or biting. This is an example from the experiments of SCHIØRRING (95) comprising 13 rats treated with d-amphetamine sulphate (5 mg/kg s.c.) and 10 rats given placebo.

The items of behaviour performed thus differ among species and in the higher species also among individuals. What is common to all mammalian species investigated, is the stereotyped feature of the behavioural pattern elicited by higher doses of amphetamine.

The selective stimulation by amphetamines stands in contrast to the more generalized stimulation of rats by 1—2 mg/kg of morphine. With morphine there is increase of locomotion and rearing as with amphetamine but also increase of all grooming responses as well as eating, drinking and social activities, which are inhibited by amphetamine (30, own unpublished observations).

Also simple "neurological" movements, such as movements of tongue and lips are elicited by amphetamine in monkeys and humans (25, 49, 80). DOPA produces similar movements (and also stereotyped behaviour and psychosis) as a side effect in the treatment of Parkinson's disease (6, 12, 45, 51, 83). Mouth and tongue movements of anaestetized rats as studied by BIEGER et al. (7) may be related to these neurological phenomena.

In the following we shall discuss the mechanisms by which amphetamine selectively affects various kinds of behaviour and produces stereotypy. It seems that amphetamines excite the dopaminergic systems in the forebrain, and that these systems influence many, perhaps all kinds of behaviour and also certain neurological functions. At the same time, however, each kind of behaviour, e.g. locomotion, items of aggressive behaviour, eating, etc. is also influenced or mediated by various other systems in the brain. Some of these systems, such as noradrenergic and serotonergic systems, are affected by amphetamines.

Most of the dopamine in the brain is found in corpus striatum and adjacent structures. The concept of the function of the dopamine systems given here agrees with ideas about the function of the striatum based on experiments with brain lesions (104).

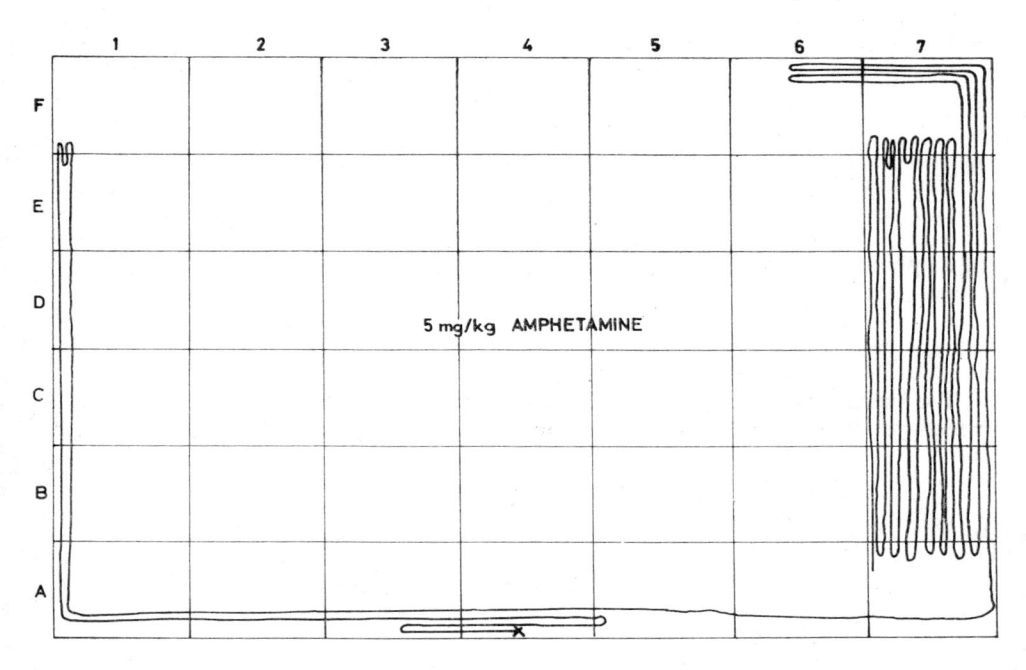

Fig. 2. Route of an amphetaminized rat in a 3×3.5 m^2 cage. There is a period with apparently normal exploration (left in the figure) and a period with repetitive running forth and back (right). The floor of the cage was divided in squares numbered after the chessboard principle as indicated in the figure. The observer followed the rat through a one-way screen and recorded its route of locomotion by speaking into a tape recorder. The figure is a representative example from an experiment by SCHIØRRING (95, 97) comprising 13 rats given 5 mg/kg d-amphetamine sulphate and 10 placebo rats. The locomotion of the amphetamine rat was recorded in the pre-phase (compare Fig. 1). All the locomotion shown in the figure was along the walls of the cage.

BIOCHEMICAL FINDINGS RELATED TO BEHAVIOURAL EFFECTS

Amphetamine affects both dopamine, noradrenaline and serotonin in the brain.

With dopamine amphetamine seems to exert a releasing action at the presynaptic site of synthesis and affect the pathway to the postsynaptic receptor in such a way that more dopamine reaches the receptor. There is evidence indicating a shift in the metabolism of dopamine (formation of less of the oxidized and more of the O-methylated metabolite) and a change in the turnover in certain subcellular pools (13, 18, 34, 35, 41, 54, 55, 57, 81, 86, 91, 110). Certain amphetamines e.g. pipradrol have similar actions but release dopamine from the site of storage rather than from the site of synthesis (90).

The effect on noradrenaline appears to be similar. Amphetamine, however, also reduces the amount of noradrenaline in the brain, an effect which is partially due to displacement of noradrenaline by the amphetamine metabolite, p-hydroxynorephedrine. (14, 19, 35, 56, 91, 109, 121).

Amphetamine causes increased turnover of serotonin in the brain (53, 85, 99, 100). Possibly this effect is secondary to the rise in body temperature (85). Other amphetamines, e.g. p-chloroamphetamine and fenfluramine, cause depletion of brain serotonin (46, 74, 92).

Apomorphine seems mainly to exert a direct action on the dopamine receptor. In the spinal cord, where there is no dopamine, amphetamine stimulates a noradrenergic mechanism causing increase of a flexor reflex, but apomorphine does not give this effect (1). Apomorphine therefore seems to be the most specific stimulant of the dopamine system.

The dopaminergic, noradrenergic and serotonergic nerve systems in the brain are clearly separated anatomically (114) and it seems highly probable that their functions are also different. In the following we shall discuss the association of some behavioural effect of amphetamines with the biochemical effects just mentioned.

Stereotypy

The extremely stereotyped pattern of behaviour, continuous sniffing, licking or biting, which rats show after higher doses of amphetamines (e.g. 10 mg/kg of d-amphetamine,

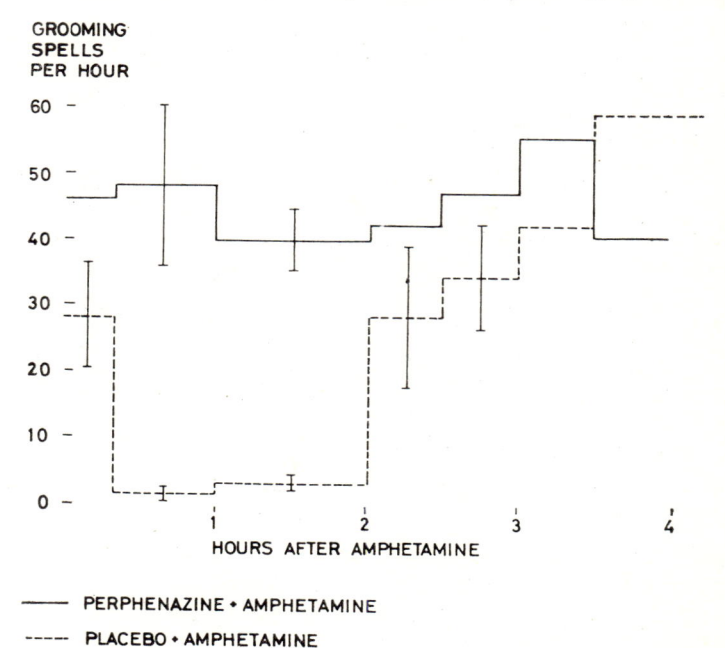

Fig. 3. Number of grooming spells from injection of amphetamine until the animals fall asleep. Cross-over design, 2×3 animals and two weeks between the two experimental days. The curve in broken line shows a strong depression of grooming activity 1/2 to 2 hrs. after the amphetamine injection; during the same period continuous stereotyped sniffing — licking — biting was observed. Perphenazine inhibited the stereotyped activity and concurrently increased the grooming, as shown in the graph. Locomotion was influenced in a way similar to grooming by both amphetamine and perphenazine (77).

0.8 mg/kg of apomorphine) is specifically antagonized by neuroleptic drugs (42, 43, 61, 77). Smaller doses of neuroleptic drugs reduce the sniffing, licking and biting and at the same time cause reappearance of other activities which were inhibited by the amphetamines, e.g. grooming (see Fig. 3), locomotion and lever-pressing under certain schedules (11, 72, 77, 87). The pattern of behaviour therefore becomes more varied, less stereotyped. Dopamine antagonism seems to be the characteristic and only common property of all neuroleptics and some of the neuroleptics are rather specific antagonists of dopamine (3, 8, 15, 33, 36, 44, 62, 67, 93, 101, 107, 108, 111, 120). This indicates that the extreme stereotypy of this behavioural pattern is due to the action of the amphetamines upon dopamine in the brain; other evidence supports this indication (22, 29, 31, 71, 80, 81, 84, 86, 113, 115).

Various features of the stereotyped behaviour may be changed by other drugs or by environmental changes, but in these cases the stereotypy of the behavioural pattern is retained. For example high doses of the antiserotonins deseril and cyproheptadine caused some reappearance of forward locomotion in the amphetaminized rats, but sniffing — licking — biting remained completely continuous (76). Drugs blocking noradrenaline or inhibiting its synthesis cause reduction of general motor activity of amphetaminized rats

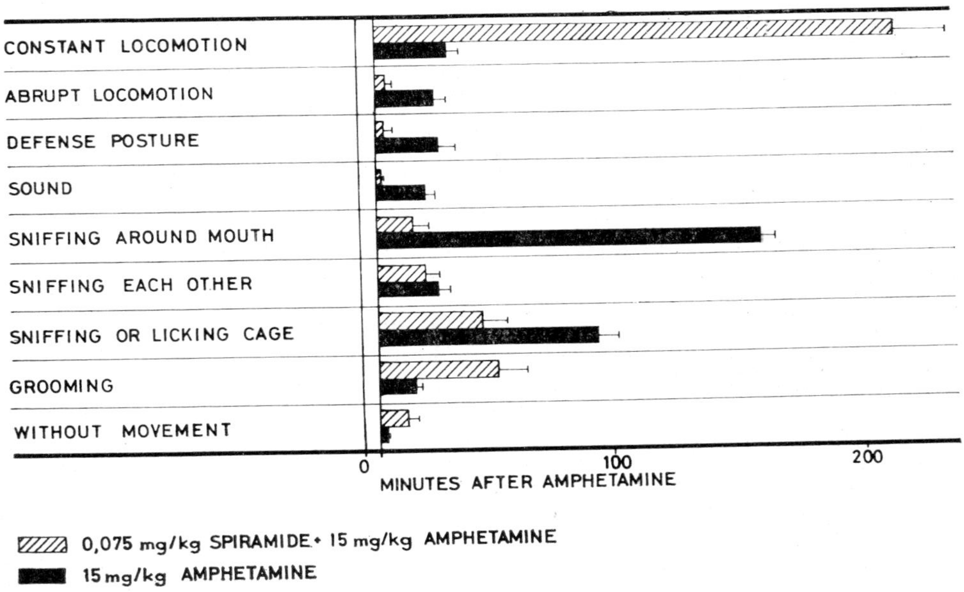

Fig. 4. Effects of spiramide, a neuroleptic, on times of amphetamine-induced aggressive behaviour of mice. Note the different effect upon the two forms of locomotion. "Constant locomotion" means locomotion performed at constant moderate speed, "abrupt locomotion" designated spells of sudden, rapid locomotion often involving several mice which may whirl or roll around each other "Abrupt locomotion", „defense posture" (two or more mice rearing against each other) and "sound" (vocalization) are regarded as items of aggressive behaviour. The experiments were made with groups of four male mice, each group in a small cage $10 \times 10 \times 10$ cm^3. The momentary behaviour of the mice was observed every second minute, and the number of mice showing each of the nine behavioural items was recorded. The diagram shows mean counts and standard deviation of the mean per cage for the whole observation period 0—180 min after the injection of amphetamine (40).

(e.g. head- and paw-movements, righting reflex, ambulation, rearing) but continuous licking or biting remains (43, 61, 78).

Anticholinergic drugs prolong and potentiate the stereotypy producing effect of amphetamine (5, 89).

Locomotion

Forward locomotion is increased by smaller doses of amphetamine and abolished by larger doses. Both effects are antagonized by small doses of neuroleptics and it therefore seems probable that a smaller increase in dopaminergic activity in the brain enhances locomotion while a further increase has the opposite effect. (40, 72, 77).

Drugs antagonizing noradrenaline cause reduction of locomotion of amphetaminized as well as untreated rats and mice, and the effect of amphetamine on noradrenaline would therefore seem to contribute in the cases where the drug causes increase of locomotion (2, 13, 43, 61, 78).

Aggression and other social activities

When four male mice were put together in a small cage we produced by 5 mg/kg of d-amphetamine a stereotyped behaviour consisting in continuous sniffing combined with much locomotion at constant, moderate speed. Raising the dose to 15 mg/kg resulted in sniffing — licking — biting stereotypy interrupted by spells of aggressive activities (defense posture, vocalization, abrupt locomotion with mice whirling or rolling around each other). At the same time the locomotion at constant moderate speed was reduced. Small doses of specific neuroleptics (spiramide, trifluperazine) counteracted the changes brought about by the higher amphetamine dose (see Fig. 4), so that the mice with neuroleptic + 15 mg/kg amphetamine behaved similar to those having received 5 mg/kg of amphetamine alone. The neuroleptics thus specifically antagonized the items of aggressive behaviour without causing a general reduction in motor activity, and this indicates that the further increase in dopaminergic activity caused by raising the dose of amphetamine from 5 to 15 mg/kg was a major cause of the aggressive behaviour. Aceperone, a noradrenaline α-blocker, also tended to reduce the aggressive activities but only in parallel with a general reduction of motor activity (40).

Another social activity, sniffing around the mouth of another mouse, was also increased by 15 mg/kg of amphetamine and specifically reduced by the neuroleptics; this behaviour was increased by aceperone (40).

In some couples of rats apomorphine elicits prolonged defense postures (the rats rearing against each other with vocalization and boxing movements of the forepaws). This stereotyped form of aggressive activity alternates with the usual sniffing — licking — biting stereotypy, which is seen all the time when these rats are put in individual cages. (58, 102; own unpublished observations). SENAULT, (102) found that atropine reduced the aggressive activity, and since anticholinergics potentiate the sniffing — licking — biting stereotypy (5, 89) the balance between dopamine and acetylcholine in the brain may be one of the factors which determine whether the stereotypy will be of the aggressive or of the usual type.

In monkeys we have observed that several forms of social activities are reduced by amphetamine even in small doses (48, 50, 96). Pretreatment with the specific neuroleptic, pimozide, appeared to cause social activities to return earlier, but during the first two hours after amphetamine the neuroleptic had no effect (48, 84).

Eating and drinking

UNGERSTEDT (112) produced by 6-hydroxydopamine specific lesions in the nigro-striatal dopaminergic nerve system and found that these produced aphagia and adipsia. Also experiments with lesions in the striatum showed the involvement of this brain structure in eating and drinking behaviour (104).

In our laboratory it was found that the amphetamine-induced reduction of drinking by rats kept on a deprivation schedule, could be partially but not completely reversed by small doses of the specific dopamine antagonist pimozide. Pimozide given alone did not increase but rather inhibited drinking (64). Likewise SCHULZ and FREY (100) found that the anorexigenic effect of amphetamine could be antagonized by small doses of haloperidol.

The effect of amphetamines on brain dopamine may therefore contribute to the inhibitory effects of amphetamines on eating and drinking.

Effects on noradrenaline may also contribute, since eating and drinking are also influenced by noradrenergic systems in the hypothalamus (10, 37, 112) and the anorexigenic effect of d-amphetamine could be antagonized by phentolamine and disulfiram (100).

Further contribution to the anorexigenic effect of certain amphetamines, e.g. fenfluramine and p-chloroamphetamine, seems to come from the effect of these drugs on brain serotonin (46, 100).

Mood

GUNNE and coworkers (39) recorded euphoric effect after intravenous injections of 200 mg d,l-amphetamine in humans. A self rating procedure was used. The effect was reduced to 50 per cent by pretreatment with the specific dopamine blocker pimozide, while noradrenergic blocking agents gave no reduction. Pretreatment with α-methyl-tyrosine also caused reduction of the euphoric response (4, 38, 39, 47).

In depressed patients VAN PRAAG et al. (74) found antidepressive effect of p-chloroamphetamine and p-chloromethylamphetamine. Their experiments were inspired by the hypothesis that the antidepressive effect was mediated by increased serotonergic activity produced by these drugs. The results, however, did not fit all their expectations based on this hypothesis. Later SCHEEL-KRÜGER (92) has shown that p-chloroamphetamine also exerts amphetamine-like effects on dopamine and noradrenaline in the brain. In view of the experiments on euphoric effects mentioned above it seems possible that brain dopamine may contribute to the antidepressive effect of p-chloroamphetamine. Other evidence supports this contention, i.a. the finding of low values of homovanillic acid (dopamine metabolite) as well as 5-hydroxyindole acetic acid (serotonin metabolite) in the cerebrospinal fluid of depressed patients (69, 73).

ANATOMICAL FINDINGS RELATED TO BEHAVIOURAL EFFECTS

The largest dopamine system in the brain is the nigro-striatal, and there is considerable evidence indicating that this system is involved in the production of the extremely stereotyped behaviour by larger doses of amphetamines. The stereotyped behaviour could be elicited by micro-injections of dopamine or amphetamines into the striatum, and it could be abolished by lesions or by micro-injection of neuroleptic drugs in this area (20, 22, 29, 34, 63, 80, 81, 84).

Some of the most recent experiments have shown lacking effect of lesions in the nucleus caudatus-putamen upon apomorphine-stereotypy (59) and lesions in the substantia nigra upon amphetamine-stereotypy (21, 103). For the evaluation of such apparently conflicting results we think it is important to consider carefully the size of the lesions since both Fog et al. (30) and Fuxe and Ungerstedt (34) found that the amphetamine-stereotypy is abolished by large lesions in the striatum but only modified by smaller lesions. Besides the histological or histochemical evaluation of the size of the lesion, it is important to watch the feeding of the animals, since large lesions seem to render the rats aphagic and adipsic (21, 112).

Another important feature is the recovery (compensation) of the lesioned animals, which progresses during several weeks after the operation (112). Fog et al. (30) found the same lesion-effects in experiment with amphetamine 2—3 hours, 3—5 days and 5 weeks after removal of the corpus striatum by suction, but after other lesions there may be changes during the recovery period.

For the evaluation of lesion experiments we also think it is important to consider the behavioural concepts outlined in the present paper, particularly the concept of stereotypy as a *pattern* of behaviour which can consist in the repetition of *various* types or fractions of normal behaviour. Thus Naylor and Olley (63) found after a unilateral lesion in the caudate-putamen of rats a marked reduction in the sniffing — licking — biting stereotypy, which was replaced by a characteristic circling at its height shown as an incessant and rapid twisting of the body. This incessant circling activity (113) may be regarded as a stereotyped behaviour and we therefore think that the unilateral lesion cause a qualitative change rather than a reduction in stereotypy. Likewise the subthalamic lesions of Boissier et al. (9) seem to cause a qualitative change in amphetamine stereotypy from "stereotyped movements of the head and forepaws" (probably sniffing — 61) to "compulsive gnawing". Schoenfeld and Uretsky (98) report that intraventricular injection of 6-hydroxydopamine causes both an increase and a modification of apomorphine stereotypy of rats. Instead of a pattern of sniffing, licking and gnawing there was locomotion and "wall climbing". This behaviour was, however, "repetitive, exaggerated and uninterrupted by normal behavioural elements such as grooming or sleeping" and was consequently considered stereotyped by the authors. Fuxe and Ungerstedt (34) report stereotyped sniffing, biting *or walking* after intrastriatal injections of apomorphine.

Ungerstedt (112) found that after 6-hydroxydopamine-induced lesions in the nigrostriatal pathway, apomorphine produced very violent compulsive gnawing, but Costall et al. (21) found little effect of apomorphine and no gnawing after electrolytic coagulation in the substantia nigra. These results are at present difficult to reconcile. Ungerstedt's result agrees with other experiments indicating that apomorphine acts directly on dopamine receptors and with experiments on unilateral lesions in the nigrostriatal pathway (21, 98).

The dopaminergic area in the forebrain comprises besides the striatum also the nucleus accumbens and the tuberculum olfactorium, and in higher mammals (but not in rats) the caudate nucleus and the putamen are clearly separated anatomically. Investigation of the roles of each of these parts of the dopaminergic area in behaviour and particularly in amphetamine stereotypy is only at its beginning. Interesting experiments were made by McKenzie (58, 59) who studied the effect of lesions in the tuberculum olfactorium upon apomorphine-induced stereotypy. The lesions abolished sniffing and chewing behaviour completely in 9 out of 20 rats while another 6 became "hyperexcitable, aggressive and performed the stereotyped behaviour intermittently". Comparison of these latter animals with unlesioned rats becoming aggressive under apomorphine would be interesting, perhaps the lesion in the tuberculum olfactorium affects both the occurrence of stereotypy and the balance between the aggressive and the usual form of apomorphine stereotypy of rats (compare the discussion of apomorphine and aggression in the previous section).

The results of Costall et al. (20) and Naylor and Olley (63) indicate that also globus pallidus exerts an effect on locomotor activity and stereotypy. According to UNGERSTEDT (114) the dopaminergic fibers from the substantia nigra pass through this brain region on their way to the caudate-putamen; other systems in the globus pallidus may also be involved.

APPLICATION OF ANIMAL DATA TO CLINICAL PROBLEMS

As mentioned in the introduction amphetamines produce selective stimulation of certain behavioural items and extremely stereotyped behaviour patterns in humans as well as in other mammals (24, 28, 79, 81, 84).

In the human species subjective experiences accompanying these behavioural changes can be studied. Thus ELLINWOOD (24, 25, 28) describes amphetamine-induced grooming stereotypies (incessant examining, rubbing and picking of certain areas of the skin) in rhesus monkeys and humans. Many of the humans, ELLINWOOD states, developed marked delusions of parasitosis and spent many hours examining their skin and digging out imagined encysted parasites. Similar cases are described in the older German literature about methamphetamine abuse (23, 88, 105).

The "amphetamine psychosis" observed in humans is often described as being very similar to schizophrenia particularly in the paranoid form. The similarity is such that misdiagnoses have been made (see reviews cited at the beginning of this section). Cases of amphetamine psychosis reminiscent of manio-depressive psychosis or with mixed manic-depressive and schizophrenic symptomatology are also reported (84). Therefore, the studies of the mechanisms by which amphetamines produce abnormal behaviour is supposed to have some bearing on psychosis research.

The inhibitory effect on brain dopamine by neuroleptics shows high correlation with antipsychotic effect in the clinic (8, 31, 67, 93, 101, 107, 108) and antagonism of amphetamine, apomorphine and methyl-phenidate stereotypies of rats and mice has been used successfully for preclinical screening of antipsychotic drugs (42, 43, 70, 71, 77).

It now seems possible that in these screening procedures further information about the antipsychotic drugs can be obtained by more detailed observations of the behaviour of the animals. One example is the above-mentioned antagonism of amphetamine-induced aggressive behaviour of mice which appears to parallel antagonism of aggression in schizophrenic patients by neuroleptic drugs. Other possibilities seem to arise from the observation that neuroleptics not only antagonize the activities of mice and rats, which are increased by amphetamines but also cause recovery of some normal activities inhibited by amphetamines e.g. locomotion and grooming (72, 77, 87). This results in a more varied, less stereotyped pattern of behaviour, and seems to parallel the revival of normal functions observed in schizophrenic patients treated with neuroleptics.

In the patients, however, there is often only partial recovery of normal functions. Many patients are reported to remain socially isolated and unable to care for themselves economically so that they must be given disablement pension after discharge from the hospital (60, 106). Parallelly we found that the inhibition of social behaviour of monkeys by amphetamine could only be little influenced by neuroleptics (48, 84 and unpublished results). In rats we found that all grooming activity was inhibited by amphetamine, but while grooming with the forepaws and with the mouth could be brought back by neuroleptics, grooming with the hind paws was recovered much more poorly (77, and unpublished results). BROWN (11) found partial but not complete restoration by chlorpromazine of lever pressing (operant) activity suppressed by amphetamine, and we have made similar observations (LYON et al., unpublished).

It thus seems possible that further studies along these lines can lead to better understanding of the limitations and shortcomings of the present neuroleptic treatment of psychoses and furnish models for preclinical testing of new drugs or other potential means for improved therapy.

As mentioned above, antagonism of dopamine appears to be the common property of neuroleptic drugs, but it may be that additional biochemical effects (e.g. on noradrenaline) can help to shape a more normal behaviour in certain types of psychotic patients. It may also be that anatomical specificity within the dopamine area in the forebrain, and the biochemical mechanism (presynaptic, postsynaptic etc.) by which dopamine is affected, are factors which modulate the resultant antipsychotic effect.

SUMMARY

The dopaminergic systems in the forebrain (nucleus caudatus, putamen and some adjacent areas) appear to have effects, in mammals, on many perhaps all types of behaviour, and these effects tend in the extreme to change the whole pattern of behaviour into a stereotyped, apparently aimless one.

At the same time each type of behaviour e.g. locomotion, aggressive and other social activities, drinking etc. appear to be influenced also by other brain systems. The behavioural effects of a drug, which like amphetamines acts on several brain systems (dopaminergic, noradrenergic, serotonergic and possibly others) are therefore bound to be complicated. For example: smaller doses of d-amphetamine cause increase in locomotion of rats while larger doses cause inhibition. The increased locomotion can be stereotyped, consisting in repetition of a fixed route in a restricted part of the cage. Brain dopamine plays a role in these locomotor effects, but locomotion is also influenced by brain noradrenaline.

Recent findings about the mechanisms by which amphetamines produce their behavioural effects are reviewed. Real and apparent contradictions in the most recent publications about experiments with brain lesions are discussed; the extent of lesions in the striatum and the slow recovery of behaviour after such lesions seem to be important items in this context. Clinical implications of the animal experiments are suggested.

REFERENCES

1. ANDÉN, N. E., RUBENSON, A., FUXE, K. and HÖKFELT, T. (1967) Evidence for dopamine receptor stimulation by apomorphine. J. Pharmacol. **19**, 627.
2. ANDÉN, N. E. (1970) Effects of amphetamine and some other drugs on central catecholamine mechanisms. In: Amphetamines and Related Compounds (Eds. E. COSTA and S. GARATTINI), p. 447, Raven Press, New York.
3. ANDÉN, N. E., BUTCHER, S. G., CORRODI, H., FUXE, K. and UNGERSTEDT, U. (1970) Receptor activity and turnover of dopamine and noradrenaline after neuroleptics. Europ. J. Pharmacol. **11**, 303.
4. ÄNGGÅRD, E., JÖNSSON, L. E. and GUNNE, L. M. (1971) Pharmacological blockade of amphetamine effects in subjects dependent on central stimulants. Acta pharmacol. toxicol. **29**, suppl. 4, 2.
5. ARNFRED, T. and RANDRUP, A. (1968) Cholinergic mechanism in brain inhibiting amphetamine-induced stereotyped behaviour. Acta pharmacol. (Kbh.) **26**, 384.
6. BARBEAU, A. (1970) Dopamine and disease. Can. med. Ass. J. **103**, 824.
7. BIEGER, D., LAROCHELLE, L. and HORNYKIEWICZ, O. (1972) A model for the quantitative study of central dopaminergic and serotoninergic activity. Europ. J. Pharmacol. **18**, 128.
8. BOBON, D., JANSSEN, P. and BOBON, J. (Eds.) (1970) The Neuroleptics. See i.a. papers by v. Rossum et al.; Randrup; v. Rossum. S. Karger, Basel.

9. BOISSIER, J. R., ETEVENON, P., PIARROUX, M. C. and SIMON, P. (1971) Effects of apomorphine and amphetamine in rats with a permanent catalepsy induced by diencephalic lesion. Res. Comm. chem. Pathol. Pharmacol. **2**, 829.
10. BOOTH, D. A. (1968) Mechanism of action of norepinephrine in eliciting an eating response on injection into the rat hypothalamus. J. Pharmacol. exp. Ther. **160**, 336.
11. BROWN, H. (1963) D-amphetamine-chlorpromazine antagonism in a food reinforced operant. J. exp. Analysis Behav. **6**, 395.
12. CALNE, D. B. (1970) L-dopa in the treatment of parkinsonism. Clin Pharmacol. Ther. **11**, 789.
13. CARLSSON, A. (1970) Amphetamine and brain catecholamines. In: Amphetamines and Related Compounds (Eds.: E. Costa and S. Garattini), p. 289, Raven Press, New York.
14. COOK, J. D. and SCHANBERG, S. M. (1970) The effects of methamphetamine on behavior and on the uptake, release and metabolism of norepinephrine. Biochem. Pharmacol. **19**, 1165.
15. COOLS, A. R. and VAN ROSSUM, J. M. (1970) Caudal dopamine and stereotype behaviour of cats. Arch. int. Pharmacodyn. **187**, 163.
16. COOLS, A. R. (1971) The function of dopamine and its antagonism in the caudate nucleus of cats in relation to the stereotyped behaviour. Arch. int. Pharmacodyn **194**, 259.
17. CORSON, S. A., CORSON, O'LEARY, E., KIRILČUK, V., KIRILČUK, J., KNOPP, W. and ARNOLD, L. E. (1972) Differential effects of amphetamines on clinically relevant dog models of hyperkinesis and stereotypy: relevance to Huntington's disease. Centennial Symp. on Huntington's chorea, Raven Press, In press.
18. COSTA, E. and GROPETTI, A. (1970) Biosynthesis and storage of catecholamines in tissues of rats injected with various doses of d-amphetamine. In: Amphetamines and Related Compounds (Eds.: E. Costa and S. Garattini), p. 231. Raven Press, New York.
19. COSTA, E. and GARANTINI, S. (Eds.) (1970) Amphetamines and Related Compounds. Raven Press, New York.
20. COSTALL, B., NAYLOR, R. J. and OLLEY, J. E. (1972) Stereotypic and anticataleptic activities of amphetamine after intracerebral injections. Europ. J. Pharmacol. **18**, 83.
21. COSTALL, B., NAYLOR, R. J. and OLLEY, J. E. (1972) The substantia nigra and stereotyped behaviour. Europ. J. Pharmacol. **18**, 95.
22. CROW, T. J. (1972) A map of the rat mesencephalon for electrical self-stimulation. Brain. Res. **36**, 265.
23. DAUBE, H. (1942) Pervitinpsychosen. Nervenarzt **15**, 20.
24. ELLINWOOD. E. H. (1969) Amphetamine Psychosis: A multi-dimensional process. Seminars in Psychiatry **1**, 208.
25. ELLINWOOD, E. H. (1971) Comparative methamphetamine intoxication in experimental animals. Pharmako.-Psychiat. **4**, 357.
26. ELLINWOOD, E. H. (1971) "Accidental conditioning" with chronic methamphetamine intoxications: Implications for a theory of drug habituation. Psychopharmacologia, **21**, 131.
27. ELLINWOOD, E. H., SUDILOVSKY, A. and NELSON, L. (1972) Behavioral analysis of chronic amphetamine intoxication. Biol. Psychiat. **4**, 215.
28. ELLINWOOD, E. H. and SUDILOVSKY, A. (1972) Chronic amphetamine intoxication: behavioral model of psychoses. Amer. psychopathol. Assoc. Proc. (in press).
29. ERNST, A. M. (1971) Chemical stimulation of central dopaminergic receptors in the striatal body of rats. In: The Correlation of Adverse Effects in Man with Observations in Animals (Ed. S. B. DE BAKER), p. 18. Excerpta Medica Internat. Congress Series no. 220, Amsterdam.
30. FOG, R., RANDRUP, A. and PAKKENBERG, H. (1970) Lesions in corpus striatum and cortex of rat brains and the effect on pharmacologically induced stereotyped, aggressive and cataleptic behaviour. Psychopharmacologia, **18**, 346.
31. FOG, R., RANDRUP, A. and PAKKENBERG, H. (1971) Intrastriatal injection of quaternary butyrophenones and oxypertine: neuroleptic effect in rats. Psychopharmacologia, **19**, 224.
32. FOG, R. (1970) Behavioural effects in rats of morphine and amphetamine and of a combination of the two drugs. Psychopharmacologia, **16**, 305.
33. FOG, R. (1972) On stereotypy and catalepsy: studies of the effect of amphetamines and neuroleptics in rats. Thesis. University of Copenhagen. Munksgaard.
34. FUXE, K. and UNGERSTEDT, U. (1970) Histochemical, biochemical and functional studies on central monoamine Neurons after acute and chronic amphetamine administration. In: Amphetamines and Related Compounds (Eds. E. Costa and S. Garattini), p. 257, Raven Press, New York.
35. GLOWINSKY, J. (1970) Effects of amphetamine on various aspects of catecholamine metabolism in the central nervous system of the rat. In: Amphetamines and Related Compounds (Eds. E. COSTA and S. GARATTINI), p. 301, Raven Press, New York.

36. GOLDBERG, L. I. (1972) Cardiovascular and renal actions of dopamine: potential clinical applications. Pharmacol. Rev. **24**, 1.
37. GROSSMAN, S. P. (1967) The central regulation of food and water intake. In: The Chemical Senses and nutrition (Eds. M. R. KARE and O. MALLER), p. 293. The Johns Hopkins Press, Baltimore, U.S.A.
38. GUNNE, L. M., ÄNGGÅRD, E. and JÖNSSON, L. E. (1970) Blockade of amphetamine effects in human subjects. In: International Institute on the Prevention and Treatment of Drug Dependence, I.C.A.A. (Eds. A. TONGUE and E. TONGUE), p. 249. Lausanne.
39. GUNNE, L. M., ÄNGGÅRD, E. and JÖNSSON, L. E. (1972) Clinical trials with amphetamine-blocking drugs. Psychiat., Neurol., Neurochir. (Amst.) **75**, 225.
40. HASSELAGER, E., ROLINSKI, Z. and RANDRUP, A. (1972) Specific antagonism by dopamine inhibitors of items of amphetamine induced aggressive behaviour. Psychopharmacologia, **24**, 485.
41. HITZEMANN, R. J., LOH, H. H. and DOMINO, E. F. (1971) Effect of para-methoxyamphetamine on catecholamine metabolism in the mouse brain. Life Sci. **10**, 1087.
42. JANSSEN, P., NIEMEGEERS, C. and SCHELLEKENS, K. (1965) Is it possible to predict the clinical effects of neuroleptic drugs (major tranquillizers) from animal data. Arzneim.-Forsch. **15**, 104.
43. JANSSEN, P., NIEMEGEERS, C., SCHELLEKENS, K. and LENAERTS, F. (1967) Is it possible to predict the clinical effects of neuroleptic drugs (major tranquillizers) from animal data. Arzneim.-Forsch. **17**, 841.
44. JANSSEN, P., NIEMEGEERS, C., SCHELLEKENS, K., DRESSE, A., LENAERTS, F., PINCHARD, A., SCHAPER, W., VAN NUETEN, J. and VERBRUGGEN, F. (1968) Pimozide, a chemically novel, highly potent and orally longacting neuroleptic drug. Arzneim.-Forsch. **18**, 261.
45. JENKINS, R. B. and GROH, R. H. (1970) Mental symptoms in Parkinsonian patients treated with L-dopa. Lancet, **II**, 177.
46. JESPERSEN, S. and SCHEEL-KRÜGER, J. (1973) Evidence for a difference in mechanism of action between fenfluramine and amphetamine induced anorexia. J. Pharm. Pharmacol. **25**, 49.
47. JÖNSSON. L.-E., ÄNGÅRD, E. and GUNNE, L.-M. (1971) Blockade of intravenous amphetamine euphoria in man. Clin. Pharmacol. Ther. **12**, 889.
48. KJELLBERG, B. and RANDRUP, A. (1971) The effects of amphetamine and pimozide, a neuroleptic, on the social behaviour of vervet monkeys (cercopithecus sp.). In: Advances in Neuro-Psychopharmacology (Eds. O. VINAŘ, Z. VOTAVA, and P. B. BRADLEY), p. 305. North-Holland Publ. Comp., Amsterdam, Avicenum, Czechoslovak Medical Press, Prague.
49. KJELLBERG, B. and RANDRUP, A. (1972) Stereotypy with selective stimulation of certain items of behaviour observed in amphetamine-treated monkeys (cercopithecus). Pharmakopsychiat. **5**, 1.
50. KJELLBERG, B. and RANDRUP, A. (1972) Changes in social behaviour in pairs of vervet monkeys (cercopithecus) produced by single, low doses of amphetamine. This meeting.
51. KNOPP, W. (1971) Pharmacopsychiatry, L-dopa and Parkinson's disease In: Abstracts from VII CINP Congress, Prague 1970, Vol. I, p. 244.
52. LÁT, J. (1965) The spontaneous exploratory reactions as a tool for psychopharmacological studies. In: Proceedings of the 2. International Pharmacological Meeting (Eds. M. MIKHELSON and V. LONGO), p. 47, Pergamon Press, Oxford.
53. LEONARD, B. E. (1971) A study of the effects of some amphetamines on brain monoamines and their precursors. In: First Congress of the Hungarian Pharmacological Society. (Ed. J. KNOLL), p. 134, Budapest, Abstracts of papers.
54. LEWANDER, T. (1970) Catecholamine turn-over studies in chronic amphetamine intoxication. In: Amphetamines and Related Compounds (Eds. E. COSTA and S. GARATTINI), p. 317, Raven Press, New York.
55. LEWANDER, T. (1971) Effects of chronic amphetamine intoxication on the accumulation in the rat brain of labelled catecholamines synthesized from circulating tyrosine-^{14}C and dopa-^{3}H. Naunyn-Schmiedeberg's Arch. Pharmak. **271**, 211.
56. LEWANDER, T. (1971a) On the presence of p-hydroxynorephedrine in the rat brain and heart in relation to changes in catecholamine levels after administration of amphetamine. Acta pharmacol. toxicol. **29**, 33.
57. McKENZIE, G. M. and SZERB, J. C. (1968) The effect of dihydroxyphenylalanine, pheniprazine and dextroamphetamine on the in vivo release of dopamine from the caudate nucleus. J. Pharmacol. exp. Ther. **162**, 302.
58. McKENZIE, G. M. (1971) Apomorphine-induced aggression in the rat. Brain Res. **34**, 323.
59. McKENZIE, G. M. (1972) Role of the tuberculum olfactorium in stereotyped behaviour induced by apomorphine in the rat. Psychopharmacologia, **23**, 212.
60. MOSHER, L., and FEINSILVER, D. (1971) Special report: Schizophrenia. National Institute of Mental Health, Rockville, Maryland, U.S.A. (Publication no. (HSM) 72-9042).

61. MUNKVAD, I. and RANDRUP, A. (1966) The persistence of amphetamine stereotypies of rats in spite of strong sedation. Acta psychiat. scand. suppl. **191** (ad vol. 42), 178.
62. MUNKVAD, I., PAKKENBERG, H. and RANDRUP, A. (1968) Aminergic systems in basal ganglia associated with stereotyped hyperactive behavior and catalepsy. Brain Behav. Evol. **1**, 89.
63. NAYLOR, R. J. and OLLEY, J. E. (1972) Modification of the behavioural changes induced by amphetamine in the rat by lesions in the caudate nucleus, the caudate-putamen and globus pallidus. Neuropharmacology, **11**, 91.
64. NIELSEN, E. B. and LYON, M.: Drinking behaviour and brain dopamine: antagonistic effect of a neuroleptic drug (Pimozide) upon amphetamine-induced hypodipsia. In preparation.
65. NORTON, S. (1967) An analysis of cat behaviour using chlorpromazine and amphetamine. Int. J. Neuropharmacol. **6**, 307.
66. NORTON, S. (1969) The effects of psychoactive drugs on cat behaviour. Ann. N.Y. Acad. Sci. **159**, 915.
67. NYBÄCK, H. (1971) Effects of neuroleptic drugs on brain catecholamine neurons. Thesis from the Department of Pharmacology, Karolinska Institutet, Stockholm, Sweden.
68. NYMARK, M. Apomorphine provoked stereotypy in the dog. Psychopharmacologia 1972. In press.
69. PAPESCHI, R. and MCCLURE, D. J. (1971) Homovanillic and 5-hydroxyindoleacetic acid in cerebrospinal fluid of depressed patients. Arch. gen. Psychiat. **25**, 352.
70. PEDERSEN, V. and CHRISTENSEN, A. V. (1971) Methylphenidate antagonism in mice as a rapid screening test for neuroleptic drugs. Acta pharmacol. toxicol. **29**, suppl. 4, 44.
71. PEDERSEN, V. and CHRISTENSEN, S. V.: Antagonism of methylphenidate-induced stereotyped gnawing in mice. Acta pharmacol. toxicol. In press.
72. PHILLIPS, M. I. and BRADLEY, P. B. (1969) The effect of chlorpromazine and d-amphetamine mixtures on spontaneous behaviour. Int. J. Neuropharmac. **8**, 169.
73. PRAAG, H. M. VAN and KORF, J. (1971) Retarded depression and the dopamine metabolism. Psychopharmacologia, **19**, 199.
74. PRAAG, H. M. VAN, SCHUT, T., BOSMA, E. and BERGH, R. VAN DEN (1971) A comparative study of the therapeutic effects of some 4-chlorinated amphetamine derivatives in depressive patients. Psychopharmacologia, **20**, 66.
75. RANDRUP, A., MUNKVAD, I. and UDSEN, P. (1963) Adrenergic mechanisms and amphetamine induced abnormal behaviour. Acta pharmacol. toxicol. **20**, 145.
76. RANDRUP, A. and MUNKVAD, I. (1964) On the relation of tryptaminic and serotonergic mechanism to amphetamine induced abnormal behaviour. Acta pharmacol. toxicol. **21**, 272.
77. RANDRUP, A. and MUNKVAD, I. (1965) Special antagonism of amphetamine-induced abnormal behaviour. Psychopharmacologia, **7**, 416.
78. RANDRUP, A. and SCHEEL-KRÜGER, J. (1966) Diethyldithiocarbamate and amphetamine stereotype behaviour. J. Pharm. Pharmacol. **18**, 752.
79. RANDRUP, A. and MUNKVAD, I. (1967) Stereotyped activities produced by amphetamine in several animal species and man. Psychopharmacologia, **11**, 300.
80. RANDRUP, A. and MUNKVAD, I. (1968) Behavioural stereotypies induced by pharmacological agents. Pharmakopsychiat. **1**, 18.
81. RANDRUP, A. and MUNKVAD, I. (1970) Biochemical, anatomical and psychological investigations of stereotyped behavior induced by amphetamines. In: Amphetamines and Related Compounds (Eds. E. COSTA and S. GARATTINI), p. 695. Raven Press, New York.
82. RANDRUP, A. and MUNKVAD, I. (1971) Behavioural toxicity of amphetamines studied in animal experiments. In: The Correlation of Adverse Effects in Man with Observations in Animals (Ed. S. B. DE BAKER), pp. 6—17. Excerpta Medica Internat. Congress Series No. 220, Amsterdam.
83. RANDRUP, A. and MUNKVAD, I. (1972) Association between schizophrenia and dopaminergic hyperactivity. Orthomolecular Psychiatry, **1**, 2.
84. RANDRUP, A. and MUNKVAD, I. Stereotyped Behavior. In: Section 25, International Encyclopedia of Pharmacology and Therapeutics (Ed. O. HORNYKIEWICZ). Pergamon Press. Toronto. In press.
85. REID, W. D. (1970) Turnover rate of brain 5-hydroxytryptamine increased by d-amphetamine. Brit. J. Pharmacol. **40**, 483.
86. RIDDELL, D. and SZERB, J. C. (1971) The release *in vivo* of dopamine synthesized from labelled precursors in the caudate nucleus of the cat. J. Neurochem. **18**, 989.
87. RIO, J. DEL and FUENTES, J. A. (1969) Further studies on the antagonism of stereotyped behaviour induced by amphetamine. Europ. J. Pharmacol. **8**, 73.
88. RYLANDER, G. (1971) Stereotype behaviour in man following amphetamine abuse. In: The Correlation of Adverse Effects in Man with Observations in animals (Ed. S. B. DE BAKER), p. 28, Excerpta Medica Internat. Congress Series No. 220, Amsterdam.

89. SCHEEL-KRÜGER, J. (1970) Central effects of anticholinergic drugs measured by the apomorphine gnawing test in mice. Acta pharmacol. toxicol. **28**, 1.
90. SCHEEL-KRÜGER, J. (1971) Comparative studies of various amphetamine analogues demonstrating different interactions with the metabolism of the catecholamines in the brain. Europ. J. Pharmacol. **14**, 47.
91. SCHEEL-KRÜGER, J. (1972a) Some aspects of the mechanism of action of various stimulant amphetamine analogues. Psychiat. Neurol. Neurochir. **75**, 179.
92. SCHEEL-KRÜGER, J. (1972b) Behavioural and biochemical comparison of amphetamine derivatives, cocaine, benztropine and tricyclic anti-depressant drugs. Europ. J. Pharmacol. **18**, 63.
93. SCHEEL-KRÜGER, J. (1972c) Studies on the accumulation of O-methylated dopamine and noradrenaline in the rat brain following various neuroleptics, thymoleptics and aceperone. Arch. int. Pharmacodyn. **195**, 372.
94. SCHELKUNOV, E. L. (1964) The technique of "phenamine stereotypy" for evaluating the effect produced by remedial agents on the central adrenergic processes. Pharmacologica et Toxicologica (Moscow) **27**, 628.
95. SCHIØRRING, E. (1971) Amphetamine induced selective stimulation of certain behaviour items with concurrent inhibition of others in an open-field test with rats. Behaviour, **39**, 1.
96. SCHIØRRING, E. Social isolation and other behavioural changes in a group of three vervet monkeys (cercopithecus) produced by single, low doses of amphetamine. This meeting.
97. SCHIØRRING, E. An open-field study on spontaneous locomotion with amphetamine treated rats. In preparation.
98. SCHOENFELD, R. and URETSKY, N. (1972) Altered response to apomorphine in 6-hydroxydopamine-treated rats. Europ. J. Pharmacol. **19**, 115.
99. SCHROLD, J. and SQUIRES, R. F. (1971) Behavioural effects of d-amphetamine in young chicks treated with p-Cl-phenylalanine. Psychopharmacologia, **20**, 85.
100. SCHULZ, R. and FREY, H.-H. (1972) Study into the mechanism of the anorectic action of amphetamine and its p-chloro analogue. Acta pharmacol. toxicol. 31, suppl. I, 12.
101. SEDVALL, G. and NYBÄCK, H. Neuroleptikabehandling ved schizofreni. Nord. psykiat. T. In press.
102. SENAULT, B. (1970) Comportement d'agressivité intraspécifique induit par l'apomorphine chez le rat. Psychopharmacologia, **18**, 271.
103. SIMPSON, B. A. and IVERSEN, S. D. (1971) Effects of substantia nigra lesions on the locomotor and stereotypy responses to amphetamine. Nature, New Biology, **230**, 30.
104. SORENSON, C. A. and ELLISON, G. D. (1970) Striatal organization of feeding behavior in the decorticate rat. Exp. Neurol. **29**, 162.
105. STAEHELIN, J. E. (1941) Pervitin-Psychose. Z. ges. Neurol. Psychiat. **173**, 598.
106. STEINESS, E. (1971) Antipsykotiske medikamenters betydning for skizofrene patienters sociale tilpasning. Nord. Med. **7**, 14.
107. STILLE, G. (1971) Zur Pharmakologie katatonigener Stoffe. Editio Cantor/Aulendorf i. Württ.
108. STILLE, G., LAUENER, H. and EICHENBERG, E. (1971) The pharmacology of 8-chloro-11-(4-methyl 1 piperazinyl)-5H-dibenzo (b, e) (1,4) diazepine (clozapine). Farmaco, **26**, 603.
109. STRADA, S. J. and SULSER, F. (1971) Comparative effects of p-chloroamphetamine and amphetamine on metabolism and in vivo release of ^{3}H-norepinephrine in the hypothalamus. Europ. J. Pharmacol. **15**, 45.
110. ROFFLER-TARLOV, S., SHARMAN, D. F. and TEGERDINE, P. (1971) 3,4-dihydroxyphenylacetic acid and 4-hydroxy-3-methoxyphenylacetic acid in the mouse striatum: a reflection of intra- and extraneuronal metabolism of dopamine? Brit. J. Pharmacol. **42**, 343.
111. UNGERSTEDT, U., BUTCHER, L., BUTCHER, S., ANDÉN, N.-E. and FUXE, K. (1969) Direct chemical stimulation of dopaminergic mechanisms in the neostriatum of the rat. Brain Res. **14**, 461.
112. UNGERSTEDT, U. (1971) Adipsia and aphagia after 6-hydroxydopamine induced degeneration of the nigro-striatal dopamine system. Acta physiol. scand., suppl. **367**, 95.
113. UNGERSTEDT, U. (1971a) Striatal dopamine release after amphetamine or nerve degeneration revealed by rotational behaviour. Acta physiol. scand., suppl. **367**, 49.
114. UNGERSTEDT, U. (1971b) Stereotaxic mapping of the monoamine pathway in the rat brain. Acta physiol. scand., suppl. **367**, 1.
115. UNGERSTEDT, U. (1971c) Postsynaptic supersensitivity after 6-hydroxydopamine induced degeneration of the nigro-striatal dopamine system. Acta physiol. scand., suppl. **367**, 69.
116. WALLACH, M. B. and GERSHON, S. (1971) A neuropsychopharmacological comparison of d-amphetamine, L-dopa and cocaine. Neuropharmacology, **10**, 743.
117. WALLACH, M. B. and GERSHON, S. (1972) The induction and antagonism of central nervous system stimulant-induced stereotyped behavior in the cat. Europ. J. Pharmacol. **18**, 22.

118. WALLACH, M. B., ANGRIST, B. M. and GERSHON, S. (1971) The comparison of the stereotyped behavior-inducing effect of d-and l-amphetamine in dogs. Commun. behav. Biol. **6**, 93.
119. WILLNER, J. H., SAMACH, ANGRIST, B. M., WALLACH, M. B. and GERSHON, S. (1970) Drug-induced stereotyped behavior and its antagonism in dogs. Commun. behav. Biol. **5**, 135.
120. YEH, B. K., MCNAY, J. L. and GOLDBERG, L. I. (1969) Attenuation of dopamine renal and mesenteric vasodilation by haloperidol: Evidence for a specific dopamine receptor. J. Pharmacol. exp. Ther. **168**, 303.
121. ZIANCE, R. J. and RUTLEDGE, C. O. (1972) A comparison of the effects of fenfluramine and amphetamine on uptake, release and catabolism of norepinephrine in rat brain. J. Pharmacol. exp. Ther. **180**, 118.

A.R., Psychopharmacological Laboratory, E Sct. Hans Hospital, 4000 Roskilde, Denmark

THE PSYCHOPHARMACOLOGY OF METHYLPHENIDATE IN MAN*)

J. M. DAVIS, D. S. JANOWSKY, M. KHALED EL-YOUSEF and H. J. SEKERKE

Department of Psychiatry and Pharmacology, Vanderbilt University School of Medicine, Nashville, Tennessee

This symposium focuses on the pharmacology of the amphetamine type drugs. This class of pharmacologic agents are thought to produce their pharmacological effects on behavior through their release of the biogenic amines, dopamine or norepinepherine (or through more complex interactions of these drugs with the amines such as those involving false transmitters etc.). This paper will present data on the human pharmacology of these drugs. It will show first that methylphenidate, an amphetamine type psychostimulant, can activate the schizophrenic process. Secondly this paper will present the concept that many of the behavioral processes thought to be under control of central adrenergic (dopamine, norepinepherine) systems may in fact be controlled by a balance between these systems and a central cholinergic system. The second section of this paper will present data which suggests that several types of behavior such as the methylphenidate activated psychosis, as well as psychomotor stimulation or cholinomimetic induced inhibition, are controlled by a central adrenergic/cholinergic balance.

Stereotyped gnawing and sniffing behavior, produced by amphetaminelike psychostimulants and thought to be caused by dopaminergic mechanisms, has been used as an animal model for schizophrenia (10). Furthermore, all antipsychotic drugs cause extrapyramidal side effects, probably mediated by their blockade of central dopamine receptor sites. This raises a question as to whether dopamine or a related substance may be involved in the schizophrenic process. One of methylphenidate's pharmacologic actions is to release dopamine and to block released dopamine's reuptake into the neuron (10, 11). If dopamine, or a similar compound, were involved in the etiology of schizophrenia, schizophrenics might be expected to respond differently to injections of methylphenidate than would normals (3, 4).

Our initial study concerned the use of intravenous methylphenidate as a provocative test for schizophrenia (3, 4). A total of 51 subjects were studied (39 psychiatric patients and 12 normal controls). A double blind rating and drug administration technique was used in all studies. In each study, a single intravenous injection of either placebo or methylphenidate 0.5 mg/kg was administered over a 30 second period. Behavior was

---

*)This research was supported in part by grant GM 15431, from the National Institutes of Health, Grant HM 11468, from the National Institute of Mental Health, and by research support from the State of Tennessee Department of Mental Health.

rated at 5 minute intervals by a rater who was blind as to whether placebo or methylphenidate was being administered. The modified Bunney-Hamburg rating technique was used, with 0—5 representing mild symptoms, 6—10 representing moderate symptoms, and 11—15 representing extreme symptoms. The symptoms rated were (1) psychosis, (2) interaction, (3) anxiety, and (4) depression. At the time of each rating, a sitting blood pressure and pulse were obtained.

Within minutes following the methylphenidate infusion, a very dramatic increase in psychosis ratings occurred in the actively ill schizophrenic patients. No increase in psychosis ratings occurred following the placebo injections, and no significant increase in psychosis rating occurred in normal patients. For the 22 actively ill schizophrenic patients evaluated, there was a clinically dramatic and statistically significant intensification of pre-existing psychotic symptoms, such as hallucinations, catatonic posturing, delusions, and inappropriate affect (baseline psychosis score = 6.5 ± 0.8; 15 minute post methylphenidate score = 10.0 ± 0.5, $p < .00003$). When the schizophrenic subjects were admitted on the research ward they often had florid psychotic symptoms. On the ward, even though drugs had been discontinued, the supportive atmosphere and milieu program often resulted in achievement of a modest decrease in these psychotic symptoms. Following methylphenidate administration, the patients changed from having an active illness in moderate control to a state where they manifested severe and florid psychotic symptoms. Qualitatively, they generally reverted to a clinical state equal to that which they showed during the most severe phase of their illness. That is, if the patient was originally delusional, he became more intensely delusional and lost insight after receiving methylphenidate. If the patient was originally catatonic, with methylphenidate his catatonic symptomatology became worse. If a patient originally had hallucinations, following the methylphenidate infusion he showed a marked intensification of his hallucinations. The activation of symptoms occurred within one or two minutes of injection and reached a peak after 10 to 30 minutes. Symptoms then gradually decreased to their baseline level over a 2 to 6 hour period of time. In general, the peripheral autonomic changes and the changes in the psychosis ratings paralleled each other significantly. Some patients studied during the acute phase of their illness were treated with anti-psychotic drugs such as chlorpromazine (when chlorpromazine was countraindicated, haloperidol was used). When subsequently given methylphenidate, these antipsychotic drug treated patients experienced a reactivation of their psychotic symptoms equal in intensity to that experienced when they were not treated with antipsychotic drugs.

After the schizophrenic process had eventually remitted and the patients were substantially recovered and ready to return home, some were studied again. At this time, infusion of methylphenidate 0.5 mg/kg did not cause a significant increase in the psychosis ratings in the 16 remitted patients studied (increase in psychosis ratings between baseline and 15 minute post methylphenidate infusion = 1.1 ± 0.9, $P = N.S.$). These patients did experience an increase in their interaction scores, as did the normal volunteers and the acutely psychotic patients. As with the actively ill schizophrenics, the remitted patients were evaluated both on and off antipsychotic medications; and in either case, methylphenidate failed to activate psychotic symptoms after remission had occurred.

The reaction of the twelve normal controls to methylphenidate infusions was similar to that of the remitted schizophrenic patients. Although there was no increase in psychosis ratings observed, most normal controls showed increased talkativeness, interactions and thoughts with some showing mild anxiety and others showing euphoria. Thus, in these studies, we found that a small dose of i.v. methylphenidate consistently intensifies psychotic symptoms for one or more hours in those schizophrenics in whom symptoms are initially present, and that this effect is clinically very dramatic. Our data further indicates that following remission, methylphenidate no longer causes an activation of the psychosis (3.4).

Thus methylphenidate, presumably by releasing dopamine and/or norepinephrine, can activate the schizophrenic process. In this symposium, a number of pharmacologic actions of amphetamine type drugs have been discussed. The emphasis of this research has been placed on the property of amphetamine to interact with amines such as norepinephrine and dopamine to produce its pharmacologic effect. The purpose of the second section of the paper is to raise to question that these pharmacologic effects are not just under the control of one amine, but rather controlled by a balance between norepinephrine or dopamine and the central cholinergic system.

Most of the animal and human studies concerning the effects of agents which alter the dopaminergic system have focussed only on this one neurotransmitter. However, there is an increasing amount of evidence reviewed elsewhere that certain behaviors are actually controlled by a balance between dopaminergic and cholinergic substances. That a balance between cholinergic and adrenergic factors regulates somatic functions is well known. Much indirect evidence exists suggesting that, as in the periphery, functionally significant antagonistic adrenergic and cholinergic systems exist centrally and that these systems are among those that regulate behavior (1, 8). Increasing central cholinergic tone causes decreased self stimulation, decreased conditioned responses of a number of types, and decreased locomotor activity; and all these behaviors are activated by increasing central adrenergic activity (8, 11). Centrally acting anticholinergic agents block inhibitory cholinergic effects (8), and themselves increase locomotion and other forms of behavioral excitation (8). Subthreshold doses of atropine and amphetamine are synergistic in inducing avoidance responses in rats and amphetamines and anticholinergic agents exhibit synergistic effects on locomotor activity in mice (8). CARLTON postulated that this synergistic effect occurs because the anticholinergic agent blocks cholinergic antagonism of increased adrenergic activity (4).

We have previously shown that methylphenidate (Ritalin) induced increases in locomotor activity and stereotyped gnawing behavior in rats are antagonized or prevented by physostigmine, a centrally active acetylcholinesterase inhibitor, but not by neostigmine, a peripherally active acetylcholinesterase inhibitor (5).

We pretreated Sprague Dawley male rats (200—250 g) with 0.5 mg/kg methylscopolamine. Thirty minutes later the rats either received physostigmine 1.0 mg/kg i.p., neostigmine 0.25 mg/kg i.p. or saline. Ten minutes later all received methylphenidate 50 mg/kg i.p. In a second study rats received methylscopolamine as described above. Thirty minutes later all received 50 mg/kg methylphenidate i.p. Thirty minutes after receiving methylphenidate, the rats received either 1.0 mg/kg physostigmine i.p., 0.25 mg/kg neostigmine, or saline. In both studies, rats were rated at five minute intervals on a 5 point scale (0 = no stereotyped behavior, 5 = maximum stereotyped behavior) for stereotyped sniffing and gnawing behavior. Physostigmine, but not neostigmine, prevented methylphenidate induced stereotyped behavior changes (physostigmine = $= 0.46 \pm 0.24$, neostigmine $= 3.23 \pm 0.34$). Physostigmine, but not neostigmine, stopped methylphenidate induced stereotyped behavior (physostigmine $= 1.0 \pm 0.45$, neostigmine $= 4.8 \pm 0.20$).

Although there is considerable evidence from our own and other animal studies that cholinergic and adrenergic influences exhibit behaviorally antagonistic effects, little such information has been reported in humans. We recently have explored interactions in man between methylphenidate and physostigmine (6—9). We have administered methylphenidate followed by physostigmine to one group of subjects and physostigmine followed by methylphenidate to another group of subjects; hypothesizing that the effects of each drug would be antagonistic (6, 7, 9). The subject group consisted of a total of 10 manic and 24 actively ill schizophrenic patients.

To evaluate the effects of methylphenidate and physostigmine on manic symptoms in the manic patients, a modification of the Beigel-Murphy manic rating scale was used (9), with items rated on a 0 to 5 point continuum (0 = none, 1 = very mild, 2 = mild, 3 = moderate, 4 = severe, 5 = extremely severe). A total "manic intensity score" was calculated from the sum of the 11 ratings noted by Beigel and Murphy to best characterize manic severity. The Beigel-Murphy manic "elation-grandiosity" subscale also was used to evaluate each patient, with each item rated on a five point continuum. Schizophrenic patients were also specifically rated for (1) psychosis and (2) interaction.

On the basis of pilot data in normals, schizophrenics and manics, we noted that "anergic-inhibitory" effects of physostigmine exist which appear to cross diagnostic categories. We therefore developed scales to be described below with which we have rated all our subjects regardless of diagnosis. A 15 point rating scale was developed to evaluate the general effects of methylphenidate and physostigmine in all subjects. Subjects were rated on a 15 point continuum every 10 minutes by a blind rater on a number of items which included: "irritable, lethargic, dysphoric, slow thoughts, wants to say nothing, hostile, withdrawn, wants to be alone, apathetic, crying, sad, lacks energy, sleepy, drained, hyperactive, lacks thoughts, depressed, motor retarded, angry, emotional withdrawal, unusual thoughts, conceptual disorganization, and blunted affect". They were also rated on cheerfulness, friendliness, interacting, and talkativeness. A "psychomotor inhibitory score" was derived from the sum of the scores of each patient's lethargic, slow thoughts, wants to say nothing, withdrawn, apathetic, lacks energy, drained, hyperactive, lacks thoughts, motor retarded, and emotionally withdrawn scores. An "activation score", based on the sum of each patient's cheerfulness, friendliness, interacting, and talkativeness scores, also was derived.

In our first study we investigated general effects of physostigmine, neostigmine and methylphenidate (6). Manic patients and schizophrenic patients received by intravenous infusion two or more placebo injections followed either by (1) methylphenidate 0.5 mg/kg; (2) neostigmine 0.25 mg every 5 minutes to a total of 1.25 mg; or (3) physostigmine 0.5 mg every 5 minutes to a total of 2.50 mg or until "inhibition" occurred. Prior to the experiment, patients who were to receive a cholinomimetic agent received i.m. 1 mg methylscopolamine (a peripheral anticholinergic agent). Those who were to receive methylphenidate received a placebo injection. Following administration of active compound, placebo was administered every 5 minutes for 30 more minutes. Patients were rated on a double blind basis every 10 minutes as to the effects of the drugs administered using the "activation scale" and "inhibitory scale" subitems. Psychosis ratings were done on the schizophrenics and various Beigel-Murphy mania rating sperformed on the manics.

In the 8 schizophrenics studied physostigmine increased the "inhibitory scale" score (change score = $+8.87 \pm 2.04$, $p < .002$) and decreased the "activation scale" score (change score = $-2.80 \pm .99$, $p < .02$) and the related subitems. This contrasted with the lack of effects of neostigmine (N = 7). In the schizophrenic patient group, physostigmine did not cause a specific decrease in psychosis ratings. However, schizophrenic patients all became more withdrawn and quiet, although their delusions persisted. In contrast, methylphenidate in these patients decreased "inhibitory scores" (change score = -4.43 ± 2.40, $p < .06$) and increased the schizophrenic's psychosis ratings (change score = 1.19 ± 0.16, $p < .0002$) causing symptoms to become more florid. Similar contrasting effects occurred in the manics in terms of changes in activation scores (methylphenidate induced increase in activation score = 3.48 ± 0.27, $p < .00001$, N = 5). Significantly, an increase in the depression ratings and sadness ratings occurred in the manic patients after physostigmine administration (depression change score = = 0.50 ± 0.22, p < .03). Furthermore, physostigmine decreased the Beigel-Murphy manic intensity score (change score = −9.57 ± 2.2, p < .002), and methylphenidate caused an increase in these scores (change score = 4.92 ± 1.68, p < .02). Neostigmine did not significantly alter any of the variables measured in the schizophrenic or manic patient groups.

In a second study a total of 24 schizophrenic patients received a series of placebo injections every 5 minutes followed by injection of 0.5 mg/kg methylphenidate over a 30 second period of time. Two placebo injections at 5 minute intervals were followed by a series of either: (1) every 5 minute placebo injections; (2) 0.5 mg physostigmine injections every 5 minutes until methylphenidate antagonism occurred or 2.50 mg had been given; or (3) neostigmine 0.25 mg injection given every 5 minutes until 1.25 mg had been given. After the above series had been given, placebos were injected every 5 minutes for 30 minutes.

The data were analyzed to determine whether physostigmine antagonized methylphenidate-induced increases in psychosis scores and interaction scores. Forty-five minutes after methylphenidate injection, an increase in psychosis ratings and interaction ratings still persisted in the placebo treated subjects. In contrast, by 45 minutes physostigmine had antagonized methylphenidate-increased psychosis ratings and interaction ratings. Furthermore, the methylphenidate-induced increase in the schizophrenic patient's "activation scale" score and the decrease in the "inhibitory scale" score was reversed with physostigmine.

Similarly, in the 5 manics tested, methylphenidate-induced increases in activation scores and decreases in inhibition scores were reversed by physostigmine.

In a third experiment, the effects of methylphenidate in reversing physostigmine induced "inhibitory" symptoms was evaluated in schizophrenics and manics. Patients were pretreated with 1.0 mg methylscopolamine. A variable number of placebo injections were followed every 5 minutes by 0.5 mg physostigmine until a physostigmine inhibitory state was elicited or 2.50 mg had been given. After this state occurred, two placebo injections were given at 5 minute intervals followed after 5 minutes by 10 mg methylphenidate followed by 30 minutes of placebo injections occurring every 5 minutes. A limited number of patients (N = 5) received 0.25 mg neostigmine in place of the 0.5 mg physostigmine injections.

For the 7 schizophrenics studied, i.v. methylphenidate reversed the physostigmine-induced increase in "inhibitory scale" score and reversed the decrease in "activation scale" scores. Furthermore, physostigmine prevented the methylphenidate-induced increase in activation and partially prevented the methylphenidate-induced increase in psychosis ratings.

In the 5 manic patients studied the physostigmine-induced increase in the "inhibitory scale" score and the decrease in the "activation" scale score was reversed by the administration of methylphenidate. Physostigmine, but not neostigmine, prevented a decrease in the "inhibitory scale" score by methylphenidate in schizophrenics and prevented a methylphenidate-induced increase in the "activation scale" score.

Discussion

The data indicate that methylphenidate, an adrenergic agent, and physostigmine, a reversible cholinomimetic agent, exhibit opposite and antagonistic effects. Methylphenidate intensifies manic symptoms and increases psychic "activation," causing increased talkativeness and interactions, while physostigmine causes a decrease in manic symptoms, a decrease in activation, and an increase in psychic "inhibition." In schizophrenics, similarly, psychotic symptoms, interactions, and talkativeness are increased by methylphenidate. Physostigmine decreases psychic activation and increases psychic inhibition in schizophrenics, but alone does not significantly decrease psychotic thinking. Although physostigmine does not decrease psychosis ratings in those schizophrenics treated with it alone, it is significant that all schizophrenics receiving it became grossly "inhibited," with associated slowed thoughts, lethargy, and psychomotor retardation. Furthermore, in manics and schizophrenics, methylphenidate reversed physostigmine's inhibitory effects and physostigmine reversed methylphenidate's activating effects. Also, methylphenidate induced increases in psychosis ratings were reversed by physostigmine, as were methylphenidate-increases in mania ratings.

The above information is consistent with the concept that one component of behavior is a continuum between "psychic activation" and "psychic inhibition," with a given behavior existing, in part, on this continuum, (8). Mania may then represent, in part, an adrenergic predominance and retarded depression may represent a cholinergic predominance. In the case of schizophrenic patients, the degree of agitation or withdrawal may be a function of adrenergic-cholinergic balance and this parameter may be independent of variables concerned with the presence of delusions, hallucinations, autistic thinking, and inappropriate or blunted affect.

It is likely that the phenomena described above correspond to the activation caused by psychostimulants and the inhibition caused by centrally acting cholinominetics in animals receiving these agents. As reviewed elsewhere, a number of other facts suggest that activity level may be due in part to a balance between adrenergic and cholinergic factors; and that acetylcholine may have inhibitory-depressant effects (8). Reserpine, traditionally viewed as a drug which decreases adrenergic activity and causes depression and motor inhibition, as well as having antipsychotic properties, has been reported to have central cholinergic properties, as well as adrenergic depleting effects. Tricyclic antidepressants, which have been viewed as working by increasing adrenergic tone and anticholinergic agents such as scopolamine, have euphoriant properties. Furthermore, tricyclic antidepressants have been known to precipitate manic episodes and to intensify schizophrenic symptoms. Anticholinergic agents are reported to intensify schizophrenic symptoms (8).

At a clinical level we wish to note that physostigmine is a dangerous drug with numerous contraindications and side effects. It should be used with extreme caution.

In conclusion, we have found that increasing acetylcholine activity with physostigmine reverses mania, increases depression, antagonizes methylphenidate induced central activation and psychosis activation, and causes an anergic syndrome consisting of drained feelings, apathy, lethargy, and decreased thoughts and sometimes depression in most subjects to whom it is administered. Methylphenidate, an amphetamine-like psychostimulant, causes the opposite effects. On this basis we feel that it is reasonable to consider that there may be a dimension in man which goes from an excited-activated-euphoric state to an inhibited-retarded-depressed state, and that these behavioral states may have as their basis a balance between adrenergic and cholinergic factors.

REFERENCES

1. CARLTON, P. L. (1963) Cholinergic Mechanisms in the Control of Behavior by the Brain. Psychol. Rev. **70**, 19.
2. GOODMAN, L. S. and GILMAN, A. (1970) The Pharmacologic Basic of Therapeutics, Section IV, 4th Ed. COLLIER-MACMILLAN, Canada, Limited, Toronto.

3. JANOWSKY, D. S. EL-YOUSEF, M. K. and DAVIS, J. M. (1972) The Elicitation of Psychotic Symptomatology by Methylphenidate. Comprehens. Psychiat. 13, 83.
4. JANOWSKY, D. S., EL-YOUSEF, M. K., DAVIS, J. M. and SEKERKE, H. J. (1973) Provocation of Schizophrenia Symptoms with Methylphenidate. Arch. gen. Psychiat. 28, 185.
5. JANOWSKY, D. S. EL-YOUSEF, M. K., DAVIS, J. M. amd SEKERKE, H. J. (1973) Cholinergic Antagonism of Methylphenidate-Induced Stereotyped Behavior. Psychopharmacologia, 24, 295.
6. JANOWSKY, D. S., EL-YOUSEF, M. K., DAVIS, J. M. and HUBBARD, B., Cholinergic-Adrenergic Balance and Affect, presented at the "New Research Program" section of the 125th Annual Meeting of The American Psychiatric Association, May, 1972.
7. JANOWSKY, D. S., EL-YOUSEF, M. K., DAVIS, J. M., HUBBARD, B. and SEKERKE, H. J. (1972) Cholinergic Reversal of Manic Symptoms. Lancet, 1, 1236.
8. JANOWSKY, D. S., EL-YOUSEF, M. K., DAVIS, J. M. and SEKERKE, H. J. (1972) A Cholinergic-Adrenergic Hypothesis of Mania and Depression. Lancet 2, 732.
9. JANOWSKY, D. S., EL-YOUSEF, M. K. and DAVIS, J. M. (1973) The Alleviation of Manic Symptoms with Physostigmine. Arch. gen. Psychiat. 28, 542.
10. RANDRUP, A. and MAKVOD (1967) Behavioral Stereotypes Induced by Pharmacologic Agents, Pharmokopsychiat. 1, 18.
11. SCHEEL-KRUGER (1971) Comparative Studies of Various Amphetamine Analogues Demonstrating Different Interactions with the Metabolism of Catecholamines in Brain. Europ. J. Pharmacol. 14, 47.

J.M.D., Department of Psychiatry and Pharmacology,
Vanderbilt University School of Medicine,
Nashville, Tennessee, U.S.A.

PSYCHOPHARMACOLOGY OF CANNABIS

Chairman: L. Hollister

Associate chairman: S. E. Møller

THE COMMISSION'S EXPERIMENTAL STUDIES OF ACUTE EFFECTS OF MARIJUANA, Δ^9-THC AND ALCOHOL IN HUMANS

R. D. MILLER, R. W. HANSTEEN, H. E. LEHMANN, L. REID, L. LONERO, C. ADAMEC, L. THEODORE and B. JONES

Commission of Inquiry into the Non-Medical Use of Drugs, Ottawa

The Commission has undertaken four experimental projects concerning the acute effects of cannabis and, in some cases, of alcohol on humans. Subjects were all experienced with alcohol and cannabis, but not heavy users of either, and had had minimal experience with other psychoactive drugs.

EXPERIMENT 1: A COMPARISON OF Δ^9-THC AND MARIJUANA EFFECTS IN HUMANS

Fourteen male subjects each attended eight weekly experimental sessions which were six hours in duration. After a no-drug practice session, seven experimental conditions were given to all subjects in a double-blind Latin square design as follows: placebo (extracted alfalfa); three levels of marijuana (9, 21, and 88 μg Δ^9-THC per kg body weight, giving average doses of 0.7, 1.5 and 6.2 mg Δ^9-THC); three equivalent doses of high-purity synthetic Δ^9-THC on extracted alfalfa. Cigarettes were smoked following a carefully controlled procedure which apparently resulted in the delivery and retention of approximately 50% of the originally available THC. A condensed test battery was constructed to assess most of the major acute cannabis effects previously indicated in the literature. The time required to complete the test battery was just over two hours, and with the exception of a few measures, the battery was repeated four hours after smoking.

The natural marijuana and the pure Δ^9-THC both resulted in an increase in pulse rate, conjunctival injection, visual imagery, autokinetic movement, estimated passage of time and subjective effects ratings; and reductions in salivation, finger temperature, short-term memory and, to a lesser degree, two flash threshold and sustained finger grip. In general, the cannabis effects increased with increased dose, with the maximal effects occurring during the period directly following smoking, and minimal effects occurring by the end of the session. Overall, the data show no consistent quantitative or qualitative differences between the marijuana and the pure Δ^9-THC. These data support the hypothesis that Δ^9-THC is the major active constituent of marijuana in humans.

No reliable drug effects were found on tonic skin conductance, momentary maximum strength of hand grip, maximum speed of stylus tapping, digit symbol substitution, 15-second time interval production, duration of spiral after-image or finger painting measures.

Experiment 2: effects of marijuana and alcohol on some automobile driving tasks

The project is divided into two separate but related studies. In the main experiment, 16 licensed drivers (4 females and 12 males) each attended four weekly experimental sessions in addition to a preliminary no-drug practice session. The four experimental conditions, given to all subjects in a double-blind Latin square design, were: placebo (extracted marijuana, and a non-alcoholic drink); two levels of marijuana (21 and 88 μg Δ^9-THC per kg body weight); and one dose of ethanol (producing an average blood alcohol level of 0.07% – the equivalent of about three cocktails).

Subjects began the first driving trial, consisting of six course laps (about 6 minutes each), directly after smoking. Each lap involved driving through a 1.1 mile course which included both slow forward and backward manoeuvering and higher speed (about 25 mph) straight and curved sections, marked out with wooden poles and plastic cones. A second trial (three laps) started three hours after smoking. The subject's driving was scored on: hits of cones and poles, rough handling (superfluous or awkward movements) and speed. Supplementary physiological and psychological measures were also obtained during the session. A separate sample of 12 subjects (three females, nine males), experienced with alcohol but not cannabis, were given only the alcohol and placebo drink conditions, and were tested on only one trial consisting of six laps. Course and rating conditions and practice trials were the same as described for the main study.

Both the alcohol dose and the higher dose of cannabis were found to result in poorer car handling performance. During the first trial, significantly more hits (of cones and poles) resulted when subjects received alcohol or the higher dose of cannabis than when they received only the placebos. There was no difference between the number of hits made in the low cannabis and placebo conditions. In the second trial, given three hours after smoking, the number of hits in the alcohol and higher marijuana conditions had decreased to a level approaching that of the placebo condition. Rough handling tended to be greater after drug treatment than in the placebo condition, although only the alcohol scores appeared significant. Driving speed, on the other hand, was affected only by the higher dose of cannabis. In the first trial, subjects drove slower in that condition than when no drug was given. The difference was small (about 1.5 miles per hour or 7%) but consistent. Driving speeds in the alcohol and low cannabis conditions were not significantly different from placebo. In the second trial, differences in driving speed among the four experimental conditions were only slight. The subjects in the second study, who were given only the alcohol and placebo conditions, showed alcohol effects which were similar to those found in the main experiment.

It would be premature to predict from these results whether or not cannabis does or will have serious effects on traffic safety. This initial study only measures car handling in rather artificial circumstances. However, these results do serve to point out the possibility that cannabis may adversely affect traffic safety and to underline the urgent need for extensive research into this question.

Experiment 3: effects of marijuana and alcohol on psychomotor tracking performance

Twenty-two male subjects each attended six weekly experimental sessions in addition to two preliminary no-drug practice sessions. The six experimental conditions (given to all subjects in a double-blind Latin square design) were: placebo (extracted marijuana and a non-alcoholic drink), two levels of marijuana (21 and 88 μg Δ^9-THC/kg), two levels of alcohol (0.07 and 0.03% blood alcohol level), and the low marijuana and low alcohol doses combined. Following smoking, subjects began the first trial consisting of six tracking runs (three minutes each). A 20-minute break occurred between the third and fourth runs, during which supplementary measures were taken. In four of the six tracking runs the subject was required only to perform the compensatory tracking (simple tracking). In the other two runs (complex tracking) additional psychomotor complications were added to the task. A second trial consisting of two simple tracking runs and one complex run was started four hours after drug administration.

In the first trial, the alcohol and, less consistently, the upper cannabis dose, resulted in an increase in tracking error scores, indicating impairment in both simple and complex tracking. The effect was greater for the higher doses than for the lower doses of each drug. The high alcohol dose resulted in significantly more tracking error than resulted from cannabis. The combination of low cannabis and low alcohol produced greater error scores in complex tracking than resulted from the corresponding doses of each drug given alone. As in Experiment I, marijuana significantly affected scores on the visual imagery, heart rate, conjunctival injection, time estimation and subjective measures. Again, no consistent effects were seen on tonic skin conductance. In addition, marijuana resulted in a transient increase in diastolic blood pressure, and there was a suggestion that accuracy of depth perception decreased slightly. Visual acuity measures were not affected by the drugs. Alcohol resulted in significant increases in heart rate, conjunctival injection and subjective effects ratings, and a slight decrease in imagery. The combined alcohol-cannabis treatment was found to have an additive effect on heart rate and conjunctival injection, but not on the subjective measures, and were possibly antagonistic on visual imagery. Blood alcohol was measured (with a Breathalyzer) at three times over the course of each session. Estimates obtained after the administration of the low alcohol dose alone were not different from the corresponding measures in the low alcohol-cannabis combination condition. This suggests that at the low doses studied, cannabis does not have a significant effect on the rate of alcohol appearance in and disappearance from the blood.

The mechanism for the interaction of alcohol and cannabis effects is not clear. It would appear that cannabis can enhance certain alcohol effects in the absence of discernible alteration of alcohol absorption, metabolism or excretion. We were not, of course, able to assess the possible effects of alcohol on blood levels of THC and its metabolites. The differential pattern of effects of the alcohol, cannabis, and combination conditions suggest that these drugs do not interact solely by one simply enhancing the general effects of the other.

EXPERIMENT 4: EFFECTS OF MARIJUANA ON VISUAL SIGNAL DETECTION AND GLARE RECOVERY

Five male subjects were trained for six practice runs (over three days) and tested in two placebo (extracted marijuana) and two marijuana sessions each. The four experimental sessions were given in a balanced alternating order (single blind) with one week between drug treatments. A single dose of marijuana was used (66 μg Δ^9-THC/kg). Immediately after smoking, subjects were given a test battery in which the major focus was on the assessment of sustained attention and vigilance (signal detection). The signal was a brief offset (gap) in a point of light that was otherwise continuously on. The tests were run in a dimly lit room. Five blocks of 100 trials each, separated by 30—60 seconds, were given over a 40-minute period. Subjects were asked to indicate on each trial the presence or absence of a temporal gap in the light, and to rate their confidence in their decision.

A warning tone was presented before each trial. A "signal" occurred in only 50% of the trials, in a random sequence. After the signal detection task (approximately three-quarters of an hour after drug administration) dim-light visual acuity was measured. A forced-choice procedure was employed using *Landolt C* test figures. Subjects were then exposed to a bright-glare light (440-L) for five seconds, and the time required to recover to the previous visual acuity level was recorded. This procedure was then immediately repeated.

Signal detection. The subjects were generally less accurate in identifying the signal after marijuana and there was a reliable decrement in d' (a measure of sensitivity to the signal) in all subjects for the drug condition. Furthermore, subjects were less confident in identifying a true signal after the drug. Subjects did not fail to respond in any more trials when under the influence of marijuana than in the placebo condition, and there were no systematic changes in the response criteria employed. There were no drug-related shifts in performance over blocks of trials within sessions. The significant decrease in d' was interpreted as an attentional decrement. The performance decrements correlated significantly with the individuals' subjective ratings of the magnitude of the drug-induced 'high'.

Visual acuity and glare recovery. There was a suggestion of reduced dim-light acuity under the drug condition in some individuals, but this trend was not consistent over sessions or subjects. No significant marijuana effect on glare recovery time was found. The possible confounding effect of a decrease in attention during this task cannot be separated out from the primary variables of interest.

H.E.L., Douglas Hospital, 6875 LaSalle Blvd., Montreal, 204 Quebec, Canada

CANNABIS AND ALCOHOL: EFFECTS ON SIMULATED CAR DRIVING AND PSYCHOLOGICAL TESTS. CORRELATION WITH URINARY METABOLITES

O. J. RAFAELSEN, P. BECH, J. CHRISTIANSEN and L. RAFAELSEN

Psychochemistry Institute, University of Copenhagen

The present study had 2 objectives: 1. to study the effect of cannabis and alcohol on driving performance in a car simulator and in series of psychological tests; 2. to compare psychological effects with individual variations in urinary metabolite excretion. The latter part of the study was unsuccessful. The analytical work-up has now been completed, and it was not possible to demonstrate positive or negative correlations between excretion of cannabis metabolites and changes in psychological function.

I will therefore concentrate on simulated driving and the psychological test battery.

The research design included principles of placebo, double-blindness, dose-response, tests for reproducibility and training effects, the volunteers acting as their own controls.

General research plan

The subjects were 8 male volunteers between the age of 21 and 29, in good physical and psychic health. MMPI (Minnesota Multiphasic Personality Inventory) showed normal profiles, and they had no excessive use of cannabis or alcohol. 3 had never tried cannabis, 5 from 1 to 15 times, no one more than once a week. The study lasted three months. After a training period each subject was tested on nine experiment days with weekly intervals. Each experiment day included three sessions: 1. before drug administration ('pre-test'); 2. under drug influence ('drug-test'); 3. the following morning ('post-test').

Cannabis was baked into small brown cakes in amounts of 200, 300, or 400 mg of a resin containing 4% Δ^1-tetrahydrocannabinol (THC). For placebo cakes cannabis with a minimal content of THC was used.

Alcohol was given in fruit juice in a dose of 70 g, leading to blood alcohol concentrations around 100 mg/100 ml one hour later.

The combined administration of alcohol and cannabis was not undertaken, but the subjects were unaware of this precaution. The use of placebo technique is not synonymous with achievement of blindness, and it is doubtful whether this can be obtained with alcohol; on the other hand, we have indications that it was probably obtained with cannabis. None of the subjects could differentiate by taste between cakes containing active and inactive cannabis, and they had difficulties assessing the various doses.

The whole experimental period fell into three parts:

In *Part I* all subjects were tested on three days with one pure placebo day, one day with cannabis 300 mg, and one day with alcohol administration.

Part II was an exact repetition of Part I, except that randomization led to a different order of treatment days for the individual subjects.

Finally in *Part III* the interest was on dose-response for cannabis, the subjects obtaining the three different doses of 200, 300, and 400 mg ($\sim$8, 12 and 16 mg THC) in randomized order. Placebo drink was here given on all days.

As the subjects were their own controls, results obtained before drug administration ('pre-test') were compared with results obtained while the subjects were under the influence of drug ('drug-test'), and with results obtained the following morning ('post-test'). For the comparisons were used non-parametric statistics. In general, the differences between pre-test values and post-test values were minimal and without statistical significance. Also, no statistically significant changes were found on placebo days. Most of the presentation will therefore be concerned with a comparison of pre-test and drug-test results.

The 300 mg of cannabis resin used was in a pilot study judged by experienced volunteers as an average cannabis dose, and it was therefore chosen for comparison with the alcohol dose used throughout Part I and Part II of the research programme.

SIMULATED CAR DRIVING

The car-simulator was a Redifon Auto-Tutor. This test model is built up like the front half of a car, and a picture from a movable cyclorama is continuously projected on the windshield giving the subject the impression of driving on a variable test course. Light signals appear at arbitrary intervals. Extra equipment made it possible to record a number of functions electronically, among these brake time, start time, number of gear changes, time, distance, and speed.

Brake time: Time from red light to the subject activates the brake pedal.

Start time: Time from green light to the subject activates the accelerator.

Subjects' estimate of time, distance, and speed: The subjects were trained to estimate time, distance, and speed in two different ways: a) 'objectively' or 'intellectually' (using cognitive and outer clues): 'how long and how far do you really *think* you have been driving?' and b) 'subjectively' or 'emotionally': 'how long and how far do you really *feel* you have been driving?'.

Both cannabis and alcohol influenced average brake time and start time in the car simulator.

A dose-response type of effect was seen on cannabis, and the effect of alcohol was more pronounced than 300 mg cannabis resin and less than 400 mg cannabis resin. The effect of both cannabis and alcohol had disappeared at the post-test the following morning.

The effect of both cannabis and alcohol was somewhat less marked on start time, and here only the increase after the highest cannabis dose obtained statistical significance. However, the pattern and relative effect of cannabis and of alcohol was similar to the brake time findings. In Part III the group on 300 mg cannabis resin only contains 7 and not the usual 8 subjects, the reason being that on this occasion one of the subjects drove through 8 of the 10 red lights without activating the brake pedal, let alone making a full stop.

The subjects' estimations of time and distance showed a much stronger effect of cannabis than of alcohol. It is noteworthy that the effect of cannabis was much more marked on the 'subjective' than on the 'objective' estimations, and on the 'subjective' estimations increase above 100% and even up to 300% were seen.

Psychological tests

The psychological tests preceded each driving period in the car-simulator and thus were administered three times on each experiment day. The psychological test battery included:

A. *Memory and concentration tests*: Digit span; reproduction of sentences; addition and subtraction tests; finger labyrinths; Bourdon's letter test; and a test of sentence construction.

B. *Consciousness and mood scales*: Subjective rating (Smith and Beecher's 12 items mood questionnaire), and objective rating (similar items rated by psychologist).

These tests all fulfilled the following criteria:

They should be replicable in 27 parallel versions according to the research design; they should only place a limited demand on the subjects in order to secure proper motivation; they should all have little or a controllable practice effect.

In a general view of the psychological tests, the effect of cannabis and of alcohol on *cognitive* functions were qualitatively alike although quantitative differencies were found on some tests. Comparing 70 g of alcohol and 300 mg of the cannabis resin used, more results obtained statistical significance after cannabis than after alcohol administration. The impairment on cannabis was only moderate in tests of sustained attention and attention span where the task is fairly simple requiring repetitive reactions of a uniform kind, but no alternating reactions or operations. In the task where every step depends on the previous one, the effect of cannabis was most clearly seen.

Comparing the results of the mood questionnaire and of the objective rating showed a very marked agreement between subjects and experimenters as to quality of intoxication. 8 out of 8 subjects rated themselves intoxicated by alcohol after alcohol administration, and the objective ratings were in complete agreement with this. Whereas wrong classifications after placebo was seen for one subject after alcohol, three subjects rated themselves intoxicated by cannabis after placebo administration. An experimenter rated one subject intoxicated by cannabis after placebo. As to degree of cannabis intoxication both mood questionnaire (subjective rating) and the objective rating by psychologist showed a clear and virtually identical dose-response pattern.

Summary

1. Cannabis and alcohol produce two different kinds of intoxication.
2. Dose-response effects of cannabis was seen on behavioural and phenomenological aspects.
3. Cannabis has pronounced effects on skills and judgments essential for driving.
4. No correlation was demonstrated between simulated car driving and psychological test performance on the one hand and urinary excretion of cannabis metabolites on the other hand.

O.J.R., Psychochemistry Institute, University of Copenhagen, Rigshospitalet, Blegdamsvej 9, 2100 Copenhagen, Denmark

THE EFFECTS OF Δ^9-THC ON SIMULATED DRIVING PERFORMANCE

D. LADEWIG and V. HOBI

Department of Psychiatry, University of Basle

Since 1967, an increasing number of experimental studies on the effect of THC has been done (1, 2, 3). Since we know that people drive cars under the influence of CNS stimulants and hallucinogenic drugs, we studied the influence of cannabis on driving fitness by a series of experiments which followed up earlier investigations on the effect of alcohol and/or tranquilizers or sedatives on driving performance.

These studies were started in 1966 by open field experiments (4) and were reproduced in 1970 by a driving simulator with surprisingly similar results (5, 6).

Methods

In the present investigation, 54 healthy subjects of both sex (mostly doctors and psychologists, average age 34 years) who had had no previous experience of cannabis were examined in a double-blind study.

In order to determine a possible dose relation curve 350, 500 and 450 µg/kg Δ^9-THC as well as an inactive placebo were dissolved in equal parts of olive oil and administered orally in capsules.

The investigation consisted of a neuro-psychiatric status including the half relaxation time (HRT), the sublingual temperature, a self-assessment scale (DWM-scale), a scale for somatical complaints, a personality inventory, a subjective report all subjects were asked to write and a battery of tests measuring some parameters of driving capacity. In this connection we used a series of performance and perception tests (d-2-Brickenkamp), 2 plate tapping tests, tracking apparatus (Spoerli and Gubser), compensation device (Spoerli and Gubser), a figure field test (Spoerli and Gubser), and the Exner-Spiral.

Each study began at 11 a.m. and continued for 24 hours. A total of four tests was made:

1. before substance,
2. one hour afterwards,
3. four hours afterwards and
4. 18—22 hours afterwards.

To include the important group factor in the test procedure, four subjects were put through the test procedure on the same day in a standardized way. Every subject had constantly his own examiner.

Psychomotor Behaviour and Driving Variables — Results

Since we had no way of distinguishing between the different doses given, we treated all three dose groups as a single THC group when processing the dates.

In the following only the results of 4 performance procedures we used (tapping, Exner-spiral, compensation device and tracking apparatus) will be described.

Tapping

In accordance with two different sets of instructions the subjects had to tap on 2 plates with a stylo at a rate they found comfortable and then as fast as possible (stress). The taps were recorded electronically. This test was performed with the left, right, and then both hands. In this way we wanted to investigate the differences between the personal working rate and the extreme variant referred to as "stress". In factor analysis investigations the latter is held to be a very good marking variable of the "wrist-finger speed" factor.

The changes in the *placebo group* were ill-defined and lacking in uniformity and for this reason no interpretation was attempted. There was only a trend of improvement from the 1.—4. test under stress (Table 1).

TABLE 1

Tapping: placebo group (tappings per 32 s) arithmetic means per examination

Examination		I	II	III	IV
Agreeable					
Single-handed	right	99,05	98,10	104.80	92,45
					⎣____S____⎦
	left	97,00	92,35	98.95	92.10
					⎣____S____⎦
		⎣_____S_____⎦
Ambidextrous	left	91,25	93,30	93.95	89.25
	right	93.65	90,65	96,75	89.85
Stress					
Single-handed	right	185.20	188,50	189.80	189.20
	left	164.10	171,30	165.70	172.80
			⎣____SS____⎦	
		⎣_____S_____⎦
Ambidextrous	left	157.00	158.30	157.10	156.80
	right	164.40	170.90	170.60	169.80

$n = 20$ $S = P \leq 0{,}05$
$SS = P \leq 0{,}025$
$SSS = P \leq 0.01$

TABLE 2

Tapping: THC group (tappings per 32 s) arithmetic means per examination

Examination		I	II	III	IV
Agreeable					
Single-handed	right	86.13	86.65	90.61	91.93
	left	81.57	87.17	86.13	90.52
Ambidextrous	left	80.43	85.83	84.09	84.48
	right	83.22	89.09	86.61	85.78
Stress					
Single-handed	right	198.90	188.50	186.10	194.60
			___SSS___		___S___	
	left	178.80	168.30	168.80	178.00
			___SSS___		___SS___	
Ambidextrous	left	172.30	161.50	159.00	168.30
			___SSS___		___SSS___	
	right	187.40	176.30	172.50	178.30
		|___SSS___|		
			_____SS_____	

n = S = P ≤ 0,05
SS = P ≤ 0.025
SSS = P ≤ 0.01

While operating at a comfortable speed, the *THC group* remained constant in all four test measurements (Table 2). In the stress test, however, it shows a statistically significant reduction under acute action of the substance. Whereas the placebo group under stress showed a trend of improvement in their performance from the first to the fourth test, we observed in the THC group a statistically significant and continuous diminution in performance from the first to the third test. Although there was a significant improvement from the third to the fourth test, the subjects never again equalled their initial performance. Thus one hour and four hours after ingestion, there is a definite THC effect which seems to be present in the subjects' performance even in the fourth test (18—22 hours later).

The result might be interpreted in terms of cannabis having a stimulating action which does not take effect in a stress situation. This correlated with the results of the DWM scale. The subjects described even 18—22 hours after ingestion a discrete distortion of autonomic functions (7).

Tracking apparatus

This instrument measures important components of specific performances of the kind required of the driver on the road. A film is projected demonstrating a track in different traffic situations. The driver has to pilot a while ball inside of his track and is asked to react on different signals. 6 errors are to be recorded.

1. Frequency with which the subject deviated outside the track to the right or left.
2. Effective time outside the track.
3., 4. Reaction time in seconds with regard to pressing on the pedal with the left or the right foot.
5., 6. Faulty pedal performance left or right.

Under the pressure of an increasing complexity of information we obtain objective information on "stress resistance" and the way the test performance (standard performance) declines (Fig. 1). The results are statistically significant enough to warrant the

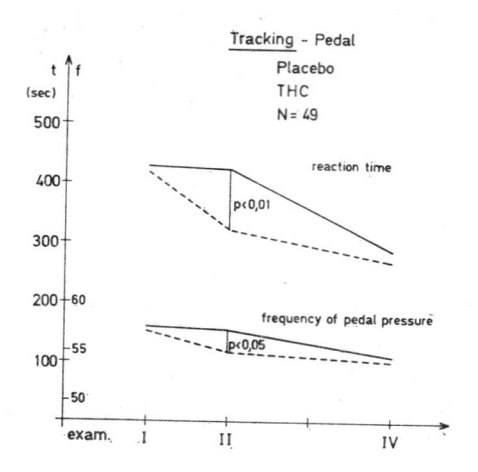

Fig. 1. Results of tests with the tracking apparatus under the influence of tetrahydrocannabinol (THC).

interpretation that the actual driving (tracking) ability of the THC group remains unaffected whereas in complex situations, i.e. in phases involving a multiplicity of stimuli, there is a (a) prolongation of reaction time and (b) an increased number of reaction errors.

This applied to the whole THC group. But there again the personality factors were important. The "inhibited" the "emotionally unstable" and the "depressives" all showed again inferior reaction performances.

Exner-spiral

The Exner-spiral is a black spiral on a white fundus which is rotated by an electromotor. After 30 sec the spiral is stopped but the subject has the impression that the spiral is still rotating. The duration of this after-image is to be measured.

This instrument, which has a long history of use in the measurement of attention and vigilance, has been utilized more particularly since Eysenck's investigations to assess variables of personality like extraversion (lowered) and introversion (raised). The correlations with flicker fusion frequency also suggest that sedating substances, such as phenobarbital, shorten the after-image while stimulating substances (benzedrine and dexedrine) prolong it. No statistically significant changes were detectable under THC in subjects with either higher or lower after-image durations. This could be clarified by a correlation with the FPI. "Excited" subjects (FPI-4), which means extraverted people in sensu Eysenck, had a shorter after-image.

Compensation device

The subject is asked to balance a ball into a notch. The tension of two springs has to be compensated by anticipating. The time the subject needs to balance the ball into the notch is a measure of the subjects to learn basic "deflection and correction movements" is examined. This calls for coordination involving both optical (eye/hand) and also proprioceptive (hand/hand) feedback signals. Hence this apparatus can be utilized for measuring driving variables as earlier studies demonstrated.

Whereas in the first measurement made in the THC group, before ingestion of the substance, a tendency to improved adaption with time was apparent, precisely the reverse situation was found in the second measurement (acute action of substance). The THC group displayed retardation, less control, and an unsteadier performance (Fig. 2).

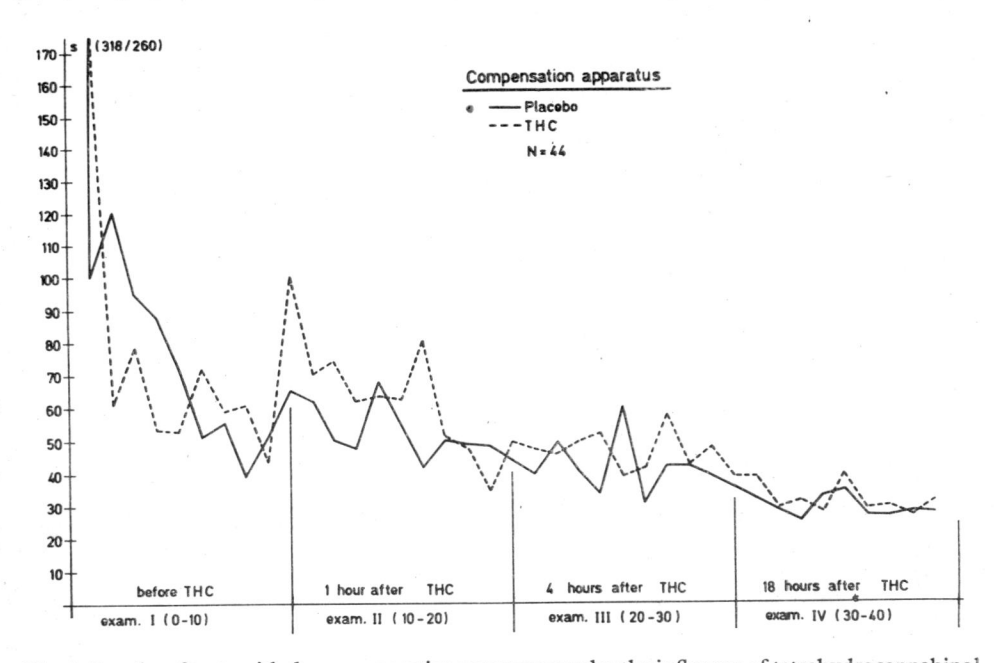

Fig. 2. Results of tests with the compensation apparatus under the influence of tetrahydrocannabinol (THC). Mean value of the time needed for each individual attempt in seconds (Drive = 10 attempts).

REFERENCES

1. HOLLISTER, L. E. (1971) Marihuana in man: three years later. Science, **172**, 21.
2. Interim Report of the Commission of Enquiry into the Non-Medical Use of Drugs, Queen's Printer for Canada Ottawa (1970) Le Dain-Report.
3. Interim Report of the Commission of Enquiry into the Non-Medical Use of Drugs, Queen's Printer for Canada Ottawa (1972) Le Dain-Report.

4. KIELHOLZ, P. and GOLDBERG, L. J. (1969) In: OBERSTEG, W. PÖLDINGER, A. RAMSEYER, P. SCHMID: Fahrversuche zur Frage der Beeinträchtigung der Verkehrstüchtigkeit durch Alkohol, Tranquilizer und Hypnotica. Dtsch. med. Wschr. **94**, 301.
5. KIELHOLZ P., GOLDBERG, L., HOBI, V. and REGGIANI, G. (1971) Teilsimulation zur Beeinträchtigung der Fahrtüchtigkeit unter Alkohol. Schweiz. med. Wschr. **101**, 1725.
6. KIELHOLZ, GOLDBERG, L., HOBI, V., LADEWIG, D. REGGIANI, G. and RICHTER, R. (1972) Haschisch und Fahrverhalten, eine experimentalle Untersuchung. Dtsch. med. Wschr. **97**, 789.
7. KIELHOLZ, P., GOLDBERG, L., HOBI, V., LADEWIG, D., REGGIANI, G. and RICHTER, R. (1972) Zur quantitativen Erfassung psychischer Erlebnissänderungen unter Delta-9-Tetrahydrocannabiol. Pharmakopsychiatria (in press).

D.L., Department of Psychiatry of the University, Basel Switzerland

HYPNOTIC SUSCEPTIBILITY DURING CANNABIS INTOXICATION[*]

S. FISHER, R. C. PILLARD and R. W. BOTTO

Psychopharmacology Laboratory, Division of Psychiatry, Boston University School of Medicine, Boston, Massachusetts

This exploratory study is, to the best of our knowledge, the first attempt to determine whether hypnotic susceptibility — as measured by standardized instruments — is modified during marijuana intoxication.

Subjects

From an original group of 90 male volunteers, 20 participated in the marijuana experiment. They were selected because: (a) they were over 21 years of age, (b) they had all reported prior experience with marijuana, and (c) they had also shown relatively stable hypnotic susceptibility scores in two previous group hypnotic sessions (Harvard Group Scale, Forms A and B, spaced two weeks apart) (1).

Procedure

These 20 subjects were subsequently retested for hypnotic susceptibility in three individual sessions (using the Stanford Scale of Hypnotic Susceptibility, Form C) (2):

(1) A baseline, "dry-run" control period, with no marijuana.
(2) Approximately two weeks later, an "ad lib" dose marijuana session, where each subject smoked sufficient marijuana (1.4% Δ^9-THC) to reach a good "social high."
(3) A final control session between two and four weeks later consisting only of a third administration of the Stanford scale.

No attempt was made to include any placebo controls in this initial study.

---

[*] This study was supported by MH-20484 from the National Institute of Mental Health, U.S. Public Health Service.

Results

From Fig. 1, a comparison of the mean Stanford scores obtained during acute intoxication with the means obtained during the two individual control sessions provides no evidence of any systematic influence of the drug upon hypnotic susceptibility. Subjects

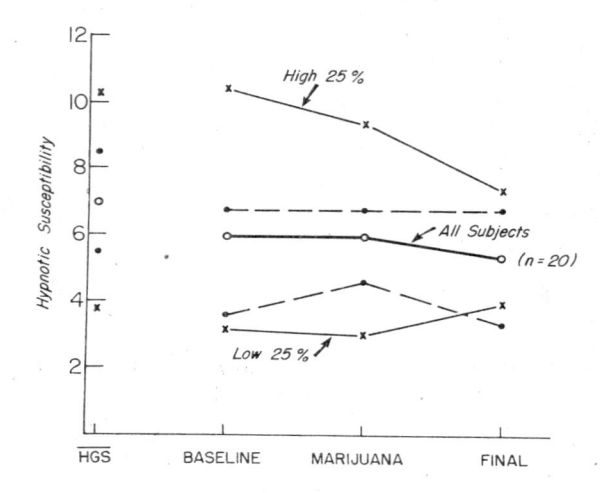

Fig. 1. Mean hypnotic susceptibility scores. ($\overline{\text{HGS}}$ refers to the mean of the two Harvard Group Scale scores obtained initially on each subject.)

who were initially resistant (extremely or moderately, as defined by lower quartiles) to the hypnotic suggestions showed no tendency to be more receptive when tested under marijuana; nor were any other hypnotic susceptibility changes observed which could reasonably be attributed to the drug.

References

1. SHOR, R. E. and ORNE, E. C. (1962) Harvard Group Scale of Hypnotic Susceptibility. Palo Alto, Calif.: Consulting Psychologists Press.
2. WEITZENHOFFER, A. M. and HILGARD, E. R. (1962) Stanford Hypnotic Susceptibility Scale. Palo Alto, Calif.: Consulting Psychologists Press.

S.F., Psychopharmacology Laboratory, Division of Psychiatry Boston University School of Medicine, Boston, Massachusetts, U.S.A.

EXPERIMENTAL STUDIES WITH Δ⁹-TETRAHYDROCANNABINOL IN VOLUNTEERS — SUBJECTIVE SYNDROMES, PHYSIOLOGICAL CHANGES AND AFTER-EFFECTS

A. DITTRICH and B. WOGGON

Psychiatric University Clinic Burghölzli, Division of Research, Zürich

Introduction

Two double-blind trials were performed on the acute effects of Δ⁹-tetrahydrocannabinol (Δ⁹-THC) in man. In order to assess the subjective Δ⁹-THC effects reliably we constructed self-rating scales for the dimensions of the Δ⁹-THC experience based on factoranalytical results. These psychological dimensions were correlated with physiological changes during the Δ⁹-THC intoxication. The after-effects of Δ⁹-THC were studied systematically.

Methods

In the first study on average 23.5 mg Δ⁹-THC (i.e. 350 µg/kg) dissolved in olive oil were administered orally to 18 volunteers with no prior experience of cannabis. The control group of 18 subjects received pure olive oil as placebo. Each subject was tested alone in a neutral setting. In the second trial 37 subjects were treated together in a lecture room by administering orally 15 mg Δ⁹-THC dissolved in ethyl alcohol, placebo and "no drug" in a cross-over design. 15 of these subjects had taken cannabis before, but only four of them more than 25 times.

When drug effects in most subjects had diminished, i.e. at a minimum of three hours after application, all subjects of both trials were required to compare their own experience during the experiment with 54 statements likely to be descriptive of Δ⁹-THC effects. In the first trial we measured pulse-rate, systolic and diastolic blood-pressure, sublingual body temperature and pH of saliva before and twice at hourly intervals after drug administration. In addition, most of the subjects of the first study were asked to fill in a semantic differential on their mood daily for several days after the experiment in order to assess after-effects.

RESULTS

Factor-analyses yielded the following three dimensions of the Δ^9-THC experience:
a) "derealization of self and surroundings",
b) "anxious-depressive state" and
c) "euphoric-stimulated state" (1).

We attempted to establish the validity of the three corresponding scales by comparing the Δ^9-THC to the placebo effects in both studies. For the first study we found statistically significant differences for all three scales. In the second study a statistically significant difference between Δ^9-THC and placebo was found only in the first dimension. The intercorrelations between the scales "anxious-depressive state" and "euphoric-stimulated state" were not significantly negative, which indicates that Δ^9-THC like LSD (2) may produce strong but opposing emotions at approximately the same time and/or at different times during one intoxication. An oral dosage of 23.5 mg Δ^9-THC caused the following physiological changes:

1. The variance of changes from the predrug level of the diastolic blood-pressure was significantly increased.
2. The pulse-rate did not change significantly which was probably due to the very high predrug pulse-rate of the subjects.
3. The body temperature decreased.
4. The pH of saliva was significantly lowered.

Anxious-depressive states during the Δ^9-THC intoxication were correlated with a relative increase in systolic blood pressure.

25 subjects of the first study completed a semantic differential on their mood daily for 9 days after the experiment. Those subjects who had received Δ^9-THC felt ill at ease and constrained on the day after the experiment. No such after-effects were found on the following days.

REFERENCES

1. DITTRICH, A., BAETTIG, K., WOGGON, B. and VON ZEPPELIN, I. (1972) Entwicklung einer Selbsteinschätzungsskala (DAE-Skala I) zur Erfassung von Cannabiseffekten Pharmakopsychiat. (In press).
2. KATZ, M. M., WASKOW, I. E. and OLSSON, J. (1967) Characterizing the Psychological State Produced by LSD. In: BRILL, H. et al. (Ed.) Neuro-Psycho-Pharmacology, p. 398 International Congress Series No. 129, Amsterdam etc.

A.D., Psychiatrische Universitätsklinik Burghölzli, Forschungsdirektion, CH-8029 Zürich, Switzerland

EFFECTS OF CANNABIS ON HUMAN EEG AND HEART RATE — EVIDENCE OF TOLERANCE DEVELOPMENT ON CHRONIC USE[*]

M. FINK, J. VOLAVKA, R. DORNBUSH and P. CROWN

Division of Biological Psychiatry, Department of Psychiatry, New York Medical College, New York City

The isolation of active constituents of cannabis provides the opportunity to assess the clinical pharmacology of different formulations, as marijuana and hashish, and that of its constituents, notably Δ^9-THC. In studies in young male volunteers with at least a one-year history of marijuana use (no less frequent than one exposure each month), we have studied the effects of smoking different doses of marijuana, hashish, and Δ^9-THC, in single sessions and in daily dosages to 22 days. We have recorded the behavioral (mood), EEG, heart rate, and memory effects. The techniques are described in prior reports (1—4). We focussed on two questions.

1. What are the CNS effects of marijuana, hashish, and Δ^9-THC?

In a study of two doses of marijuana equivalent to 22.5 and 7.5 mg Δ^9-THC, we observed dose-related, rapid central effects of increased alpha activity and decreased beta and theta EEG activities. Performance on short-term memory and reaction time tasks was impaired; and heart rate was increased.

In a second study, we injected 10 and 20 mg Δ^9-THC into oregano cigarettes. When smoked, dose-related increases in EEG alpha activity and decreased beta and theta quantities were observed. Heart rate increased and reached a peak during the first 8 minutes of smoking. We concluded that Δ^9-THC replicated the CNS and heart rate effects of marijuana.

In a recent study we directly compared marijuana, Δ^9-THC, and hashish equivalent to 20 mg Δ^9-THC and again observed similar CNS effects for these substances when equated for the amount of Δ^9-THC.

2. Can tolerance be demonstrated?

Much discussion has focussed on the problem of inverse tolerance — an increased responsivity reported by some experienced cannabis users to successive doses of cannabis, so that doses can be decreased and yet achieve the same clinical effects. Using the EEG

---

[*] Aided, in part, by NIMH grants 13358 and 18172.

and heart rate as indices, we examined the effects of smoking marijuana (equivalent to 14 mg Δ^9-THC) for 22 days.

The heart rate increased during each smoking session, but the amount of response, in beats per minute, progressively decreased.

While the alpha percent-time increased during each smoking session, the amount of increase became progressively smaller with succeeding sessions. Also, post-smoking levels were successively lower at the end of each experiment than at the beginning of each experiment.

In memory tasks, the decrement in performance with cannabis became progressively less with increased exposure, again suggesting the development of tolerance.

(These data for tolerance are also supported by observations in chronic hashish users in Greece where we have observed men able to smoke marijuana, hashish, and Δ^9-THC impregnated cigarettes containing between 75 and 140 mg equivalent Δ^9-THC with behavioral and physiological effects equivalent to much lower dosages [= 10—20 mg Δ^9-THC] in our U.S. volunteers).

SUMMARY

In studies of cannabis smoking in non-naive volunteer users we have observed dose-related EEG increases in alpha activity and decreased beta and theta activities; increased heart rate; and increased errors on memory tasks. In chronic studies, these effects show a progressively smaller response on successive days — changes that are consistent with the development of tolerance in the classic sense.

REFERENCES

1. DORNSBUSH, R., FINK, M. and FREEDMAN, A. (1971). Marijuana, Memory and Perception. Amer. J. Psychiat. **128**, 194.
2. DORNBUSH, R., VOLAVKA, J., CLARE, G., ZAKS, A. and FINK, M. (1972) 21-Day Administration of Marijuana in Male Volunteers. In: Current Research in Marijuana. M. F. LEWIS (Ed.), Academic Press, New York and London, p. 115.
3. VOLAVKA, J., DORNBUSH, R., FELDSTEIN, S., CLARE, G., ZAKS, A., FINK, M. and FREEDMAN, A. (1971). Marijuana, EEG, and Behavior. Ann. N.Y. Acad. Sci. **191**, 206.
4. VOLAVKA, J., DORNBUSH, R., FELDSTEIN, S., CROWN, P. and FINK, M. Δ^9-Tetrahydrocannabinol Effects on Human Electroencephalogram and Heart Rate. Psychopharmacologia (in press).

M.F., Department of Psychiatry, Health Sciences Center, Suny at Stony Brook, Stony Brook, N.Y. 11790.

HUMAN PHARMACOLOGY OF MARIHUANA: WHAT NEXT?[*]

L. E. HOLLISTER

Veterans Administration Hospital, Palo Alto, California

A number of questions of pharmacological and therapeutic interest are likely to be answered in the near future, as research with marihuana in man continues to increase. Some of these are:

1. *Are materials other than Δ^9-tetrahydrocannabinol (THC) active in marihuana?* — Very likely any component of marihuana resembling THC in structure will be active. The Δ^{6a}-THC isomer, as well as its synthetic side-chain homolog, synhexyl, has about 1/3 to 1/6 the activity of Δ^9-THC (3). Recent work in our laboratory indicates that Δ^8-THC has about 2/3 the activity of the Δ^9-THC isomer, while both cannabinol and cannabidiol are inactive. So far, there is no evidence that any active material is qualitatively different from Δ^9-THC. Although many other materials have been found in various species of marihuana, unless some should prove to be active in ways markedly different, their small quantities should mitigate against their having any discernible influence of their own. It appears that marihuana effects can be ascribed to THC-like materials.

2. *How is the drug metabolized in man and are metabolites active?* — The primary route of metabolism is to the 11-hydroxy metabolite, which apparently has activity in man (6). This compound is probably inactivated by further hydroxylations. Other monohydroxy metabolites, such as 8-hydroxy-THC, may also be active, but their potency is not yet established. The question of whether THC must be metabolized to become active is still uncertain. We have tried to impair hydroxylation by pretreatment with methylphenidate but have not yet been able to show any attenuation of the action of Δ^9-THC.

3. *Does chronic use lead to tolerance or sensitization?* — Experience with subchronic oral doses in our laboratory provides little evidence for either phenomenon, as judged by the clinical syndromes elicited by the same challenge doses of drug after a placebo or drug-treatment interval. Some evidence of tolerance to the tachycardic action, to dizziness and to memory deficit may occur. Patterns of excretion of metabolites provide no clear basis for any accumulation of drug, but show rather great differences between subjects (5). Some still unpublished studies of chronic marihuana smoking also provide little evidence to support the development of tolerance or sensitization. These results are consistent with experience derived from social use of the drug.

---

[*] Work cited as the author's was supported in part by grant MH-03030, U.S. Public Health Service.

4. *How does marihuana interact with other drugs?* — When marihuana or THC is combined with alcohol, the effects are additive, and largely in the area of increased sedation. One would expect that soon interactions with other social drugs, such as LSD, amphetamines and barbiturates will be studied. Interactions with alpha-methyl-para-tyrosine, an inhibitor of tyrosine hydroxylase, have been studied in our laboratory to determine if depletion of newly synthesized catecholamines alters the responses to THC. So far the evidence is negative. The failure of the beta-adrenergic blocking drug, propranolol, to attenuate the mental effects of marihuana also tends to rule out central adrenergic mechanisms of action (1). Recent reports of the attenuation of effects of marihuana intoxication by physostigmine suggest that a central cholinergic mechanism of action is more likely. The interesting possibility has been raised that THC may interact with cannabidiol, a normally inactive component of marihuana. The latter blocks hydroxylations of drugs and could possibly alter either the degree or duration of effect of THC when the two compounds are taken together.

5. *Does marihuana have any therapeutic uses?* — Single dose studies indicate some degree of appetite stimulation, but it remains to be seen if this can be applied to clinical disturbances of appetite (4). Anorexia nervosa might be a good place to try first. The euphoriant effects of marihuana have suggested its use as an antidepressant, but initial trials have not been very encouraging. Although the drug has hypnotic effects, and in single doses will prolong sleep time, like other conventional sedatives, it decreases rapid eye-movement sleep (7). Fragmentary evidence from studies of chronic use of the drug suggest a disruptive influence on sleep patterns. At the moment, it is not a good candidate for a hypnotic drug. Lowering of intraocular pressure was a totally unexpected finding and one that is now being exploited in the treatment of glaucoma (2). In the near future we should have information regarding the possible use of the drug for treating hypertension, migraine, pain of dying patients and as a sexual stimulant. It should be remembered that the very effects which are desired socially in the use of the drug may be regarded as side effects when the drug is used therapeutically.

References

1. DREW, W. G., KIPLINGER, G. F., MILLER, L. L. and MARK, M. (1972) Effects of propranolol on marihuana-induced cognitive dysfunctioning. Clin. Pharmacol. Ther. **13**, 526.
2. HEPLER, R. S. and FRANK, I. M. (1971) Marihuana smoking and intraocular pressure. J. Amer. med. Ass. **217**, 1392.
3. HOLLISTER, L. E. (1970) Tetrahydrocannabinol isomers and homologues: Contrasted effects of smoking. Nature, **227**, 968.
4. HOLLISTER, L. E. (1971) Hunger and appetite after single doses of marihuana, alcohol and dextroamphetamine. Clin. Pharmacol. Ther. **12**, 44.
5. HOLLISTER, L. E., KANTER, S. L., MOORE, F. and GREEN, D. E. (1972) Marihuana metabolites in urine of man. Clin. Pharmacol. Ther. **13**, 849.
6. LEMBERGER, L., CRABTREE, R. E. and ROWE, H. M. (1972) 11-Hydroxy-Δ^9-tetrahydrocannabinol: Pharmacology, disposition and metabolism of a major metabolite of marihuana in man. Science, **177**, 62.
7. PIVIK, R. T., ZARCONE, V., DEMENT, W. C. and HOLLISTER, L. E. (1972) Delta-9-tetrahydrocannabinol and synhexyl: Effects on human sleep patterns. Clin. Pharmacol. Ther. **13**, 426.

L.E.H., Veterans Administration Hospital, 3801 Miranda Avenue, Palo Alto 94304 California, U.S.A.

The name "False Hormone" only implies the hypothesis that some kind of interference is suspected between some THC metabolites and the normal regulatory action of the mentioned hormones.

For example, "False Hormones"*) may affect the induction of gluconeogenic enzymes in the liver by glucocorticoids thus interfering with the regulation of blood glucose levels. We also know that corticosteroids as well as sex hormones can affect the central nervous system by selectively binding to specific receptors in the hypothalamus and hippocampus (2). If false hormones interfere with such bindings, they may have profound effect on behavior, especially in youngsters whose developing nervous system in especially sensitive to hormonal influences. And, perhaps, even the so-called "amotivational syndrome" could have a basis in chronically altered hormonal balance as a result of the effects of the hypothetical false hormones.

Since hormones may have different "receptors" in different organs, it will probably be necessary to study the interaction of the "False Hormones" with the natural ones on all possible target organs, and not only in the brain, before a comprehensive picture of the overall result of the hypothetical interaction can be elucidated.

REFERENCES

1. BURSTEIN, S., ROSENFELD, J. and WITTSTRUCK, T. (1971) Isolation and Characterization of Two Major Urinary Metabolites of Delta-1-Tetrahydrocannabinol. Science, **176**, 422.
2. GERLACH, J. and MCEWEN, B. S. (1972) Rat Brain Binds Adrenal Steroid Hormone: Radioautography of Hippocampus with Corticosterone. Science, **175**, 1133.
3. HO, B. T., ESTEVEZ, V., ENGLERT, L. F. and MCISAAC, W. M. (1972) Delta-9-Tetrahydrocannabinol and its Metabolites in Monkey Brains. J. Pharm. Pharmacol. **24**, 414.
4. HOLLISTER, L. E. (1971) Marihuana in Man: Three Years Later. Science, **172**, 21.
5. LEMBERGER, L., CRABTREE, R. E. and ROWE, H. M. (1972) 11-Hydroxy-Delta-9-Tetrahydrocannabinol: Pharmacology Disposition, and Metabolism of a Major Metabolite of Marihuana in Man. Science, **177**, 62.
6. LEMBERGER, L., TAMARKIN, N. R., AXELROD and KOPIN, I. (1971) Delta-9-THC: Metabolism and Disposition in Long-Term Marihuana Smokers. Science **173**, 72.
7. MECHOULAM, R., and GAONI, Y. (1965) A Total Synthesis of dl-Delta-1-Tetra-hydrocannabinol, the Active Constituent of Hashish. J. Amer. chem. Soc. **87**, 3273.
8. THOMPSON, G. R., ROSENKRANTZ, H. and BRAUDE, M. C. (1971) Neurotoxicity of Cannabinoids in Chronically Treated Rats and Monkeys, Pharmacologist, **13**, 297.
9. WALL, M. E. (1971) The *In Vitro* and *In Vivo* Metabolism of Tetrahydrocannabinol (THC). Ann. N. Y. Acad. Sci. **191**, 23.
10. *Marihuana and Health Report*, Second Annual Report to Congress (1972) U.S. Government Printing Office, No. 75 — 724 O, Washington.

S.S., *Clinical Drug Studies Section, Center for Studies of Narcotic and Drug Abuse, NIMH, 5600 Fishers Lane, Rockville, Maryland 20825, U.S.A.*

---

*) The "False Hormones" themselves coud probably be prepared from 8β-hydroxy Δ^9-THC (3) by further enzymatic hydroxylation of the side chain for experimental purposes.

AUTHOR INDEX

Adamec C., 685
Albrecht F., 171
Andén N. E., 407
Arnold O. H., 69

Baastrup P. C., 65
Ban T. A., 99, 293
Baum E., 395
Bech P., 689
Benkert O., 489
Bente D., 149
Berlet H. H., 209
Bock Elisabeth, 205
Boháček N., 75
Boissier J. R., 43, 49, 395
Böszörményi Z., 85, 177
Botto R. W., 699

Caldwell J., 577
Carruba M., 517
Cattabeni F., 585
Christiansen J., 689
Cochin J., 369
Corrodi H., 407
Costa E., 585, 637
Crown P., 703

Daigle L., 323
Da Prada M., 517
Davis J. M., 675
De Buck R. P., 265
Deniker P., 43, 441
Dietsch P., 171
Dittrich A., 701
Dixon K., 143
Dornbush R., 703
Dring L. G., 577

Eckmann F., 257
Edel W., 273
Eliasson M., 463
Ellinwood E. H. Jr., 189
Emson P. C., 555
Etevenon P., 49

Fieve P. R., 301, 309
Fink M., 703
Fisher S., 699
Fjalland B., 383
Fleiss J. L., 301
Fonnum F., 555
Fuller R. W., 615
Fuxe K., 407

Gautier J., 431
Gessa G. L., 451

Ginestet D., 441
Grof P., 323

Hansen E., 391
Hansteen R. W., 685
Heilbronn E., 551
Heimann H., 127
Helmchen H., 105
Henderson P. Th., 595
Hobi V., 693
Hollister L. E., 705
Holmstedt B., 525
Hordern A., 81
Huber H. P., 165
Hunter D. L., 119

Inanaga K., 229
Israel M., 547
Itil T. M., 13, 279

Janke W., 157
Janowsky D. S., 675
Jones B., 685,
Jonsson J., 625
Jungk R., 59
Jus A., 431
Jus K., 431

Kanowski S., 335
Karlén B., 525
Kaufman Joyce J., 31
Khaled El-Yousef M., 675
Kielholz P., 109
Knaack M., 273
Knop W., 119
Koella W. P., 135
Kordon C., 481
Kühne G. E., 55

Ladewig D., 693
Laduron P., 235
Laschet L., 497
Laschet Ursula 497
Lehmann H. E., 293, 685
Lewander T., 625
Lichtensteiger W., 473
Linden K. J., 273
Lindström L., 463
Lonero L., 685
Loughrey E., 323
Lopez-Ibor Aliño J. J., 115
Lopez-Ibor J. J., 115
Lundgren G., 525

Mako R., 119
Mellerup E. T., 319

Mendlewicz J., 301, 309
Metyšová J., 387
Meyerson B. J., 463
Michanek A., 463
Miller R. D., 585
Mönikes H. J., 171
Møller-Nielsen I., 383
Molloy B. B., 615
Munkvad I., 415, 659
Müller-Oerlinghausen B., 105, 335

Neuman F., 503
Nistri A., 563
Nordgren I., 525
Nymark M., 383

O'Brien R. A., 517

Papeschi R., 415
Parli C. J., 615
Pedersen V., 383
Pepeu G., 563
Pillard R. C., 699
Plenge P., 319
Pletscher A., 3, 517

Quesnell J., 323

Racagni G., 585
Rafaelsen L., 589
Rafaelsen O. J., 113, 205, 319, 689
Randrup A., 659
Ravn J., 391
Reid L., 685
Rennert H., 55
Richter D., 185
Ris M. M., 355
Ropert R., 91
Rud C., 391

Saletu B., 279
Saletu M., 279
Sanders-Bush Elaine, 607
Saner A., 517
Saxena B., 323
Scheel-Krüger J., 659
Schou M., 65
Schuberth J., 533
Sekerke H. J., 675
Simeon J., 279
Smeltzer D. J., 119
Smeltzer F. M., 119
Söderlund A. Ch., 463
Solti Gy., 177

AUTHOR INDEX

Stallone F., 309
Steinbeck H., 503
Steinberg Hannah, 343
Stille G., 143
Sudilovsky A., 189
Sulser F., 607
Sundwall A., 533
Szara S., 707

Tagliamonte A., 451

Tanaka M., 229
Tesařová O., 363
Theodore L., 685
Tomkiewicz M., 343

Ungerstedt V., 407

van der Logt J. Th. M., 595
van Rossum J. M., 595
Viamontes G., 279

Villeneuve A., 431
Vinař O., 247
Volavka J., 703
von Wartburg J. P., 355
Votava Z., 377
Vree T. B., 595

Werner W., 329
White T. G., 355
Woggon B., 701

SUBJECT INDEX

A-35, 616 see Dipotassium clorazepate 23
Acetylcholine
 biosynthesis in brain 533, 539
 biosynthesis in nerve electroplaque junctions in *Torpedo marmorata* 547
 bound fraction in brain homogenates and slices 533
 bound fraction in nerve homogenates from *Torpedo marmorata* 547
 effects of drugs on its CNS distribution 563
 endogenous and newly synthesized, compartmentation in brain 533, 541
 enzymatic release from isolated synaptic vesicles 553
 estimation after chemical demethylation 526
 estimation by pyrolysis 526
 estimation in tissues 525
 free fraction in brain homogenates and slices 533
 free fraction in nerve homogenates from *Torpedo marmorata* 547
 its function as neurohumoral transmitter 3
 precursors in brain 536
 release from cholinergic vesicles 551
 release from CNS, drug-induced 563, 567
Acetylcholinesterase
 activity in single neurons of *Helix aspersa* snail 560
ACTH
 role in animal sexual activity 456
ACTH tests
 use in assessing pituitary ACTH capacity 499
Activation level
 use of EEG in its assessment 133
Acute dystonia
 drug-induced 416
Addictive drugs
 increase of consume 83
S-Adenosylmethionine
 use as methyl donor *in vitro* 239
Adverse Reaction Monitoring Service 101
Affective disorders
 lithium stabilization and weight gain 323
Aggressive behavior
 amphetamine-induced in mice. Its antagonism by neuroleptics (spiramide, trifluperazine) 664
Aggressivity tests
 use of psychotropic drugs, correlation with human behavior 145
Akathisia
 drug-induced 417, 444
Akinetic syndrome
 neuroleptic drug-induced, its psychologic correlates 443

Alcohol
 acute effects in man. Driving tasks, psychomotor tracking performance 686
 effects on psychological tests 689
 interaction with marijuana 705
Alcohol dehydrogenase
 transformation of alcohol to aldehyde 357
Aldehyde dehydrogenase
 oxidation of aldehydes to acids 357
Aldehyde reductase
 reduction of aldehydes to alcohol 357
Amantadine
 liberation of dopamine from intraneuronal stores 3
Amino acids
 relation to schizophrenia 217
γ-Aminobutyric acid
 its activity as neurohumoral transmitter 3
Aminorex
 effect on motor activity in rats 651
 effect on steady state concentrations of brain monoamines 650
Amitriptyline
 use in healthy volunteers, comparison with benzodiazepine derivative Tofizopam 177
Amphetamine
 brain monoamine turnover changes induced by 637
 chronic intoxication in animals and humans, model psychosis 191
 determination in tissues 626
 disappearance rate. Influence of age, sex and other factors on it 628
 drugs interfering with its metabolism and excretion in rats 625
 experimental intoxication induced 189
 p-hydroxylation 625
 mass fragmentographic identification of its metabolites 585
 metabolic interactions 626
 metabolism in rats 625
 mixture with barbiturate, after-effects in rats 344
 psychosis induced by 189
 urinary metabolites 626
(+) Amphetamine
 brain norepinephrine depletion induced by 638
 combination with thioridazine 279
 food intake reduction 637
 hyperthermic effect 637
 motor activity enhancement 637, 645
 psychotic episodes in abusers 645
(—) Amphetamine
 effect on brain norepinephrine turnover as compared with cocaine 647

SUBJECT INDEX

Amphetamine antagonism
  development of tolerance to neuroleptics in rats 383
Amphetamines
  antidepressive activity 665
  binding affinity 601
  β, β-difluoro substituted 615
  effect of β, β-difluoro substitution on metabolism 615
  excretion in man 596
  hydroxy metabolites 598
  mechanism of stereotyped and aggressive behavior produced by 659
  metabolism in animals 577, 615
  metabolism in comparison with that of cyclohexyl isopropylamines 595
  metabolism in man 577, 595
  oxidative deamination 621
  partition coefficients 600
  psychotic episodes in abusers 667
  stereoisomers, metabolic behavior 597
Amygdala
  stimulation, search for areas influencing dopaminergic neurons 477
Analeptic drugs
  quantitative EEG analysis, use in discrimination between analeptic and hypnotic drugs 52
Androgen target areas
  inhibition by antiandrogens 497
Animal behavior
  biochemical aspects 661
  CNS anatomical findings 665
  correlation with EEG recordings after perphenazine in rabbits 380
  long-term effects of psychotropic drugs 343
"Antiaggressive" drugs
  use of computerized EEG in prediction 24
Antiandrogens
  use in sexual disorders in man 497
Anticholinergic drugs
  decrease of brain acetylcholine in animals in cortex and caudate nucleus 566
  use in neuroleptic drug-induced catalepsy 408
Antidepressant drugs
  discovery 43
  EEG prediction 23
  interference with metabolic disposition of amphetamine 630
Antiparkinsonic drugs
  simultaneous use with neuroleptics 445
Antisocial behavior
  combined treatment in children with thioridazine and d-amphetamine 283
Anxiety
  correlation between pharmacological and clinical aspects 128
  environmental causes 81
  worsening after thioridazine withdrawal in behavioral disorders treated with thioridazine — d-amphetamine combination 283

Anxiolytic drugs
  investigation of a new drug — Tofizopam 86
Apomorphine
  gnawing induced in rats 400
  stereotyped running induced in dogs 384
Apomorphine antagonism
  development of tolerance to neuroleptics in rats 383
Arcuate nucleus
  increase in LH secretion after electric stimulation 474
Arousal reaction
  neocortical and hippocampal EEG recordings 137
  testing in perphenazine-treated rabbits after sensory stimulation 379
ATP
  release from synaptic vesicles 553
Atropine
  blockade of stimulatory response of dopamine neurons 475
  decrease in brain acetylcholine in animals in cortex and caudate nucleus 566
  role in animal sexual behavior 459
Audiovisual methods
  use in psychopharmacological training 109
Automatic rat hypnogram plot
  ratios of integrated EEG vs. integrated EMG values, similarity to human "sleep prints" 52
Automobile driving tasks
  influenced by marijuana and alcohol 686
Avoidance response
  use in neuroleptic drug testing in healthy volunteers 171

Barbiturates
  inhibition of aldehyde reductase 359
Barron ego-strength scale
  use in ego-strength changes assessment during pharmacotherapy 85
Behavior
  models in man 127
  neurophysiological basis 135
Behavioral disorders
  correlation with urinary indoles 212
  in children, treatment by thioridazine — d-amphetamine combination 279
Behavioral patterns
  overt and non-overt mental aspects 135
Benzodiazepine derivative (SCH-12,041)
  structure relationship to minor tranquillizers (chlordiazepoxide, diazepam, oxazepam) 21
Biochemical errors
  role in origin of schizophrenia and its mental symptoms 185
Biogenic aldehydes
  role in long-term effects of drugs 355
Biogenic amines
  conformational similarity with neuroleptics 33
  N-methylation 235
  scheme of catabolism 356

SUBJECT INDEX

Bipolar manic-depressive illness
  genetic aspects of lithium prophylaxis 309
Bisexuality
  androstenedione-induced during the critical period of psychic differentiation 505
Brain dopamine
  turnover rate in rats after amphetamine 637
Brain — gonads relationship
  regulation of sexual behavior 503
Brain — mind unity 135
Brain monoamines
  role in controlling sexual behavior in male animals 451
  turnover rate in rats after amphetamine 637
Brain norepinephrine
  depletion induced by amphetamine 638
Brain of *Helix aspersa* snail
  enzymatic analysis of its neurons 555
Brain serotonin
  effects on male sexual activity 452
Brain tissue
  choline uptake, role in acetylcholine biosynthesis 538
Brain — stem structures
  involvement in schizophrenia-like psychoses 187
Brainstorming sessions
  use in evaluation of psychotropic drugs 177
Brengelman-Eysenck questionnaire
  use in assessment of ego-strength and neuroticism 87
Brief Psychiatric Rating Scale (BPRS)
  as an aid in predicting therapeutic response to chlorpromazine 249
  rating of improvement and degree of illness in fluphenazine-HCl treatment 266
  use in evaluation of niacin effects in schizophrenia 297
Bufotenin
  formation in plasma of schizophrenics after incubation with serotonin 214
Butyrophenones
  blockade of DA receptors in neostriatum 407

Calcium metabolism
  lithium-induced changes 321
Cannabidiol
  component of marijuana, comparison with with Δ^9-THC 705
Cannabinol
  component of marijuana, comparison with Δ^9-THC 705
Cannabis
  development of tolerance 703
  effects on heart rate in man 703
  effects on human EEG 703
  effects on memory in man 703
  effects on psychological tests 689
  interaction with alcohol 687
  intoxication induced in man 699
  urinary metabolites 689

Carbohydrate metabolism
  lithium-induced changes 319
Castration in males
  influence on sexual motivation and libido 508
Catalepsy
  drug-induced 384, 387, 398, 408, 420, 425
Catatonia
  amphetamine-induced, resemblance to catatonic schizophrenia 189, 197
  drug-induced by chronic and acute administration of amphetamine, disulfiram, bulbocapnine, mescaline, and apomorphine 200
Catecholamines
  amphetamine-induced liberation from nerve endings 3
  enhanced turnover 5
  influence on ovulation 483
  role in male sexual behavior 458
Central adrenergic/cholinergic balance
  role in human behavior 675
Central cholinergic synapses
  influencing by atropine 476
Central cholinergic system
  relation to extrapyramidal system 395, 401
  role in animal sexual behavior 459
Central Consultation Service
  levels of proposed organization of psychiatric services 100
Central dopaminergic system
  activity of neostriatum after neuroleptics 407
  interactions with pituitary-gonadal axis 473
  role in eating and drinking behavior in animals 665
  role in functioning of extrapyramidal structures 398, 401
  role in origin of parkinsonian symptoms 417, 435
  role in stereotyped behavior 646
  use in animal models of schizophrenia (stereotyped gnawing and sniffing behavior) 675
Central noradrenergic system
  coordination of behavioral and hormonal state 473
  influence on exploratory activity in animals 646
Central serotoninergic system
  coordination of behavioral and hormonal state 473
  influence on ovulation 484
Cerebral serotonin
  effects induced by p-chloroamphetamine 607
Cerebrospinal fluid
  levels of 5-hydroxyindoles in schizophrenia and endogenous depression 212
Ceruloplasmin
  blood levels in psychotic patients and in healthy controls 205
Chlorazepam
  EEG changes and clinical anxiolytic effects 20

SUBJECT INDEX

Chlordiazepoxide
  mixture with dexamphetamine, use in long-term effects analysis of drugs 346
p-Chlormethamphetamine
  effect on brain monoamine concentrations 650
p-Chloroamphetamine
  biochemical mechanism of its action on brain serotonin 607
  comparison with amphetamine β, β-difluorinated analogs 618
  effect on brain monoamine concentrations 650
  long-term effects 611
p-Chlorophenylalanine
  combination with pargyline, effects on oestradiol + progesterone-activated copulatory behavior in ovariectomized rats 466
  effect on male sexual activity 452
  mounting behavior in animals 491
  serotonin synthesis inhibition 484
  species differences in activity 454
Chlorphentermine
  effects on brain monoamine concentrations 650
Chlorpromazine
  predictability of therapeutic response 249
Choline
  uptake in brain tissue 538
Choline acetyltransferase
  regional distribution 557
  single cell studies 558
  subcellular distribution 535
Cholinergic nerve endings
  in central nervous system, pharmacological properties 568
  in peripheral nervous system, pharmacological properties 568
Cholinergic neurons
  functional significance in regional distribution and release of acetylcholine under drug influence 563
Cholinergic stereotypies
  pilocarpine and eserine-induced in rats 400
Cholinergic vesicles
  release of low molecular substances 551
Cholinesterase
  diminution in neostriatum after substantia nigra lesions 401
Choreo-athetoid syndrome
  drug-induced 409
Chronicity of mental illness
  definition problems 248
Civilization hazards 82
Classification of depressions
  problems of masked depressions, impact on depression treatment 117
Clinical experimentation
  basic principles 46
Clinical psychopharmacology
  postgraduate training 105
  use of computers 120

Clopenthixol
  long-term treatment, analysis of laboratory tests (hematology, liver and kidney functions, proteins, ECG) 391
Clozapine
  dopaminergic receptor blockade, neuroleptic activity 410
  neuroleptic activity 418
CNS depressants
  effects on regional brain acetylcholine 565
  effects on whole brain acetylcholine 564
CNS stimulants
  effects on regional brain acetylcholine 565
  effects on whole brain acetylcholine 564
Cocaine
  effects on motor activity, body temperature and food intake in rats 647
  reduction of acetylcholine output from cholinergic nerve endings 568
Compensation device
  use in Δ^9-THC-influenced driving performance 697
Computers
  use in clinical psychopharmacology 120
  use in clinical training 119
Concentration tests
  use in cannabis and alcohol influence assessment on car driving 691
Conditioned avoidance response
  inhibition by flupenthixol 385
Conduct
  changes in behavioral disturbances in children during thioridazine and d-amphetamine treatment 284
Consciousness and mood scales
  use in cannabis and alcohol influence assessment on car driving 691
Continuing Treatment Service
  levels of proposed psychiatric service organization 100
Continuous lithium takers 329
Copulatory behavior
  activation by oestradiol benzoate and progesterone in animals 464
Cortical acetylcholine
  drug-induced variations 568
Cortical hypovariability
  in EEG recordings after droperidol in baboons 53
Cortical spreading depression
  influence on cerebral neurotransmitters 6
Corticosterone
  similarity with "false hormones" 708
Crisis of participation
  and social implications of psychopharmacology 60
Cross-tolerance to neuroleptics
  relation to amphetamine antagonism in rats 383
N-Cycloheptylamphetamine
  metabolism of amphetamines, attack by cytochrome P-450 604

SUBJECT INDEX

Cycloheximide
  protein synthesis inhibition 355, 374
N-Cyclohexylamphetamine
  metabolism of amphetamines, attack by cytochrome P-450 603
Cyclohexylisopropylamines
  metabolism in man, comparison with amphetamine metabolism 595
Cyclopentamine
  demethylation and excretion in urine 602
N-Cyclopentylamphetamine
  metabolism of amphetamines, attack by cytochrome P-450 603
Cyproterone acetate
  influence on human neuro-endocrine system, antiandrogenic activity 497
Cytochrome P-450
  binding affinities of amphetamines to it 601

Decarboxylase inhibitor Ro 4-4602
  combination with L-DOPA to induce mounting behavior 492
  inhibition of extracerebral catecholamine formation from L-DOPA 519
Depressive disturbances
  apomorphine-induced 363
  phenoharmane-induced 363
  role of personality factors 363
Depressive experience
  lithium-influenced 69
Depressive syndrome
  induced by neuroleptic treatment 444
Desmethylimipramine
  enhancement of amphetamine levels in rat brain 619, 625, 640
Dexamphetamine
  mixture with chlordiazepoxide 346
Diazepam
  comparison with Tofizopam using Barron ego-strength scale 87
Diazepines
  low incidence of extrapyramidal side effects in Clozapine 445
Diethyldithiocarbamate
  disulfiram metabolite, effects on amphetamine metabolite distribution changes 628
Differential diagnosis
  its importance before psychopharmacological treatment 116
Differential effects of sedatives
  differentiation of barbiturates and chlorpromazine 129
β, β-Difluoroamphetamine
  distribution and metabolism in rats 616, 618
10, 11-Dihydrodibenzo (b, f) thiepines
  changes of sedative and cataleptogenic effects in mice and rats (octoclothepin and oxyprothepin) 387
5,6-Dihydroxytryptamine
  effects on sexual behavior 517
3,4-Dimethoxyphenylethylamine (DMPEA)
  role in psychopathological changes 293

Diphenylbutylpiperidines
  neuroleptics with low incidence of extrapyramidal side effects 445
Dipotassium clorazepate (A-35,616)
  anxiolytic effects, EEG character as minor tranquillizer 23
Disulfiram
  combination with amphetamine in producing experimental catatonia 196, 200
Dominant inheritance
  role in the origin of manic-depressive psychosis 306
L-DOPA
  combination with α-methyl-p-tyrosine and Ro 4-4602 423
  combination with Ro 4-4602, effects on sexual behavior in rats 519
  effects on sexual behavior 451, 458, 491, 517
  mania-like symptoms induced in Parkinson's disease treatment 219
  role as precursor of dopamine 4, 219
  simultaneous use with neuroleptics 229
  use in schizophrenia 229
  use in treatment of Parkinson's disease 435
Dopamine
  N-methylation 235
  role in mechanism of psychotropic drug action (amantadine, neuroleptics, L-DOPA, lithium) 3, 407
  role in neostriatum 407, 416
  role in producing stereotypy and bizarre postures in animals 193
Dopaminergic receptors
  blockade by haloperidol and thiopropazate 416
  blockade by pimozide and fluspirilene 410
Drug abuse
  relapse tendencies 350
Drug after-effects
  single drug experience, influence on animal behavior 344
Drug dependence
  its long-term duration aspects 369
  self-administration of opiates in rats 350
  social aspects of psychopharmacology 60
Drug identification
  in brain homogenates 585
Drug withdrawal
  in childhood behavioral disorders 279
Dysesthetic crises
  appearance during neuroleptic treatment 443
Dyskinesias
  induced by neuroleptic drugs 431
Dysphoria
  changes of mood under lithium long-term treatment 70
Dyssynchrony
  drug-induced; head-neck, shoulder-foreleg, hip-hindleg asynchronous movements 195

Early Clinical Drug Evaluation Units (ECDEU)
  use in childhood behavioral disorders 280

Early dyskinesias
  induced by butyrophenones and piperazine phenothiazines 442
EEG
  activated pattern 379
  alpha activity in man 703
  arousal level 129
  beta activity in man 703
  digital computer period analysis 280, 287
  drug-induced changes 13, 52, 287
  indication of learning ability 138
  quantitative analysis 13, 47, 49, 52, 280, 287
  reaction types 13
  resting pattern 379
  theta activity in man 703
  use in discrimination between hypnotic and analeptic drugs 52
Ego-strength
  changes during pharmacotherapy (anxiolytic drugs) 85
  concept, personality structure, age and somatic conditions 86
  weakening effect of anxiolytic drugs, relationship with drug addiction 89
Electroencephalography
  coefficient of variability changes 52
  discriminant analysis 51
  period analysis 49
  statistical spectral analysis 49
Electronic charge distribution
  as an aid for understanding of psychotropic drug mode of action 31
EMD 16, 139
  neuroleptic activity, use in healthy volunteers 171
Emotional withdrawal
  changes in manic-depressive psychosis under long-term lithium treatment 70
Encephalitis
  involvement in schizop.-like psychoses 188
Environmental temperature
  effect on norepinephrine turnover 643
Epinine
  conversion of dopamine to it in presence of N-methyltransferase 238
Eserine salicylate
  use in producing experimental catalepsy and stereotypy 398
Etifoxin
  influence on human EEG in healthy volunteers 150
  personality specific effects 166
Examining behavior
  see exploratory activity
Exhibitionism
  treatment with cyproterone acetate 500
Exner-spiral
  use in assessment of extraversion and introversion 696
Exploratory activity
  amphetamine-induced in animals, correlation with behavior in human abusers 190
  influenced by (+)amphetamine in rats 646
  influenced by α-methyl-p-tyrosine in rats 420
Extrapyramidal syndrome
  drug-induced 270, 415, 431, 441
Extrapyramidal system
  cholinergic aspects of its anatomy and physiology 395
Extraversion
  role in psychotropic drug effects 165
  use of Exner-spiral in its assessment 696

"False hormones"
  Δ^9-tetrahydrocannabinol as their potential precursor 707
False neurotransmitters
  metabolites of amphetamine and metamphetamine 580, 586
Feedback information
  modulation of the neuronal pool activity 136
Feedback system
  cortico-subcortico-cortical 138
Feminization
  cyproterone acetate-induced in dogs 509
Fenfluramine
  action on monoamine stores of rat tissues 653
  EEG profiles 29
  identification in rat brain homogenates 585
  metabolites 585
Film
  use in psychopharmacological training 109
Fluorinated amphetamines
  distribution and metabolism in rats 616
Flupenthixol
  development of tolerance with respect to amphetamine antagonism in rats 383
Fluphenazine decanoate
  social aspects of its use 92
Fluphenazine enanthate
  social aspects of its use 92
Fluphenazine hydrochloride
  high dose administration 265
  incidence of side-effects 265
  low dose administration 265
  use in psychotic patients 265
Fluspirilene
  objectivization and quantification of neuroleptic effects, double-blind study 273
Food intake
  influence of nigro-striatal dopaminergic system, role of amphetamines 665
Free fatty acids
  mobilization induced by amphetamine and difluoroamphetamine 622
FSH levels
  in men treated with cyproterone acetate 499

Gas chromatography
  combination with mass spectrometry in determination of amphetamines in brain tissue 585
  use in amphetamine metabolite determination 579

SUBJECT INDEX

use in choline and choline esters determination in tissues 525
Gender orientation development
  role of androgens and antiandrogens 507
General Monitoring Service
  role in psychopharmacological education 101
Genetic transmission
  role in pathogenesis of manic-depressive psychosis 301
Glare recovery
  effects of marijuana in humans 687
Glycogen metabolism
  lithium-induced changes, role of carbohydrate metabolism enzymes 319
Gnawing
  apomorphine-induced 400
Gonadotropic activity
  total, in men treated with cyproterone acetate 499
Gonadotropin releaser function
  regulatory mechanism of pure antiandrogens, androgens with progestogenic action and antigonadotropins without antiandrogen action 497
Gonadotropins
  effect of CNS electrical stimulation on secretion 474
  effect of drugs on tonic levels 482
Group information flow
  effects of placebo and benzodiazepine derivative Tofizopam 180

Hallucinogens
  influence on EEG 148
  influence on head tremor in mice 146
Haloperidol
  development of tolerance with respect to amphetamine antagonism in rats 383
Handwriting test
  combination with rating scales, use in objectivization and quantification of neuroleptic drug effects 273
Haptoglobin
  cerebrospinal fluid levels in schizophrenic patients 206
Hashish
  effects on human EEG, comparison with marijuana and Δ^9-THC 703
Head tremor in mice
  induced by hallucinogens, comparison with hallucinogenic effects in man 146
Helix aspersa snail
  its brain neurons used in determination of acetylcholine esterase and choline acetylase activities 555
Hemopexin
  plasmatic levels in manic-depressive psychosis and schizophrenia 206
Heredity
  role in pathogenesis of manic-depressive psychosis 301

Hippocampus
  EEG theta rhythm triggering during movements 137
  role in neuroendocrine regulations 478
Hole board test
  use in assessment of long-term effects of single drug experience 346
Homovanillic acid (HVA)
  correlation of its content in CSF with akinesia in parkinsonian patients 417
Hormonal regulation
  long-term vs. short-term effects of drugs 484
Hormonal regulation of sexuality
  activational phase 507
  organizational phase 507
Hot-plate test
  use in the study of tolerance to drugs (narcotic analgesics) 370
Hunger and satiety
  neurophysiological correlates 138
p-Hydroxyamphetamine
  study of amphetamine metabolites in rat 587, 626
11-β-Hydroxy-androstendione
  as hypothetical Δ^9-THC metabolite and "false hormone" 708
6-Hydroxydopamine
  lesions induced in the dopaminergic pathways in rat brain 408
5-Hydroxyindole acetic acid (5-HIAA)
  cerebral levels after p-chloroamphetamine in rats 610
  CSF levels in schizophrenic and depressive patients 212
β-Hydroxylation
  concept of false neurotransmitters 580
p-Hydroxynorephedrine
  as amphetamine metabolite in man and laboratory animals 577, 582, 587, 639
  implications of its accumulation in neurons 645
  neuronal localization and efflux from tissues during sympathetic stimulation 642
L-5-Hydroxytryptophan
  role in regulation of sexual behavior in male rats 453
Hyperkinetic syndrome
  as side effect of butyrophenone and phenothiazine treatment 442
Hyperthermia
  induced by difluoroamphetamine in comparison with amphetamine 622
Hypnotic drugs
  influence on EEG 52
Hypnotic susceptibility
  influenced by marijuana 699
Hypokinesia
  neuroleptic drug-induced 417
Hypophysis
  role in p-chlorophenylalanine activity 455
Hypothalamus
  participation in the regulation of pituitary functions 481

SUBJECT INDEX

Iceberg phenomenon
  treatment of depressions by non-psychiatric physicians 117
ICSH levels
  determination in men treated with cyproterone acetate 499
Immunoglobulin M
  levels in plasma of psychotic patients 205
Impulsivity
  worsening after d-amphetamine withdrawal in behaviorally disturbed children 283
Inactivation of indoleamines
  role in schizophrenic psychoses 216
Inborn metabolic errors
  role in pathogenesis of schizophrenia 209
Increasing barrier technique
  use in oestrogen activated sexual motivation study in ovariectomized female rat 470
Indolealkylamines
  relation to schizophrenia 209, 216
Intermittent lithium takers 329
Introversion
  role in psychotropic drug effects 165
  use of Exner-spiral in its assessment 696
Ion-exchange chromatography
  use in purification of amphetamine 626
Ion pair extraction
  use for estimation of acetylcholine in tissues 525
Ionization
  role in drug effects 615

Latent depressivity
  involvement in depression induced by apomorphine and phenoharmane in neurotic patients 363
Learning
  neurophysiological correlates 139
Learning problems
  occurrence in behaviorally disturbed children 283
Levels of biological organization
  correlation with pharmacodynamic effects 143
LH levels
  regulation by dopamine 483
LH secretion
  induced by preoptic area and arcuate nucleus stimulation 474
Libido
  influenced by L-DOPA administration 491
Limbic system
  action on tubero-infundibular dopaminergic neurons 478
Lithium
  combined treatment with antidepressants 336
  combined treatment with antidepressants and neuroleptics 336
  combined treatment with neuroleptics 336
  effects on carbohydrate metabolism 319
  effects on electrolyte metabolism 319
  enhancement of noradrenaline reuptake into CNS adrenergic nerve endings 4
  long-term treatment 69
  maintenance treatment 65
  serum levels 337
  social implications of treatment 65
Lithium non-responders
  biological reasons 314
  correlation with weight gain 324
Lithium prophylaxis
  genetic aspects 309
  incidence of affective psychosis relapses 338
  need for additional medication 335
  personal and social implications 65
  side effects 338
  "technical failures" 329
Lithium responders
  correlation with weight gain 324
Lithium stoppers
  comparison with lithium takers (continuous and intermittent) 330, 331
Lithium treatment
  non-responders, need of other psychotropic drugs 335
  response in humans 323
  side effects 323
Locomotor activity
  influence of amphetamine and neuroleptics 664
Long-acting neuroleptics
  double-blind trial with Fluspirilene and Penfluridol 274
  nursing team's attitude 94
  patient's attitude 92
  physician's attitude 93
  social aspects 91
Long-term effects of drugs
  observations made with psychotropic drugs in animal behavior 343
  role of biogenic aldehydes 355
  tolerance to narcotic analgesics 369
Lordosis response
  inhibition by LSD 466
Low molecular substances
  release from cholinergic vesicles after phospholipase A_2 attack 551

Magnesium metabolism
  lithium-induced changes 321
Major tranquilizers
  EEG prediction 20
  EEG profiles 17
Malignant neuro-vegetative syndrome
  due to neuroleptic treatment 443
Mania
  activation by methylphenidate 678
Manic-depressive patients
  determination of blood and CSF proteins 205
Manic-depressive psychosis
  changes of long-term course 69
  dominant X-linked transmission 301
  genetic aspects of lithium prophylaxis in bipolar form 309
  heredity factors 301

SUBJECT INDEX

lithium stabilization and weight gain, lithium responders and non-responders 324
lithium takers (continuous and intermittent) vs. lithium stoppers 330
mixed states 70
need for additional medication in lithium prophylactic treatment 335
use of lithium maintenance treatment 65
Marijuana
  acute effects in man 685
  adverse reactions 707
  chronic effects 707
  comparison with hashish and Δ^9-THC in effects on human EEG and heart rate 703
  comparison with Δ^9-THC in man 685
  development of tolerance 705
  drug interactions 706
  effects on attention 687
  effects on driving 686
  human pharmacology 705
  interaction with alcohol 706
  modification of hypnotic susceptibility 699
Marital relations
  positive and negative effects of lithium treatment 66
Masculinization
  in human fetuses by synthetic progestins 505
  in rats, neonatally androgenized 505
Mass fragmentography
  use in acetylcholine analysis 525
  use in identification of amphetamine, methamphetamine and fenfluramine metabolites 585
Mass spectrometry
  combination with gas chromatography in analysis of biological samples 579, 585
Mating behavior
  in feminized dogs treated with cyproterone acetate 509
Maudsley Medical Questionnaire
  use in limiting personality-specific variance in psychobiological comparison 129
Medial preoptic area
  increase in LH secretion after electrical stimulation 474
Medical education
  use of computers 119
Membrane structure
  hydrophobic protein — phospholipid interaction 553
Memory
  neurophysiological correlates 138
Memory tests
  use in simulated car driving, influence of cannabis and alcohol 691
Mental performance levels
  effects of psychostimulant and sedative drugs 133
Mental unemployment
  role in drug dependency origin in consume society 60

Mesorgydine
  combination with testosterone, effect on mounting behavior in animals 493
Mesterolone
  combination with L-DOPA, effects on human sexual behavior 492
  effects on human sexual behavior and libido 492
Methamphetamine
  as amphetamine metabolite, drug dependency aspects 577
  biochemical pharmacology in rats 648
  metabolism, identification of metabolites in rat brain homogenates 585
Methodology of psychobiology
  comparison of psychotropic drug effects 128
N-Methylation
  and biogenic amines in brain, implications in schizophrenia 235
  role in tryptophan metabolism and schizophrenia 214
O-Methylation
  role in molecular modification of indoleamines 215
Methylphenidate
  psychopharmacology in man 675
  tolerance to neuroleptics with respect to methylphenidate antagonism in mice 383
5-Methyltetrahydrofolic acid
  as methyl donor in biogenic amine N-methylation 235
N-Methyltransferase
  activity in rat brain 239
  role in pathogenesis of schizophrenia 214
α-Methyl-p-tyrosine
  behavioral effects; decrease of exploratory activity, inducing of catalepsy in rats 420
Methysergide
  effect on mounting behavior in rats in combination with testosterone 493
Mianserin hydrochloride
  antidepressive amitriptyline-like effects 27
  antiserotonin activity 25
  EEG amitriptyline-like effects 26
Microchemical analysis
  characterization of mollusc brain neurons 555
Microsomes
  oxidative deamination of amphetamines in rat liver 621
Minnesota Multiphasic Personality Inventory
  use in testing effects of cannabis and alcohol on simulated car driving and psychological tests 689
Minor tranquilizers
  EEG prediction 20
  EEG profiles 16
Mirror drawing
  use in personality specific drug effect testing 167
Molecular quantum chemical calculation
  basis for psychotropic drug action understanding 31

SUBJECT INDEX

Monoamine oxidase
  role in tissue indoleamine inactivation 216
Monoamine oxidase inhibitors
  role in cerebral monoamine increase 4
  role in copulatory behavior in animals 453, 465
Monoaminergic tone
  effects on female copulatory behavior 468
Monoamines
  role in female sexual behavior 463
Morphine
  influence on acetylcholine content in and output from rat central and peripheral nervous system 569
  use in hot-plate test in study of tolerance to narcotics 370
Motor activity
  as model of neuro-behavioral relations 136
Mounting behavior
  induced in rats by decarboxylase inhibitor Ro 4-4602 and L-DOPA 492
  induced in rats by repeated administration of L-DOPA 518
Multifactorial pathogenetic concept 55
Multiple regression analysis
  use in prediction of psychotropic drug treatment outcome 252
Muscarinic compounds
  effects on female copulatory behavior 469

Naja nigricollis
  phospholipase A_2 content in its venom, study of cholinergic synapses 551
Narcotic analgesics
  classification and common characteristic features 39
  influence on norepinephrine pathway 39
  system analysis 39
  tolerance as long-term phenomenon 369
  topological analysis 39
Neostigmine
  administration to schizophrenic and manic-depressive patients 678
Neostriatum
  dopaminergic-cholinergic mechanisms after neuroleptics 407
Nerve electroplaque junctions
  synthesis and release of acetylcholine 547
Neuro-endocrine system
  in man, influenced by cyproterone acetate 497
Neurohumoral transmitters
  role in CNS function, use in study of new psychotropic drugs 3
Neuroleptic drugs
  action on nigro-neostriatal dopaminergic pathway 407
  as help for schizophrenic patients 247
  cataleptogenic effects 387
  catacholamine turnover enhancement 4
  changes in central effects after repeated administration 387
  chlorpromazine type 418
  conformational similarity with biogenic amines 33
  cross-tolerance 383
  discovery 43
  electronic structure 32
  EMD 16, 139 (2-hydroxy-2-ethyl-1, 2, 3, 4, 6, 7-hexahydro-11 bH-benzo [a] chinolizine malonate) 172
  extrapyramidal side effects 409, 415, 431, 441
  haloperidol type 418
  influence on EEG 52
  inhibition of amphetamine stereotypy 663
  long-term treatment 257
  medium-acting 171
  metabolic interactions with amphetamine in rats 630
  pimozide-fluspirilene type 418
  relation of neuroleptic effect in animals to pharmacological parkinsonism and antipsychotic activity in man 415
  repeated administration 387
  reserpine type 418
  sedative effects 387
  simultaneous use with L-DOPA 229
  structu — reactivity relationship 33
  subacute oral administration in mice 388
  testing in healthy subjects 171
  tolerance and cross-tolerance in animals after repeated administration 383
  use in schizophrenia 229, 257
Neuroleptic effects
  objectivization 273
  quantification 273
Neuroleptic treatment
  analysis of laboratory tests 391
  side effects 392
Neuronal activities
  EEG patterns, evoked potentials, arousal reaction 137
Neurosis
  role of drugs in its evolution 117
Neuroticism
  role in psychotropic drug effects, personality-dependent drug effects 161, 165
Neurotics
  drug-induced experimental depression 363
Neurotransmitters
  involvement in drug interference with pituitary gonadotropic regulation 481
  involvement in narcotic addiction 40
Neurotropic viruses
  role in pathogenesis of schizophrenia 188
Niacin
  use in combination treatment of schizophrenia 293
  use in schizophrenia 293
Nicotinamide adenine nucleotide (NAD)
  inhibition of aminochrome formation, role in pathogenesis of schizophrenia 293
Nigro-neostriatal dopaminergic pathway
  influencing by neuroleptics 407

SUBJECT INDEX

Noise stress
  testing of psychotropic drugs 174
Nomifensin
  effects on EEG in man in comparison with Etifoxin 150
Non-ionic diffusion
  acceleration of renal amphetamine excretion 629
Non-REM sleep
  effects on tardive dyskinesia and rabbit syndrome in schizophrenics 434
Norephedrine
  involvement in amphetamine metabolism in man and laboratory animals 577
Norepinephrine
  depletion in amphetamine intoxication 193
  increased CNS turnover in neuroleptic treatment 410
  role as neurohumoral transmitter 3
Norepinephrine receptor blockade
  role in neuroleptic-induced sedation (chlorpromazine, thioridazine, clozapine) 410
Norfenfluramine
  as brain metabolite of fenfluramine, subcellular localization 588
  involvement in telencephalic serotonin decrease 654
Nosological models
  contribution of pharmacopsychiatry to their development 55
Nurses' Observation Scale for Inpatient Evaluation (NOSIE)
  use in safety and efficacy testing of fluphenazine-HCl 266
  use in testing of niacin effects in schizophrenia 297

Obesity
  drug-induced 323
Octoclothepin
  changes of central effects after repeated administration 387
Organization of psychiatric services
  structural levels 100
Oxidative deamination of amphetamines
  involvement of rat liver microsomes 621
Oxotremorine
  effects on acetyl-CoA and free choline in brain 536
  involvement in rise of brain acetylcholine 566, 570
Oxyprothepin
  changes of central effects after repeated administration 387

Paedophilia
  treatment with cyproterone acetate, gonadotropin excretion values 500
Pallidum
  anatomy in man and animals, physiological correlates 397

Paper chromatography
  use in determination of urinary metabolites of amphetamine 626
Paranoid psychosis
  chronic amphetamine intoxication as model 189, 197
Paranoid thinking
  in depressive patients treated with lithium 70
Pargyline
  role in copulatory behavior in rats 453
Parkinsonism
  drug-induced 409, 415, 432
Patterns of sexual behavior
  changes after castration 508
Penfluridol
  use of rating scales and handwriting test in objectivization of its neuroleptic effects 273
Penile erection
  effect of L-DOPA in man 491
Perphenazine
  changes in central effects after repeated administration 387
  tolerance and withdrawal effects in rabbits 377
Pharmacodynamic effects
  behavioral level 144
  cellular level 143
  cerebral and spinal level 144
  correlation between animal and human experimentation 143
  subcellular level 143
Pharmacopsychiatry
  contribution to nosology 55
Pharmacopsychology
  relevance of effects 158
  relevance of methods 158
Pharmacotherapeutic quantification of psychoses 251
Phenmetrazine
  effects on steady state concentrations of brain monoamines 650
Phenothiazines
  action on nigro-neostriatal dopaminergic pathway 407
  influence on EEG 14
  involvement in adrenergic mechanisms 37
Phosphate metabolism
  lithium-induced changes 321
Phospholipase A_2
  as tool in cholinergic synapse study 551
Phospholipids
  role in synaptosomal membrane and cholinergic vesicle structure 553
Physostigmine
  effects on manic symptoms together with methylphenidate 678
Pilocarpine
  cataleptogenic effects in rats 398
Pimozide
  dopamine receptor blockade, behavioral effects 407

SUBJECT INDEX

Pincer grasp
  induced in primates by amphetamines 190
Pineal gland
  role in p-chlorophenylalanine activity 455
Pipothiazine derivatives
  social aspects of long-acting neuroleptic use 92
Pituitary-adrenal system
  impairment induced by high doses of Δ^9-THC in animals 707
Pituitary-gonadal axis
  interactions with tubero-infundibular dopamine neurons 473
Pituitary gonadotropic regulation
  effects of drugs interfering with central neurotransmitters 481
Placebo
  use in evaluation of psychotropic drug effects in healthy volunteers 172, 177
  use in the study of genetic aspects of lithium prophylaxis 312
  use with Etifoxin and Nomifensin in controlled trial, effects on human EEG 150
Plasma proteins
  variations during acute phase of psychosis (schizophrenia, manic-depressive psychosis) 206
Pleasure
  neurophysiological correlates 138
Polygraphic studies in schizophrenics 433
Postural-motor-attitudinal sets
  common features of paranoid and catatonic pathways of psychotic processes 190
Primary Hospitalization Service
  levels of structural organization of psychiatric services 100
Prochlorperazine
  inhibition of apomorphine-induced stereotypy in rats 400
Psychiatric admissions
  diminished rate 75
Psychiatric discharges
  increasing rate, involvement in "revolving-door psychiatry" 76
Psychiatric education
  psychopharmacological approach 102
Psychiatry
  scope and structure 99
Psychoactive drugs see Psychotropic drugs
Psychoanalysis
  stress on training 115
Psychobiological levels of organization
  importance for psychotropic drug effects 127
Psychomotor behavior
  testing in evaluating Δ^9-THC effects on driving performance 694
Psychomotor tracking performance
  influenced by marijuana and alcohol 686
Psychopharmacological Consultation Service
  involvement in psychopharmacological education 101

Psychopharmacological curriculum
  in WHO training course in psychopharmacology 113
Psychopharmacological research
  chemical level 45
  co-operation between pharmacologist and clinician 106
  physiological level 45
  psychological level 45
  screening of new drugs, pharmaco-clinical correlations 44
Psychopharmacology
  course for medical teachers sponsored by WHO 113
  futurological aspects 59
  postgraduate training 105
  social aspects 59, 75
  training models 109, 115
Psychopharmacotherapy
  depressive side effects 363
Psychosexual differentiation
  role of gonadal hormones in regulation of sexual behavior 503
Psychotomimetic drugs
  role in pathogenesis of schizophrenia 214
Psychotropic drugs
  amphetamine-like 3
  biochemical approaches 3
  classification 13, 14
  clinical testing 106
  combinations 344
  comparison of effects in healthy and mentally ill subjects 158
  correlation of effects with patient's personality 161
  differential EEG effects 149
  discovery 3, 13
  effects on animal aggressivity 145
  general EEG effects 149
  group testing 177
  increase of consumption 77
  increase of prescription 83
  influence of non-specific factors on effects 165
  influence on human EEG 149
  molecular orbital calculations 35
  personality-specific effects 165
  prophylactic use 65
  psychobiological comparison of effects 127
  quantum chemical techniques for understanding of mode of action 31
  reserpine-like 3
  testing in healthy subjects 177

"Rabbit syndrome"
  neuroleptic drug-induced 431
Rapid-reading test
  use in neuroleptic drug testing in healthy subjects 171
Rat heart
  levels of p-hydroxynorephedrine 642
Rat salivary gland
  levels of p-hydroxynorephedrine 642

SUBJECT INDEX

Rating scales, questionnaires
  Barron ego-strength scale 85
  Brief Psychiatric Rating Scale 249, 266, 297
  Clinical Global Impression Rating Scale 280
  combination with handwriting test 273
  consciousness and mood scales (Smith and Beecher's mood questionnaire), subjective and objective rating 691
  Early Clinical Drug Evaluation Units (ECDEU) 280
  Maudsley Medical Questionnaire 129
  Minnesota Multiphasic Personality Inventory (MMPI) 689
  Nurses' Observation Scale for Inpatient Evaluation (NOSIE) 266, 297
  Side Effects Rating Scale 266
  Taylor-Manifest Anxiety Scale 87
  Wittenborn Psychiatric Rating Scale 273
Reaction time tasks
  impairment of performance after marijuana 703
Receptivity behavior
  induction on spayed rats by estradiol benzoate and progesterone 512
Recurrent affective psychosis
  bipolar 336
  unipolar 336
Rehabilitation in psychiatry
  relation to psychopharmacology 117
Rehabilitation Facilities
  levels of psychiatric services' structural organization 100
REM sleep
  influence on drug-induced tardive dyskinesia in schizophrenics 434
Repeated drug administration
  changes induced in central effects of some neuroleptics 387
  effects on animal behavior 343
Reserpine
  antagonizing effects on drug-induced tardive dyskinesia 431
  effect on male sexual activity 451
"Revolving-door psychiatry"
  due to increased psychiatric discharge rate 76
Righting reflexes
  influenced by chronic amphetamine intoxication with disulfiram pretreatment 199

SCH – 12,041
  benzodiazepine derivative, effects on EEG in man 21
Schizophrenia
  activation by methylphenidate 675
  biochemical hypotheses of pathogenesis 185
  blood proteins 205
  cerebrospinal fluid proteins 205
  effects of L-DOPA 229
  endocrine factors 187
  genetic factors 187
  metabolic aspects 235
  prediction of neuroleptic treatment outcome 249
  productive vs. non-productive forms 261
  relation to inborn errors of metabolism 209
  relation to N-methylation 235
  relationship to amphetamine model psychosis 189
  treatment by fluphenazine hydrochloride 265
  treatment by neuroleptics 261
  treatment by niacin 293
  tryptophan metabolism 209
Schizophrenia-like psychoses
  pathogenetic conditions (tissue damage, toxic agents, metabolic disorders, functional disorders) 186
Schizophrenics
  competence status 260
  contact with family members 261
  discharges from hospital 257
  level of education 260
  marital status 259
  parents' social position 258
  readmissions to hospital 257
  social position 259
Sedation
  difficulties in assessment of criteria due to different approach to the concept 128
Self-administration of drugs
  after-effects in long-term experiment in rats 349
Self-observation
  use in psychopharmacotherapy 158
Serotonin
  cerebral; biochemical mechanism of p-chloroamphetamine action on it 607
  decrease in brain 517
  enzymatic modifications 213
  role in female sexual behavior 466
  role in sexual activity 451
Serotonin antagonists
  inducing of mounting behavior in rats 493
Sex-specific urinating position in dogs 510
Sexual behavior
  in animals 8, 451, 517
  in female animals 463
  in humans 489
  regulation by castration and/or hormone stimulation in animals 503
Sexual disorders
  use of antiandrogens 497
  use of sexual stimulating substances 489
Sexual motivation
  endocrinological aspects in female animals 463
  role of monoamines 469
Side-Effects Rating Scale
  use in safety and efficacy assessment of fluphenazine-HCl in psychotics 266
Signal-to-noise ratio
  increase after LSD treatment, EEG studies 53
Simulated car driving
  influenced by cannabis and/or alcohol 689, 693

SUBJECT INDEX

Single drug administration
  long-term effects of psychotropic drugs 343
Sleep stages
  influence on tardive dyskinesia 433
Social behavior in rats
  influenced by amylobarbitone administration 348
Specialized Treatment Service
  levels of psychiatric services' structural organization 100
Spiramide
  influence on amphetamine-induced aggressive behavior in mice 663
State-dependent learning
  use in psychopharmacological investigations in healthy subjects 162
Stereotyped behavior
  amphetamine-induced in animals, effect of dose on its character 189, 646, 659
  amphetamine-induced in rats, inhibition by neuroleptics 662
  drug-induced in rats (apomorphine, amphetamine, anticholinergic drugs, cholinergic drugs) 400
  methylphenidate-induced in rats, inhibition by physostigmine 677
Stereotyped running
  apomorphine-induced in dogs 384
Stress situation
  testing of simulated driving under Δ^9-THC influence 695
Striatum
  anatomical and physiological aspects 396
  turnover rate of catecholamines in correlation with amphetamine-influenced locomotor activity 646
Subcellular localization of drugs
  use of chromatographic and spectrometric methods 585
Subjective feeling
  in investigation of neuroticism correlated with drug effects 168
Substantia nigra lesions
  stereotypies induced in rats; correlation with cholinesterase content in neostriatum 402
Sulpiride
  neuroleptic activity with psychostimulant features 446
Supersensitive dopamine receptors
  involvement in nigro-neostriatal DA pathway lesions 409
Synhexyl
  marijuana-like activity in terms of Δ^9-THC effects 705
System analysis
  involvement in theoretical and quantum studies of antipsychotics 36

Tapping
  use in testing of Δ^9-THC effects on simulated driving 694

Tardive dyskinesias
  drug-induced 442, 444
  drug-induced, inhibition by dopamine depleting agents 416
  drug-induced; negative effects of antiparkinsonic medication, positive effects of neuroleptics 431
Taylor-manifest anxiety scale
  use in clinical anxiolytic drug testing 87
Teaching of psychiatry
  role of psychopharmacology 99
Television
  as non-pharmaceutical tranquillizer 83
  use in psychopharmacological training 109
Testosterone
  role in p-chlorophenylalanine activity 456
Tetrabenazine
  effect on male sexual activity 451
  inhibitory effect on drug-induced tardive dyskinesia 431
Δ^9-Tetrahydrocannabinol
  acute effects in man 685
  after-effects 701
  as potential precursor of "false hormones" 707
  comparison with marijuana in human EEG and heart rate effects 703
  comparison with marijuana in man 685
  derealization evoked after its administration 702
  effect on blood pressure 702
  effect on body temperature 702
  effect on pH of saliva 702
  effect on pulse rate 702
  effects on simulated car driving 693
  euphoric-stimulated state evoked by its administration 702
  involvement in producing anxious-depressive state 702
  metabolism 705
  use in volunteers 701
Tetrodotoxin
  reduction of acetylcholine output from cholinergic nerve endings 568
Thiaxanthenes
  neuroleptics with low incidence of extrapyramidal side effects 445
Thioridazine
  combination with d-amphetamine 279
Thought processes
  neurophysiological aspects 136
Thymoleptic drugs
  EEG profiles 18
Time estimation
  testing in labile vs. stabile personality types under Etifoxin vs. placebo administration 167
Tofizopam
  ego-strength changes assessment 86
  evaluation of effects in healthy subjects in comparison with amitriptyline and placebo 177

SUBJECT INDEX

Tolerance to narcotics
  its long duration; role of single drug dose 396
Tolerance to neuroleptics
  development after one week administration in rabbits, EEG and behavioral evidence 377
  development after repeated administration in animals 383
Topographical conformational similarity 33
Torpedo marmorata
  nerve electroplaque junctions, acetylcholine synthesis and release 547
Tracking apparatus
  use in testing Δ^9-THC effects on driving performance 695
Training program in psychiatry 99
Tranquillizers
  testing under experimental stress 160
Transfer of drug tolerance
  morphine administration to female rats, testing of their offspring for drug tolerance 373
Tremor
  drug-induced 419
Tremorine
  rise in brain acetylcholine induced by its administration 566
Triazolobenzodiazepine derivative (U-31, 889)
  anxiolytic effects 23
Tricyclic antidepressants
  interference with catecholamine and serotonin uptake in CNS 4
  long-term treatment 71
Tryptophan
  metabolites of body fluids 211
  relationship to behavior 218
  role in pathogenesis of schizophrenia, its metabolism 209
Tryptophan hydroxylase
  modification by *p*-chloroamphetamine in rat brain 607
Tubero-infundibular dopamine neurons 473

U-31, 889
  see triazolobenzodiazepine derivative
Unipolar depression
  problem of genetic difference of bipolar affective psychosis 302
Unit discharge
  in basal ganglia, relations to learned movements of limbs 137
Urinary metabolites of cannabis 689

Validation problems
  in computer-assisted psychopharmacological study 123
Vigilance
  aspects of neuronal-behavioral relations 137
Visual evoked potentials
  assessment in behaviorally disturbed children during d-amphetamine-thioridazine treatment (withdrawal and rerteatment experiments) 284
Visual signal detection
  influencing by marijuana 687

Wakefulness
  influence on tardive dyskinesia 433
Withdrawal symptoms
  after perphenazine treatment in rabbits 377
Wittenborn Psychiatric Rating Scales
  use in objectivization and quantification neuroleptic effects 273
World Health Organization
  as sponsor of training course in psychopharmacology 113

X-chromosome
  transmission of manic-depressive psychosis 301
XGa blood group
  statistically significant linkage with manic-depressive psychosis 301, 303

Y-maze
  use in testing after-effects of single drug experience 344